Disorders of the Neonatal Airway

Janet Lioy • Steven E. Sobol
Editors

Disorders of the Neonatal Airway

Fundamentals for Practice

Springer

Editors
Janet Lioy, MD, FAAP
Attending Neonatologist
Director Neonatal Outreach
Medical Director, Neonatal Airway Program
The Children's Hospital of Philadelphia
Associate Professor of Clinical Pediatrics
The University of Pennsylvania Perelman School of Medicine
Philadelphia, PA, USA

Steven E. Sobol, MD, MSc, FRCS(C)
Attending Surgeon
Fellowship Director, Pediatric Otolaryngology
The Center for Pediatric Airway Disorders
The Children's Hospital of Philadelphia
Associate Professor
Department of Otorhinolaryngology-Head and Neck Surgery
University of Pennsylvania Perelman School of Medicine
Philadelphia, PA, USA

Videos to this book can be accessed at http://www.springerimages.com/videos/978-1-4939-1609-2

ISBN 978-1-4939-1609-2 ISBN 978-1-4939-1610-8 (eBook)
DOI 10.1007/978-1-4939-1610-8
Springer New York Heidelberg Dordrecht London

Library of Congress Control Number: 2014957164

Printed on acid-free paper

Springer is part of Springer Science+Business Media (www.springer.com)

I would like to dedicate this book to Isabella Schneeman, whose life as a precious and fragile 24-week infant was afflicted with all the dreaded complications of prematurity. Although successful in overcoming her chronic lung disease, she remained intubated for many months and struggled many times to survive without a breathing tube. Unfortunately, she developed severe subglottic stenosis and needed a tracheostomy. Given those details, Isabella beat the odds, went home with a wonderfully capable, loving family, and was able to successfully decannulate a few years later after reconstructive surgery. Subsequently, she has managed to live the life of a normal 6-year-old. Isabella has taught many of the neonatologists caring for her that courage, perseverance, and determination are the essential elements needed for her family to overcome the long hospitalization and a technology-dependent medical home. Without Isabella teaching me how to continue to search for ways to allow her damaged neonatal airway to heal and grow, I would not have realized the need for this book and how it can enlighten others when there seems to be no hope amidst a dim light.

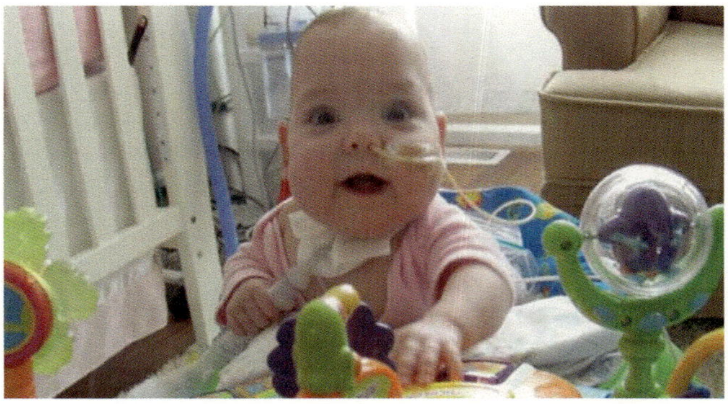

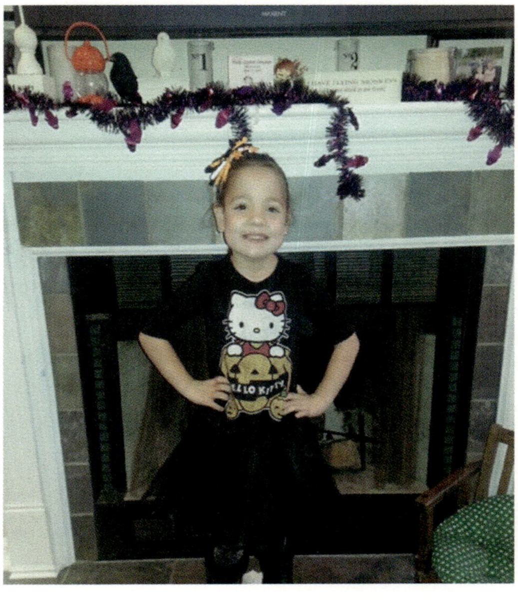

Janet Lioy, MD

As I progress through my career, I find myself reflecting on individuals who have played a major role in my professional and personal development. As a young resident, my hero was Dr. Martin Black, a head and neck surgeon who taught me that at the end of the day it is only about the patient. Dr. Saul Frenkiel, my former program director, taught me the value of treating every individual on my team as if they are part of my own family. I am indebted to Dr. Mel Schloss, one of the fathers of our subspecialty, who introduced and encouraged me to pursue a career in pediatric otolaryngology. I am grateful to continue to have the opportunity to work with Dr. Bill Potsic and Dr. Ralph Wetmore who exemplify what it takes to work at one of our country's best children's hospitals.

I owe a debt of gratitude to my parents, Rhona and Joey Sobol, who gave me everything that I needed in life to ensure my success. Lastly, I dedicate this text to my beautiful wife, Jennifer, and my daughters, Lexi and Ella, who provide me with unconditional support and continue to make every day of my life a joy.

Steven E. Sobol, MD, MSc, FRCS(C)

Preface

Over the past three decades, the field of pediatric otolaryngology has grown from a small group of individuals who understood that children are not just small adults, into its own distinct subspecialty. The collaborative efforts of this subspecialty with other pediatric providers have allowed for the emergence of the exciting field of pediatric airway surgery. With advances in airway management algorithms and techniques, the child born with a critically obstructed airway is no longer condemned to death or a life defined by a tracheostomy tube. This book is a testament to the efforts put in by our pioneers and represents the state of the art of neonatal airway management in the twenty-first century.

Neonatal airway emergencies seem to be a relatively new concept within many neonatal units. Previously, conditions such as preterm respiratory distress syndrome and meconium aspiration in term infants were two common reasons for airway management. Lately, many large-scale children's hospitals, like our own, have created Fetal Medicine programs that deliver neonates with more complex and life-threatening congenital airway anomalies that would otherwise result in instant death. These neonates are populating many expanding children's hospitals and require airway expertise 24 h a day. Alternatively, a growing number of extremely low birth weight preterm infants are surviving with long-term chronic airway and lung issues such as subglottic stenosis, severe tracheobronchomalacia, and significant micrognathia-induced airway obstruction requiring a tracheostomy. Subsequently, the referrals for these types of infants are growing exponentially, necessitating that pediatric otorhinolaryngologists trained for special airways are readily available.

Managing pediatric airway emergencies is certainly not limited to one specialty. As part of the necessary multidisciplinary approach, neonatologists work alongside pediatric ORL as well as pediatric anesthesiologists in a well-coordinated response. Each of these specialties also relies upon innovative equipment designed specifically for neonatal and infant applications. Videolaryngoscopy with small-sized equipment is now available for the smallest neonates and these techniques alone have a variety of cameras and scopes that can be tailored to patient and situation. Consequently, having portable equipment readily available and organized in a predetermined arrangement improves the team's ability to effectively respond to neonatal airway emergencies at the bedside.

Ultimately, a change in the profile of neonatal patients has created a need for preparation in responding to neonatal airway emergencies. As our neonatal patients get smaller and live longer, airway damage and compromise can become an integral part of the total hospital care. Many centers are now delivering neonates with airway disorders once felt to be incompatible with life. This shift in perinatal medicine has significantly increased the burden of long hospitalizations with technology dependency far beyond what was common 20 years ago.

Philadelphia, PA, USA

Steven E. Sobol, MD, MSc, FRCS(C)
Janet Lioy, MD

Acknowledgments

I would like to especially thank and recognize Dr. Hitesh Deshmuhk, author, friend, and former CHOP neonatal fellow, for his expertise and steadfast help in organizing and formatting many of the figures in our book. Without his daily help I would not have been able to be as organized in getting everything in on time.

Other thanks to author Dr. David (Andrew) Mong for his expertise in radiological imaging preparation and to CHOP neonatal fellow, Dr. Shaon Sengupta, for assisting with early chapter preparation.

Contents

Part II Assessment, Evaluation and Treatment

Part III Education, Simulation and Quality Improvement

Contributors

Saima Aftab, MD Division of Neonatology, Floating Hospital for Children, Tufts University School of Medicine, Boston, MA, USA

Henry Akinbi, MD Division of Neonatology, Cincinnati Children's Hospital Medical Center, University of Cincinnati School of Medicine, Cincinnati, OH, USA

Jacqueline Anderson, MD Department of Otolaryngology—Head and Neck Surgery, Madigan Army Medical Center, Tacoma, WA, USA

Steven Andreoli, MD Division of Otolaryngology, The Children's Hospital of Philadelphia, Philadelphia, PA, USA

Christina Baldasseri, MD Department of Otolaryngology, Children's Hospital of The King's Daughters, Eastern Virginia Medical School, Norfolk, VA, USA

Eric E. Berg, MD Division of Pediatric Otolaryngology, Department of Otolaryngology—Head & Neck Surgery, University of Texas Southwestern Medical Center, Dallas, TX, USA

Thane Blinman, MD, FACS Division of General, Thoracic, and Fetal Surgery, The Children's Hospital of Philadelphia, Philadelphia, PA, USA

University of Pennsylvania, Perelman School of Medicine, Philadelphia, PA, USA

Gian-Marco Busato, MD, MSc Department of Otolaryngology—Head and Neck Surgery, University of Toronto, Toronto, ON, Canada

Paolo Campisi, MSc, MD, FRCS(C) Department of Otolaryngology—Head and Neck Surgery, Hospital for Sick Children, University of Toronto, Toronto, ON, Canada

Jeffrey Cheng, MD Division of Pediatric Otolaryngology, The Children's Hospital of Philadelphia, Philadelphia, PA, USA

John Chuo, MD, MS Division of Neonatology, The Children's Hospital of Philadelphia, The Perelman School of Medicine at the University of Pennsylvania, Philadelphia, PA, USA

Timothy M. Crombleholme, MD Division of Pediatric General, Thoracic and Fetal Surgery, Colorado Fetal Care Center and the Colorado Institute for Maternal and Fetal Health, Children's Hospital Colorado, Aurora, CO, USA

David H. Darrow, MD, DDS Department of Otolaryngology, Children's Hospital of The King's Daughters, Eastern Virginia Medical School, Norfolk, VA, USA

Alessandro deAlarcón, MD, MPH Division of Pediatric Otolaryngology—Head and Neck Surgery, Cincinnati Children's Hospital Medical Center, Cincinnati, OH, USA

Department of Otolaryngology—Head and Neck Surgery, University of Cincinnati College of Medicine, Cincinnati, OH, USA

Sara B. DeMauro, MD, MSCE Division of Neonatology, The Children's Hospital of Philadelphia, Philadelphia, PA, USA

University of Pennsylvania, Perelman School of Medicine, Philadelphia, PA, USA

Craig Derkay, MD Department of Otolaryngology, Children's Hospital of The King's Daughters, Eastern Virginia Medical School, Norfolk, VA, USA

Hitesh Deshmuhk, MD, PhD Division of Neonatology, Pulmonary Biology, Cincinnati Children's Hospital Medical Center, University of Cincinnati School of Medicine, Cincinnati, OH, USA

Kevin Dysart, MD Division of Neonatology, The Children's Hospital of Philadelphia, University of Pennsylvania, Perelman School of Medicine, Philadelphia, PA, USA

Monica Epelman, MD Department of Radiology, Nemours Children's Hospital, University of Central Florida and Florida State University, Orlando, FL, USA

John Fiadjoe, MD Department of Anesthesiology & Critical Care Medicine, The Children's Hospital of Philadelphia, Philadelphia, PA, USA

University of Pennsylvania, Perelman School of Medicine, Philadelphia, PA, USA

Heather M. French, MD Division of Neonatology, The Children's Hospital of Philadelphia, University of Pennsylvania, Perelman School of Medicine, Philadelphia, PA, USA

Stephanie Fuller, MD The Division of Cardiothoracic Surgery, The Children's Hospital of Philadelphia, Philadelphia, PA, USA

University of Pennsylvania, Perelman School of Medicine, Philadelphia, PA, USA

Jason Gien, MD The Children's Hospital of Colorado, University of Colorado School of Medicine, Aurora, CO, USA

Jesse A. Goldstein, MD Division of Plastic Surgery, Children's Hospital of Philadelphia, University of Pennsylvania, Perelman School of Medicine, Philadelphia, PA, USA

Megan Gray, MD Division of Neonatology, The Children's Hospital of Philadelphia, University of Pennsylvania, Perelman School of Medicine, Philadelphia, PA, USA

David A. Gudis, MD Department of Otolaryngology—Head and Neck Surgery, Medical University of South Carolina, Charleston, SC, USA

Matt Harrison, MD Division of Cardiology, The Children's Hospital of Philadelphia, Philadelphia, PA, USA

Holly L. Hedrick, MD Division of General, Fetal and Thoracic Surgery, The Children's Hospital of Philadelphia, Philadelphia, PA, USA

University of Pennsylvania, Perelman School of Medicine, Philadelphia, PA, USA

Rebecca Isserman Department of Anesthesiology & Critical Care Medicine, The Children's Hospital of Philadelphia, Philadelphia, PA, USA

University of Pennsylvania, Perelman School of Medicine, Philadelphia, PA, USA

Ian N. Jacobs, MD Division of Otolaryngology, The Children's Hospital of Philadelphia, Department of Otorhinolaryngology—Head and Neck Surgery, University of Pennsylvania, Perelman School of Medicine, Philadelphia, PA, USA

Luv R. Javia, MD Division of Otolaryngology, The Children's Hospital of Philadelphia, Department of Otorhinolaryngology—Head and Neck Surgery, University of Pennsylvania, Perelman School of Medicine, Philadelphia, PA, USA

Jessica Kurian, MD Department of Radiology, Montefiore Medical Center, Albert Einstein College of Medicine, Bronx, NY, USA

Pablo Laje, MD Division of General, Fetal and Thoracic Surgery, The Children's Hospital of Philadelphia, Philadelphia, PA, USA

University of Pennsylvania, Perelman School of Medicine, Philadelphia, PA, USA

April Landry, MD Department of Pediatric Otolaryngology Head and Neck Surgery, Cincinnati Children's Hospital Medical Center, The University of Cincinnati College of Medicine, Cincinnati, OH, USA

Bryan Liming, MD Department of Otolaryngology—Head and Neck Surgery, Madigan Army Medical Center, Tacoma, WA, USA

Richard Lin, MD, FAAP Departments of Anesthesiology and Critical Care Medicine, The Children's Hospital of Philadelphia, University of Pennsylvania, Perelman School of Medicine, Philadelphia, PA, USA

Janet Lioy Attending Neonatologist, Director Neonatal Outreach, Medical Director, Neonatal Airway Program, The Children's Hospital of Philadelphia, Associate Professor of Clinical Pediatrics, The University of Pennsylvania Perelman School of Medicine, Philadelphia, PA, USA

Kathryn Maschhoff, MD, PhD Division of Neonatology, The Children's Hospital of Philadelphia, Philadelphia, PA, USA

University of Pennsylvania, Perelman School of Medicine, Philadelphia, PA, USA

John McClay, MD Frisco ENT for Children, Dallas, TX, USA

John McCloskey, MD Department of Anesthesiology & Critical Care Medicine, The Children's Hospital of Philadelphia, Philadelphia, PA, USA

The Perelman School of Medicine at the University of Pennsylvania, Philadelphia, PA, USA

Nathan W. Mick, MD, FACEP Associate Chief, Department of Emergency Medicine, Associate Professor, Tufts University School of Medicine Director, Clinical Operations Maine Medical Center, Portland, MA, USA

David A. Mong Department of Radiology, The Children's Hospital of Philadelphia, Philadelphia, PA USA

University of Pennsylvania, Perelman School of Medicine, Philadelphia, PA, USA

Pamela Mudd, MD Division of Otolaryngology, The Children's Hospital of Philadelphia, Philadelphia, PA, USA

Joshua Nagler, MD, MHPEd Department of Pediatrics, Harvard Medical School, Fellowship Director, Division of Emergency Medicine, Boston Children's Hospital, Boston, MA, USA

Carolyn V. Nguyen, MD Staff Otolaryngologist, Kaiser Permanente, Los Angeles, CA, USA

Melissa Ortiz, MD Department of Surgery Otolaryngology—Head and Neck Surgery, University of Puerto Rico-Medical Sciences Campus, San Juan, PR, USA

J. Thomas Paliga Division of Plastic Surgery, Department of Surgery, The Children's Hospital of Philadelphia, Philadelphia, PA, USA

Duke University School of Medicine, Durham, NC, USA

Sanjay R. Parikh, MD Department of Otolaryngology—Head and Neck Surgery, University of Washington, Seattle, WA, USA

Kara K. Prickett, MD Division of Otolaryngology, The Children's Hospital of Philadelphia, Philadelphia, PA, USA

J. Drew Prosser, MD Division of Pediatric Otolaryngology—Head and Neck Surgery, Cincinnati Children's Hospital Medical Center, Cincinnati, OH, USA

Gresham T. Richter, MD Arkansas Children's Hospital, University of Arkansas Medical School, Little Rock, AR, USA

Michael J. Rutter, MB ChB, FRACS Division of Pediatric Otolaryngology—Head and Neck Surgery, Cincinnati Children's Hospital Medical Center, Cincinnati, OH, USA

Department of Otolaryngology—Head and Neck Surgery, University of Cincinnati College of Medicine, Cincinnati, OH, USA

Sulagna C. Saitta, MD, PhD Clinical Genetics, Cedars-Sinai Medical Center Department of Pediatrics, David Geffen School of Medicine at UCLA, Los Angeles, CA, USA

Scott R. Schoem, MD, FAAP Division of Otolaryngology—Head and Neck Surgery, University of Connecticut, Connecticut Children's Medical Center, Hartford, CT, USA

Lynn Shesser, RN, MSN, MBA The Children's Hospital of Philadelphia Home Care, The Children's Hospital of Philadelphia, Philadelphia, King of Prussia, PA, USA

Nicholas Smith, MD Department of Otolaryngology—Head and Neck Surgery, University of Alabama at Birmingham, Pediatric ENT Associates, Children's of Alabama, Birmingham, AB, USA

Steven E. Sobol, MD, MSc, FRCS(C) Attending Surgeon, Fellowship Director, Pediatric Otolaryngology, The Center for Pediatric Airway Disorders, The Children's Hospital of Philadelphia, Associate Professor, Department of Otorhinolaryngology-Head and Neck Surgery, University of Pennsylvania Perelman School of Medicine, Philadelphia, PA, USA

Stig Somme, MD Department of Surgery, The Children's Hospital of Colorado, University of Colorado School of Medicine, Aurora, CO, USA

Aseem Srivastava, MD The Division of Cardiothoracic Surgery, The Children's Hospital of Philadelphia, Philadelphia, PA, USA

Joanne Stow, PPCNP-BC, CORLN Division of Otorhinolarygology, The Children's Hospital of Philadelphia, Philadelphia, PA, USA

Daniel T. Swarr, MD Divisions of Neonatology, Department of Human Genetics, The Children's Hospital of Philadelphia, University of Pennsylvania, Perelman School of Medicine, Philadelphia, PA, USA

John Tamasitis, RRT-NPS Children's Hospital Home Care, The Children's Hospital of Philadelphia, Philadelphia, King of Prussia, PA, USA

Jesse A. Taylor, MD Department of Plastic, Reconstructive, and Craniofacial Surgery, The Children's Hospital of Philadelphia, University of Pennsylvania, Perelman School of Medicine, Philadelphia, PA, USA

Dana M. Thompson, MD, MS Department of Pediatric Otolaryngology Head and Neck Surgery, Ann & Robert H. Lurie Children's Hospital of Chicago, Northwestern University Feinberg School of Medicine, Chicago, IL, USA

Nicholas Tsarouhas, MD Department of Pediatrics, The Children's Hospital of Philadelphia, University of Pennsylvania, Perelman School of Medicine, Philadelphia, PA, USA

David E. Tunkel, MD Department of Otolaryngology—Head and Neck Surgery, Johns Hopkins School of Medicine, Johns Hopkins Outpatient Center, Baltimore, MD, USA

Elliott M. Weiss, MD Division of Neonatology, The Children's Hospital of Philadelphia, Philadelphia, PA, USA

Department of Medical Ethics & Health Policy, University of Pennsylvania, Philadelphia, PA, USA

David R. White, MD Department of Otolaryngology—Head and Neck Surgery, Medical University of South Carolina, Charleston, SC, USA

Brian J. Wiatrak, MD Department of Otolaryngology-Head and Neck Surgery, University of Alabama at Birmingham, Pediatric ENT Associates, Children's of Alabama, Birmingham, AB, USA

Huayan Zhang, MD Division of Neonatology, Medical Director, Chronic Lung Disease Program The Children's Hospital of Philadelphia, University of Pennsylvania, Perelman School of Medicine, Philadelphia, PA, USA

Karen B. Zur, MD Division of Otolaryngology, The Children's Hospital of Philadelphia, Department of Otorhinolaryngology—Head and Neck Surgery, University of Pennsylvania, Perelman School of Medicine, Philadelphia, PA, USA

Part I

Malformations, Deformations and Disorders

Embryology of Congenital Airway Disorders

Paolo Campisi and Gian-Marco Busato

Congenital Nasal Airway Disorders

Congenital nasal airway obstruction is a common cause of respiratory distress in newborns and infants as they remain obligate nasal breathers for the first few months of life. The respiratory distress may be apparent immediately after birth or may become evident when the child is challenged by an upper respiratory tract infection or secondary airway anomaly. Obstruction can occur at different regions of the nasal airway including the piriform aperture, mid-nasal vault, and choana. The differential diagnosis of congenital nasal airway obstruction is varied (Table 1) but this section of the chapter will focus on congenital nasal piriform aperture stenosis (CNPAS) and choanal atresia.

Congenital Nasal Piriform Aperture Stenosis

The piriform aperture is the most anterior aspect of the bony nasal airway. It has a pear shape and anatomically distinct bones contribute to the aperture. The horizontal processes of the maxilla contribute inferiorly. The frontal processes of the maxilla (inferiorly) and nasal bones (superiorly) constitute the lateral aspect of the aperture. The aperture is divided in the midline by the anterior nasal spine and septum. CNPAS is defined as horizontal narrowing of the lateral walls resulting in a smaller aperture. The narrowing is typically measured at the level of the inferior meatus.

P. Campisi, M.Sc., M.D., F.R.C.S.(C) (✉)
Department of Otolaryngology—Head and Neck Surgery, Hospital for Sick Children, University of Toronto, 555 University Avenue, Toronto, ON, Canada M5G 1X8
e-mail: sobols@email.chop.edu

G.-M. Busato, M.D., M.Sc.
Department of Otolaryngology—Head and Neck Surgery, University of Toronto, Toronto, ON, Canada M5G 1X8

Etiology

Embryologically, the piriform aperture is derived from fusion of the medial nasal prominences (floor of the aperture) and fusion of the lateral nasal prominences and maxillary prominences (lateral bones of aperture). Therefore, it has been hypothesized that CNPAS can be caused by either a deficiency in the primary palate (floor of the aperture) or bony overgrowth/dysplasia of the nasal processes of the maxilla. Both etiologies would result in horizontal narrowing of the lateral walls of the piriform aperture.

Epidemiology

CNPAS is an uncommon cause of congenital nasal airway obstruction and the true incidence is unknown.

Pathogenesis

The embryological development of the nose begins early in the fourth week of gestation [4]. The nose is derived from the single median frontonasal prominence and the paired maxillary prominences. The prominences arise from the proliferation and migration of neural crest cells during the fourth week.

The frontonasal prominence gives rise to bilateral nasal placodes by the end of the fourth week. The mesenchyme at the periphery of the placodes proliferates creating medial and lateral nasal prominences and central depressions called nasal pits. The nasal pits are the primordium of the nostrils and nasal cavities.

With medial migration of the maxillary prominences, the medial nasal prominences begin to fuse and form the primary palate (Fig. 1a, b). Concurrent fusion of the lateral nasal prominences with the maxillary prominences forms the lateral bones of the piriform aperture.

A deficiency in the bulk of the primary palate primordium may result in CNPAS by allowing medial migration of the palatal shelves during the 6th week of gestation that is closer to the midline than usual. The deficient primary palate would account for the narrow aperture, triangular shaped palate, and single central incisor associated with CNPAS (Fig. 2). The resultant "over-migration" of the palatal shelves may

J. Lioy and S.E. Sobol (eds.), *Disorders of the Neonatal Airway: Fundamentals for Practice*,
DOI 10.1007/978-1-4939-1610-8_1, © Springer Science+Business Media New York 2015

Table 1 Differential diagnosis of congenital nasal airway obstruction

Choanal stenosis and atresia
Congenital nasal piriform aperture stenosis
Midnasal stenosis
Nasal masses
Dermoid cyst
Encephalocele
Glioma
Hemangioma
Nasolacrimal duct cyst
Deviated nasal septum
Rhinitis of the newborn

account for the observed ridge of bone along the inferior aspect of the palate.

The other possible cause of CNPAS is the overgrowth of the medial maxillary bones. Imaging studies frequently show thickened bone in this region.

Clinical Presentation

The clinical presentation of CNPAS is similar to the presentation of any condition that causes nasal obstruction. Typical signs and symptoms include stertor, tachypnea, obstructive apnea, feeding difficulty, respiratory distress, and cyclical and paradoxical cyanosis. Crying usually relieves the respiratory symptoms as the infant shifts their breathing from nasal to oral routes.

On physical examination, the nasal inlet is visibly narrow and there may be difficulty passing a suction catheter or small endoscope. There may be other craniofacial abnormalities noted during the routine head and neck examination such as a triangular shaped palate, a bony ridge under the palate, and other maxillary abnormalities.

Diagnosis

Although the suspicion for CNPAS is initiated by the clinical presentation and physical examination, the diagnosis is typically confirmed with computed tomography scanning of the craniofacial skeleton. The width of the piriform aperture is less than 11 mm [1], there may be bony thickening of the medial maxilla and there may be a single central incisor tooth bud (Figs. 3 and 4). The presence of a central incisor is pathognomonic for CNPAS and requires further investigations to rule out other midline brain anomalies.

Management

The management of CNPAS primarily depends on the severity of the respiratory symptoms of the patient. Management options include observation, nasal hygiene, topical steroids and decongestants, serial nasal dilatation, nasal stenting, and surgical correction. The medical literature contains several small case series describing all of the management options listed above.

The larger case series by Van Den Abbeele et al. [3] and Visvanathan and Wynn [2] confirm that conservative or surgical intervention depends on the severity of symptoms. Both studies recommend an initial conservative approach with nasal steroids and topical decongestants for 2 weeks before considering surgery. Their criteria for surgical intervention included sleep apnea, failure to thrive, and persistent dependency on airway assistance at the end of the 2-week trial.

The most common surgical approach employed in the correction of CNPAS is a sublabial incision and mucosal elevation to reveal the piriform aperture. A drill is then used to expand the aperture inferiorly and laterally. Care is taken to avoid injury to the nasolacrimal duct laterally and tooth buds inferiorly. Postoperative nasal stenting for several weeks is used to prevent restenosis.

Multidisciplinary Considerations

CNPAS may occur in isolation or as part of the holoprosencephaly spectrum. The suspicion for other central anomalies is increased if there is a single central incisor (Figs. 2 and 3). Specifically, patients require an endocrinological assessment for pituitary hormone deficiency, an MRI of the brain to assess the corpus callosum and pituitary gland, and a genetics consultation if there are other congenital anomalies. Patients may also require dental and orthodontic consultation following the eruption of the secondary dentition.

Choanal Atresia

Choanal atresia is the end result of a failure to establish communication between the nasal cavity and nasopharynx during embryological development. In essence, an atretic plate remains that obstructs the region of one or both choanae. The choanae are bounded by the sphenoid superiorly, the medial pterygoid plate laterally, the vomer medially and the horizontal portion of the palate inferiorly. The choanae may be stenosed or completely blocked (atresia) by bone and membranous tissue (70 % of cases) or by bone only (30 % of cases). In addition to the atretic plate of bone and/or membranous tissue, medialization of the medial pterygoid plate and thickening of the posterior vomer often contribute to the stenosis and atresia.

Etiology

Many theories have been proposed to explain the development of choanal atresia. The four most popular theories include: (1) persistence of the bucconasal membrane of Hochstetter; (2) misdirection of neural crest cell migration; (3) persistence of the buccopharyngeal membrane from the foregut; and (4) abnormal persistence or location of mesodermal adhesions in the naso-choanal region [6].

Molecular models have also been linked to the development of choanal atresia. For example, it has been shown that mice with a retinaldehyde dehydrogenase 3 (Raldh3) knockout mutation develop choanal atresia. This work suggests that

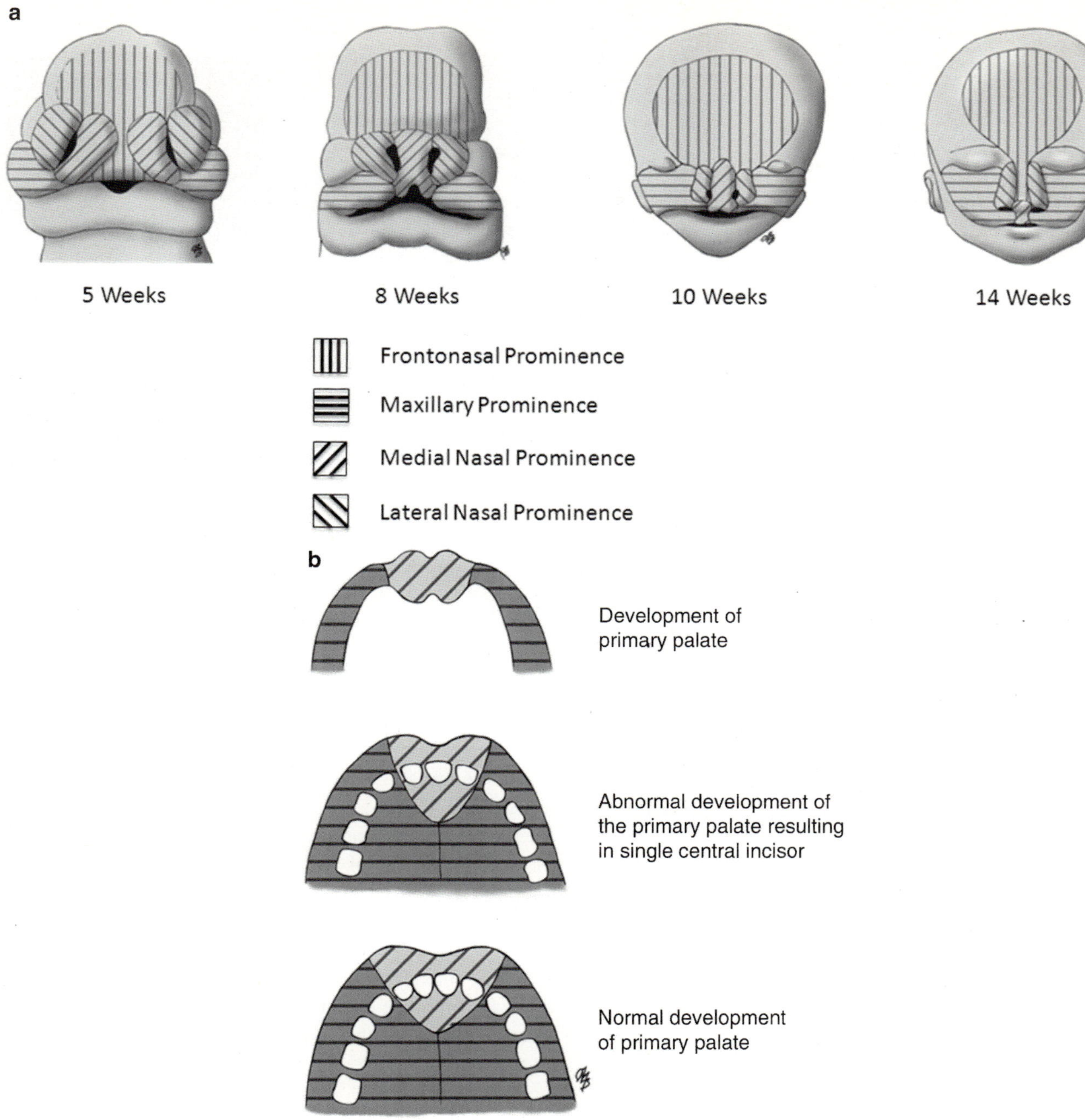

Fig. 1 (**a**, **b**) Drawings illustrating the embryological development of the piriform aperture and primary palate

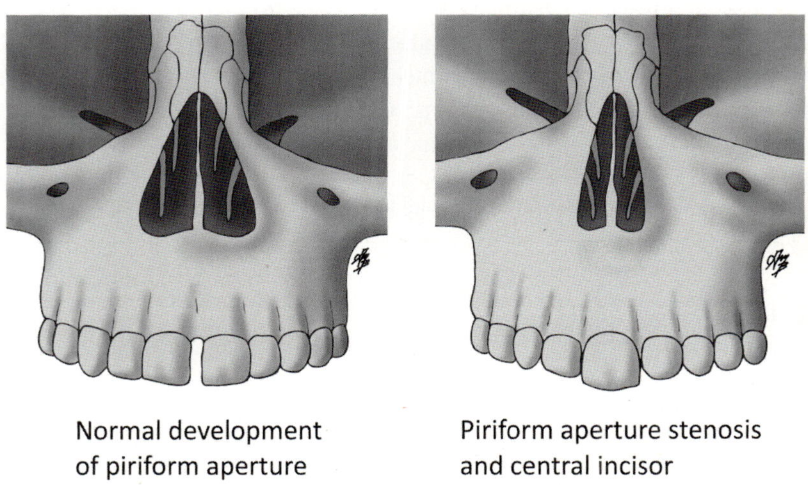

Fig. 2 Drawing illustrating the normal and abnormal size and shape of the piriform aperture

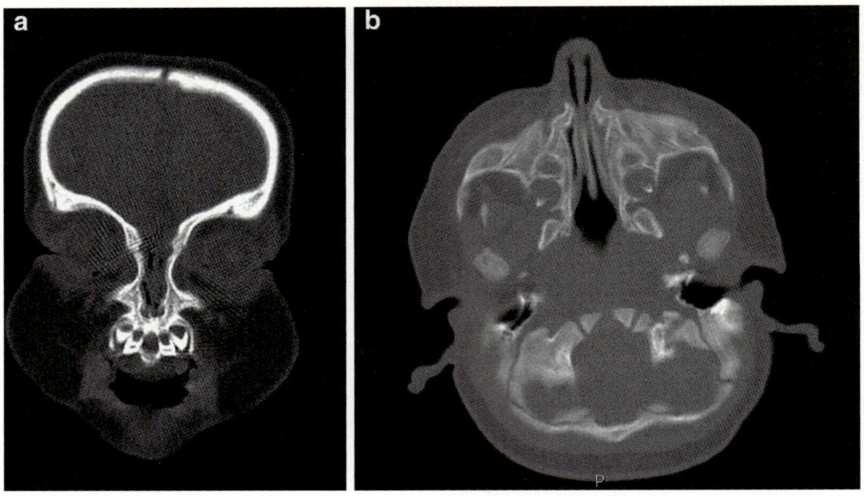

Fig. 3 Computed tomography imaging of a child with congenital nasal piriform aperture stenosis. (**a**) Coronal image demonstrating the central incisor tooth bud. (**b**) Axial image demonstrating the narrow aperture and prominence of the maxillary bone

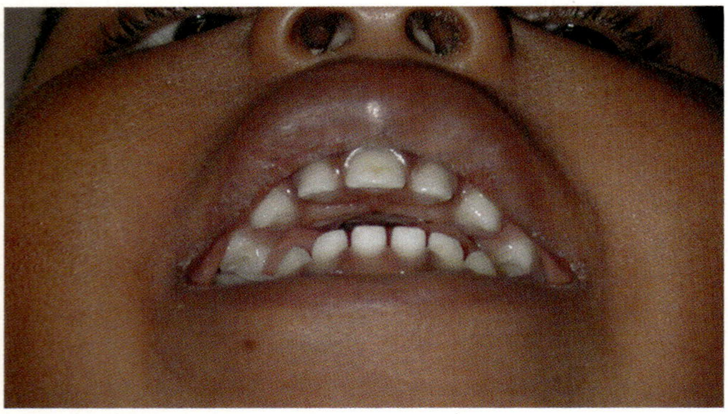

Fig. 4 Clinical photograph of an older child with a central incisor

retinoic acid metabolism is linked to fibroblast growth factor (FGF) expression and eventual perforation of the nasobuccal membrane. Another example is the observed increased incidence of non-syndromic choanal atresia in the children of mothers treated for hyperthyroidism with thionamides. Subsequent animal studies have demonstrated that elevation of thyrotropin alters the expression of FGF, FGF receptors which may play a role in the development of choanal atresia.

Choanal atresia is a hallmark feature of CHARGE syndrome. A mutation in the chromodomain helicase DNA-binding protein 7 (Chd7), located on chromosome 8q12.1, is identified in 60–80 % of children with CHARGE syndrome. Chd7 regulates other genes that control cell-lineage specification and rRNA biogenesis in the nucleolus. The pathogenic mechanism on organ systems such as choanal development is not fully understood.

Epidemiology

Choanal atresia is the most common congenital nasal anomaly with an estimated incidence of 1 in 5,000–8,000 live births. Choanal atresia is more likely to occur in females and be unilateral. When unilateral, the right choana is twice as likely to be affected. Choanal atresia can occur in isolation or be associated with several other conditions such as CHARGE, Apert, Crouzon, Pfeiffer, Antley–Bixler, Marshall–Smith, Schinzel–Giedion, and Treacher Collins syndromes. Approximately 30 % of children with choanal atresia have CHARGE syndrome based on clinical criteria.

Pathogenesis

During the fourth week of gestation, the nasal placodes become depressed and form nasal pits. From the fourth to sixth week, the nasal pits deepen to form primitive nasal sacs. The nasal sacs grow dorsally and remain separate from the oral cavity by the bucconasal membrane of Hochstetter (Fig. 5). By 7 weeks, the bucconasal membrane ruptures allowing communication of the oral and nasal cavities. The resultant primitive choanae are located just posterior to the primary palate. As the secondary palate develops by fusion of the lateral palatine processes, the choanae assume a more posterior location [4].

The pathogenesis of choanal atresia is poorly understood. However, the description of the embryological development provided above renders the theory of failure to disrupt the bucconasal membrane of Hoschstetter plausible (Fig. 5). Further elucidation of the molecular and genetic theories may help to explain the mechanism by which the bucconasal membrane fails to rupture.

Clinical Presentation

The clinical presentation of choanal stenosis and atresia is consistent with the presentation of any condition that causes nasal obstruction: stertor, obstructive apnea, cyclical cyanosis, etc. Newborns with bilateral choanal atresia present with immediate respiratory distress and require prompt securing of the airway with intubation. The suspicion for choanal atresia in these instances is reinforced by the inability to pass a

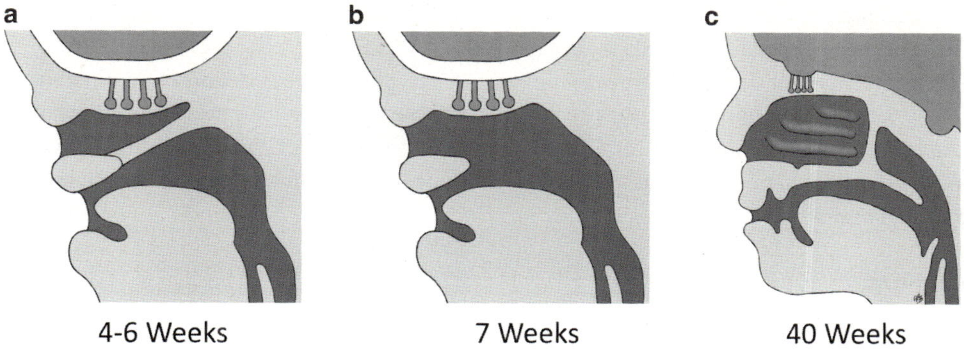

Fig. 5 Drawings illustrating the normal and failed embryological development of the nasal choanae. (**a**) The nasal and oral cavities are separated by the bucconasal membrane. (**b**) The normal rupture of the bucconasal membrane. (**c**) Persistence of the bucconasal membrane at birth

suction catheter into the nasopharynx. Children with unilateral choanal atresia are often diagnosed later in life as they present with complaints of persistent unilateral nasal obstruction and rhinorrhea [5].

Infants and children with isolated choanal atresia typically have a normal physical examination (excluding the signs and symptoms of nasal obstruction). However, if the child presents with other anomalies, the clinician should determine if the choanal atresia is part of a genetic syndrome. The most commonly associated condition is CHARGE syndrome (*C*oloboma of the eye, *H*eart malformations, *A*tresia of choanae, *R*etardation in growth and development, *G*enital hypoplasia, *E*ar anomalies).

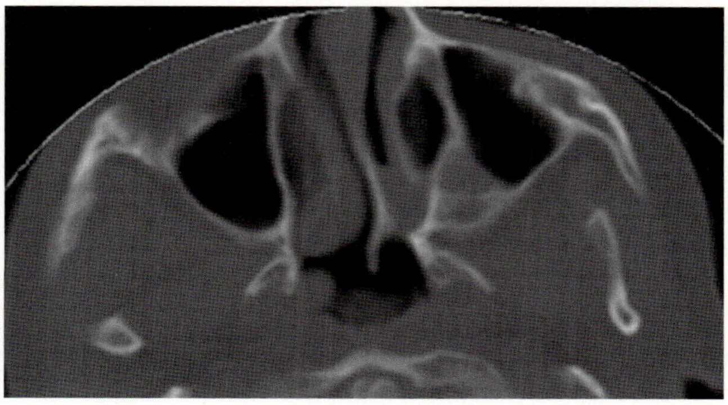

Fig. 6 Computed tomography image (axial view) of a child with unilateral (*left*) choanal atresia. The image demonstrates a combined bony and membranous atretic plate, deviated vomer, and medialized left medial pterygoid plate

Diagnosis

Choanal atresia can be diagnosed with a thorough clinical examination of the nose. The failure to observe fogging of a cold metal speculum placed in front of the nostrils, the movement of a wisp of cotton wool, or the inability to auscultate air flow with the bell of a stethoscope suggests a blocked nasal passage. The visualization of a blind ended nasal cavity with endoscopy confirms the diagnosis of choanal atresia.

The diagnosis is further confirmed with computed tomography scanning of the nose, paranasal sinuses, and skull base (Fig. 6). The images are used to characterize the location and nature of the atresia (bony versus bony and membranous). The images may also demonstrate thickening of the posterior vomer and medialization of the medial pterygoid plate.

Genetic testing may also be warranted if the child presents with other craniofacial anomalies or features of CHARGE syndrome.

Management

The definitive management of choanal atresia requires surgical intervention. The timing of the surgery depends on the severity of the respiratory compromise. Newborns with bilateral choanal atresia undergo surgery in the first few days of life to promptly reestablish the obligatory nasal airway and initiate oral feeding. The surgical correction of unilateral choanal atresia is preferably delayed for 2–4 years. A delayed repair allows for growth of the nasal airway which facilitates surgical access to the atretic plate and may mitigate the clinical significance of partial restenosis of the repaired site.

Many surgical techniques have been described for the correction of choanal atresia. The surgical techniques can be broadly categorized as trans-nasal puncture, endoscopic resection, and trans-palatal resection of the atretic plate. Each approach has its inherent advantages and disadvantages. A thorough review of the nuances of each approach is beyond the scope of this chapter.

The use of postoperative nasal stenting, the type of stent used, the technique used to fix the stent in place, and the duration of stenting is highly variable and contentious. Due to a lack of consensus, the issues surrounding stent use remain highly dependent on surgeon preference. The routine application of mitomycin C to the repair site to prevent restenosis is similarly contentious.

It should be noted that children with complex craniofacial abnormalities, beyond isolated choanal atresia, may require tracheostomy to establish a secure airway.

Multidisciplinary Considerations

As mentioned above, choanal atresia can occur in isolation or be associated with several other genetic syndromes, most notably CHARGE syndrome. All children diagnosed with choanal atresia, therefore, should be assessed for CHARGE syndrome. If confirmed, consultation with ophthalmology, cardiology, urology, and audiology services is required.

Future Considerations

With the discovery of Chd7 gene mutations in 60–80 % of patients with CHARGE syndrome, recently published studies exploring the role of Chd7 in animal models may have profound implications for the elucidation of the pathogenesis of choanal atresia. A mouse model with a spontaneous deletion mutation in the Chd7 gene exhibits morphological alteration in the Eustachian tubes, dysregulation of epithelial proliferation, and hearing loss [7]. Multi-organ system dysfunction has also been demonstrated in zebrafish with Chd7 knockdown mutations [8].

Congenital Laryngeal Disorders

There are several congenital disorders that can affect the development of the laryngo(tracheal) complex. Some of these disorders are very common and others are exceedingly rare. The clinical presentation is similarly variable as laryngeal disorders may be innocuous and self-resolving or incompatible with life. Laryngeal disorders may have an impact on a child's ability to breathe comfortably, protect the airway during swallowing and phonate normally. A list of congenital laryngeal disorders is summarized in Table 2. This section of the chapter will focus on disorders resulting from incomplete closure or recanalization of the laryngo(tracheal) complex during embryological development.

Table 2 Differential diagnosis of congenital laryngeal disorders

Laryngomalacia
Congenital vocal fold insufficiency
Laryngeal cysts
Saccular cyst
Vallecular cyst
Thyroglossal duct cyst
Ductal cyst
Duplication cyst
Laryngocele
Laryngeal web
Laryngeal atresia and stenosis
Congenital subglottic stenosis
Congenital subglottic hemangioma

Laryngeal Clefts

A laryngeal cleft is defined as an incomplete midline fusion of the posterior aspect of the larynx (and upper trachea) resulting in direct communication between the laryngeal and upper tracheal lumen and the esophagus.

Etiology

The specific cause of laryngeal clefts is unknown. However, prematurity and maternal polyhydramnios have been associated with their development. Genetic causes have also been implicated as laryngeal clefts are associated with genetic syndromes (Pallister–Hall and Opitz–Frias) and affected families demonstrate an autosomal dominant pattern of inheritance. Irrespective of the cause, the common embryological anomaly is the incomplete development of the tracheoesophageal septum.

Epidemiology

Congenital laryngeal clefts have an estimated incidence of 1 in 10,000–20,000 live births. They are more common in males than females with an observed ratio of 5:3. In one review, children with congenital laryngeal clefts had an observed overall mortality rate of 46 % when all subtypes of clefts were included in the analysis.

Pathogenesis

The larynx, trachea, bronchi, and lung buds begin to form during the fourth week of gestation [4]. The process begins with the development of a laryngotracheal groove on the ventral wall of the primitive pharynx. By the end of the fourth week, the laryngotracheal groove evaginates to form a laryngotracheal diverticulum (Fig. 7). As the diverticulum elongates, the distal end forms the lung buds. The diverticulum also gradually separates from the primitive pharynx with the development of longitudinal tracheoesophageal folds on both sides. As the folds approximate in the midline, they fuse and form a partition known as the tracheoesophageal septum. The septum develops in a caudal to cranial direction to separate the diverticulum from the primitive pharynx. When separated, the diverticulum is referred to as the laryngotracheal tube. The opening at the proximal/cranial end of the laryngotracheal tube forms the laryngeal inlet (or aditus).

It is the incomplete development of the tracheoesophageal septum that results in laryngeal clefts. The length (severity) of the cleft depends on the distance the tracheoesophageal septum developed in the caudal to cranial direction.

Clinical Presentation

A diagnosis of congenital laryngeal cleft should be considered in a newborn or infant presenting with dysphagia or refusal to feed, unexplained repeated aspiration and intermittent

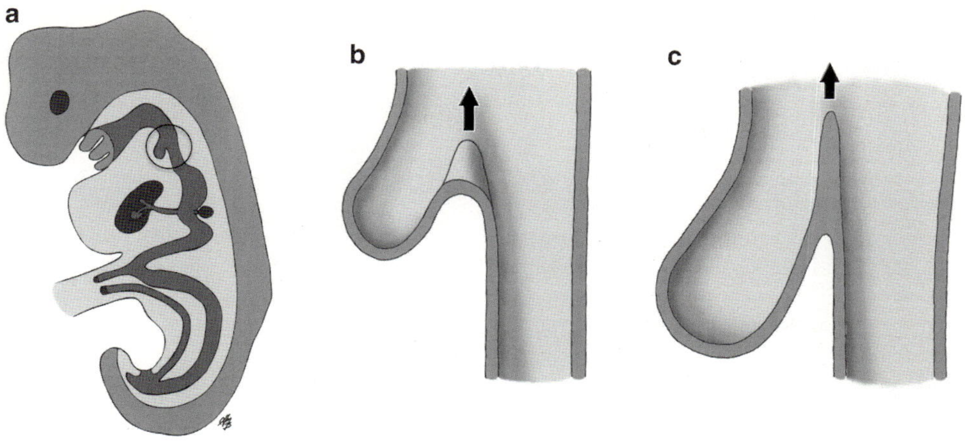

Fig. 7 Drawings illustrating the development of the laryngotracheal diverticulum and tracheoesophageal septum in a caudal to cranial direction

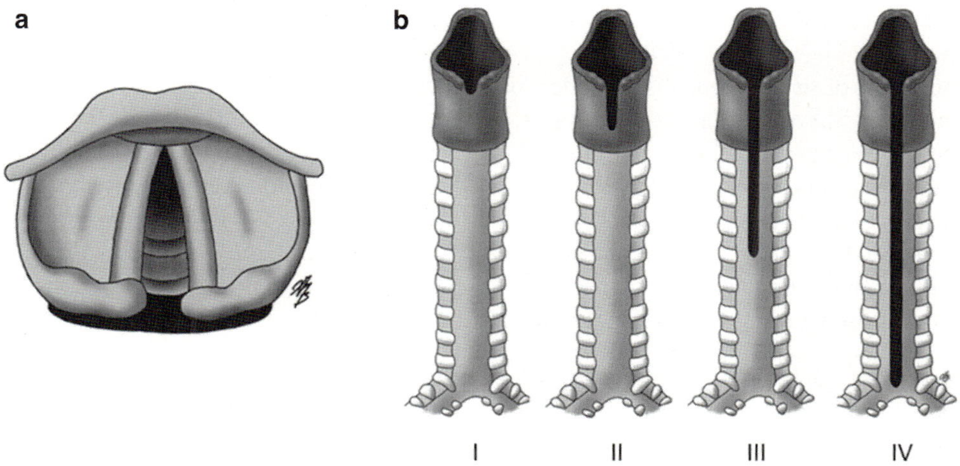

Fig. 8 Drawings illustrating incomplete fusion of the posterior glottis (**a**) and the classification of laryngeal clefts as described by Benjamin and Inglis (**b**)

respiratory distress. Stridor, cough, cyanosis, and regurgitation are particularly evident during feeds.

The most commonly used classification system for congenital laryngeal clefts was introduced by Benjamin and Inglis in 1989 [9] (Fig. 8). Type I clefts result from incomplete fusion of the inter-arytenoid soft tissue with an inferior extension no further than the level of the vocal folds. Type I clefts may not result in symptoms and may be identified incidentally during laryngobronchoscopy. Type II clefts extend beyond the level of the vocal folds and into the cricoid lamina. Type III clefts extend completely through the cricoid cartilage and into the upper trachea. Type IV clefts involve the posterior wall of the trachea and may extend to the carina.

Diagnosis

Newborns and infants presenting with dysphagia and respiratory distress are investigated initially with flexible laryngoscopy and video fluoroscopic swallow studies. The swallow studies typically confirm the suspicion of laryngeal penetration and aspiration of feeds. However, flexible endoscopy frequently fails to reveal laryngeal clefts as redundant mucosa from the posterior larynx or upper esophagus may obscure the cleft. As such, direct laryngoscopy and instrument palpation of the posterior larynx are required to confidently diagnose laryngeal clefts. Rigid bronchoscopy should also be performed to determine the extent of the cleft and to search for secondary airway anomalies which can be found in more than 50 % of patients. The most common secondary airway anomalies are tracheomalacia and tracheoesophageal fistula [10].

Management

The initial priority in the management of children diagnosed with a laryngeal cleft is to prevent aspiration pneumonia. Children with clinically significant dysphagia should not be fed by mouth but rather by nasogastric tube.

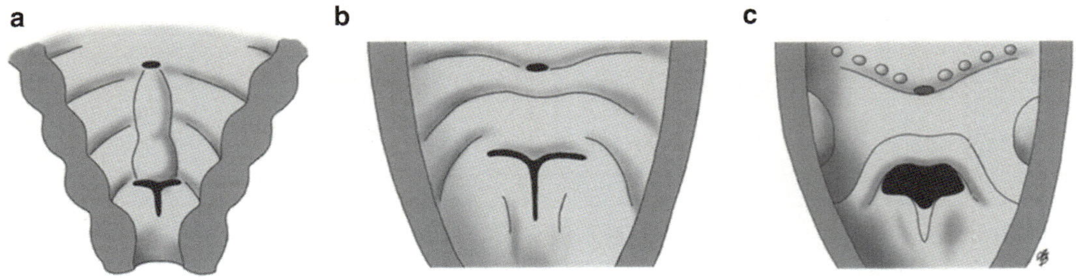

Fig. 9 Drawings illustrating the normal development of the laryngeal inlet

Anti-reflux measures should also be initiated to prevent regurgitation. A thorough assessment of other organ systems is required before proceeding to surgical correction of the cleft. A genetics consultation should also be requested as laryngeal clefts have been associated with Pallister–Hall and Opitz–Frias syndromes.

The need for and timing of surgical repair is dependent on the severity of symptoms, the extent of the cleft, and the overall medical stability of the child. Incidental and minimally symptomatic type I clefts may not require surgical management. In general, symptomatic type I and II clefts are repaired endoscopically and type III and IV clefts are repaired with open surgery. The open surgical repairs can be performed through an anterior laryngotracheal fissure or lateral pharyngotomy approach. Closure of the cleft must be meticulous and multilayered [10].

Multidisciplinary Considerations

Congenital laryngeal clefts may occur in isolation but are often associated with other anomalies of the gastrointestinal, genitourinary, and cardiovascular systems. As such, consultation with a geneticist, pediatrician, and other surgical specialties is required. Occupational therapy and speech-language pathology services are also required for ongoing swallowing and voice concerns.

Laryngeal Webs and Atresia

Laryngeal webs and atresia result from the incomplete recanalization of the larynx during embryological development.

Etiology

The specific cause of laryngeal webs and atresia is unknown. There is likely a genetic cause as laryngeal webs are associated with 22q11.2 deletion syndrome. Laryngeal atresia has been associated with partial trisomy of chromosomes 9 and 16 and chromosome 5p deletion. Embryologically, laryngeal webs and atresia are the result of incomplete recanalization of the larynx that normally occurs during the 10th week of gestation.

Epidemiology

The incidence of laryngeal webs and atresia is unknown.

Pathogenesis

At 5 weeks gestation, the mesenchyme at the laryngeal inlet (cranial end of the laryngotracheal tube) rapidly proliferates to form arytenoid swellings [4] (Fig. 9a). The arytenoid swellings change the shape of the laryngeal inlet from a vertical slit-like appearance to a T-shaped appearance (Fig. 9b). The laryngeal epithelium also proliferates rapidly and temporarily occludes the laryngeal lumen by the eighth week. By the 10th week, the epithelium is resorbed and the laryngeal lumen is recanalized (Fig. 9c). Laryngeal webs and atresia are the result of incomplete recanalization of the larynx during the 10th week of gestation. The laryngeal obstruction may be in the form of a thin membranous web at the glottic level or a thick trans-glottic atresia.

Clinical Presentation

Children with laryngeal webs may present with stridor, croup-like cough, recurrent atypical croup, and a high-pitched voice. Children may present at any age depending on the severity of the airway symptoms. Children that present at an older age typically have an isolated concern of high-pitched voice. If the child has cardiac anomalies, learning disabilities, thyroid and parathyroid dysfunction or immunologic disorders, the laryngeal web may be a component of an underlying 22q11.2 deletion syndrome.

Complete laryngeal atresia is usually incompatible with life. Failure to recanalize the larynx usually results in fetal demise due to the development of fetal hydrops. If the fetus survives the pregnancy, immediate respiratory distress develops at birth. Failure to establish an airway immediately after birth results in death. Laryngeal atresia can occur in isolation or in association with tracheoesophageal fistula.

Laryngeal atresia can be detected antenatally with ultrasound and magnetic resonance imaging studies. In these instances, a fetus that survives the pregnancy should be delivered by ex-utero intrapartum treatment (EXIT) procedure and receive a tracheostomy prior to clamping of the umbilical cord to enhance survival.

Diagnosis

Laryngeal webs are diagnosed by endoscopic visualization of the larynx (Fig. 10). Webs are usually anteriorly based and partially compromise the airway lumen. Asymptomatic webs may be detected incidentally during direct laryngoscopy and intubation for an unrelated surgical intervention. All children diagnosed with a laryngeal web should undergo genetic testing for 22q11.2 deletion syndrome.

As described above, laryngeal atresia can be diagnosed antenatally or during resuscitative efforts at birth. Attempts to place an endotracheal tube fail due to the absence of a lumen and normal glottic anatomy.

Management

Congenital laryngeal webs require surgical intervention to relieve airway symptoms and normalize vocal pitch. Surgical correction by an endoscopic or open approach depends on the vertical length of the web. Thick webs typically require an open approach and the temporary insertion of a keel or stent to maintain patency of the lumen. A thorough discussion of the nuances of surgical correction of laryngeal webs is beyond the scope of this chapter.

Children with laryngeal atresia that were successfully tracheotomized at birth require laryngotracheal reconstructive procedures to establish a stable lumen and eventual decannulation.

Multidisciplinary Considerations

Children with laryngeal webs are best managed in a hospital-based voice clinic with access to speech-language pathology services for diagnosis and ongoing postoperative voice therapy.

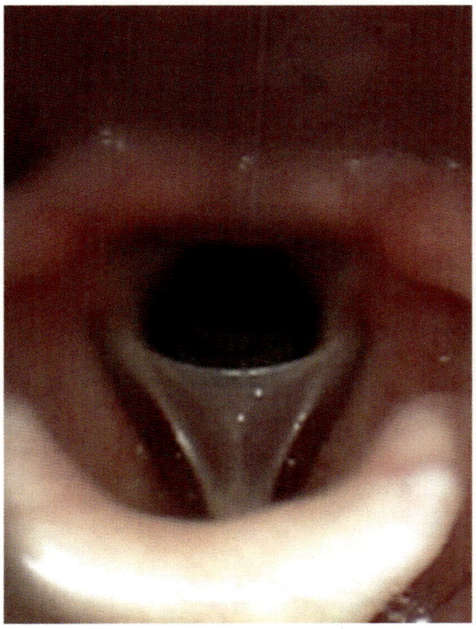

Fig. 10 Endoscopic view of a congenital laryngeal web

Genetics testing for 22q11.2 deletion syndrome should also be requested.

The antenatal diagnosis and management of laryngeal atresia requires a well-established multidisciplinary team of medical professionals that includes fetal diagnostic imaging, maternal–fetal medicine, neonatology, anesthesia, and pediatric otolaryngology. The successful EXIT procedure, in particular, requires precise and efficient coordination of resources and experienced individuals.

Future Considerations

Advances in fetal endoscopic surgery may enable the antenatal treatment of laryngeal atresia to avoid complications such as fetal hydrops and the need for EXIT procedures. The application of balloons and lasers to correct a laryngeal web and atresia has been described in the literature (Kohl et al. [12]).

Congenital Subglottic Stenosis

The subglottis, the narrowest part of the pediatric airway, is formed by the cricoid cartilage ring. Congenital abnormalities in the size or shape of the cricoid cartilage, therefore, result in significant airway compromise.

Etiology

Congenital subglottic stenosis is usually the result of an abnormally small cricoid cartilage ring. A normal-sized cricoid ring, however, may also cause stenosis if it is abnormally shaped. An elliptical cricoid is the most common abnormal shape to cause subglottic stenosis. The cricoid may also be flattened or have a thickened anterior or posterior lamina. A first tracheal ring that is trapped within the cricoid ring is yet another cause of congenital subglottic stenosis [11].

Epidemiology

An incidence rate for congenital subglottic stenosis has not been reported.

Pathogenesis

The pathogenesis of congenital subglottic stenosis has not been well described in the literature. Abnormalities in the size or shape of the cricoid cartilage ring may be due to anomalous proliferation of mesenchyme at the cranial end of the laryngotracheal tube during the 5th week of gestation or incomplete recanalization of the laryngotracheal lumen at the 10th week of gestation.

Clinical Presentation

Infants and children with congenital subglottic stenosis present with inspiratory or biphasic stridor, croup-like cough and atypical, recurring croup. The recurrent croup may occur in children younger than 6 months of age and does not readily respond to standard treatment with steroids and nebulized epinephrine.

Diagnosis

Subglottic stenosis can be diagnosed on plain radiographs of the neck, especially on anterior–posterior views. The diagnosis is confirmed and severity staged with direct laryngoscopy and bronchoscopy in the operating room.

Management

Congenital subglottic stenosis can be managed expectantly if the stenosis is minimal and the airway symptoms reversible with medical treatment. On the other hand, children with chronic and frequently recurrent symptoms require surgical correction with cartilage augmentation of the cricoid ring.

Congenital Tracheal Disorders

There are several congenital anomalies that affect the trachea including tracheal stenosis and atresia, tracheoesophageal fistula, vascular rings and slings, tracheomalacia, tracheal duplication, complete tracheal rings, and cartilaginous sleeve trachea. Fortunately, these anomalies are rare as they cause significant morbidity and are potentially life threatening.

Congenital Tracheal Stenosis

Congenital tracheal stenosis is defined as a narrowing of the tracheal lumen. The stenosis is commonly associated with complete tracheal rings. It may involve a single ring, a segment of rings, or the entire trachea.

Etiology

The direct cause of congenital tracheal stenosis is unknown but it is associated with genetic syndromes and associations (e.g., Down syndrome, VACTERL and VATER association). Complete tracheal rings may also represent an adaptive or protective response to external compression from vascular rings or slings.

Small rodent animal models have demonstrated tracheal anomalies when exposed prenatally to medications (Adriamycin, doxorubicin, and nitrofen) or genetic manipulations (sonic hedgehog, FGF 18 expression). This research, however, may not be applicable to humans.

Epidemiology

Congenital tracheal stenosis is very rare. The incidence has not been reported previously.

Pathogenesis

It has been hypothesized that congenital tracheal stenosis is the result of unequal partitioning of the primitive foregut into the esophagus and trachea by the tracheoesophageal folds. This may result in the abnormal fusion of the posterior aspect of the tracheal rings.

Clinical Presentation

Antenatally, the mothers of children with congenital tracheal stenosis commonly present with polyhydramnios. Immediately after birth, children with severe stenosis present with respiratory distress and attempts to intubate the newborn are unsuccessful as the endotracheal tube cannot be advanced beyond the vocal folds.

With milder degrees of stenosis, the child may remain asymptomatic for several months until they are affected by an upper respiratory tract infection. These children present with respiratory distress, biphasic stridor, and a prolonged expiratory phase of the respiratory cycle.

Diagnosis

A diagnosis of congenital tracheal stenosis is established with rigid bronchoscopy. Care must be taken to avoid trauma to the mucosal lining that may cause edema. The bronchoscopy should be performed with a small telescope to assess the full length of the trachea if possible. If the stenosis does not allow the passage of a small telescope, a computed tomography scan of the chest will provide important information regarding the length of the stenosis and if it extends to the bronchi (Fig. 11). The scan also characterizes the cardiopulmonary vasculature which may require simultaneous repair.

Management

The management of congenital tracheal stenosis includes a period of observation, avoidance of viral contacts and supportive care. A subset of children will not require surgical intervention and may outgrow their mild form of tracheal stenosis. The remaining children require surgical intervention that may include segmental tracheal resection or slide tracheoplasty, depending on the length of the stenosis.

Slide tracheoplasty is delayed as long as possible as this procedure requires the use of cardiopulmonary bypass which is associated with a low survival in very young children. It should also be noted that tracheostomy is not helpful with long segment tracheal stenosis and should be avoided.

Multidisciplinary Considerations

The care of children with congenital tracheal stenosis requires a multidisciplinary approach with input from medical services (respirology, critical care medicine, and anesthesia) and surgical services (cardiothoracic surgery and otolaryngology).

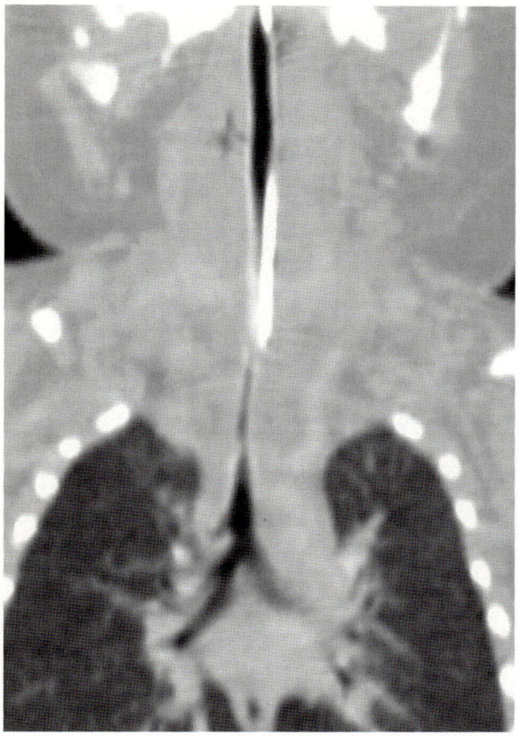

Fig. 11 Computed tomography coronal image of a child with long segment congenital tracheal stenosis. The endotracheal tube cannot be passed beyond the stenotic segment

Future Considerations

There are several exciting new prospects in tissue engineering and tracheal transplantation that may provide hope to children affected with severe forms of stenosis that are not amenable to traditional forms of surgery.

References

1. Belden CJ, Mancuso AA, Schmalfuss IM. CT features of congenital nasal piriform aperture stenosis: initial experience. Radiology. 1999;213:495–501.
2. Visvanathan V, Wynne DM. Congenital nasal pyriform aperture stenosis: a report of 10 cases and literature review. Int J Pediatr Otorhinolaryngol. 2012;76:28–30.
3. Van Den Abbeele T, Triglia JM, Francois M, Narcy P. Congenital nasal pyriform aperture stenosis: diagnosis and management of 20 cases. Ann Otol Rhinol Laryngol. 2001;110:70–5.
4. Moore KL, Persaud TVN. The developing human: clinically oriented embryology. 5th ed. Philadelphia: W.B. Sauders Company; 1993.
5. Ramsden JD, Campisi P, Forte V. Choanal atresia and choanal stenosis. Otolaryngol Clin North Am. 2009;42:339–52.
6. Hengerer AS, Brickman TM, Jeyakumar A. Choanal atresia: embryologic analysis and evolution of treatment, a 30-year experience. Laryngoscope. 2008;118:862–6.
7. Tian C, Yu H, Yang B, Han F, Zheng Y, Bartels CF, Schelling D, Arnold JE, Scacheri PC, Zheng QY. Otitis media in a new mouse model for CHARGE syndrome with a deletionin the Chd7 gene. PLoS One. 2012;7:e34944.
8. Patten SA, Jacobs-McDaniels NL, Zaouter C, Drapeau P, Alberton RC, Moldovan F. Role of Chd7 in zebrafish: a model for CHARGE syndrome. PLoS One. 2012;7:e31650.
9. Benjamin B, Inglis A. Minor congenital laryngeal clefts: diagnosis and classification. Ann Otol Rhinol Laryngol. 1989;98:417–20.
10. Rahbar R, Rouillon I, Roger G, Lin A, Nuss RC, Denoyelle F, McGill TJ, Healy GB, Garabedian EN. The presentation and management of laryngeal cleft. A 10-year experience. Arch Otolaryngol Head Neck Surg. 2006;132:1335–41.
11. Holinger LD. Histopathology of congenital subglottic stenosis. Ann Otol Rhinol Laryngol. 1999;108:101–11.
12. Kohl T, et al. Fetal Diagn Ther. 2009;25(1):67–71.

Craniofacial Syndromes with Airway Anomalies: An Overview

Craniofacial Syndromes with Airway Anomalies: An Overview

Carolyn V. Nguyen and Luv R. Javia

Abnormal craniofacial development can cause airway anomalies in the neonate at multiple levels (Table 1). While evaluating a neonate with a craniofacial syndrome, it is imperative that airway concerns are taken into account. This consideration is important for treating any immediate and evident airway problems and for identifying any nascent airway pathology to avert avoidable airway emergencies. In one study, 65 % of patients with craniofacial abnormalities required some airway management ranging from positioning to tracheotomy, and 80 % of interventions occurred within the first month of life [29]. This chapter provides an introduction to several craniofacial syndromes commonly associated with airway pathologies (Table 2). These syndromes will be discussed in detail in the subsequent chapters.

Nasal Cavity and Midface

Nasal obstruction can cause respiratory distress immediately after birth in the neonate who is an obligate nasal breather. It has been suggested that this phenomenon is due to the prominent soft palate and relatively higher epiglottis in the neonate with a resultant smaller oropharyngeal airway. The neonate can have cyclical breathing in which he/she initially has nasal obstruction, develops cyanosis and hypercapnia, and then begins to cry and ventilate orally. When the cyanosis subsides, the neonate calms and attempts to breathe nasally, thus starting the cycle over again. These cyanotic episodes and ineffective ventilation can result in death if not discovered quickly. Neonates gradually outgrow this sole reliance on nasal breathing by about 4–6 months of age. Obstruction at the nasal level is commonly due to nasal pyriform aperture stenosis, choanal stenosis or atresia, and midface hypoplasia.

C.V. Nguyen
Staff Otolaryngologist, Kaiser Permanente, Los Angeles, CA, USA

L.R. Javia, MD (✉)
Division of Otolaryngology, The Children's Hospital of Philadelphia, Department of Otorhinolaryngology—Head and Neck Surgery, University of Pennsylvania, Perelman School of Medicine, Philadelphia, PA, USA
e-mail: Javia@email.chop.edu

Congenital Nasal Pyriform Aperture Stenosis

Etiology. Congenital nasal pyriform aperture stenosis (CNPAS), first described in 1989, is believed to occur when bony overgrowth of the nasal processes of the maxilla narrows or obstructs the nasal cavities [12]. CNPAS can occur in isolation, but there are frequently additional findings suggestive of a microform holoprosencephaly (HPE). The full spectrum of HPE has been linked to many chromosomal abnormalities.

Epidemiology. The true incidence of CNPAS is unknown but occurs less commonly than choanal stenosis or atresia.

Pathogenesis. HPE, the abnormal division of the forebrain, varies widely in severity. A single central maxillary incisor, present in approximately 60 % of CNPAS, is considered the least severe form of HPE [5, 43]. Additional findings linked with CNPAS can include abnormal development of the brain and the pituitary gland leading to endocrine dysfunction.

Clinical presentation. CNPAS causes symptoms of nasal obstruction, which develop shortly after birth. In mild cases, the patient may present with "noisy breathing," aggravated with feeding and agitation. In severe cases, cyclical breathing may be present with cyanotic episodes.

Diagnosis. The inability to pass a suction catheter larger than 5 Fr through the anterior nares is suspicious for CNPAS and should be confirmed by an otolaryngologist with nasal endoscopy. CT imaging can help evaluate for other contemporaneous midline defects such as a single central maxillary incisor (Fig. 1). A pyriform aperture width, as viewed on CT axial imaging, of less than 11 mm in a term infant is considered to be diagnostic for CNPAS [7]. Careful evaluation is

J. Lioy and S.E. Sobol (eds.), *Disorders of the Neonatal Airway: Fundamentals for Practice*, DOI 10.1007/978-1-4939-1610-8_2, © Springer Science+Business Media New York 2015

necessary to distinguish CNPAS from choanal atresia, which can present in a similar fashion.

Management. Neonates with CNPAS often require airway monitoring in the intensive care unit. Conservative management, including support with special feeding techniques and monitoring until the airway grows, is indicated in mildly symptomatic neonates. Nasal decongestants, humidification, and nasal continuous positive airway pressure (CPAP) may be sufficient. Surgery to widen the nasal pyriform aperture, accessed through a sublabial incision, is often required in the more severely afflicted neonates. Some feel that CNPAS is associated with an overall narrowing of the width of bilateral nasal cavities. Thus, dilation of the nasal cavities with inferior turbinate outfracturing may be required with possible temporary nasal stent placement.

Table 1 Overview of sites of primary airway anomalies and associated craniofacial syndromes

Site of primary airway anomaly	Syndrome
Nasal Cavity and Midface	Congenital nasal pyriform aperture stenosis
	CHARGE syndrome
	Craniosynostosis syndromes (Crouzon, Apert, Pfeiffer)
Oromandibular	Stickler syndrome
	Treacher Collins syndrome
	Craniofacial microsomia
Laryngotracheal	Complete tracheal rings in Down syndrome (Trisomy 21)
	Tracheal cartilaginous sleeve in craniosynostosis syndromes

Table 2 Specific airway concerns with craniofacial syndromes

Craniofacial syndrome	Specific airway concerns
Congenital nasal pyriform aperture stenosis	Narrow pyriform aperture width
	Can have associated narrow nasal cavities
CHARGE syndrome	Unilateral choanal atresia
	Bilateral choanal atresia
	Laryngomalacia
	Pharyngolaryngeal hypotonia
Craniosynostosis syndromes	Midface hypoplasia—nasopharyngeal and oropharyngeal obstruction
	Obstructive sleep apnea
	Nasal cavity stenosis
	Choanal atresia
	Tracheal anomalies—tracheal cartilaginous sleeve
Stickler syndrome	Macroglossia
	Micrognathia
Treacher Collins syndrome	Severe micrognathia
	Unilateral choanal atresia
	Bilateral choanal atresia
	Obstructive sleep apnea
Craniofacial microsomia	Mandibular hypoplasia
Down syndrome	Complete tracheal rings resulting in tracheal stenosis
	Subglottic stenosis
	Laryngomalacia
	Tracheobronchomalacia
	Macroglossia
	Midfacial hypoplasia
	Obstructive sleep apnea
	Pharyngeal hypotonia

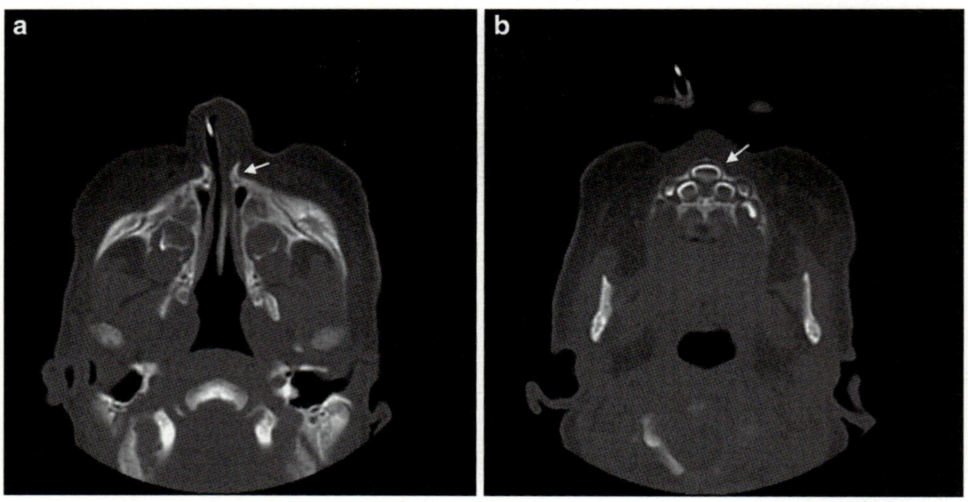

Fig. 1 Congenital nasal pyriform aperture stenosis (CNPAS). (**a**) Axial computed tomographic (CT) image showing a narrow 4 mm pyriform aperture width. (**b**) Concurrent single central maxillary incisor

Multidisciplinary considerations. A brain MRI and blood tests for pituitary hormone levels should be considered to assess for pituitary dysfunction. The need for consultation of specialists, such as endocrinology and neurology, depends on the constellation of HPE-associated findings. Developmental delay of variable severity may occur in children with HPE and patients should be followed long-term.

CHARGE Syndrome

Etiology. The CHARGE acronym stands for *C*oloboma of the eye, *H*eart defects, *A*tresia of the choanae, *R*estricted growth, *G*enital anomalies, and *E*ar anomalies. CHARGE syndrome, also known as Hall Hittner syndrome, was first described in 1979. CHARGE is associated with mutations in the *CHD7* gene, but approximately one-third of cases have no identified mutation [24]. Most cases arise *de novo* and represent a single occurrence in a family, but an autosomal dominant inheritance pattern is seen in familial CHARGE syndrome.

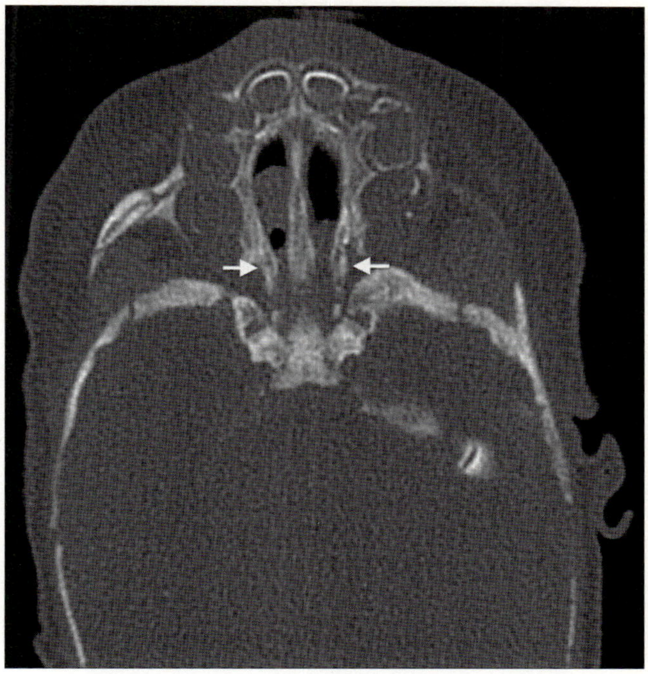

Fig. 2 Bilateral mixed membranous and bony choanal atresia in a patient with CHARGE syndrome

Epidemiology. Approximately between 1:8,500 and 1:12,000 [14, 24].

Pathogenesis. CHD7 gene mutations affect the protein involved in chromatin remodeling, which disrupts the regulation of gene expression [13].

Clinical presentation. Choanal stenosis or atresia can cause life-threatening respiratory distress in neonates (Fig. 2). Unilateral or bilateral choanal atresia is present in 50–60 % of patients [24]. Laryngomalacia is a major cause of upper airway obstruction and can be present in 8–37 % of patients with CHARGE [27]. Pharyngolaryngeal hypotonia can result in additional upper airway obstruction. Patients may also have cranial neuropathies involving cranial nerves V, VII, VIII, IX, and X [27]. Cardiovascular instability and feeding issues such as dysphagia and aspiration can present additional significant challenges in the neonatal period. As many as 80 % of children with CHARGE may have gastroesophageal reflux disease [27], which can further exacerbate airway obstruction.

Diagnosis. Mutations in the *CHD7* gene are identified by genetic testing in approximately 67 % of individuals with a phenotype consistent with CHARGE [38]. Four major defining characteristics in CHARGE are ocular coloboma, choanal stenosis or atresia, cranial nerve dysfunction (varies from dysphagia, sensorineural hearing loss, hyposmia, or facial palsy), and anomalies of the middle or inner ear. The minor characteristics that are less specific but commonly seen in CHARGE are cardiovascular anomalies, growth delays, developmental delay and genital hypoplasia, which are more apparent in males. A clinical diagnosis can be made if an individual has four major characteristics or three major with one minor characteristic [10].

Management. Airway and cardiac evaluations are required immediately. Airway management may require intubation, transnasal or transpalatal surgical repair of choanal stenosis or atresia, or tracheotomy. A tracheotomy may need to be performed in as many as 10–60 % of patients [27]. A supraglottoplasty for management of severe laryngomalacia should be performed only after a thorough airway evaluation as children with CHARGE syndrome have poorer outcomes likely due to concurrent airway pathology. Feeding difficulties can be a major source of morbidity requiring speech and swallow therapy.

Multidisciplinary considerations. Specialist consultations of cardiology, otolaryngology, ophthalmology, audiology, and speech pathology services are usually needed. Individuals with CHARGE usually have feeding issues and variable learning disabilities worsened by dual visual and hearing impairment. Serial audiologic and ophthalmologic exams are recommended. Hypogonadism may disrupt progression into puberty.

Craniosynostosis Syndromes

Etiology. Mutations in the fibroblast growth factor receptor (*FGFR*) genes account for many craniosynostosis syndromes including Crouzon, Apert and Pfeiffer syndromes. *FGFR* genes encode different fibroblast growth factor receptors that

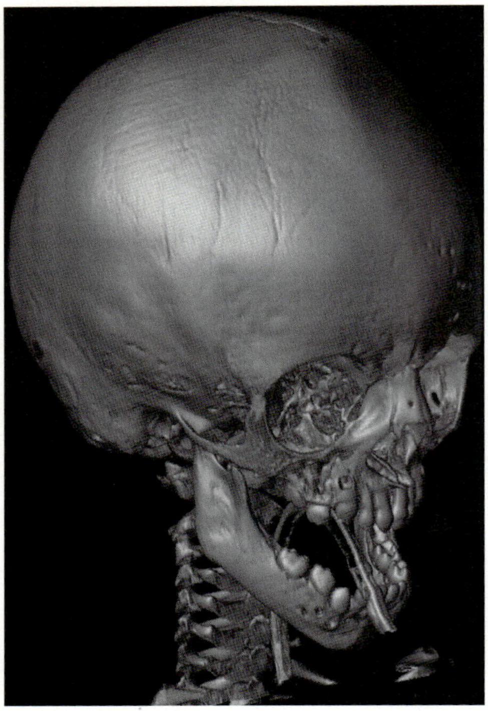

Fig. 3 Patient with Crouzon syndrome with premature fusion of the cranial sutures. Three-dimensional reconstructed image from CT images shows ridge in the midline of the frontal bone which results from early fusion of the metopic suture

regulate cell growth and embryonic development. The *FGFR* mutations are transmitted in an autosomal dominant inheritance pattern [36].

Epidemiology. Crouzon syndrome affects 16 per million newborns [15]. Apert syndrome affects between 1:65,000 and 1:88,000 newborns [3], and Pfeiffer syndrome affects 1:100,000 newborns [45].

Pathogenesis. Mutations in the *FGFR* protein affect the development of bone cells and cause premature fusion of the sutures of the skull (Fig. 3). Craniosynostosis can cause airway obstruction from midface hypoplasia or tracheal abnormalities.

Clinical presentation. An abnormally shaped skull is apparent at birth in a neonate with craniosynostosis. The degree of airway compromise secondary to midface hypoplasia is variable, and almost half of children with Crouzon, Apert and Pfeiffer syndromes develop obstructive sleep apnea [6]. Nasal cavity stenosis or choanal atresia may also be present in this population. Additionally, neonates with Crouzon, Apert and Pfeiffer syndromes may have stridor and respiratory distress secondary to tracheal abnormalities, which are discussed later in this chapter. In one large retrospective review, children with craniofacial synostosis syndromes had the highest rate of tracheotomy at 48 % [39].

Diagnosis. Genetic testing is available, but a clinical diagnosis is frequently possible for most of the *FGFR*-related craniosynostosis syndromes based on facial features, distinguishing anomalies of the hands and feet, and the cranial sutures affected. These three craniosynostosis syndromes share common features of maxillary hypoplasia, shallow orbits causing proptosis, wide set eyes and a beaked nose. Apert syndrome is notable for syndactyly of the fingers and toes whereas normal hands and feet are typical for Crouzon syndrome [4, 16, 35]. Individuals with Pfeiffer syndrome tend to have partial syndactyly and medially displaced, broad and short thumbs and big toes [30, 45].

Management. Expansion of the cranial vault and midface advancement require staged surgeries. Tracheotomy may be needed for airway management especially when multiple surgeries are often needed to address the craniofacial abnormalities. Midface advancement can help alleviate obstruction of the nasopharyngeal and oropharyngeal airway. Choanal atresia repair or nasal splints may be needed to address nasal obstruction. Adenotonsillectomy may partially alleviate OSA if hypertrophy of these structures develops later in childhood.

Multidisciplinary considerations. Long-term care should be managed by a craniofacial team involving neurosurgery, plastic surgery, otolaryngology, ophthalmology, genetics, and developmental pediatrics. Intellectual disability affects individuals in certain types of *FGFR*-related craniosynostosis. Cognitive function is normal in Crouzon syndrome, but variable intellectual disability is common in Apert and Pfeiffer syndromes [23]. Individuals with craniosynostosis may require lifelong monitoring for hydrocephalus.

Oromandibular

An underdeveloped mandible can cause upper airway obstruction due to the resulting posterior or downward displacement of the tongue.

Stickler Syndrome

Etiology. Stickler syndrome is a group of connective tissue disorders characterized by distinctive orofacial features, hearing loss, premature degenerative joint disease, progressive myopia, and retinal detachment [41]. The subtypes of Stickler syndrome (types I through V) are associated with mutations in the genes *COL2A1*, *COL11A1*, *COL11A2*, *COL9A1*, and *COL9A2*, respectively, with types I through III being most common [41]. The inheritance pattern could be either autosomal dominant or recessive depending on the subtype.

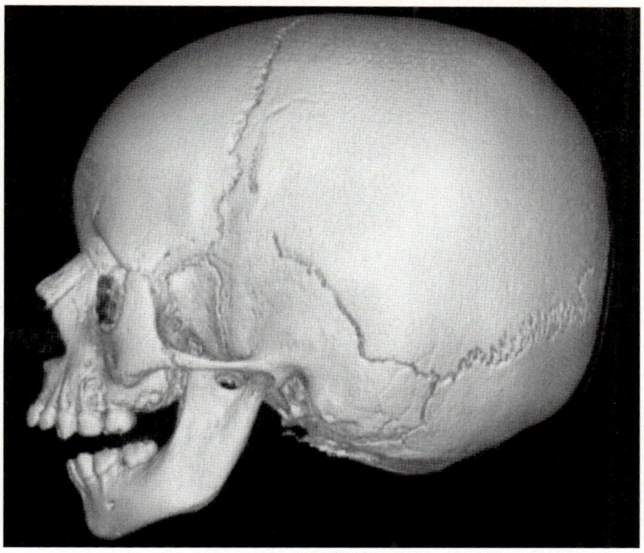

Fig. 4 Patient with Pierre Robin sequence. Three-dimensional reconstructed image from CT images shows retrognathia

Epidemiology. The estimated incidence of Stickler syndrome is between 1:7,500 and 1:9,000 [35]. Approximately 35 % of newborns with Pierre Robin sequence develop features of Stickler syndrome.

Pathogenesis. Mutations in any of these genes affect the production of collagen types II, IX, and XI. Connective tissues containing these collagen fibers do not develop normally.

Clinical presentation. Common orofacial findings include the Pierre Robin sequence of macroglossia, cleft palate, and micrognathia (Fig. 4). Some neonates may present with airway distress requiring intubation in severe cases of micrognathia. Cleft palate occurs in about 40 % and causes feeding difficulties [37]. Additional facial characteristics, such as a hypoplastic flattened midface with a depressed nasal bridge, are more prominent in younger children than in adults [40]. Hearing loss affects approximately 63 % of individuals and is predominantly sensorineural (67.8 %) from abnormal collagen in the inner ear [1]. A mixed or conductive hearing loss is common in individuals with a cleft palate from chronic Eustachian tube dysfunction. Common eye problems include myopia and vitreous abnormalities. The different subtypes of Stickler syndrome have specific associated features for each genotype, but phenotypic variability is common even within families with the same genotype.

Diagnosis. Genetic testing is available, but the diagnosis is considered when this combination of orofacial, ocular, auditory, and musculoskeletal manifestations are present.

Management. The feeding and airway problems present in the neonatal period often require care coordination to determine the timing of cleft palate repair and airway management. Airway management is aimed at relieving base of tongue obstruction at the level of the oropharynx. Non-operative management includes prone positioning, oral airway placement, nasopharyngeal stenting, and short-term intubation. Operative management includes tongue-lip adhesion and mandibular distraction osteogenesis [34]. Tracheotomy is reserved for severe airway obstruction.

Multidisciplinary considerations. Long-term care should be coordinated by a craniofacial team including plastic surgery, oromaxillofacial surgery, otolaryngology, and genetics. Children with Stickler syndrome should have an eye exam performed annually by a vitreoretinal specialist and a hearing test biannually until age five then annually thereafter [35]. Screening for mitral valve prolapse should be performed during routine physicals. Contact sports should be avoided due to the underlying risk of retinal detachment.

Treacher Collins Syndrome

Etiology. Abnormal development of the facial bones and soft tissues is a hallmark of Treacher Collins syndrome. Three genes have been identified. Mutations in the *TCOF1* gene account for more than 80 % of cases, often arise *de novo* and have an autosomal dominant inheritance pattern [22]. Mutations in the *POLR1C* or *POLR1D* genes account for about 8 % of cases [22].

Epidemiology. Approximately between 1:10,000 and 1:50,000 [42].

Pathogenesis. Mutations in these genes reduce the production of ribosomal RNA, which is essential in the assembly of proteins that regulate cell function and cell death. Abnormal cellular death disrupts the development of the facial bones and soft tissues bilaterally. It is not known why the abnormal development is limited to structures originating from the nasal placode and the first and second branchial arches [32].

Clinical presentation. There is significant phenotypic variability in Treacher Collins syndrome. Symmetrical characteristic features are apparent at birth. The underdevelopment of the zygoma causes downward slanting eyes, a prominent appearing nose, and a convex-appearing facial profile bilaterally. Severe mandibular hypoplasia can cause airway distress in the neonate. Choanal atresia, either unilateral or bilateral, can be present and exacerbate neonatal respiratory distress. More than half of children with Treacher Collins syndrome develop obstructive sleep apnea [31]. Microtia, notching of the lower eyelids, and the paucity of medial lower eyelashes are also classic findings. Conductive hearing loss is common from anomalies of the outer ear (microtia and aural atresia) and middle ear (ossicular anomalies and hypoplasia of the middle ear). The inner ear is rarely affected [22].

Diagnosis. Distinguishing clinical features and radiographic findings (malar hypoplasia, hypoplasia of the zygoma on CT scan or X-rays) are sufficient for diagnosis. Genetic testing is available.

Management. An airway evaluation is often required to assess for obstruction secondary to micrognathia. Airway management is aimed at relieving base of tongue obstruction at the level of the oropharynx. Non-operative management includes prone positioning, oral airway placement, nasopharyngeal stenting, and short-term intubation. Operative management includes tongue-lip adhesion and mandibular distraction osteogenesis [34]. Tracheotomy is reserved for severe airway obstruction and provides a secure airway for the multiple surgeries that are usually needed to address the craniofacial abnormalities. Bilateral choanal atresia may require early neonatal surgical repair, whereas surgical repair of unilateral choanal atresia usually can be delayed. Swallowing difficulties present in the neonatal period and may require speech and swallow therapy.

Multidisciplinary considerations. Long-term care should be coordinated by a craniofacial team including plastic surgery, oromaxillofacial surgery, orthodontics, and otolaryngology. Ophthalmologic care and hearing amplification are often necessary. Intellect is usually normal although children are at risk for developmental delay from hearing loss and visual problems. Dental anomalies and malocclusion are addressed at an older age.

Craniofacial Microsomia

Etiology. Craniofacial microsomia is characterized by the abnormal development of structures derived from the embryologic first and second branchial arches and results in maxillary and mandibular hypoplasia. The term craniofacial microsomia is used broadly to encompass a spectrum of syndromes with asymmetric facial development including hemifacial microsomia and Goldenhar syndrome. No frequently occurring genetic mutation has been identified. One suspected cause may be a disruption of the blood supply to the first and second branchial arches early in pregnancy. Several environmental risk factors including maternal diabetes, multiple gestation, exposure to vasoactive drugs, and the use of assisted reproductive technology have been associated with craniofacial microsomia [9].

Epidemiology. The incidence for craniofacial microsomia is estimated to be between 1:3,000 and 1:5,000, and it is the second most common facial birth defect after cleft lip and palate [9]. The reported male-to-female ratio is approximately between 1.2:1 and 1.6:1 [26, 33].

Pathogenesis. The asymmetric facial anomalies in craniofacial microsomia are due to the disruption of the embryologic development of the nerves, muscles, blood vessels, cartilages, and bones derived from the first and second branchial arches.

Clinical presentation. Craniofacial microsomia commonly affects only one side of the face, but approximately 10–15 % have bilateral involvement to varying degrees causing facial asymmetry [26]. The ratio of right-to-left sided involvement is 3:2 [19]. One classification system, *OMENS-Plus*, is used to rate the severity of *O*rbital distortion, *M*andibular hypoplasia, *E*ar anomaly, *N*erve involvement, *S*oft tissue deficiency, and extra-craniofacial anomalies ("*Plus*") [21, 44]. Mandibular hypoplasia is the most apparent feature and can cause respiratory distress (Fig. 5). The common ear anomalies include preauricular skin tags, microtia, anotia, or external auditory canal atresia. Facial nerve palsy is the most frequently observed nerve anomaly. Soft tissue deficiencies of the face and macrostomia can occur. Cleft lip and/or palate affect approximately 25 % of individuals [26]. Additional craniofacial abnormalities and extra-craniofacial abnormalities, such as vertebral, renal, limb, cardiac, and central nervous system deformities, have been associated with craniofacial microsomia [19].

Diagnosis. The distinctive facial findings characteristic for craniofacial microsomia help distinguish it from other craniofacial syndromes. Facial asymmetry is one key component of craniofacial microsomia that separates it from the symmetrical anomalies seen in Treacher Collins syndrome.

Management. In severe cases of mandibular hypoplasia, the initial neonatal airway management is aimed at relieving base of tongue obstruction at the level of the oropharynx. Non-operative management includes prone positioning, oral airway placement, nasopharyngeal stenting, and short-term intubation. Operative management includes tongue-lip adhesion and mandibular distraction osteogenesis. Tracheotomy is reserved for severe airway obstruction and provides a secure airway for the multiple surgeries that are usually needed to address the craniofacial abnormalities.

Multidisciplinary considerations. Long-term care should be coordinated by a craniofacial team including plastic surgery, maxillofacial surgery, orthodontics, and otolaryngology.

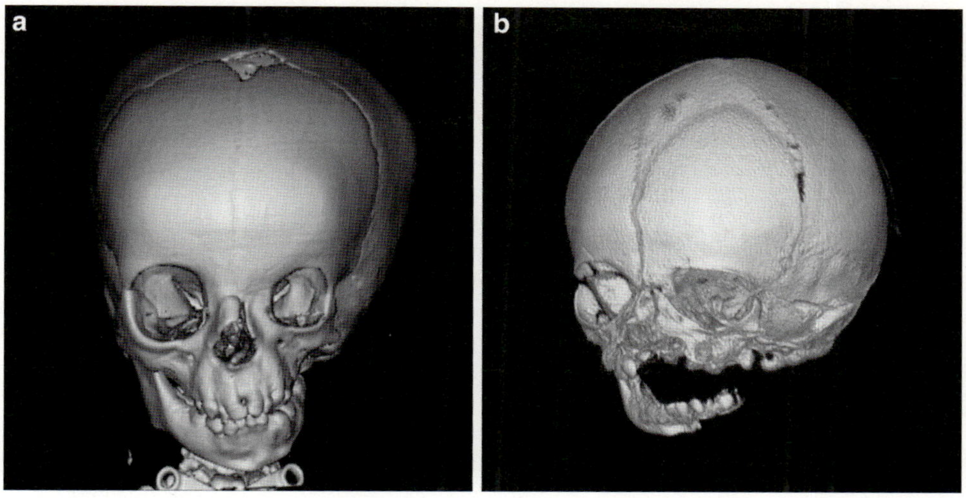

Fig. 5 Craniofacial microsomia. (**a**) Three-dimensional reconstructed image from CT images shows left sided maxillary and mandibular hypoplasia resulting in facial asymmetry and airway narrowing-note the tracheotomy tube flange in the inferior aspect of the image. (**b**) Three-dimensional reconstructed image from CT images from another patient shows left sided mandibular body, ramus, and condylar agenesis

Feeding difficulties may require additional support. Hearing amplification may be necessary if the ear anomalies cause hearing loss, which can be conductive, sensorineural, or mixed. Intellect is usually normal although children are at risk for developmental delay from hearing loss. Further surgeries to improve facial asymmetry, ear anomalies, and jaw malocclusion are usually performed at an older age.

Laryngotracheal

Anomalies of the laryngotracheal complex can complicate management of the airway when using standard options such as intubation or tracheotomy. A select few anomalies are discussed below.

Complete Tracheal Rings in Down Syndrome (Trisomy 21)

Etiology. Complete tracheal rings causing tracheal stenosis have been associated with Down syndrome [8, 11, 47]. No specific factor has been identified that causes the formation of complete tracheal rings. Down syndrome occurs when an individual has three copies of chromosome 21 instead of the normal two copies. This occurs most commonly from a random nondisjunction error in cell division that results in an egg or sperm with an extra chromosome. Less commonly, Down syndrome can occur from translocation (inheriting an extra copy of chromosome 21 that is attached to another chromosome) or from mosaicism (an error of cell division that occurs during embryonic development resulting in only some cells carrying three copies) [18].

Epidemiology. Down syndrome is the most common chromosomal abnormality and affects approximately 1 in 600–800 newborns [8]. The incidence of complete tracheal rings in children with Down syndrome is unknown.

Pathogenesis. It is unclear how the extra copy of chromosome 21 results in intellectual disability and the diverse effects on multiple organ systems. Laryngotracheal airway anomalies in Down syndrome include complete tracheal rings, subglottic stenosis, laryngomalacia, tracheal bronchus, and tracheobronchomalacia [8, 46]. Tracheal stenosis from complete tracheal rings can involve either a short-segment or a long-segment of the tracheobronchial tree (Fig. 6).

Clinical presentation. Down syndrome is associated with a characteristic facies including low-set ears, up-slanting palpebral fissures, a flat nasal bridge, and a tendency to protrude the enlarged tongue. Discussion of the numerous medical issues commonly associated with Down syndrome is beyond the scope of this book. Respiratory difficulty in a newborn should raise the concern for tracheal stenosis, particularly when there is a history of a difficult intubation or persistent airway instability after intubation. Respiratory symptoms can range from mild stridor with exertion to the complete inability to ventilate necessitating the use of extra-corporeal membrane oxygenation (ECMO).

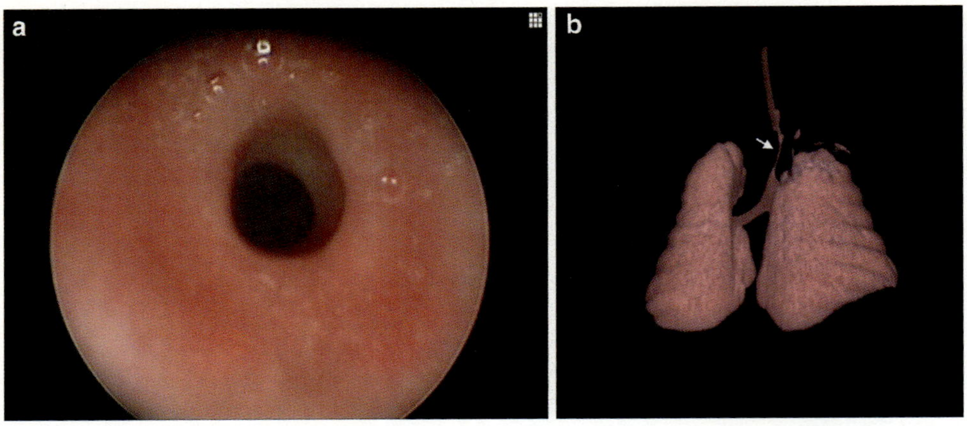

Fig. 6 Complete tracheal rings and tracheal stenosis. (**a**) Endoscopic view of airway during bronchoscopy shows complete tracheal rings with the absence of trachealis muscle posteriorly and a narrowed tracheal lumen. (**b**) Three-dimensional image of trachea and lungs reconstructed from CT images from a patient with long segment tracheal stenosis. Note the segment of the distal trachea marked with the arrow where the airway narrows to 1 mm

Diagnosis. Down syndrome can usually be diagnosed based on clinical findings, and chromosomal analysis is available for uncertain cases. Prenatal testing for Down syndrome is widely available. If tracheal stenosis is suspected, a tracheobronchoscopy is essential to evaluate the airway for complete tracheal rings or other airway anomalies. Tracheobronchoscopy permits characterization of the type, location, length, and severity of stenosis under dynamic conditions. Additionally, CT or MRI imaging can provide helpful information about the airway and evaluate for other cardiovascular anomalies [2].

Management. Respiratory distress secondary to tracheal stenosis can range from mild to life threatening. In one institution's experience, the overall mortality rate was 21 % for all children with tracheal stenosis in the study period [2]. Observation with medical management may be sufficient in mild cases, and symptoms will improve as the affected airway grows over time. In severe cases, intubation or tracheotomy may help provide temporary airway stability. When surgical repair is necessary, a partial tracheal resection with end-to-end anastomosis is preferred for short-segment stenosis; whereas, slide tracheoplasty is preferred for long-segment stenosis.

Multidisciplinary considerations. Otolaryngology should be consulted for a complete airway evaluation in symptomatic children with Down syndrome because airway compromise may be multifactorial. Obstructive sleep apnea later in childhood is commonly multifactorial due to macroglossia and midface hypoplasia in addition to adenotonsillar hypertrophy. Cardiothoracic surgery should be consulted in cases that may require intraoperative cardiopulmonary bypass. Long-term, children with Down syndrome require care coordination to monitor and support special needs including developmental and intellectual delay, hearing loss, immune compromise, endocrine dysfunction, and monitoring for leukemia.

Tracheal Cartilaginous Sleeve in Craniosynostosis Syndromes

Etiology. Tracheal cartilaginous sleeve (TCS), a rare airway malformation in which the normally discrete tracheal rings are replaced by a continuous cartilaginous segment, has been associated with multiple craniosynostosis syndromes but most commonly in Crouzon, Pfeiffer and Apert syndromes [25]. Please refer to the earlier section for an overview of mutations in the fibroblast growth factor receptor (*FGFR*) gene in these craniosynostosis syndromes.

Epidemiology. The incidence of TCS in *FGFR*-related craniosynostosis syndromes is unknown but is rare.

Pathogenesis. Mutations in the *FGFR* protein affect the development of bone cells and cause premature fusion of the sutures of the skull. The premature fusion of preformed cartilaginous structures is the suspected cause of the additional anatomic abnormalities in craniosynostosis [28]. In TCS, the continuous cartilaginous segment is formed by the vertical fusion of either C- or O-shaped cartilaginous tracheal rings. TCS can affect a few tracheal rings in length, involve the entire trachea or even extend into the bronchial airways. The diagnosis of TCS in children with craniosynostosis portends a poor prognosis with a reported 90 % mortality rate by age 2 years of age [28].

Clinical presentation. Upper airway obstruction from midface hypoplasia is frequently present in the craniosynostosis population and may necessitate tracheotomy. TCS may in fact first become apparent at the time of tracheotomy. In other patients, biphasic stridor, cough, recurrent croup, failure to thrive and cyanotic episodes may necessitate an endoscopic airway evaluation, which can reveal TCS. TCS greatly diminishes the normal elasticity present in the tracheal airway, and the trachea may not grow adequately to support the ventilation needs as a child grows [20].

Diagnosis. Previously reported TCS cases have been diagnosed postmortem, during endoscopic airway evaluation and during tracheotomy. Persistent airway distress in a neonate with craniosynostosis should raise suspicion for TCS when significant midface and pharyngeal obstruction have been ruled out. Endoscopy findings include the visible absence of discrete tracheal rings, complete or almost complete absence of the posterior membranous septum, little tracheal motion with respiration, and an abnormal carina [17, 20].

Management. In a neonate with craniosynostosis, a thorough airway evaluation is required to evaluate for multiple levels of obstruction from possible choanal stenosis or atresia, midface hypoplasia, and tracheal anomalies. Tracheotomy may help to increase life expectancy, but the rigidity of the involved segment appears to be a risk factor for the tendency to form granulation tissue [25]. Intraluminal granulation tissue can be problematic and may require the need for multiple bronchoscopic interventions to prevent secondary airway obstruction [20, 25]. Short-segment TCS may be amenable to tracheal resection with primary anastomosis.

Multidisciplinary considerations. Craniosynostosis syndromes often require collaboration between the neurosurgeon, otolaryngologist, and plastic surgeon.

Summary

Children with craniofacial syndromes may have several airway anomalies that contribute to airway obstruction at multiple levels. A comprehensive airway evaluation is essential for identifying the possible causes of obstruction and for formulating an optimal plan to manage the compromised neonatal airway. Being familiar with the characteristic airway anomalies in these syndromes serves as a useful guide, but there must be an awareness of the diverse phenotypic variability that exists in these syndromes. A familiarity of possible airway anomalies that can occur with craniofacial syndromes can allow clinicians to anticipate potential airway issues and institute earlier evaluation and management.

References

1. Acke FR, Dhooge IJ, Malfait F, De Leenheer EM. Hearing impairment in Stickler syndrome: a systematic review. Orphanet J Rare Dis. 2012;7:84. doi:10.1186/1750-1172-7-84.
2. Antón-Pacheco JL, Cano I, Comas J, Galletti L, Polo L, García A, López M, Cabezalí D. Management of congenital tracheal stenosis in infancy. Eur J Cardiothorac Surg. 2006;29(6):991–6. Epub 2006 May 3.
3. Apert syndrome. Genetics Home Reference. February 2008. Available from: http://ghr.nlm.nih.gov/condition/apert-syndrome. Accessed 3 Feb 2014.
4. Apert syndrome. OMIM. Updated 5/16/2013. Available from: http://www.omim.org/entry/101200?search=apert&highlight=apert. Accessed 4 Feb 2014.
5. Arlis H, Ward RF. Congenital nasal pyriform aperture stenosis. Isolated abnormality vs developmental field defect. Arch Otolaryngol Head Neck Surg. 1992;118(9):989–91.
6. Bannink N, Nout E, Wolvius EB, Hoeve HL, Joosten KF, Mathijssen IM. Obstructive sleep apnea in children with syndromic craniosynostosis: long-term respiratory outcome of midface advancement. Int J Oral Maxillofac Surg. 2010;39(2):115–21. doi:10.1016/j.ijom.2009.11.021. Epub 2010 Jan 6.
7. Belden CJ, Mancuso AA, Schmalfuss IM. CT features of congenital nasal piriform aperture stenosis: initial experience. Radiology. 1999;213(2):495–501.
8. Bertrand P, Navarro H, Caussade S, Holmgren N, Sánchez I. Airway anomalies in children with down syndrome: endoscopic findings. Pediatr Pulmonol. 2003;36(2):137–41.
9. Birgfeld CB, Heike C. Craniofacial microsomia. Semin Plast Surg. 2012;26(2):91–104. doi:10.1055/s-0032-1320067.
10. Blake KD, Davenport SL, Hall BD, Hefner MA, Pagon RA, Williams MS, Lin AE, Graham Jr JM. CHARGE association: an update and review for the primary pediatrician. Clin Pediatr (Phila). 1998;37(3):159–73.
11. Bravo MN, Kaul A, Rutter MJ, Elluru RG. Down syndrome and complete tracheal rings. J Pediatr. 2006;148(3):392–5.
12. Brown OE, Myer 3rd CM, Manning SC. Congenital nasal pyriform aperture stenosis. Laryngoscope. 1989;99(1):86–91.
13. CHARGE syndrome. Genetics Home Reference. May 2008. Available from: http://ghr.nlm.nih.gov/condition/charge-syndrome. Accessed 3 Feb 2014.
14. CHARGE syndrome. OMIM. Updated 8/30/2013. Available from: http://www.omim.org/entry/214800?search=charge&highlight=charge. Accessed 4 Feb 2014.
15. Crouzon syndrome. Genetics Home Reference. May 2008. Available from: http://ghr.nlm.nih.gov/condition/crouzon-syndrome. Accessed 3 Feb 2014.
16. Crouzon syndrome. OMIM. Updated 1/22/2011. Available from: http://www.omim.org/entry/123500. Accessed 4 Feb 2014.
17. Devine P, Bhan I, Feingold M, Leonidas JC, Wolpert SM. Completely cartilaginous trachea in a child with Crouzon syndrome. Am J Dis Child. 1984;138(1):40–3.
18. Down syndrome. Genetics Home Reference. February 2014. Available from: http://ghr.nlm.nih.gov/condition/down-syndrome. Accessed 11 Feb 2014.
19. Heike CL, Hing AV. Craniofacial Microsomia Overview. 2009 Mar 19. In: Pagon RA, Adam MP, Bird TD, et al., editors. GeneReviews™ [Internet]. Seattle (WA): University of Washington, Seattle; 1993–2014. Available from: http://www.ncbi.nlm.nih.gov/books/NBK5199/. Accessed 6 Feb 2014.
20. Hockstein NG, McDonald-McGinn D, Zackai E, Bartlett S, Huff DS, Jacobs IN. Tracheal anomalies in Pfeiffer syndrome. Arch Otolaryngol Head Neck Surg. 2004;130(11):1298–302.

21. Horgan JE, Padwa BL, LaBrie RA, Mulliken JB. OMENS-Plus: analysis of craniofacial and extracraniofacial anomalies in hemifacial microsomia. Cleft Palate Craniofac J. 1995;32(5):405–12.
22. Katsanis SH, Jabs EW. Treacher Collins Syndrome. 2004 Jul 20 [Updated 2012 Aug 30]. In: Pagon RA, Adam MP, Bird TD, et al., (eds.) GeneReviews™ [Internet]. Seattle: University of Washington, Seattle; 1993–2014. Available from: http://www.ncbi.nlm.nih.gov/books/NBK1532/. Accessed 4 Feb 2014.
23. Kimonis V, Gold JA, Hoffman TL, Panchal J, Boyadjiev SA. Genetics of craniosynostosis. Semin Pediatr Neurol. 2007;14(3):150–61. Review.
24. Lalani SR, Hefner MA, Belmont JW, et al. CHARGE Syndrome. 2006 Oct 2 [Updated 2012 Feb 2]. In: Pagon RA, Adam MP, Bird TD, et al., editors. GeneReviews™ [Internet]. Seattle (WA): University of Washington, Seattle; 1993–2014. Available from: http://www.ncbi.nlm.nih.gov/books/NBK1117/. Accessed 3 Feb 2014.
25. Lertsburapa K, Schroeder Jr JW, Sullivan C. Tracheal cartilaginous sleeve in patients with craniosynostosis syndromes: a meta-analysis. J Pediatr Surg. 2010;45(7):1438–44. doi:10.1016/j.jpedsurg.2009.09.005.
26. McCarthy JG. Chapter 26: Craniofacial microsomia. In: Thorne CH, ed. Grabb & Smith's plastic surgery. Available from: http://www.med.unc.edu/surgery/plastic/grabb/Chapter%2026.pdf. Accessed 6 Feb 2014.
27. Naito Y, Higuchi M, Koinuma G, Aramaki M, Takahashi T, Kosaki K. Upper airway obstruction in neonates and infants with CHARGE syndrome. Am J Med Genet A. 2007;143A(16):1815–20.
28. Noorily MR, Farmer DL, Belenky WM, Philippart AI. Congenital tracheal anomalies in the craniosynostosis syndromes. J Pediatr Surg. 1999;34(6):1036–9.
29. Perkins JA, Sie KC, Milczuk H, Richardson MA. Airway management in children with craniofacial anomalies. Cleft Palate Craniofac J. 1997;34(2):135–40.
30. Pfeiffer syndrome. OMIM. Updated 5/24/2006. Available from: http://www.omim.org/entry/101600?search=pfeiffer&highlight=pfeiffer. Accessed 4 Feb 2014.
31. Plomp RG, Bredero-Boelhouwer HH, Joosten KF, Wolvius EB, Hoeve HL, Poublon RM, Mathijssen IM. Obstructive sleep apnea in Treacher Collins syndrome: prevalence, severity and cause. Int J Oral Maxillofac Surg. 2012;41(6):696–701. doi:10.1016/j.ijom.2012.01.018. Epub 2012 Apr 20.
32. Posnick JC. Treacher Collins syndrome: perspectives in evaluation and treatment. J Oral Maxillofac Surg. 1997;55(10):1120–33.
33. Poon CC, Meara JG, Heggie AA. Hemifacial microsomia: use of the OMENS-Plus classification at the Royal Children's Hospital of Melbourne. Plast Reconstr Surg. 2003;111(3):1011–8.
34. Rachmiel A, Emodi O, Aizenbud D. Management of obstructive sleep apnea in pediatric craniofacial anomalies. Ann Maxillofac Surg. 2012;2(2):111–5. doi:10.4103/2231-0746.101329.
35. Robin NH, Falk MJ, Haldeman-Englert CR. FGFR-related Craniosynostosis syndromes. 1998 Oct 20 [Updated 2011 Jun 7]. In: Pagon RA, Adam MP, Bird TD, et al., editors. GeneReviews™ [Internet]. Seattle (WA): University of Washington, Seattle; 1993–2014. Available from: http://www.ncbi.nlm.nih.gov/books/NBK1455/. Accessed 3 Feb 2014.
36. Robin NH, Moran RT, Warman M, et al. Stickler Syndrome. 2000 Jun 9 [Updated 2011 Nov 3]. In: Pagon RA, Adam MP, Bird TD, et al., editors. GeneReviews™ [Internet]. Seattle (WA): University of Washington, Seattle; 1993–2014. Available from: http://www.ncbi.nlm.nih.gov/books/NBK1302/. Accessed 4 Feb 2014.
37. Rose PS, Levy HP, Liberfarb RM, Davis J, Szymko-Bennett Y, Rubin BI, Tsilou E, Griffith AJ, Francomano CA. Stickler syndrome: clinical characteristics and diagnostic criteria. Am J Med Genet A. 2005;138A(3):199–207.
38. Sanlaville D, Verloes A. CHARGE syndrome: an update. Eur J Hum Genet. 2007;15(4):389–99. Epub 2007 Feb 14.
39. Sculerati N, Gottlieb MD, Zimbler MS, Chibbaro PD, McCarthy JG. Airway management in children with major craniofacial anomalies. Laryngoscope. 1998;108(12):1806–12.
40. Snead MP, Yates JR. Clinical and molecular genetics of Stickler syndrome. J Med Genet. 1999;36(5):353–9. Review.
41. Stickler syndrome. Genetics Home Reference. January 2013. Available from: http://ghr.nlm.nih.gov/condition/stickler-syndrome. Accessed 4 Feb 2014.
42. Treacher Collins syndrome. Genetics Home Reference. June 2012. Available from: http://ghr.nlm.nih.gov/condition/treacher-collins-syndrome. Accessed 4 Feb 2014.
43. Van Den Abbeele T, Triglia JM, François M, Narcy P. Congenital nasal pyriform aperture stenosis: diagnosis and management of 20 cases. Ann Otol Rhinol Laryngol. 2001;110(1):70–5.
44. Vento AR, LaBrie RA, Mulliken JB. The O.M.E.N.S. classification of hemifacial microsomia. Cleft Palate Craniofac J. 1991;28(1):68–76; discussion 77.
45. Vogels A, Fryns JP. Pfeiffer syndrome. Orphanet J Rare Dis. 2006;1:19.
46. Watts R, Vyas H. An overview of respiratory problems in children with Down's syndrome. Arch Dis Child. 2013;98(10):812–7. doi:10.1136/archdischild-2013-304611. Epub 2013 Jun 27.
47. Wells TR, Landing BH, Shamszadeh M, Thompson JW, Bove KE, Caron KH. Association of Down syndrome and segmental tracheal stenosis with ring tracheal cartilages: a review of nine cases. Pediatr Pathol. 1992;12(5):673–82.

Disorders of the Midface

Jacqueline Anderson, Bryan Liming, and Sanjay R. Parikh

Embryology

The face and nasal structures develop from cells of ectodermal, neural crest and mesodermal origin, which occurs during the fourth through eighth week of gestation. At 4 weeks gestation, the first sign of facial development begins with the stomodeum, a depression below the developing brain. Surrounding the stomodeum are five structures arising from neural crest cells migrating into the first pharyngeal arches. These structures, the frontonasal prominence, the paired maxillary prominences, and paired mandibular prominences, will guide the development of midface structures.

The frontonasal prominence forms during the fourth gestational week and consists of a frontal and a nasal component. The frontal part of the frontonasal prominence is the precursor to the nasal dorsum and forehead. Near the end of the fourth week, paired ectodermal thickenings on the nasal part of the frontonasal prominence called nasal placodes form. During the fifth week, mesenchymal thickenings form on the margin of the nasal placodes. These are known as the lateral nasal prominences and medial nasal prominences. This proliferation creates a central depression in the placodes called nasal pits. From the fifth week, the nasal pits deepen toward the oral cavity forming the nares and nasal cavity. This progresses until only a thin oronasal membrane separates the oral cavity from nasal cavity. This membrane is an epithelial plug that normally resorbs during the third trimester resulting in posterior choanae.

During the sixth and seventh weeks, the maxillary prominences extend medially toward each other and push the medial nasal prominences medially. The upper lip, nasal tip, columella, philtrum, primary palate, and columella are formed as fusion occurs at the junction of these processes. The nasal septum grows inferiorly from the frontonasal prominence. As the maxillary processes fuse, they form the lateral upper lip and secondary palate.

At the end of the sixth week of gestation, the lateral nasal processes fuse with the maxillary processes to form the lateral borders of the nostril. The nasolacrimal grooves form at the junction of the lateral nasal and maxillary processes. Surface ectoderm migrates from the naso-optic fissure within the nasolacrimal grooves to form epithelial cords, which canalize by the 6th month to form the nasolacrimal ducts and sacks.

The lateral nasal wall begins to take shape at 7–8 weeks gestation when the cartilaginous capsule that surrounds the nasal cavity extends from the chondrocranium of the skull bases. Pre-turbinates form as protrusions from this capsule. Between 9 and 10 weeks gestation, cartilage penetrates the pre-turbinates and the cartilaginous precursor to the uncinate process forms.

Superiorly, the nasal and frontal bones are separated by the fonticulus frontalis. As the frontal and nasal bones grow, they obliterate this space, forming the frontonasal suture. At the same time, the nasal bones and cartilaginous nasal capsule framework are separated by a prenasal space. A dural extension extends from the anterior cranial fossa through the foramen cecum where the frontal bone articulates with the ethmoid bone (maybe define this space) into the transient prenasal space where it contacts the tip of the nose prior to receding. As the nasal bones grow, they obliterate this prenasal space.

History, Physical and Imaging

In the setting of a neonate with a severely compromised airway, history taking will be secondary to assessment and stabilization. However, once the child is stabilized, a focused history should be taken (Fig. 1). It is of significance to note

J. Anderson, M.D. • B. Liming, M.D.
Department of Otolaryngology—Head and Neck Surgery, Madigan Army Medical Center, Tacoma, WA, USA

S.R. Parikh, M.D. F.A.C.S. (✉)
Department of Otolaryngology—Head and Neck Surgery, University of Washington, Seattle, WA, USA
e-mail: sanjay.parikh@seattlechildrens.org

J. Lioy and S.E. Sobol (eds.), *Disorders of the Neonatal Airway: Fundamentals for Practice*, DOI 10.1007/978-1-4939-1610-8_3, © Springer Science+Business Media New York 2015

History	Physical
Onset of symptoms (immediate vs delayed) Constant vs intermittent Exacerbating/remitting factors History of adjunctive procedures required Gestational age Route of delivery Instrumentation during delivery Prenatal complications Known nutritional deficiencies (folate) Exposures (drugs, alcohol, toxins, radiation) Family history of craniofacial syndromes Any history of prenatal screening Prenatal ultrasound results	Evidence of respiratory distress: • Cyanosis • Loud stridor/stertor • Retractions, alar flaring • Hypoxemia/hypercarbia Facial dysmorphisms Midface hypoplasia Bubbling from the nares Anterior rhinoscopy Mirror exam to look for fogging Passage of suction catheter Flexible fiberoptic nasopharyngoscopy

Fig. 1 Midfacial Disorders: History and Physical Examination

when the respiratory distress started (immediately at birth or delayed onset) and whether it is constant. Exacerbating or remitting factors such as crying, feeding, or positioning should be noted. There should be inquiry into which adjunctive airway measures were used (positive pressure, jaw thrust, nasal trumpet). One should know the gestational age of the child, whether there were any significant peripartum events, the route of delivery (Cesarean section or vaginal) and whether there was instrumentation of the child during delivery. Parental questioning should include the presence of maternal pregnancy complications, risk factors for nutritional deficiency (specifically folate), exposures to drugs, alcohol, toxins or radiation and family history of craniofacial or other syndromes. One should know whether any prenatal genetic screening was done and whether there were any abnormalities on prenatal ultrasonography.

Initial assessment of an infant with respiratory distress should focus on the ability of the child to maintain ventilation and oxygenation. Signs that may indicate the need for rapid intervention include cyanosis, loud stridor or stertor, the presence of retractions, hypoxemia or hypercarbia.

In the more stable neonate, or in the neonate with a secure airway, a more thorough physical examination can take place. With regards to midface abnormalities, one must pay attention to stigmata of craniofacial syndromes such as gross dysmorphisms or midface hypoplasia. Anterior rhinoscopy can demonstrate mass lesions obstructing nasal airflow. Signs of bubbling of nasal secretions suggest patency of the nasal airway. A mirror placed under the nares will fog if nasal airflow is present and a flexible suction catheter can be passed to assess patency of the nasal airway. Flexible fiberoptic nasopharyngoscopy and laryngoscopy allows a rapid evaluation of nasal passages as well as the nasopharynx, oropharynx, and larynx.

Imaging studies may be useful in the setting of a suspected mass or neoplasm, or if there are concerns for osseous or soft tissue obstruction of the nasal airway. Computed tomography (CT) is the imaging modality of choice to evaluate bony narrowing and osseous lesions but should be used judiciously given the concerns regarding ionizing radiation exposure in infants. Magnetic resonance imaging (MRI) may be more useful when soft tissue evaluation is needed.

Syndromic Midfacial Obstruction

Crouzon Syndrome

Etiology

Crouzon Syndrome was first described by French physician Octave Crouzon in 1912 who noted the features in a mother and daughter. It is one of the craniosynostosis syndromes that result from a mutation of the fibroblast growth factor receptor gene. It is classically associated with bicoronal synostosis, midface hypoplasia, proptosis, and normal intellect.

Epidemiology

Crouzon Syndrome is a rare disease, affecting only approximately 1.6 in every 100,000 births [1].

Pathogenesis

Crouzon syndrome is a genetic syndrome with autosomal dominant inheritance and typically complete penetrance. The majority of cases are associated with various mutations of the FGFR2 genes although one variant, Crouzon with acanthosis nigricans is associated with mutations of the FGFR3 gene [1]. Typically these are missense mutations [1].

Clinical Presentation

Patients with Crouzon's typically present at birth with classic phenotypic abnormalities that should raise the clinician's suspicions for one of the craniosynostosis disorders. These findings include craniosynostosis (i.e., bilateral coronal suture synostosis, pansynostosis, or clover leaf skull), hypertelorism, beaked nose and midface hypoplasia. There may also be limb involvement, however, the absence of syndactyly and broad thumbs can help differentiate the syndrome clinically from others such as Pfeiffer and Apert's (see below). Also, unlike patients with Pfeiffer and Apert's, patients with Crouzon's do not typically have neurocognitive impairment. Due to the presence of craniosynostosis, these patients are at high risk for development of increased intracranial pressure and should be monitored closely for signs of such.

Diagnosis

The diagnosis of Crouzon's is typically suspected based on clinical findings as noted above, however, ultimately diagnosis typically requires molecular testing and identification of mutations within the FGFR2 gene.

Management

As with all patients with midface disorders, the first step in management of these patients is the establishment of a stable airway. Midface retrusion, choanal atresia, nasopharyngeal narrowing, and tracheal/laryngeal abnormalities may all contribute to airway obstruction. Stabilization may require nasopharyngeal airway placement, intubation, and/or tracheotomy. Shallow orbits and severe proptosis require aggressive management to prevent exposure keratitis and ulcerations. Temporizing tarsorrhaphies may ultimately be required until midface reconstruction can be completed.

In patients with elevated intracranial pressures, decompression procedures are warranted on an urgent basis. Of the craniosynostosis disorders, Crouzon's has the highest risk of significant intracranial hypertension [1]. However, in the absence of these findings, cranial vault expansion has traditionally been delayed until around 6–12 months of age [2]. With the advent of endoscopic approaches however, the age to intervene is trending toward a younger age with some institutions performing elective strip craniectomies as early as 3 months [3]. Midface procedures are typically delayed until around 5 years of age [4]. Due to the underlying biology of these syndromes, high rates of reoperation have been reported [4].

Multidisciplinary Considerations

As with patients with other craniosynostosis syndromes, children with Crouzon's are typically best served at large medical institutions with multidisciplinary craniofacial teams that include pediatricians, otolaryngologists, oral maxillofacial surgeons, geneticists, and others. All patients should also be evaluated with developmental screens and management as indicated.

Apert Syndrome

Etiology

Eugene Apert, a French pediatrician, first described nine people in 1906 with the similar findings of craniosynostosis, midface hypoplasia, and syndactyly of hands and feet [5, 6]. Most cases (>98 %) are due to the mutation of chromosome bands 10q25–q26 [7].

Epidemiology

The prevalence of Apert Syndrome is roughly 1 in 65,000 newborns. It is the cause of 4.5 % of cases of craniosynostosis and is equally distributed between male and females [8].

Pathogenesis

Apert syndrome is most commonly caused by a missense substitution mutation in chromosome bands 10q25–q26. The mutation affects downstream production of adjacent amino acids (i.e., Ser252Trp, Ser252Phe, Pro253Arg) in the linker between the second and third extracellular immunoglobulin domains of fibroblast growth factor receptor 2 (FGFR2). The inheritance pattern is thought to be autosomal dominant [6].

Clinical Presentation

The typical findings of Apert syndrome are those of craniosynostosis (coronal, sagittal, metopic), midface hypoplasia, and syndactyly of the hands and/or feet. The skull appearance is a flat elongated forehead with bitemporal widening and occipital flattening. The skull may appear like a "cloverleaf" depending on the position of the temporal bones. The midface is hypoplastic with a flat nose and bulbous tip. The palate is arched with swelling of the palatine processes creating a "pseudocleft" in the midline. Soft palate clefting is found in 30 % of cases. Dentition tends to be crowded with an anterior open bite. Hand anomalies consist of variable syndactyly of the second through fourth fingers, ranging from webbing to complete fusion. Equal variability is seen between the second and fourth digits of the feet. The combination may be referred to as "mitten hand" and "sock foot" [8, 9].

Diagnosis

The majority of cases are diagnosed based on physical exam findings in keeping with Apert Syndrome. Imaging in the form of plain films and computed tomography will be required for diagnostic and therapeutic purposes. Genetic evaluation may be performed to confirm the diagnosis [8, 9].

Management

Each of the three typical components of Apert Syndrome will typically require surgical intervention. Craniotomy will be required in the first year of life for associated craniosynostoses: coronal, sagittal, and/or metopic. Syndactyly repair will be carried out soon thereafter for functional gain. Midface and frontoorbital advancement is typically performed later for cosmetic improvement while orthodontic treatment will be carried out as soon as possible to improve teeth alignment [8, 9].

Multidisciplinary Considerations

Given the cranial and extracranial manifestations of Apert syndrome, multidisciplinary care of patients is required. Ideally, in a collaborative center, surgical intervention will be staged based on functional and cosmetic goals.

Pfeiffer Syndrome

Etiology

Pfeiffer syndrome was first described in 1964 as a rare craniosynostosis syndrome associated with craniosynostosis, midface hypoplasia, broad thumbs, great toes, and variable syndactyly of the hands and feet [10]. It is caused by mutations in the fibroblast growth factor genes [10–13]. These mutations can be transmitted in an autosomal dominant fashion or arise de novo. Interestingly, the spontaneous mutation is thought to be related to advanced paternal age [13].

Epidemiology

Pfeiffer syndrome affects an estimated one in 100,000 live births [14]. Men and women are affected equally [15].

Pathogenesis

Pfeiffer syndrome is associated with more than 25 mutations on one of the two FGFR genes. Five percent of the patients have a mutation on FGFR1. These individuals are likely to present with the less severe phenotype (Type 1). The majority of patients, however, present with a mutation on the FGFR2 gene (Type 2 and 3).

Clinical Presentation

Abnormal development of structures derived from preformed cartilage appears to be at the root of many of the abnormalities seen with Pfeiffer's Syndrome [15]. These structures, which include the skull, trachea, spine, fingers, and ribs can be affected to various degrees depending on the severity of the phenotype. Type 1 "classic" Pfeiffer syndrome involves mild manifestations including brachycephaly, midface hypoplasia, and short, broad thumbs and great toes. These individuals generally have normal intelligence and good long-term prognosis. Type 2 Pfeiffer syndrome is generally associated with the classic "cloverleaf skull," extreme proptosis, finger and toe abnormalities, elbow ankylosis or synostosis, developmental delay and neurological complications. Type 3 is similar to type 2 but without a cloverleaf skull. Infants born with any craniofacial dysostosis may have moderate to severe midface hypoplasia. This may significantly narrow the nasal and nasopharyngeal airway potentially causing severe airway obstruction.

Diagnosis

The majority of cases of Pfeiffer syndrome are diagnosed clinically based on classic phenotypic findings to include craniosynostosis with a wide head and flat occiput, midface hypoplasia, ocular proptosis, short broad thumbs and great toes with deviation away from other digits, various degrees of syndactyly [16]. Molecular diagnosis may also play a role particularly in suspected, but not classic cases of Pfeiffer's. Rarely, prenatal diagnosis is possible via ultrasound. Ultrasound findings of craniosynostosis and broad thumbs and toes should raise a suspicion for Pfeiffer syndrome.

Management

Infants are obligate nasal breathers and therefore any condition affecting the midface can potentially affect their airway. Airway management is therefore a cornerstone of treatment for all neonates born with midface disorders. For infants with severe obstruction, nasopharyngeal airway placement or intubation may be necessary. Ultimately many of these children will require tracheostomy tube placement. Once the patient's airway is secure, long-term plans for reconstructive surgery can be made. Temporizing procedures such as tarsorrhaphy are often necessary due to the severe proptosis which may inhibit complete eye closure. Ultimately the synostotic sutures require release in order to decompress the brain. This procedure may take place as early as 3 months of age [16]. Subsequent surgeries typically include midface distraction osteogenesis to both improve airway dimensions as well as orbital volumes. These procedures may involve external or internal devices depending largely on the patient's age and surgeon preferences [17].

Multidisciplinary Considerations

The complexity of these patients mandates that a multidisciplinary approach be taken to their long-term management. These children are typically best served at large medical institutions with multidisciplinary craniofacial teams that include pediatricians, otolaryngologists, oral maxillofacial surgeons, geneticists, and others.

Inflammatory and Traumatic Disorders

Neonates are obligate nasal breathers so nasal obstruction may lead to respiratory distress, feeding difficulties, cyanotic episodes, and even death. Respiratory distress that improves with crying is the classic clinical scenario for nasal airway obstruction.

Neonatal Rhinitis (Rhinitis Neonatorum)

Etiology/Epidemiology

Rhinitis of infancy is a clinical entity that is seen commonly in pediatric otolaryngology practice; however, a paucity of literature exists regarding this problem. The condition is the most common cause of neonatal nasal obstruction.

The etiology is unclear although there appears to be a seasonal component with most cases presenting in the fall or winter months [25].

Clinical Presentation/Diagnosis

Presenting signs can include stertor, mucoid nasal discharge, mucosal edema, difficulty feeding and intermittent apneas. Thought to be an under-recognized problem [25], it has even been implicated in the sudden infant death syndrome [28].

There have been some questions as to whether there is an atopic component to rhinitis of infancy. Nearly 10 % of children will display symptoms of allergic rhinitis by 18 months and there seems to be an association with parental history of allergic rhinitis [24]. However, immunologic mechanisms seem unlikely to play a major role in the first weeks of life given the mechanism of allergy as it is currently understood.

Rarely, primary ciliary dyskinesia (PCD) can manifest as neonatal rhinitis causing respiratory distress [20]. Suspicion is raised when plain films demonstrate dextrocardia. Diagnosis is by electron microscopy studies demonstrating morphological abnormalities in cilia obtained by bronchial or nasal mucosal brush biopsies. Treatment aims at improving pulmonary toilet [20]

Management

Nasal saline and bulb suctioning should be utilized to clear the mucoid discharge. For severe cases, a short course of topical decongestant such as 0.125 % neosynepherine alone or in combination with topical corticosteroids such as 0.1 % dexamethasone ophthalmic drops may be considered. Dexamethasone drops can be cadministered for up to 1 month and then tapered [25]. Rarely does this condition require further intervention and most infants will respond within 12 weeks [25].

Multidisciplinary Considerations

Neonatal rhinitis can usually be managed by the primary care physician or otolaryngologist. When indicated, allergy/immunology consultation should be considered.

Nasal Septal Deviation

Etiology/Epidemiology

It has been recognized since as early as 1936 that the forces on the neonatal face encountered during the birth process may impact the morphology of the nose and face [18]. The incidence of nasal septal deviation in the newborn is described at between 1.25 and 25 % [26, 27]. Incidence may be related to intrauterine positioning of the fetus with a breech position being associated with the highest incidence [18].

Clinical Presentation/Diagnosis

Morphologically, neonatal septal deviation can take the form of anterior dislocation off of the maxillary crest or anterior/posterior septal deformity [21]. On occasion, neonatal nasal septal deviation can be so severe as to cause obstructive symptoms, with cases severe enough to present with apneas and cyanotic episodes while awake [21].

Management

Closed reduction of the anterior septum can be performed in the first days of life with good results [21]. In severe cases, formal septoplasty can be performed on infants as young as 8 days [21]. This can be done through either a transnasal or sublabial approach, either directly or with endoscopic visualization [21, 22].

Multidisciplinary Considerations

Neonatal septal deviation can usually be managed by the otolaryngologist. In cases of suspected trauma, additional consultations may be necessary.

Septal Hematoma

Septal hematoma can present either as a result of birth trauma or as the consequence of non-accidental trauma. It may be misdiagnosed as a nasal mass. Treatment is transnasal incision and drainage [19].

Congenital Nasal Masses

Intranasal Infantile Hemangiomas

Etiology/Epidemiology

Infantile hemangiomas (IH) are the most common vascular tumors of infancy and are known to present very early in life. One review article published in the NEJM in 1999 reported that in neonates with infantile hemangiomas 55 % are present at birth and the remainder develops within the first few weeks of life [31]. Older studies suggest an incidence as high as 10 %, [30] however, more recent reviews of the existing literature highlight the general lack of methodologically standardized studies and place the presumed incidence more towards 4–5 % [46].

Clinical Presentation/Diagnosis

Infantile hemangiomas are unique in that they are characterized by a rapid proliferative phase followed by a spontaneous slow involution phase [35]. Warner and colleagues [32] highlighted their propensity for growth along embryological fusion planes, which can result in nasal distortion and obstruction in the neonate. Clinically, appearance of these lesions varies based on depth, location, and stage of involution [35]. In neonates, however, they often appear as relatively pale, soft masses covered with telangectasias until they begin the proliferative phase [35]. They then may begin to appear like the classic soft, red, elevated hemangioma that we often think of. Diagnosis of IH is made based on the clinical appearance of the lesion and, when indicated, imaging of the facial soft tissues. Surveillance for additional skin or internal hemangiomas may be warranted.

Management

The primary goal of treatment, as with any nasal obstruction in the neonate, is focused around airway support. Once this is established, more definitive management of the lesion itself can be entertained. Historically, laser treatments, systemic corticosteroids, intralesional corticosteroids, and surgical resection have been the mainstay for treatment of infantile hemangiomas. However, with the introduction of propranolol as a treatment modality in 2008, there has been a dramatic shift in the management of these lesions. While the exact mechanism by which propranolol treats IH remains unknown, proposed mechanisms include induction of endothelial cell apoptosis [33], vasoconstriction, and blocking of proangiogenic signals [34]. A general paucity of high quality, prospective studies have limited recommendations on propranolol, however, the recent consensus conference on initiation and use of propranolol for IH has led to some guidelines which may help guide clinicians in their use of this medication. Currently the consensus group recommends an initiation dose of 1–3 mg/kg/day with most members advocating 2 mg/kg/day divided TID [35].

Multidisciplinary Considerations

Management of IH often requires a team approach, including input from the dermatologist, plastic surgeon, and ophthalmologist, when indicated.

Nasopharyngeal Germline Malformations

Etiology/Epidemiology

Teratomas of the head and neck account for less than 5 % of all teratomas and reportedly occur in 1 in 20,000 to 1 in 40,000 live births with a female predominance of 5–6:1 reported in the literature [36, 40]. The cervical neck is reported to be the most common head and neck site involved with the nasopharynx second [36]. Like all teratomas, they are composed of all three embryologic germ layers (ectoderm, endoderm, and mesoderm).

Clinical Presentation/Diagnosis

While the literature on nasopharyngeal teratomas is somewhat limited, clinically these lesions seem to have associations with central nervous system abnormalities [37], cleft palates [38], and cardiac abnormalities [40]. A review of 113 cases of germline malformations of the nasopharynx by Chaudhry et al. [39] reported that true teratomas are often sessile lesions while dermoids are more often pedunculated. Both most frequently present with respiratory distress, however, teratomas are associated with a higher incidence of preterm birth, delivery via Cesarean section, and neonatal distress [40].

Nasopharyngeal germline malformations may be identified on prenatal US for maternal polyhydramnios and/or elevated alpha fetoprotein. A literature review by Coppit et al. found that while polyhydramnios is identified in 18 % of patients with cervical neck lesions, it is seen much less frequently in patients with NP malformations.

Management/Multidisciplinary Considerations

When teratomas are identified prenatally, a multidisciplinary approach to perinatal management is warranted. Considerations for airway management include endotracheal intubation, tracheotomy, and even consideration for an EXIT procedure (ex utero intrapartum treatment). Once the airway is secured, treatment of both teratomas and dermoids is focused on surgical resection, which typically occurs via a transnasal approach. Recurrence rates are dependent on completeness of the surgical resection with a higher rate of recurrence in teratomas thought to be secondary to the more difficult resection of a broad-based lesion in the neonate.

Nasal Dermoid Cysts

Etiology/Epidemiology

The nasal dermoid cyst is the most common congenital midline nasal lesion and represents approximately 4–12 % of head and neck dermoids [50]. It is composed embryologically of mesoderm and ectoderm due to failed separation of dural diverticulum and the overlying ectoderm [47]. Contrary to nasopharyngeal teratomas, dermoids present with a slight male predominance.

Clinical Presentation/Diagnosis

These lesions can be located anywhere from the columella to the anterior cranial fossa and can be intranasal, extranasal, or a combination of the two [49]. Clinically, these lesions present as a noncompressible mass with a sinus tract that drains sebaceous material and can occasionally cause recurrent local infections [49]. Hair protruding through a cutaneous punctum is pathognomonic for a nasal dermoid [49]. In a retrospective chart review performed by Wardinsky et al., nasal dermoids were associated with other anomalies in 41 % of cases and with intracranial extension in 45 % of cases.

While the exact percentage of intracranial extension varies in the literature, it highlights the importance of preoperative

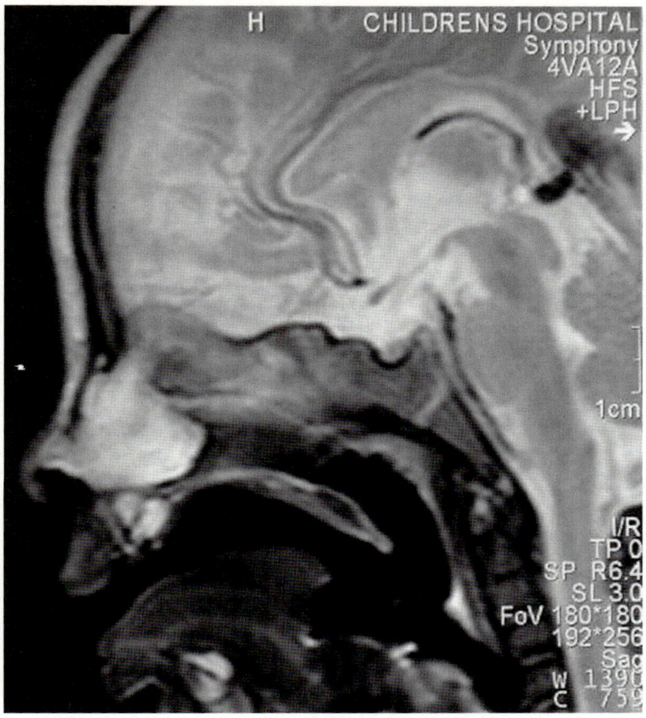

Fig. 2 Sagittal MRI of Nasal Glioma

imaging in patients with suspected dermoid cysts. Both MRI and CT scan may provide complimentary information crucial to the perioperative planning period although MRI avoids potential radiation risks. Normal anatomic variations in the pediatric patient can be easily mistaken for intracranial extension. For instance, a midline gap between the paired nasal bones, non-ossification of the cribiform plate, and the presence of the foramen cecum can all lead to false-positives (Zapata). Widening of the foramen cecum (up to 10 mm) is normal, a bony defect in the crista galli, and a bifid or dystrophic crista galli suggest intracranial extension (Posnick). Dermoids appear hyperintense on T1 and T2 images (Saettele). Contrast may be useful in helping to differentiate dermoids, which are non-enhancing, from other enhancing structures such as infantile hemangiomas, teratomas, and even normal nasal mucosa.

Management/Multidisciplinary Considerations

Treatment of nasal dermoids revolves around complete surgical excision with a high recurrence rate associated with incomplete excision. While multiple surgical approaches have been described, the open rhinoplasty remains the most widely used (Zapata). This approach allows for a single-staged intracranial–extracranial resection if indicated (Zapata). Neurosurgical consultation and involvement in the perioperative and intraoperative management is crucial if intracranial extension is suspected since craniotomy may be required for complete extirpation (Zapata).

Epidermoid

Nasal epidermoids are similar to dermoids in their embryological development but differ in the fact that they contain ectodermal tissue only and therefore never form communication with the central nervous system. Imaging is often required to differentiate epidermoid and dermoid lesions. Epidermoids are characteristically hypointense on T1 and T2 MRI imaging with restricted diffusion. CT scan shows fluid attenuation (Saettele).

Nasal Cerebral Heterotopia/Glioma

Etiology/Epidemiology

Nasal cerebral heterotopias, previously known as nasal glioma, is the least common of the midline nasal masses (Saettele). Embryologically, nasal cerebral heterotopias are similar to dermoids with the addition of rests of neural glial tissue (Saettele). The lack of subarachnoid communication helps distinguish these lesions from anterior encephaloceles (Saettele). While not in direct communication with the subarachnoid space, approximately 15 % of nasal cerebral heterotopias do maintain a stalk connection to the dura [48].

Clinical Presentation/Diagnosis

Clinically, these lesions present as firm, noncompressible masses with overlying skin telangectasias. They grow in proportion with the child and they do not transilluminate nor enlarge with crying (Saettele). They are typically isolated lesions with the most common sites for presentation being the glabella, nasomaxillary suture, and intranasally [48]. On MRI, these lesions are hypointense with T1 signal and can be hyper or hypointense on T2 depending on the degree of gliosis (Fig. 2). They appear isointense to brain matter on CT scan and rarely enhance.

Management/Multidisciplinary Considerations

Surgical resection of heterotopias is generally curative so long as the stalk is removed as well if present (Saettele). Surgery is usually performed using a transnasal approach. When indicated, neurosurgical consultation may be necessary.

Encephalocele

Etiology/Epidemiology

A bony defect in the skull with resulting protrusion or herniation of varying degrees of meninges and brain parenchyma is termed an encephalocele. In contrast to gliomas, encephaloceles maintain a patent communication with the subarachnoid space, which plays an important role in the diagnostic and therapeutic approaches to these lesions.

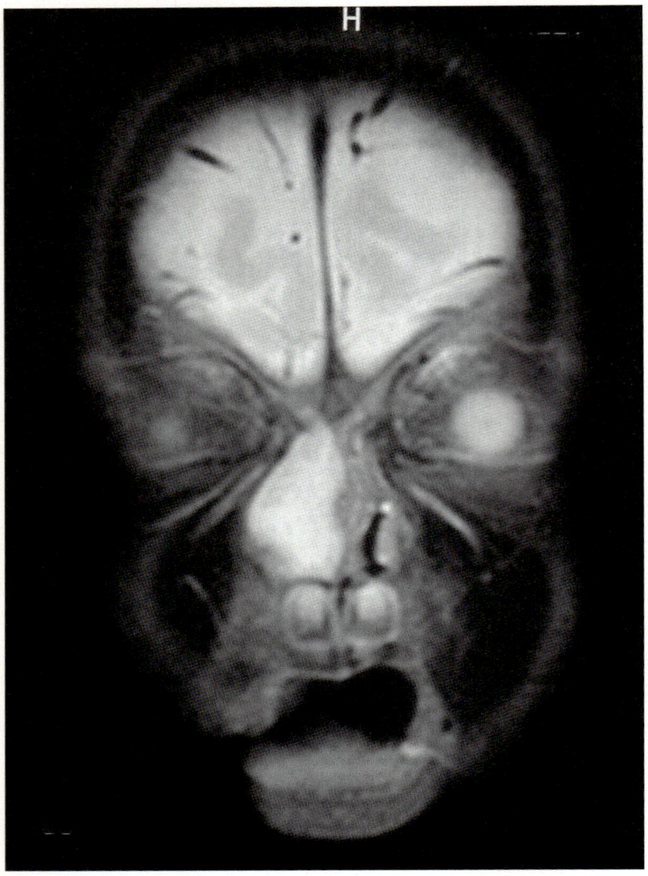

Fig. 3 Coronal MRI of Transethmoidal encephalocele

The majority of encephaloceles are posteriorly based; however, the 25 % that arise anteriorly tend to present much greater diagnostic and therapeutic challenges due to their associated functional, anatomic, and cosmetic affects. Potential complications include but are not limited to: nasal obstruction and impaired nasal function, facial disfigurement, impaired binocular vision, and risk of CNS infection [42]. These anterior, or sincipital, encephaloceles are relatively uncommon in the western hemisphere however are noted to have a high predilection for Southeast Asia with an incidence of 1:6,000 live births [44].

In the Sunwanela [45] classification was published and remains one of the more commonly used classification systems for sincipital encephaloceles. This system classified sincipital encephaloceles based on their location of skull base herniation: frontoethmoidal, interfrontal, and those associated with other craniofacial clefts. Under the umbrella of frontoethmoidal clefts, encephaloceles are further subdivided into: nasofrontal, nasoethmoidal, and nasoorbital.

In addition to their location, encephaloceles are also named based on the tissue that has herniated through the bony defect. Specifically, herniation of meningeal tissue only is referred to as a meningocele and herniation of both meningeal tissue and brain parenchyma is referred to as a meningocephalocele. In extreme cases, a portion of the ventricular system may also be protruding through the bony defect in which case it is referred to as a hydroencephalomeningocele [44].

Theories surrounding the development of encephaloceles are debated within the literature with some believing that failure of bony fusion results in prolapsed tissue whereas others believe that the preexistence of the prolapsed tissue and the resulting stalk prevents normal bony fusion [41]. Regardless of the underlying cause, the resulting prolapsed tissue creates cephalic displacement of the frontal bones, caudal displacement of the nasal bones, and anterolateral displacement of the medial orbital walls [41].

Clinical Presentation/Diagnosis

On examination, an encephalocele will present as a midline nasal mass with a bluish coloration. The mass is soft, compressible and due to its subarachnoid communication, may be visibly pulsatile [44]. Crying, Valsalva, and internal jugular vein compression will lead to enlargement of the mass, again secondary to its intracranial connection. This is referred to as a positive Furstenberg sign. Other characteristic exam findings include a long, flat, and widened nose along with the universal presence of telecanthus. Depending on the severity of these anatomic malformations, this diagnosis may be made in utero during a routine prenatal screening US or much later in life. If identified perinatally, alpha-fetal protein and acetylcholinesterase levels are typically elevated given that it is considered a neural tube defect [43].

MRI is the imaging modality of choice if an encephalocele is suspected (Fig. 3). MRI allows identification of CSF within the malformation, extent of herniated cerebral tissue, and the presence of hydrocephalus [43].

Management/Multidisciplinary Considerations

The process of herniation through the bony defect tends to be a progressive one with enlargement of the mass overtime. As a result, surgical excision is the treatment of choice. Options for surgical excision include combined intracranial/extracranial, fully extracranial, and endoscopic resections, often times in conjunction with a neurosurgical specialist. Regardless of the surgical approach, the general concepts remain the same: resect the mass, repair the skull base defect, and attempt to reconstruct the midline structures. It is important to note that the herniated neurologic tissue is unviable and can be safely removed without compromising neurologic function.

Nasolacrimal Duct Cyst

Nasolacrimal duct cysts (NLDC) arise from incomplete canalization of the epithelial cord that is the precursor to the nasolacrimal drainage system. Obstruction often occurs distally at Hasner's valve resulting in epiphora, crusting, and ocular irritation. This occurs in up to 6 % of infants. Dacrocystoceles result from cystic swellings of the lacrimal sac when both the valve of Rosenmuller and Hasner's valves are obstructed. If large enough, NLDC can cause nasal obstruction. While NLDCs are most often unilateral, bilateral lesions have been described and can lead to respiratory distress [23] In emergent cases, a simple puncture of the cyst can be performed at the bedside to relieve obstruction; however, definitive management requires marsupialization of the cyst itself. This can be done in a number of ways to include at the bedside under rigid endoscopic guidance. The mucosa is decongested with lidocaine and phenylepherine and then alligator forceps are used to strip the mucosa from the mucocele. Other techniques have been described including the use of powered instrumentation [29] and either endoscopic or external dacrocystorhinostomy for long segment occlusion of the nasolacrimal system. If the intervention is performed under general anesthesia, then the lacrimal system can be probed with nasolacrimal ducts to ensure patency of the system.

Conclusions

Midface physiologic and developmental abnormalities can cause potentially life threatening airway obstruction. Appropriate recognition of airway threats, diagnosis of the correct problem, and directed treatment can mitigate the potential impact.

References

1. Robin NH, Falk MJ, Haldeman-Englert CR. FGFR-related craniosynostosis syndromes. Gene Reviews. (http://www.ncbi.nlm.nih.gov/books/NBK1455/). 2011.
2. Brown L, Proctor MR. Endoscopically assisted correction of sagittal craniosynostosis. AORN J. 2011;93:566–79.
3. Agochukwu NB, Solomon BD. Impact of genetics on the diagnosis and clinical management of syndromic craniosynostoses. Childs Nerv Syst. 2012;28:1447–63.
4. Forrest CR, Hopper RA. Craniofacial syndromes and surgery. Plast Reconstr Surg. 2013;131(1):86–109.
5. Cohen MM. Apert syndrome, not Apert's syndrome: Apert neither had nor owned the syndrome that bears his name. Plast Reconstr Surg. 1997;100:532–3.
6. Lee DS, Chung KC. Eugene Apert and his contributions to plastic surgery. Ann Plast Surg. 2010;64:362–5.
7. Heuze Y, Singh N, Basilico C, Jabs EW, Holmes G, Rictsmeier JT. Morphological comparison of the craniofacial phenotypes of mouse models expressing the Apert FGFR2 S252W mutation in neural crest-or mesoderm-derived tissues. Bone. 2014;63:101–9.
8. Bhatia PV, Patel PS, Jani UV, Soni NC. Apert's syndrome: report of a rare case. J Oral Maxillofac Pathol. 2013;17:294–7.
9. Perlyn CA, Nichols C, Woo A, Becker D, Kane AA. Le premier siècle: one hundred years of progress in the treatment of Apert syndrome. J Craniofac Surg. 2009;20:801–6.
10. Pfeiffer RA. [Dominant hereditary acrocephalosyndactylia]. Z Kinderheilkd. 1964;90:301–20.
11. Muenke M, Schell U, Hehr A, et al. A common mutation in the fibroblast growth factor receptor 1 gene in Pfeiffer Syndrome. Nat Genet. 1994;8:269–74.
12. Rutland P, Pulleyn LJ, Reardon W, et al. Identical mutations in the FGFR2 gene cause both Pfeiffer and Crouzon syndrome phenotypes. Nat Genet. 1995;9:173–6.
13. Glaser RL, Jiang W, Boyadjiev SA, et al. Paternal origin of FGFR2 mutations in sporadic cases of Crouzon syndrome and Pfeiffer syndrome. Am J Hum Genet. 2000;66:768–77.
14. Fearon JA, Rhodes J. Pfeiffer syndrome: a treatment evaluation. Plast Reconstr Surg. 2009;123(5):1–9.
15. Aina VH, et al. Pfeiffer syndrome: analysis of a clinical series and development of a classification system. J Craniofac Surg. 2013; 24:204–15.
16. Vogels A, Fryns JP. Pfeiffer syndrome. Orphanet J Rare Dis. 2006;1:19.
17. Mitsukawa N, Kaneko T, Saiga A, Akita S, Satoh K. Early midfacial distraction for syndromic craniosynostotic patients with obstructive sleep apnoea. J Plast Reconstr Aesthet Surg. 2013;66(9):1206–11.
18. Bhattacharjee A, Uddin S, Purkaystha P. Deviated nasal septum in the newborn-A 1 year study. Indian J Otolaryngol Head Neck Surg. 2005;57(4):p304–8.
19. Bevans S. Boseley MB. Neonatal septal hematoma. Poster presentation at Combined Otolaryngological Societies meeting, April 12–14 2012. San Diego, CA.
20. Hossain T, Kappelman MD, Perez-Atayde AR, Young GJ, Huttner KM, Christou H. Primary Ciliary Dyskinesia as a cause of neonatal respiratory distress: implications for the neonatologist. J Perinatol. 2003;23:684–7.
21. Emami AJ, Brodsky L, Pizzuto M. Neonatal septoplasty: case report and review of the literature. Int J Pediatr Otorhinolaryngol. 1996;35:271–5.
22. Healy G. An approach to the nasal septum in children. Laryngoscope. 1986;96:123991242.
23. Duval M, Alsaba BH, Carpineta L, Daniel SJ. Respiratory distress secondary to bilateral nasolacrimal duct mucoceles in a newborn. Otolaryngol Head Neck Surg. 2007;137:353–4.
24. Herr M, Clarisse B, Nikasinovic L, Foucault C, Le Marec AM, Giordanella JP, Just J, Momas I. Does allergic rhinitis exist in infancy? Findings from the PARIS birth cohort. Allergy. 2011;66(2):214–21.
25. Nathan CO, Seid AB. Neonatal rhinitis. Int J Pediatr Otolaryngol. 1997;39:59–65.
26. Jazbi B. Diagnosis and treatment of nasal birth deformities. Clin Pediatr (Phila). 1974;13:1974.
27. Sooknundan M, Deka RC, Kacker SK, Verma IC. Indian J Pediatr. 1986;53:105–8.
28. Schafer AT, Lembe R, Althoff H. Airway resistance of posterior nasal pathway in sudden infant death victims. Eur J Pediatr. 1991;150(595):598.
29. Friedman NR, Luck M, Scapa VI. Excision of congenital nasolacrimal duct cyst with powered instrumentation. Laryngoscope. 2011;121:135–6.
30. Jacobs AH. Strawberry hemangiomas: the natural history of the untreated lesion. Calif Med. 1957;86:8–10.
31. Drolet BA, Esterly NB, Frieden IJ. Hemangiomas in children. N Engl J Med. 1999;341:173–81.
32. Warner NM, et al. The nonrandom distribution of facial hemangiomas. Arch Dermatol. 2003;139(7):869–75.
33. Sommers Smith SK, Smith DK. Beta blockade induces apoptosis in cultured capillary endothelial cells. In Vitro Cell Dev Biol Anim. 2002;38(5):298–304.

34. Storch CH, Hoeger PH. Propranolol for infantile hemangiomas: insights into molecular mechanisms of action. Br J Dermatol. 2010;163(2):269–74.
35. Drolet BA, et al. Initiation and Use of propranolol for infantile hemangioma: report of a consensus conference. Pediatrics. 2013;181(1):128–40.
36. Cay A, Bektas D, Imamoglu M, Bahadir O, Cobanoglu U, Sarihan H. Oral teratoma: a case report and literature review. Pediatr Surg Int. 2004;20:304–8.
37. Rybak LP, Rapp MF, McGrady MD, Schwart MR, Myers PW, Orvidas L. Obstructing nasopharyngeal teratoma in the neonate. A report of two cases. Arch Otolaryngol Head Neck Surg. 1991;117(12):1411–5.
38. Makki FM, Al-Mazrou KA. Nasopharyngeal teratoma associated with cleft palate in a newborn. Eur Arch Otorhinolaryngol. 2008;265(11):1413–5.
39. Chaudhry AP, Lore JM, Fisher JE, Gambrino AG. So-called hairy polyps or teratoid tumors of the nasopharynx. Arch Otolaryngol. 1978;104:517–25.
40. Coppit GL, Perkins JA, Manning SC. Nasopharyngeal teratomas and dermoids: a review of the literature and case series. Int J Pediatr Otorhinolaryngol. 2000;52(3):219–27.
41. Kumar A, Helling E, Guenther D, et al. Correction of frontonaso-ethmoidal encephalocele: the HULA procedure. Plast Reconstr Surg. 2009;132(2):661–9.
42. Holm C, Thu M, et al. Extracranial correction of frontoethmoidal meningoencephaloceles: feasibility and outcomes in 52 consecutive cases. Plast Reconstr Surg. 2008;121(6):386–95.
43. Kanev PM. Congenital malformations of the skull and meninges. Otolarynol Clin North Am. 2007;40(1):9–26.
44. Andrews BT, Meara JG. Reconstruction of frontoethmoidal encephalocele defects. Atlas Oral Maxillofac Surg Clin North Am. 2010;18(2):129–38.
45. Suwanwela C, Suwanwela N. A morphological classification of sincipital encephalomeningoceles. J Neurosurg. 1972;36:201–11.
46. Kilcline C, Frieden IJ. Infantile hemangiomas: how common are they? A systematic review of the medical literature. Pediatr Dermatol. 2008;25(2):168–73.
47. Saettele M, Alexander A, Markovich B, Morelli J, Lowe LH. Congenital midline nasofrontal masses. Pediatr Radiol. 2012; 42(9):1119–25.
48. Swift AC, Singh SD. The presentation and management of the nasal glioma. Int J Pediatr Otorhinolaryngol. 1985;10(3):253–61.
49. Zapata SJ, Kearns DB. Nasal dermoids. Curr Opin Otolaryngol Head Neck Surg. 2006;14(6):406–11.
50. Rahbar R, Shah P, Mulliken JB, Robson CD, Perez-Atayde AR, Proctor MR, Kenna MA, Scott MR, McGill TJ, Healy GB. The presentation and management of nasal dermoid: a 30-year experience. Arch Otolaryngol Head Neck Surg. 2003;129(4): 464–71.

Disorders of the Nasal Cavity

Scott R. Schoem

Introduction

One of the myths in otolaryngology is the notion that neonates are obligate nose breathers. This long-believed misconception still permeates our literature. The word "obligate" implies that the neonate has no choice but to breathe through the nose. The appropriate terminology is that neonates are "preferential" nasal breathers since the infant can breathe through the mouth if the nose is blocked [1–3]. However, in certain circumstances such as with bilateral choanal atresia, the child has complete nasal obstruction and must breathe through the mouth. The term cyclical cyanosis refers to this condition whereby the neonate attempts to breathe through the nose, is unable to do so resulting in hypercapnia, opens the mouth to cry, and then breathes orally temporarily resolving the cyanosis. This results in severe breathing and discoordination of feeding problems. Yet, at least one report describes bilateral choanal atresia first discovered in adulthood [4].

Some disorders may be life-threatening and not amenable to surgical correction in the neonatal period, while others are mild and self-limiting. Anatomic, structural lesions may be bilateral or unilateral. Most neonates resolve nonanatomical obstruction with medical management and growth.

Normal Nasal Physiology

The nasal cavity provides several important physiologic functions including air-conditioning, filtration of inhaled particles and microbes, maintaining mucus flow, sinus drainage, and olfaction [5, 6]. The proper physical shape of the nasal interior impacts on these functions. The nasal mucosa contains a rich supply of resistance blood vessels such as arterioles and arteriovenous anastomoses that drain into venous sinusoids. The sinusoids are innervated by sympathetic fibers which release norepinephrine leading to reduced blood flow and venous return into capacitance vessels. This results in decreased nasal congestion. Conversely, parasympathetic fibers release acetylcholine which increases nasal secretions and vasodilation. Sensory C-fibers release neurokinin A, calcitonin gene-related peptide, and substance P that downregulate sympathetic vasoconstriction and increased congestion.

Pathogenesis

On initial evaluation by an otolaryngologist, nasal obstruction in neonates and infants is generally classified as either an anatomic anomaly or congestion due to some nonanatomic problem—medication, allergy, laryngopharyngeal reflux, or some undiagnosed issue. However, the astute clinician should delve much more carefully into the pathogenesis or pathophysiology of neonatal nasal obstruction. Development of nasal obstruction is an extremely complex interplay of still not very well-defined competing sympathetic and parasympathetic triggers. Moreover, mast cells, eosinophils, basophils, and goblet cells release local inflammatory mediators including histamine, kinins, prostaglandins, arachidonic acid metabolites, and mucin that all contribute to nasal congestion [6].

Clinical Presentation and Evaluation

Rarely does a neonate have complete nasal obstruction except in the event of arhinia or bilateral choanal atresia. Usually there is at least some airflow on at least one side. For the baby with bilateral choanal atresia, the child will exhibit cyclical cyanosis marked by failed attempt to breathe nasally, eventual crying with mouth opening, oral air

S.R. Schoem, M.D., F.A.A.P. (✉)
Division of Otolaryngology—Head and Neck Surgery, University of Connecticut, Connecticut Children's Medical Center, Hartford, CT 06106, USA
e-mail: sschoem@ccmckids.org

J. Lioy and S.E. Sobol (eds.), *Disorders of the Neonatal Airway: Fundamentals for Practice*, DOI 10.1007/978-1-4939-1610-8_4, © Springer Science+Business Media New York 2015

exchange with cessation of hypoxia and cyanosis, and resumption of the cycle once the mouth closes. Placement of an oral prop eliminates the problem temporarily allowing for an orderly evaluation.

An initial overall examination includes the assessment of whether the baby has the ability to breathe nasally and if so whether this is unilateral or bilateral. Traditionally, we are taught to pass a 5–6 Fr catheter in the nose on each side to determine patency. However, the catheter often coils up in the nose or bounces against the inferior turbinate invalidating interpretation of the maneuver. Rather than the catheter test, with the mouth closed, try the mirror test by placing a laryngeal mirror in front of the nose on each side to see if nasal airflow fogs the mirror. Alternatively, if the parent has a pocket mirror, place it in front of the nose to see if two fog dots are present. In addition, listen for stertor, which is a low-pitched, inspiratory noise caused by turbulent airflow of nasal, nasopharyngeal or oropharyngeal tissue vibrations. If there is no air movement, then flexible fiberoptic endoscopy usually will help determine the site and degree of obstruction. Flexible endoscopy is very helpful to distinguish pryiform, midnasal or posterior nasal stenosis, a congenital nasal septal deviation, or mass effect either intranasally or in the nasopharynx. Rigid telescope endoscopy in the neonate is much more difficult to accomplish than flexible endoscopy.

Examination of breathing – feeding coordination is essential. If the baby is unable to feed properly due to nasal obstruction, or has discoordination of feeding with choking, this may accelerate the need for intervention. A modified barium esophagram or endoscopic evaluation of feeding may assist in the assessment of feeding.

Imaging studies may be very helpful or essential. Computed tomography (CT) is most helpful to diagnose and surgically plan bony anomalies such as pyriform stenosis and choanal atresia. Magnetic resonance imaging (MRI) is best for soft tissue obstructing masses that may have intracranial extension such as encephaloceles and nasal dermoids. Antenatal fetal MRI has been enormously helpful in establishing the extent of head and neck masses causing respiratory obstruction.

Differential Diagnosis and Management

After performing a complete history and physical examination, most diagnoses are evident and straightforward. In general, the care algorithm depends on whether the baby has generalized nasal inflammation or an anatomic/surgical entity.

Nasal Inflammation/Rhinitis

In neonates, placental blood flow transmits medications and drug metabolites that may cause nasal congestion. Several known agents may cause nasal congestion including antihypertensives, beta-blockers, antidepressants, cocaine, and gabapentin. Sometimes, obtaining a truthful maternal medication history is difficult and the clinician needs to proceed with treatment options empirically. Neonatal rhinitis is defined as mucoid or clear rhinorrhea with nasal mucosal edema in the afebrile newborn with stertor, poor feeding, and respiratory distress that responds to the use of steroid drops [7].

After establishing the diagnosis of a non-surgically correctable lesion, treatment starts with nasal saline to decongest the nasal mucosa. If unsuccessful, topical oxymetazoline may be used three times a day for 3–4 days for maximal decongestion while concurrently starting use of topical steroid and continuing with topical nasal steroids.

Birth Trauma

The reported incidence of birth trauma-related external nasal and intranasal septal deviation is reported as 1 %. However, in clinical practice, it seems much less common. Moreover, the clinician should be careful not to label the baby with a deviated nose as birth delivery-related, when the mechanism of action may be positioning of the head in the birth canal during uneventful passage. When the deviation is minor, this usually self-corrects within several weeks after birth. Rarely, the nose is so deviated that a reduction in the first week after birth is required to re-establish normal nasal breathing. Mild anterior nasal septal abnormalities are common, but rarely cause any respiratory distress.

Congenital Anatomic Anomalies

Arhinia

Congenital arhinia (or arrhinia) is a rare entity defined as absence of the external nose, nasal cavities, and olfactory apparatus. Embryologically, arhinia is due to failed fusion of the maxillary process and the lateral nasal process between the third and eighth week of gestation. Cribriform plate fusion abnormalities lead to olfactory agenesis. Tessier defines this malformation as total arrhinia, hemi-arrhinia, and proboscis lateralis [8]. Arhinia may be associated with hypertelorism, microphthalmia, palatal abnormalities, cryptorchidism, and blindness [9]. Many children with arhinia have normal intelligence Fig. 1.

Initial management of arhinia may require tracheotomy to provide a safe airway with deferred surgical planning as a child or adolescent once the degree of cognitive development has been established. For high-functioning children, a craniofacial team approach of otolaryngology, plastic surgery, and potentially neurosurgery is required to establish nasal patency followed by external nasal reconstruction. Both CT and MRI may be complementary for surgical planning.

Anterior (Pyriform) Stenosis

Congenital nasal pyriform aperture stenosis (CNPAS) is an unusual narrowing of the anterior nasal vault. Anatomically, the anterior nasal vault is defined by the nasal bones superiorly, the nasal process of the maxilla laterally and the junction of the horizontal process of the maxilla and the anterior nasal spine inferiorly.

This entity was first described in adults in 1952 [10] and in a neonate in 1989 [11]. CNPAS may be an isolated anomaly or associated with other craniofacial malformations. The most common is the holoprosencephaly spectrum including a single central upper incisor tooth, absent upper labial frenulum, and absence of the corpus callosum [12, 13]. In mild cases, the neonate may have stertor and mild difficulty coordinating breathing and feeding. In more severe cases, the child may have symptoms and signs that mimic atresia with cyclical cyanosis and respiratory distress. Often, patients will pass the mirror test since there is stenosis but not atresia.

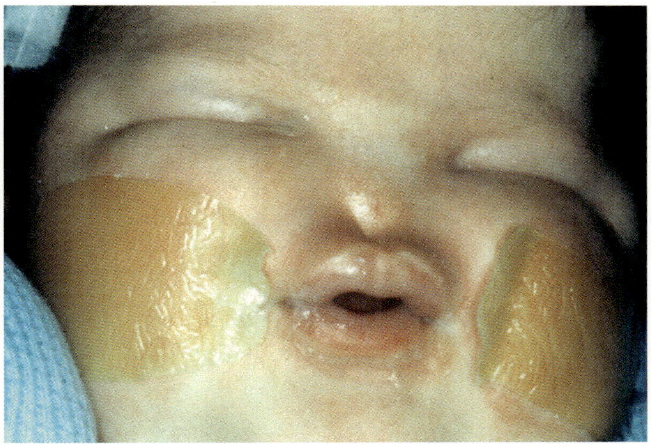

Fig. 1 Photo of arhinia

Flexible nasal endoscopy may demonstrate the inability to pass the infant fiberoptic telescope. CT scan is diagnostic and helps to rule out other midline anatomic abnormalities. Beldon performed CT analysis and determined that the normal term infant should have at least an 11 mm width across the pyriform aperture Fig. 2 [14].

Initial management depends on the degree of respiratory distress. In isolated instances, intubation is rarely necessary. However, in syndromic neonates, establishment of a safe airway may be necessary. If multiple airway anomalies are present, nasal surgery alone may not be sufficient and a tracheotomy is required. When the lesion is isolated, surgery with nasal stenting is very successful.

Mid-vault Stenosis

Rarely, a congenital thickening of the nasal septum or narrowing of the total vault may cause mid-vault stenosis premature infants. Typically, this is self-limited and responds well to topical steroid treatment.

Posterior (Choanal) Stenosis or Atresia

Choanal atresia (CA) is a relatively rare malformation occurring in approximately 1 in 7,000–8,000 births. Unilateral atresia is more common than bilateral. Previous textbooks report that CA is more common in females than males; however, more recent reviews report an equal gender distribution [15, 16]. The purported mechanism leading to CA is either failure of buccopharyngeal membrane breakdown or persistence and misdirection of mesoderm during embryogenesis. In only rare circumstances is the obstruction due to soft tissue alone. In almost all cases, there is some bony component that needs to be removed for successful surgical treatment.

Bilateral CA is diagnosed shortly after birth due to characteristic cyclical cyanosis. The mirror test or inability to pass a 5–6 Fr catheter is suspicious for CA. Flexible

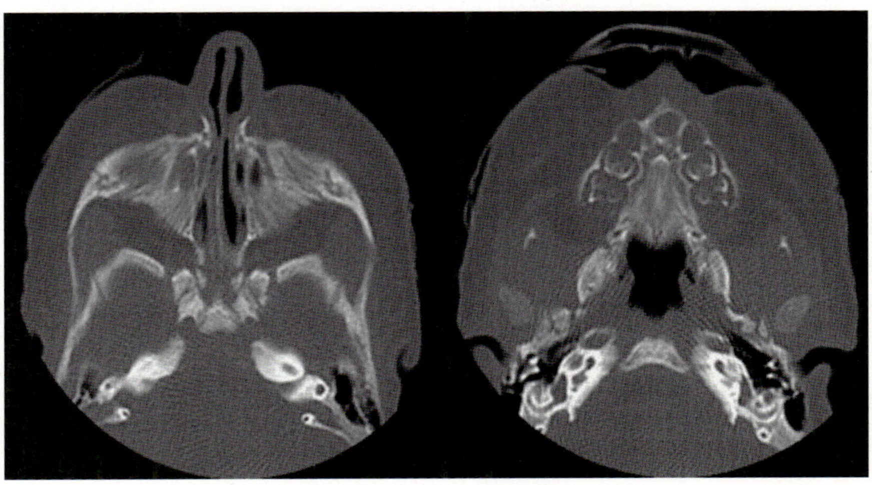

Fig. 2 CT scan of pyriform stenosis and single central incisor associated with holoprosencephaly spectrum

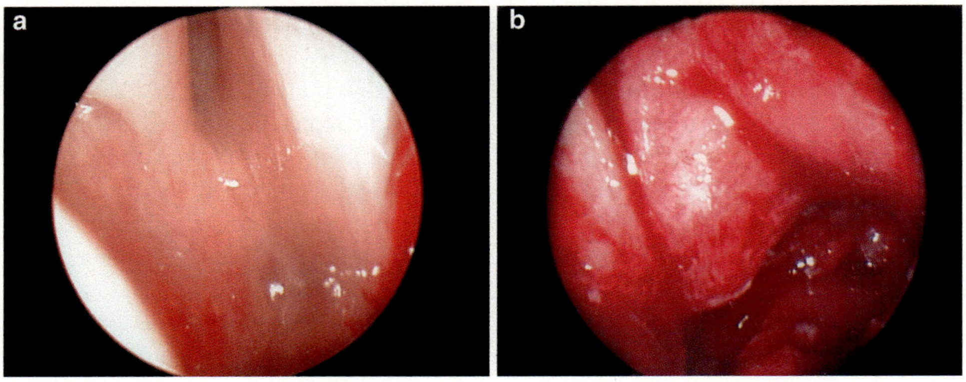

Fig. 3 (**a**) Endoscopic photo of choanal atresia preop. (**b**) Endoscopic photo of choanal atresia postop

fiberoptic endoscopy is diagnostic in most cases Fig. 3. Occasionally, an obstructing posterior nasal or nasopharyngeal growth may mimic CA. Fine cut CT scan is essential to determine the site and degree of obstruction, and image the presence of the nasopharyngeal roof and cavity. Unilateral CA may go unrecognized for years and often presents during childhood or adolescence as inability to breathe through one side of the nose with constant unilateral runny nose. Likewise, choanal stenosis as opposed to atresia may go unrecognized for years.

Every neonate with choanal atresia should be screened for CHARGE syndrome. CHARGE used to be classified as an association. However, with the discovery of the genetic marker CHD7 on Chromosome 8, which encodes the chromodomain helicase DNA binding protein, CHARGE is now classified as a syndrome [17]. CHARGE syndrome is characterized by ocular *C*olobomas, *H*eart defects, choanal *A*tresia, *R*etarded growth, *G*enitourinary hypoplasia, and *E*ar abnormalities. CHD7 analysis in CHARGE syndrome detects mutations in 65–70 % of individuals. Cardiovascular abnormalities occur in 75–85 % and tracheoesophageal fistula is present in 15–20 % of newborns with CHARGE syndrome. Ossicular malformations, cochlear anomalies, and semicircular canal hypoplasia occur in over 80 % of patients [17].

Bilateral CA is a medical urgency; however, it is not a surgical emergency. Use of an oral prop for adequate breathing and an orogastric feeding tube for nutrition allows for the orderly evaluation of other potential anomalies, proper counseling, and surgical planning. With the advent of endoscopic equipment, miniaturization of power-assisted drills and shavers, surgical repair of choanal atresia has evolved over the past 20 years. Whereas previous textbooks discuss both transpalatal and transnasal approaches, the vast majority of current repairs are performed using transnasal techniques. Whether or not to place a short-term stent is still debated in the literature [18–21]. The most difficult cases involve syndromes with severe down sloping nasopharyngeal roofs or nearly absent nasopharyngeal cavities such as Treacher Collins syndrome.

Congenital Masses

Nasolacrimal Duct Cyst (Dacryocystocele)

Obstruction of the nasolacrimal duct is a common anomaly with widely varying reported rates [22, 23]. Many duct obstructions are partial and self-correct by 1 year of age. The duct is usually obstructed at the valve of Hasner just lateral to the inferior turbinate [24]. This may lead to a round mass in the lower nasal cavity. If the proximal valve is obstructed at the common canniculus, this leads to a round facial swelling inferior to the medial canthus of the eye. This may become infected with impressive swelling and erythema mimicking acute unilateral sinusitis. Occasionally, when bitateral cysts are present, this may lead to severe nasal obstruction in the neonate and difficulty coordinating breathing and feeding similar to bilateral choanal atresia. When the clinical picture is uncertain, CT scan with contrast or MRI helps to distinguish between bilateral nasolacrimal duct obstruction, anterior pyriform stenosis, or other mass effects due to tumor.

Surgical treatment and timing varies depending on surgeon preference and severity of presentation. Unilateral dacryocystoceles rarely need urgent surgical correction. However, bilateral obstruction may require surgery within the first few weeks of life. Treatment ranges in escalation from duct probing and balloon dilation for simple duct obstruction to intranasal marsupialization and silastic stenting for large obstructing cysts [25].

Infantile Hemangioma

Infantile hemangiomas are the most common benign neoplasms of infancy. The most common site is in the head and neck primarily in the central facial region. Occasionally, a

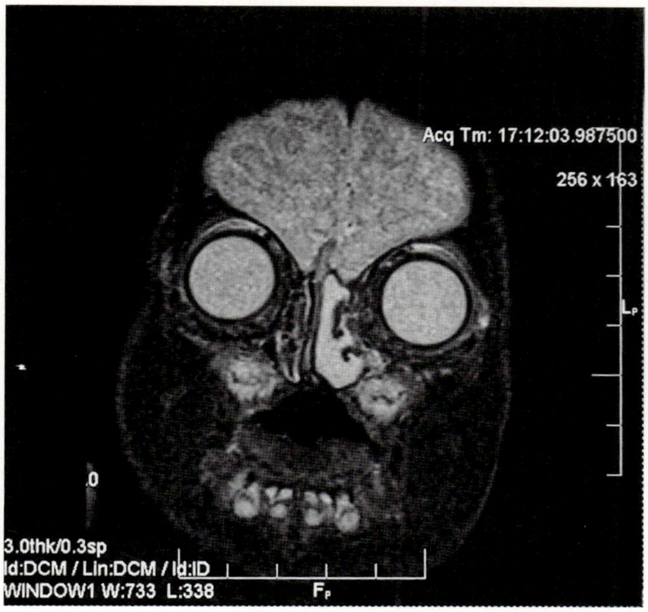

Fig. 4 CT scan of left intranasal glioma: note distinct separation from dura

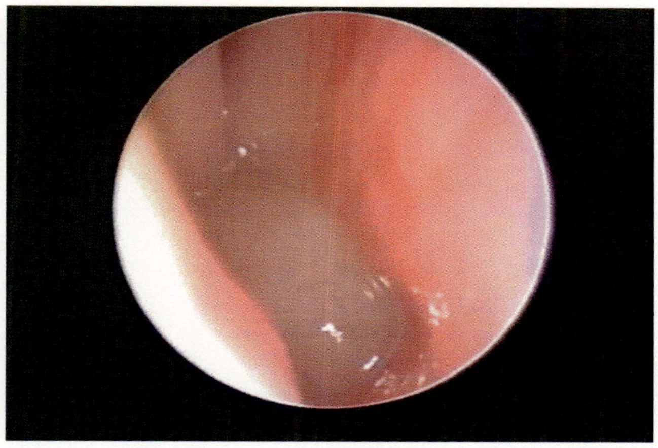

Fig. 5 Endoscopic photo of nasopharyngeal glioma

large nasal and facial hemangioma may proliferate quickly in the intranasal region leading to obstructed breathing. The traditional treatment for many years had been intralesional injection of steroids or systemic steroids with laser ablation during the proliferative phase. However, in recent years, propranolol treatment has supplanted older modalities [26, 27]. Propranolol has been identified on molecular analysis to block endothelial cell proliferation, migration, and formation of the actin cytoskeleton with alteration in vascular endothelial growth factor receptor- 2 [28]. Neonates and infants should be referred to a center familiar for multidisciplinary evaluation and management [29].

Meningocele, Meningoencephalocele, and Glioma (Heterotopic Glial Tissue)

Meningoceles, meningoencephaloceles, and gliomas are often grouped together. A meningocele represents downward displacement into the nose of only the meninges due to small defects in the floor of the intracranial cavity. A meningoencephalocele results from a larger defect that allows for herniation of both meninges and brain tissue. This may extend outward at the glabellar region or only downward with a cribiform plate defect with a large intranasal mass that resemble a polyp. By definition, a nasal glioma is sequestered or displaced neural tissue with fibrous and vascular connective tissue that increases the firmness of the mass. There may be a connecting fibrous stalk to the skull base in 10–15 %; however, it is rare to have any meningeal connection. Therefore, clinically, a meningoencephalocele is soft, compressible, pulsatile; whereas a glioma is firm, noncompressible, and non-pulsatile.

CT scan helps to identify the bony defect in the skull base. MRI is much more useful to demonstrate the characteristics of the soft tissue mass and locate the site of intracranial extension Fig. 4. On T1-weighted MRI, the intranasal component is isointense or hypointense and on T2-weighted images is hyperintense relative to brain tissue. Gliomas are 60 % extranasal, 30 % intranasal, and 10 % combined (dumbbell growth).

Surgery on a meningoencephalocele requires a neurosurgeon and otolaryngologist. Surgery is typically via anterior frontal craniotomy [30]. Glioma surgery is typically performed via the intranasal approach and usually does not require intraoperative neurosurgical involvement; however, a neurosurgeon should be available on a standby basis for any unexpected encounter or complication Fig. 5 [31, 32].

Nasal Dermoid Sinus and Cyst

Derived from ectoderm and mesoderm, a dermoid cyst or sinus may form due to a remnant in the prenasal space posterior to the nasal bones and anterior to the nasal and septal cartilages. The typical sinus tract has a pit and related small hair tuft on the nasal dorsum. This may present as an infected midline mass or with keratin discharge. The tract is usually well-defined on imaging. However, in some cases, the distal extent may project anteriorly all the way to the nasal tip altering surgical planning or increasing the likelihood of recurrence. CT scan helps to define bony skull-base defects and widening of the crista galli, which is associated with potential intracranial extension. MRI is very useful to determine the extent of the tract and mass, and serpentine extensions and intracranial extension.

If no imaging evidence of intracranial extension, surgical correction may be limited to a nasal approach with neurosurgical standby. Various options include the endoscopic-assisted closed approach for cysts without sinus tracts, external rhinoplasty, and the direct, open approach [33–35]. Even if the tract has intracranial extension, in selected cases

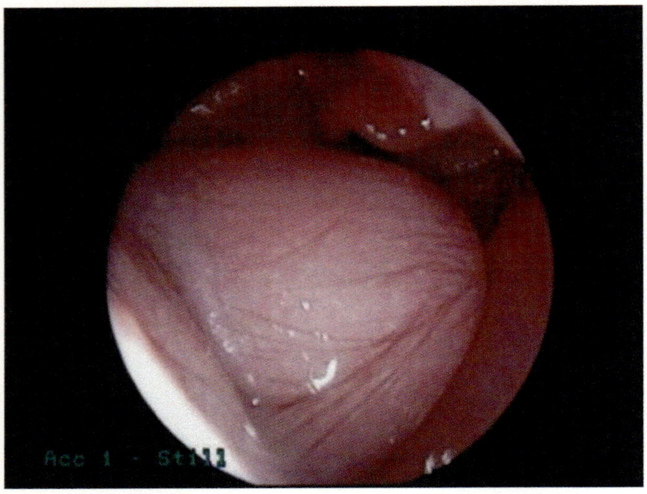

Fig. 6 Endoscopic photo of nasopharyngeal teratoma (courtesy of Tulio Valdez, MD)

the endonasal endoscopic approach may be sufficient; [36] however, neurosurgical standby is recommended for patient safety.

Rare Tumors

In rare cases, neonates are born with unrecognized nasal and nasopharyngeal tumors causing varying degrees of obstruction. These may be benign or malignant teratomas, or other unusual and aggressively growing fibrous tissue tumors Fig. 6 [37–39]. More often, these tumors are noted on fetal ultrasound during gestation with polyhydramnios due to impaired fetal swallowing. Fetal MRI delineates the site and degree of obstruction enabling an orderly evaluation and plan for management.

Multidisciplinary Considerations

The *EX*-utero *I*ntrapartum *T*reatment (EXIT) approach to management has been highly successful in many cases to provide safe initial airway management followed by tumor excision after stabilization [40]. Maternal-fetal circulation may be prolonged for up to almost 1 h providing oxygen to the baby while establishing airway control. The EXIT procedure using a combined team approach has become the best modality for optimal care of known obstruction lesions discovered during pregnancy [41].

Future Considerations

In the past decade, the newest frontier is development of operative teams for intrauterine surgery. Intrauterine surgery is a rapidly developing field. Fetal surgery for spina bifida and congenital diaphragmatic hernia has become a therapeutic alternative for expectant mothers in selected cases [42–44]. The potential exists for expansion of fetal surgery to other embryologic anomalies and tumors.

References

1. Bergeson PS, Shaw JC. Are infants really obligate nasal breathers? Clin Pediatr. 2001;40:567–9.
2. Miller M, Martin R, Carlo W, Fouke J, Strohl K, Fanaroff A. Oral breathing in newborn infants. J Pediatr. 1985;107:465–9.
3. Trabalon M, Schaal B. It takes a mouth to eat and a nose to breathe: abnormal oral respiration affects neonates' oral competence and systemic adaptation. Int J Pediatr. 2012; 2012:207605.
4. Panda N, Simhadri S, Ghosh S. Bilateral choanal atresia in an adult: is it compatible with life? J Laryngol Otol. 2004;118:244–5.
5. Wang D, Lee H, Gordon B. Impacts of fluid dynamics simulations in study of nasal airflow physiology and pathophysiology in realistic human three-dimensional nose models. Clin Exp Otorhinolaryngol. 2012;5:181–7.
6. Leong S, Chen X, Lee H, Wang D. A review of the implications of computational fluid dynamic studies on nasal airflow and physiology. Rhinology. 2010;48:139–45.
7. Nathan C, Seid A. Neonatal rhinitis. Int J Pediatr Otorhinolaryngol. 1997;14:59–65.
8. Tessier P, Ciminello F, Wolfe S. The arrhinias. Scand J Plast Reconstr Surg. 2009;43:177–96.
9. Graham J, Lee J. Bosma arhinia microphthalmia syndrome. Am J Med Genet. 2006;140:189–93.
10. Douglas B. The relief of vestibular nasal obstruction by partial resection of the nasal process of the superior maxilla. Plast Reconstr Surg. 1952;9:42–51.
11. Brown O, Myer C, Manning S. Congenital nasal pyriform aperture stenosis. Laryngoscope. 1989;99:86–91.
12. Hui Y, Friedberg J, Crysdale W. Congenital nasal pyriform aperture stenosis as a presenting feature of holoprosencephaly. Int J Pediatr Otorhinolaryngol. 1995;31:263–74.
13. Tavin E, Stecker E, Marion R. Nasal pyriform aperture stenosis and the holoprosencephaly spectrum. Int J Pediatr Otorhinolaryngol. 1994;28:199–204.
14. Belden C, Mancuso A, Schmalfuss I. CT features of congenital nasal pyriform aperture stenosis: initial experience. Radiology. 1999;213:495–501.
15. Harris J, Robert E, Kallen B. Epidemiology of choanal atresia with special reference to the CHARGE association. Pediatrics. 1997;99: 363–7.
16. Hengerer A, Brickman T, Jeyakumar A. Choanal atresia: embryologic analysis and evolution of treatment, a 30-year experience. Laryngoscope. 2008;118:862–6.
17. Bauer P, Wippold F, Goldin J, Lusk R. Cochlear implantation in children with CHARGE association. Arch Otolaryngol Head Neck Surg. 2002;128:1013–7.
18. Schoem S. Transnasal endoscopic repair of choanal atresia: why stent? Otolaryngol Head Neck Surg. 2004;131:362–6.
19. El-Ahl M, El-Anwar M. Stentless endoscopic transnasal repair of bilateral choanal atresia starting with resection of vomer. Int J Pediatr Otorhinolaryngol. 2012;76:1002–6.
20. De Freitas R, Berkowitz R. Bilateral choanal atresia repair in neonates—a single surgeon experience. Int J Pediatr Otorhinolaryngol. 2012;76:873–8.
21. Bedwell J, Choi S. Are stents necessary after choanal atresia repair? Laryngoscope. 2012;122:2365–6.

22. Cunningham M, Woog J. Endonasal endoscopic dacryocystorhinostomy in children. Arch Otolaryngol Head Neck Surg. 1998;124:328–33.
23. Guery D, Kendig E. Congenital impotency of the nasolacrimal duct. Arch Ophthalmol. 1979;97:1656–8.
24. Shashy R, Durairaj V, Holmes J, Hohberger G, Thompson D, Kasperbauer J. Congenital dacryocystocele associated with intranasal cysts: diagnosis and management. Laryngoscope. 2003; 113:37–40.
25. Leonard D, O'Keefe M, Rowley H, Hughes J. Neonatal respiratory distress secondary to bilateral intranasal dacryocystoceles. Int J Pediatr Otorhinolaryngol. 2008;72:1873–7.
26. Leaute-Labreze C, Dumas de la Roque E, Hubiche T, Boralevi F, Thambo J, Taieb A. Propranolol for severe hemangiomas of infancy. N Engl J Med. 2008;12:2649–51.
27. Sans V, Dumas de la Roque E, Berge J, Grenier N, Boralevi F, Mazereeuw-Hautier J, Lipsker D, Dupuis E, Ezzedine K, Vergnes P, Taieb A, Leaute-Labreze C. Propranolol for severe infantile hemangiomas: follow up report. Pediatrics. 2009;124:e423–31.
28. Stiles J, Amaya C, Pham R, Rowntree R, Lacaze M, Mulne A, Bischoff J, Kokta V, Boucheron L, Mitchell D, Bryan B. Propranolol treatment of infantile hemangioma endothelial cells: a molecular analysis. Exp Ther Med. 2012;4:594–604.
29. Parikh S, Darrow D, Grimmer J, Manning S, Richter G, Perkins J. Propranolol use for infantile hemangiomas: American Society of Pediatric Otolaryngology vascular anomalies task force practice patterns. JAMA Otolaryngol Head Neck Surg. 2013;139:153–6.
30. Mahapatra A, Agrawal D. Anterior encephaloceles: a series of 103 cases over 32 years. J Clin Neurosci. 2006;13:536–9.
31. Rahbar R, Resto A, Robson C, Perez-Atayde A, Goumnerova L, McGill T, Healy G. Nasal glioma and encephalocele: diagnosis and management. Laryngoscope. 2003;113:2069–77.
32. Yokoyama M, Inouye N, Mizuno F. Endoscopic management of nasal glioma in infancy. Int J Pediatr Otorhinolaryngol. 1999;51:51–4.
33. Holzmann D, Huisman T, Holzmann P, Stoeckli S. Surgical approaches for nasal dermal sinus cysts. Rhinology. 2007;45:31–5.
34. Locke R, Kubba H. The external rhinoplasty approach for congenital nasal lesions in children. Int J Pediatr Otorhinolaryngol. 2011;75:337–41.
35. Winterton R, Wilks D, Chumas P, Russell J, Liddington M. Surgical correction of midline nasal dermoid sinus cysts. J Craniofac Surg. 2010;21:295–300.
36. Re M, Tarchini P, Macri G, Pasquini E. Endonasal approach for intracranial nasal dermoid sinus cysts in children. Int J Pediatr Otorhinolaryngol. 2012;76:1217–22.
37. Klein A, Schoem S, Altman A, Eisenfeld L. Inflammatory myoblastic tumor in the neonate: a case report. Otolaryngol Head Neck Surg. 2003;128:145–7.
38. Katona G, Hirschberg J, Hosszu Z, Kiraly L. Epipharyngeal teratoma in infancy. Int J Pediatr Otorhinolaryngol. 1992;24:171–5.
39. Hansen J, Soerensen F, Christensen M. A five week old girl with inspiratory stridor due to infantile hemangiopericytoma. Eur Arch Otorhinolaryngol. 2006;263:524–7.
40. Hirose S, Farmer D, Lee H, Nobuhara K, Harrison M. The ex utero intrapartum treatment procedure: looking back at the EXIT. J Pediatr Surg. 2004;39:375–80.
41. Osborn A, Baud D, Macarthur A, Propst E, Forte V, Blaser S, Windrim R, Seaward G, Keunen J, Shah P, Ryan G, Campisi P. Multidisciplinary perinatal management of the compromised airway on placental support: lessons learned. Prenat Diagn. 2013; 18:1–8.
42. Adzick N. Fetal surgery for myelomeningocele: trials and tribulations. Isabella Forshall Lecture. J Pediatr Surg. 2012;47:273–81.
43. Diemert A, Diehl W, Glosemeyer P, Deprest J, Hecher K. Intrauterine surgery—choices and limitations. Dtsch Arztebl Int. 2012;109:603–38.
44. Adzick N. Fetal surgery for spina bifida: past, present, future. Semin Pediatr Surg. 2013;22:10–7.

Impact of Micro- and Retrognathia on the Neonatal Airway

Jesse A. Goldstein and Jesse A. Taylor

Etiology and Background

The human mandible is a unique structure that undergoes considerable anatomic changes during growth and development. In the neonatal period, the mandible is flat, with a short ramus, and poorly defined articulation with the skull base [1]. It is, therefore, prone to retroposition (retrognathia) which, when combined with insufficient mandibular sagittal projection (micrognathia), can result in posterior-inferior positioning of the tongue base. Because the tongue is anchored to the mandible, micro- or retrognathia forces the tongue posteriorly into the oropharynx and can lead to its displacement into the hypopharynx (glossoptosis) resulting in severe tongue-base obstruction of the supraglottic airway (Fig. 1).

The triad of micrognathia, glossoptosis, and tongue-based airway obstruction (TBAO) was initially described in 1939 by Dr. Pierre Robin, a French somatologist, who implicated the small mandible as the causative deformity leading ultimately to airway compromise [2, 3]. This "domino" effect is therefore known as Pierre Robin sequence (PRS). A sequence is constellation of abnormalities which are linked from an inciting anomaly or deformity. In the case of Pierre Robin sequence, failure of normal mandibular development sets off a cascade of anatomic changes in utero which result in the varying and seemingly unrelated physical findings (Fig. 2). {Figueroa 1991}.

J.A. Goldstein, M.D.
Division of Plastic Surgery, Children's Hospital of Philadelphia, University of Pennsylvania, Perelman School of Medicine, Philadelphia, PA, USA
e-mail: Goldstein.jesse@gmail.com

J.A. Taylor, M.D. (✉)
Department of Plastic, Reconstructive, and Craniofacial Surgery, The Children's Hospital of Philadelphia, University of Pennsylvania, Perelman School of Medicine, Philadelphia, PA, USA
e-mail: Taylorj5@email.chop.edu

The etiology of this mandibular deformity is the topic of much debate. Several studies have attributed the micrognathia seen in Pierre Robin sequence to intrauterine deformation or extrinsic factors rather than intrinsic growth restriction of the mandible itself [4]. From between the 6th to 12th week of gestation, the human embryo transitions from a position of extreme neck flexion where the mandible is buried in the upper thorax to a position of gradual extension [5]. This period coincides with rapid mandibular growth that allows the tongue to descend and the palatal shelves to fuse. Several factors including multiple gestation, oligohydramnios, and cervical hemivertebrae may restrict this extension [6]. These studies point to the phenomenon of "catch-up growth" as evidence that extrinsic compression plays an important role in the deformity.

Increasingly, attention has focused on genetic cause of PRS. In addition to the syndrome-associated cases of PRS such as those patients with Stickler or Treacher Collins syndromes who demonstrate intrinsic mandibular growth deficiency, non-syndromic PRS may also have a genetic component. Investigators have demonstrated increased frequency of palatal clefts in the parents of patients with PRS [7] as well as several novel genetic mutations present in a proportion of such patients [8, 9].

No matter the cause, PRS is a challenging disease process which can result in acute airway compromise, chronic obstructive sleep apnea, cor pulmonale, anoxic brain injury, and even death [10]. In the neonatal period, this entity can be particularly devastating, often necessitating emergent postnatal intubation in severe cases. Even in patients who do not require emergent airway management, chronic hypoxia, feeding intolerance, and failure to thrive may be common [11]. In one of Pierre Robin's early publications, he describes the grim prognosis of a severely affected child: "I have never seen a child live more than 16–18 months who presented hypoplasia as such the lower maxilla was pushed more than 1 cm behind the upper"[2].

J. Lioy and S.E. Sobol (eds.), *Disorders of the Neonatal Airway: Fundamentals for Practice*,
DOI 10.1007/978-1-4939-1610-8_5, © Springer Science+Business Media New York 2015

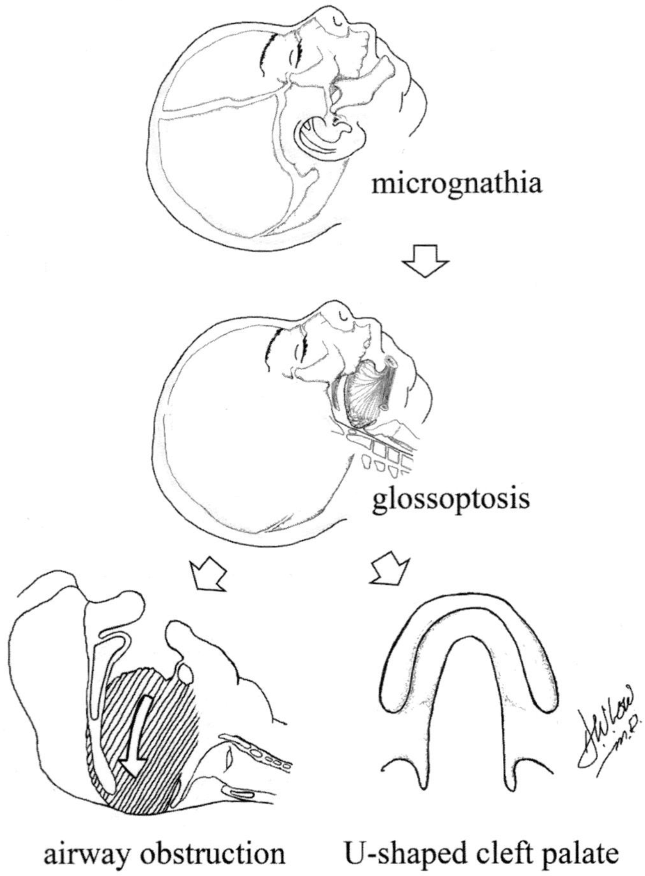

Fig. 1 The "domino effect" of Pierre Robin sequence (Courtesy of David Low, MD)

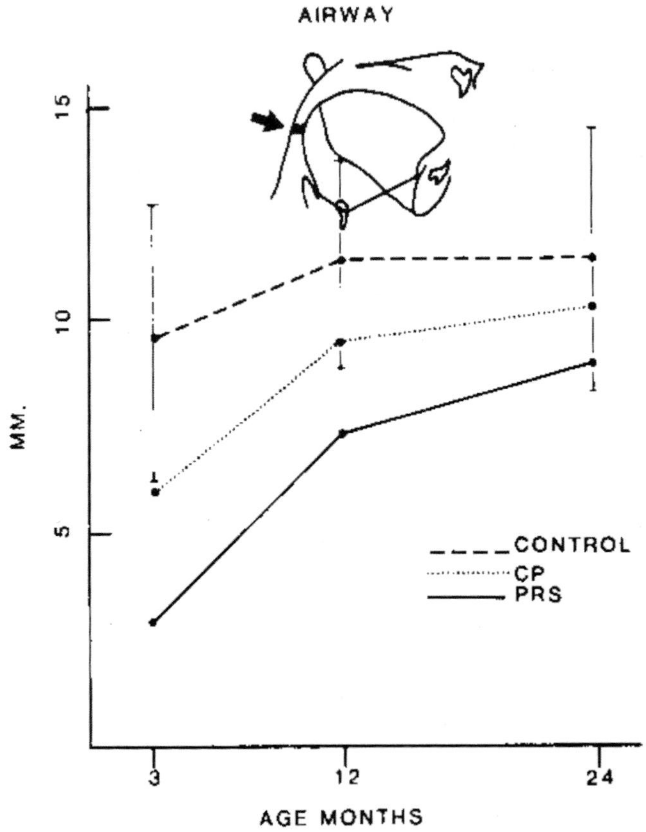

Fig. 2 Catch-up growth (Reprinted from [40] Permission granted from Allen Press Publishing Services)

Table 1 Frequency of associated syndromes

	Frequency in general population[a]	Frequency in Robin sequence[b]
Stickler	1:8,000	1:3
Velocardiofacial Syndrome	1:2,000	1:9
Fetal alcohol	1:1,000	1:10
Treacher Collins Syndrome	1:25,000	1:20
Undefined syndrome	–	1:3

[a]Per live births
[b]Per patients with Robin sequence

History and Epidemiology

Congenital micrognathia is associated with over 100 known syndromes [12]; however, in the setting of tongue-based airway obstruction as is seen with Pierre Robin sequence, it is estimated to occur in 1 in 8,500 to 1 in 14,000 live births [13]. In 40–60 % of cases, PRS occurs in isolation, as the only disease process. However, over half of patients may carry syndromic diagnoses which not only play a role in disease pathogenesis but may contribute to increased disease severity. The most common of these associated syndromes, for example, is Stickler syndrome, which has prevalence of 1 in 8,000 live births in the general population but is present in over 30 % of patients with PRS. Table 1 lists several of the major syndromes commonly associated with PRS.

Classification

There is no widely accepted classification system to stratify disease severity in patients with Pierre Robin sequence. As mentioned previously, several studies have associated worse outcomes in PRS patients who also carry syndromic diagnoses, and most centers now routinely recommend genetic screening after diagnosis. However, there is a wide variability in the severity of many syndromic diagnoses, and the simple presence or absence of a syndrome, alone, does little to differentiate such patients. Patients with Stickler or Nager syndromes often have more severe presentations than in PRS patients without accompanying syndromes, whereas many syndromes seen in these patients may contribute little or not at all to disease severity. Although many studies demonstrate worse outcomes in syndromic PRS as a whole, we caution against making management decisions based solely on the presence or absence of a syndrome.

Indeed, the key to differentiating the impact of micrognathia on the neonatal airway is to quantify its degree of deformity,

Table 2 GILLS scoring system for tongue-based airway obstruction

	GILLS Criteria
1	Presence of GER
2	Preoperative intubation
3	Late presentation (>2 weeks old)
4	Low birth weight (<2,500 g)
5	Syndromic diagnosis

Greater than two of these criteria correlate with high failure of Tongue-lip Adhesion surgery {Rogers 2011; Abramowicz 2012}

and those syndromes which adversely affect outcomes in Pierre Robin sequence are all associated with macroglossia or micrognathia. In order to assess the severity of anatomic mandibular deficiency, several authors advocate for the measurement of maxillary-mandibular discrepancy (MMD) as a simple, reliable, and reproducible method for stratification [14]. From the "worms eye" position looking superiorly, the mandible is gently closed to the maxilla and the distance between the midline mandibular alveoli and maxillary alveoli is measured. The realization that maxillary projection may also be inadequate in some forms of PRS, however, limits the utility of this tool [15]. In contrast, others recommend a clinical grading scale based on the severity of airway compromise [16].

The only validated classification system for patients with Pierre Robin system was developed as a means of determining which patients would benefit from surgical intervention. The GILLS criteria [17, 18] assesses for the presence of five factors which are shown to predict which patients might benefit from tongue-lip adhesion (TLA) surgery and which patients required direct tracheostomy (Table 2). Those patients with scores of two or less had a 100 % chance of success with the procedure whereas those patients with scores of three or more had close to a 50 % failure rate requiring tracheostomy.

Clinical Presentation

As stated previously, patients with Pierre Robin sequence demonstrate a wide spectrum of disease severity ranging from subclinical presentation to frank life-threatening respiratory compromise. Although the degree of micrognathia plays an important role in the development of respiratory symptoms, this is often a subtle finding in the neonatal period and observation for clinical signs of distress is imperative.

In the immediate postnatal period, patients with severe forms of Pierre Robin sequence will often display signs of distress such as grunting and crying, obvious apneic episodes, and even cyanosis. Those less severely affected may demonstrate increased work of breathing including supra- and substernal and intercostal retractions as well as cervical hyperextension. Symptoms are often positional with some improvement in prone position. Some neonates show few signs of respiratory compromise while awake. However, as resting tone decreases during phases of deep sleep, the tongue may assume a more posterior posture leading to obstruction.

In the first weeks of life, patients with moderate obstruction may present during an initial well child visit with inadequate weight gain, cachexia, or even failure to thrive sometimes without a history of apneic events. There are several reasons for feeding difficulties in PRS. First, the small mandible and tongue malposition as well as the presence of a palatal cleft pose significant physical restrictions on infant suckling. Indeed, primary oropharyngeal dysmotility has been noted in some patients. Second, feeding in infancy poses substantial metabolic demands, and patients with subnormal oxygenation may present with "exercise-induced" anorexia. Finally, gastroesophageal reflux (GER), although common in many infants, is especially challenging in those with Robin sequence with a reported incidence as high as 85 %. [19] As the tongue falls back, infants may increase inspiratory pressures in order to overcome the obstruction. The increased negative intrathoracic pressure then overcomes lower esophageal sphincter tone, and the gastric contents are "sucked" into the esophagus and the bronchial tree [6]. Such subclinical aspiration can be a substantial source of morbidity.

Cleft palate, although not a diagnostic criteria, occurs in the majority of patients with PRS, so much so that it is often incorrectly included among its essential characteristics. It is, however, distinct from other forms of palatal clefting with or without cleft lip [20]. The cleft palate associated with Pierre Robin sequence most often is wide and U-shaped, a result of failure of the palatal shelves to fuse in early gestation (8–12 weeks) due to the presence of an abnormally positioned tongue.

Evaluation and Clinical Approach

Timely multidisciplinary team evaluation—including Neonatology, Genetics, Pulmonology, Otolaryngology, the Feeding Team, and Plastic Surgery—is essential to maintaining adequate oxygenation and weight gain in patients with Pierre Robin sequence. A thorough history and physical exam should be performed to assess for potential syndromic association as well as evaluate overall appearance and tone. Indeed, hypotonia has the potential to exacerbate airway obstruction in affected patients and, in severe cases, may suggest poor response to interventions which address the upper airway. A complete airway exam is also an imperative first step in evaluation to determine the need for adjunctive airway support including high flow supplemental oxygen, continuous positive airway pressure, and intubation if necessary. Continuous pulse-oxymetry should also be employed early on in order to fully evaluate the number and degree of obstructive events.

Plain lateral radiographs with soft tissue windows may help characterize degree of micrognathia as well as assess for severity of glossoptosis by allowing for visualization of a patent or occluded airway stripe. In neonates the airway stripe should measure approximately 4 mm [21]. Although such an evaluation may provide insight into the degree of upper airway compromise, it is not substitution for direct visualization of the airway.

Bedside fiberoptic naso-endoscopy is an important tool to localize the level of airway obstruction and should be performed prior to any definitive intervention. In addition to a noninvasive way to visualize the lower airway, endoscopic evaluation of the entirety of the upper airway can rule out other causes of obstruction such as choanal atresia. Additionally, direct micro-laryngo-bronchoscopy (MLB) is essential to evaluate subglottic structures and to rule out the presence of laryngomalacia, tracheomalacia, and other pathologies [22]. A jaw-thrust maneuver performed under anesthesia at the time of MLB can help determine the extent to which mandibular advancement can improve tongue base position. Presence of lower airway pathology may significantly alter management decisions.

Diagnosis

The diagnosis of Pierre Robin sequence relies on the clinical finding of micrognathia in the setting of tongue-based airway obstruction. Although the presence of micrognathia is easy to establish on exam, and airway obstruction is readily apparent in severe cases, the extent to which the tongue base contributes to airway compromise can be difficult to determine. For this reason, diagnostic airway endoscopy is essential to confirm the presence of glossoptosis and rule out other sources of upper or lower airway obstruction.

Mild to moderate cases of Pierre Robin sequence, however, where profound desaturation and cyanosis are often absent, present diagnostic challenges to clinicians. In these settings, polysomnography (PSG) has been utilized to establish and characterize the presence of apneic events and to quantify the frequency and degree of airway obstruction [14]. Sixteen lead polysomnography, in particular offers a thorough evaluation of neonatal sleep and respiratory function. It consists of electroencephalographic, electrooculographic, electromyographic, electrocardiographic monitoring as well as detailed analysis of respiratory performance and tissue oxygenation throughout the sleep cycle. It is utilized to quantify the number of apnea and hypopnea events per hour (apnea–hypopnea index) as well as the severity of obstruction as measured through oxygen saturation and end tidal and transcutaneous carbon dioxide measurements (Fig. 3). Indeed, PSG plays an important role in establishing the presence of subtle obstructive events that may be overlooked clinically during wakefulness and is crucial for quantifying the severity of airway obstruction during sleep [23–25]. Additionally, PSG can differentiate central apneas secondary to brainstem dysfunction and the obstructive events that may be improved with intervention. Many practitioners now advocate for an expanded role for polysomnography beyond mild presentations of the disease citing its utility as an objective way to measure improvement after airway interventions.

Management

Neonates with tongue-based airway obstruction represent therapeutic challenges to caregivers, in part because of the diagnostic difficulties that exist for these complex patients. Another source of difficulty is the relatively poor outcomes data available to provide an evidence-based treatment framework, especially for severely affected patients. Although numerous authors have published treatment algorithms for the management of Pierre Robin sequence, prospective comparative studies are lacking. A recent systematic review of the literature highlights the dearth of high quality evidence related to the management of this challenging patient population [26]. In 126 peer-reviewed articles published between 1980 and 2010, the authors found few studies utilizing standardized diagnostic criteria, therapeutic algorithms, or outcomes measures making side-by-side comparison difficult. Nonetheless, because the repercussions of therapeutic failure so are great for patient with Pierre Robin sequence, including anoxic brain injury, cardiac and pulmonary dysfunction, malnutrition and even death, the stakes of adequate management are extremely high.

Any therapy should be tailored to the individual needs of the patient and particular concerns of the family. The gold standard treatment of TBAO has historically been tracheostomy, as this is the only intervention that completely bypasses the tongue base as the source of obstruction. However, given this procedure's high associated cost, morbidity, and mortality [27], many alternative treatment modalities have been investigated, including nonsurgical remedies such as prone positioning or nasopharyngeal airways (NPA) as well as surgical interventions such as tongue-lip adhesion (TLA) and mandibular distraction osteogenesis (MDO). No matter what treatment is planned in order to address the airway obstruction in Pierre Robin sequence, nutritional supplementation with oral, nasogastric, or gastrostomy feeding is essential to maximize growth and development.

The first-line therapy for patients with Pierre Robin sequence is conservative airway management including supplemental oxygen and positioning. Prone positioning of the patient allows the mandible and tongue to fall forward and out of the posterior pharynx, serving to minimize the obstruction caused by the tongue base. Positioning, however, requires constant vigilance and may make already tenuous feeding more difficult. It also places considerable stress on family and caregivers. Additionally, a nasopharyngeal airway

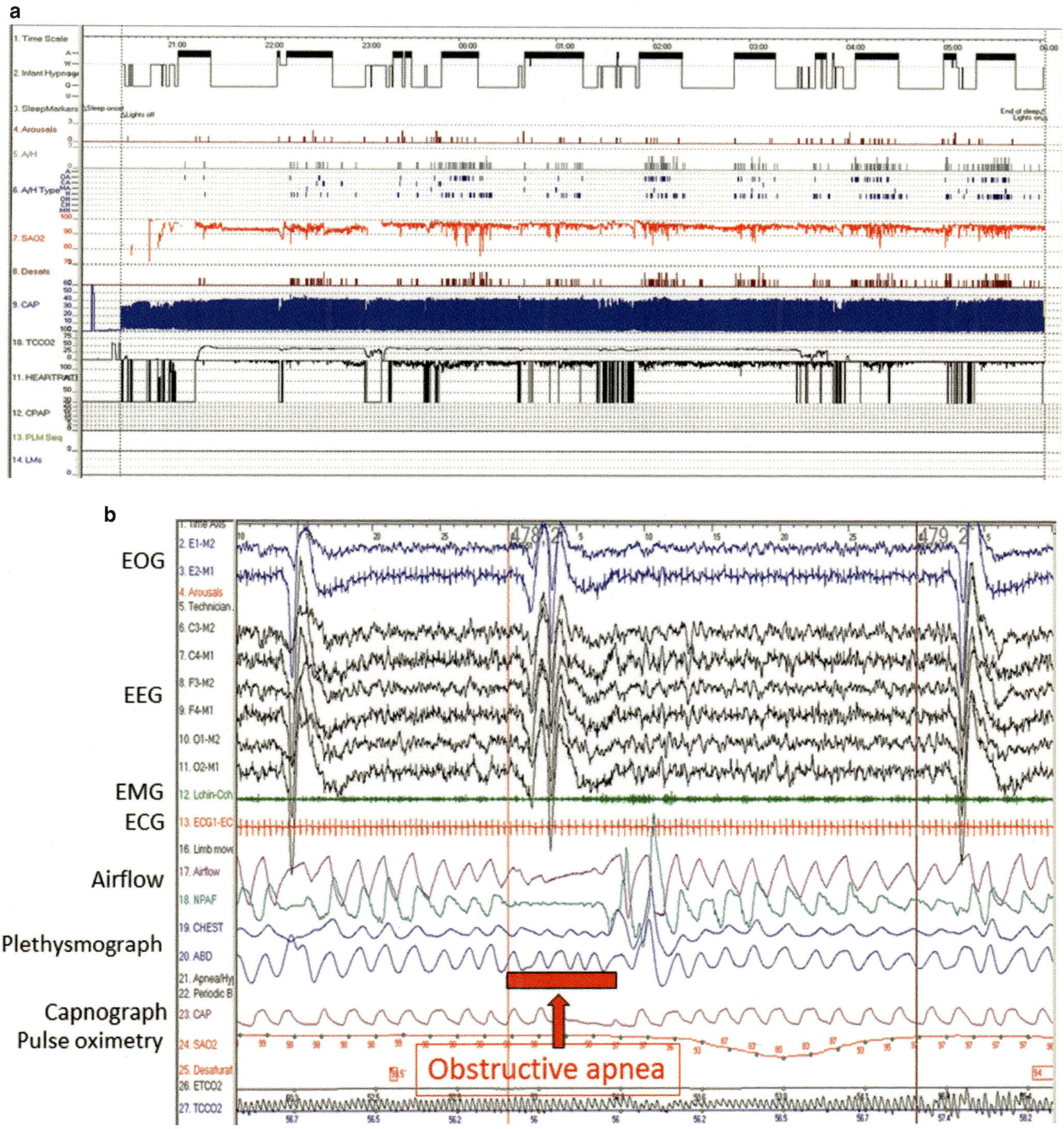

Fig. 3 (**a**)17 channel polysomnogram used to evaluate for occult obstructive apnea often seen in tongue based obstruction in neonates with micrognathia. (**b**) A closer view of the 17 channel extensive polysomnogram showing obstructive apnea in a more magnified view of airflow disruption with resultant desaturation in an infant with micrognathia. (Courtesy of Christopher Cielo, Pulmonary Medicine, The Children's Hospital of Philadelphia)

(NPA) can be fashioned from a small endotracheal tube and placed at the bedside without anesthesia. The NPA must be long enough to extend beyond the obstructing tongue base so that it can help push the retropositioned tongue out of posterior pharynx and relieve any obstruction [28, 29]. A final avenue for conservative treatment is prolonged intubation, a period of several weeks, in order to allow for improved airway tone and mandibular growth. Taken together, the success of these conservative measures has been reported to be between 50 and 85 % of patients [30–32].

Surgical intervention should be considered for persistent or severe airway obstruction that has failed or is not amenable to conservative treatment alone. The three main options for surgical airway correction include tongue-lip adhesion

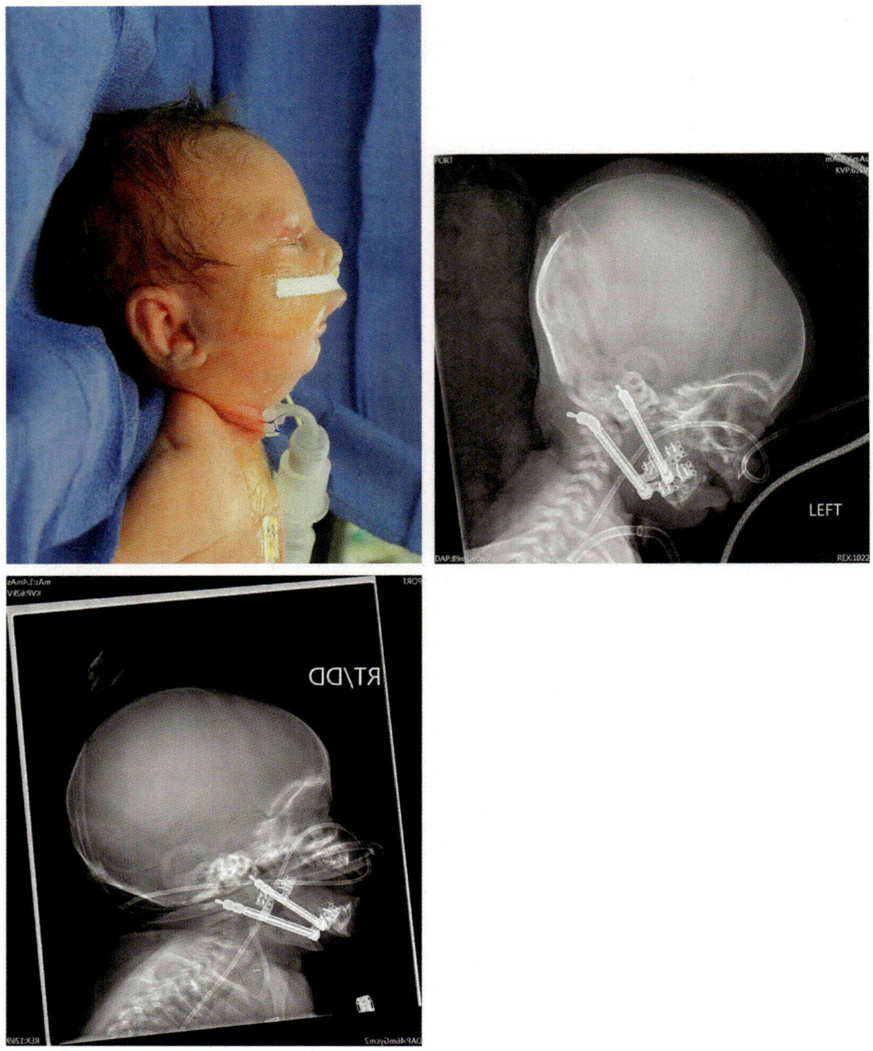

Fig. 4 (**a–d**) Pre- and postoperative photographs of patient undergoing mandibular distraction osteogenesis through a submandibular approach

(TLA), mandibular distraction osteogenesis (MDO), and tracheostomy.

Tongue-lip adhesion has been utilized for the treatment of airway obstruction associated with micrognathia for close to six decades [33]. Although variations of the procedure exist, in its simplest form, TLA approximates the muscularis proprious of the tongue and ventral mucosa to the mentalis muscle and labial mucosa. Variations include placing a permanent circum-mandibular retention suture through the body of the tongue itself. All iterations of the procedure serve to bring the tongue into a more anterior position in the mouth, preventing glossoptosis. This adhesion is left in place during the first 6–12 months of life to allow for mandibular and airway growth prior to its surgical reversal. Several centers have published on their experience using TLA as a first-line surgical treatment for patients who fail conservative management [17, 34–36]. They cite success rates ranging from 73 to 90 % while complications range from 10 to 55 %. Historically, TLA has been the most utilized surgical procedure to avoid tracheostomy in patients with PRS.

The introduction of mandibular distraction osteogenesis (MDO) to the surgical armamentarium for the treatment of Pierre Robin sequence over a decade ago has increased the treatment options for these complicated patients [37]. Although it has been over two decades since McCarthy et al. applied the principles of distraction osteogenesis to the mandible, {Mccarthy 1992} MDO has only recently developed traction as an effective and easily applied technique. Indeed, MDO remains the only currently available treatment modality that directly addresses micrognathia in patients with PRS.

In the procedure, the mandible is accessed bilaterally either through intraoral or submandibular incisions and mandibular osteotomies are made through the mandibular body. Internal or external distraction devices are then applied. After a short latency period, the devices are activated, slowly separating the mandibular segments at a rate of 1 mm/day. Once the desired advancement has been achieved, the devices are left in position for 6–8 weeks until the new space has re-ossified at which time the devices are removed.

Since its first description in 2002, only a handful of studies have been published with rigorous outcomes metrics assessing the efficacy of MDO. In two such retrospective studies, the authors report on a total of 57 patients with TBAO. {Hammoudeh 2012} (Goldstein, et al. PRS submitted 2013) Both studies demonstrate the improvement in airway parameters as measured by PSG after surgery while failure of MDO ranged from 3 to 14 % and surgical complications ranged from 14 to 28 %.

Although successful and safe, MDO is not without risks. Injury to the inferior alveolar nerve as well as developing tooth buds may theoretically occur, but long-term analyses are lacking to adequately assess such risks. Both techniques are associated with scaring, however, with the submandibular approach, such scars are generally acceptable and well hidden (Fig. 4 a–d). Additionally, there are currently no long-term data indicating the effect of MDO on mandibular growth, although growth restriction may be difficult to distinguish from that inherent to PRS itself.

Multidisciplinary Considerations

As mentioned previously, the assessment, diagnosis, and management of patients with Pierre Robin sequence requires significant input from a multitude of specialists. These infants, therefore, should be evaluated in a team setting to assess the anatomic and genetic findings, determine the cause of airway obstruction, educate caregivers on conservative measures including positioning and feeding protocols, and establish a course of treatment which minimizes obstructive events and burden to patient and family alike [6, 38]. Such a multidisciplinary team should consist of specialists from craniofacial and plastic and reconstructive surgery, pediatric/neonatal intensive care, pediatric otolaryngology, pulmonology, anesthesia, nursing, speech pathology, and genetics [30].

Future Considerations

Our understanding of Pierre Robin sequence is rapidly evolving due to improved diagnosis and treatment modalities. A better grasp of nonsurgical and surgical approaches to management has been achieved by an improved ability to characterize disease severity and accompanying disorders in these patients. As we continue to better stratify patients into more meaningful risk groups, and long-term prospective studies are performed, a cohesive treatment algorithm will begin to emerge which may help reduce the burden of care for patients, number of procedures, and time to adequate treatment in this challenging patient population.

References

1. Tonkin SL, Gunn TR, Bennet L, Vogel SA, Gunn AJ. A review of the anatomy of the upper airway in early infancy and its possible relevance to SIDS. Early Hum Dev. 2002;66(2):107–21.
2. Randall P, Krogman WM, Jahins S. Pierre Robin and the syndrome that bears his name. Cleft Palate J. 1965;36:237–46.
3. Robin P. A fall of the base of the tongue considered as a new cause of nasopharyngeal respiratory impairment: Pierre Robin sequence, a translation. 1923. Plast Reconstr Surg. 1994;93(6):1301–3.
4. Singh DJ, Bartlett SP. Congenital mandibular hypoplasia: analysis and classification. J Craniofac Surg. 2005;16(2):291–300.
5. Diewert VM. Craniofacial growth during human secondary palate formation and potential relevance of experimental cleft palate observations. J Craniofac Genet Dev Biol Suppl. 1986;22:67–76.
6. Mackay DR. Controversies in the diagnosis and management of the Robin sequence. J Craniofac Surg. 2011;22(2):415–20.
7. Jakobsen LP, Knudsen MA, Lespinasse J, García Ayuso C, Ramos C, Fryns J-P, et al. The genetic basis of the Pierre Robin Sequence. Cleft Palate Craniofac J. 2006;43(2):155–9.
8. Jakobsen LP, Ullmann R, Christensen SB, Jensen KE, Mølsted K, Henriksen KF, et al. J Med Genet. 2007;44(6):381–6.
9. Izumi K, Konczal LL, Mitchell AL, Jones MC. Underlying genetic diagnosis of Pierre Robin sequence: retrospective chart review at two children's hospitals and a systematic literature review. J Pediatr. 2012;160(4):645–50. e2.
10. Cozzi F, Pierro A. Glossoptosis-apnea syndrome in infancy. Pediatrics. 1985;75(5):836–43.
11. Marques IL, de Sousa TV, Carneiro AF, Barbieri MA, Bettiol H, Gutierrez MR. Clinical experience with infants with Robin sequence: a prospective study. Cleft Palate Craniofac J. 2001;38(2):171–8.
12. Gorlin RJ, Cohen MM, Hennekam RCM. Syndromes of the head and neck. 4th ed. New York: Oxford University Press; 2001.
13. Bush PG, Williams AJ. Incidence of the Robin Anomalad (Pierre Robin syndrome). Br J Plast Surg. 1983;36(4):434–7.
14. Schaefer RB, Stadler JA, Gosain AK. To distract or not to distract: an algorithm for airway management in isolated Pierre Robin sequence. Plast Reconstr Surg. 2004;113(4):1113–25.
15. Glander K, Cisneros GJ. Comparison of the craniofacial characteristics of two syndromes associated with the Pierre Robin sequence. Cleft Palate Craniofac J. 1992;29(3):210–9.
16. Cole A, Lynch P, Slator R. A new grading of Pierre Robin sequence. Cleft Palate Craniofac J. 2008;45(6):603–6.
17. Rogers GF, Murthy AS, Labrie RA, Mulliken JB. The GILLS score: part I. Patient selection for tongue-lip adhesion in Robin sequence. Plast Reconstr Surg. 2011;128(1):243–51.
18. Abramowicz S, Bacic JD, Mulliken JB, Rogers GF. Validation of the GILLS score for tongue-lip adhesion in Robin sequence patients. J Craniofac Surg. 2012;23(2):382–6.
19. Dudkiewicz Z, Sekuła E, Nielepiec-Jałosińska A. Gastroesophageal reflux in Pierre Robin sequence—early surgical treatment. Cleft Palate Craniofac J. 2000;37(2):205–8.
20. Caouette-Laberge L, Bayet B, Larocque Y. The Pierre Robin sequence: review of 125 cases and evolution of treatment modalities. Plast Reconstr Surg. 1994;93(5):934–42.
21. Wheeler DS, Wong HR, Shanley TP. Pediatric critical care medicine: basic science and clinical evidence. In: Mehta RL, editor.

Pediatric critical care medicine: basic science and clinical evidence. London: Springer; 2007.
22. Evans KN, Sie KC, Hopper RA, Glass RP, Hing AV, Cunningham ML. Robin sequence: from diagnosis to development of an effective management plan. Pediatrics. 2011;127(5):936–48.
23. Berry RB, Budhiraja R, Gottlieb DJ, Gozal D, Iber C, Kapur VK, et al. Rules for scoring respiratory events in sleep: update of the 2007 AASM Manual for the Scoring of Sleep and Associated Events. Deliberations of the Sleep Apnea Definitions Task Force of the American Academy of Sleep Medicine. J Clin Sleep Med. 2012;8(5):597–619.
24. Freed G, Pearlman MA, Brown AS, Barot LR. Polysomnographic indications for surgical intervention in Pierre Robin sequence: acute airway management and follow-up studies after repair and takedown of tongue-lip adhesion. Cleft Palate J. 1988;25(2):151–5.
25. Gilhooly JT, Smith JD, Howell LL, Deschaine BL, Richey SL. Bedside polysomnography as an adjunct in the management of infants with Robin sequence. Plast Reconstr Surg. 1993;92(1):23–7.
26. Bookman LB, Melton KR, Pan BS, Bender PL, Chini BA, Greenberg JM, et al. Neonates with tongue-based airway obstruction: a systematic review. Otolaryngol Head Neck Surg. 2012;146(1):8–18.
27. Hong P, Bezuhly M, Mark Taylor S, Hart RD, Kearns DB, Corsten G. Tracheostomy versus mandibular distraction osteogenesis in Canadian children with Pierre Robin sequence: a comparative cost analysis. J Otolaryngol Head Neck Surg. 2012;41(3):207–14.
28. Chang AB, Masters IB, Williams GR, Harris M, O'Neil MC. A modified nasopharyngeal tube to relieve high upper airway obstruction. Pediatr Pulmonol. 2000;29(4):299–306.
29. Anderson KD, Cole A, Chuo CB, Slator R. Home management of upper airway obstruction in Pierre Robin sequence using a nasopharyngeal airway. Cleft Palate Craniofac J. 2007;44(3):269–73.
30. Bull MJ, Givan DC, Sadove AM, Bixler D, Hearn D. Improved outcome in Pierre Robin sequence: effect of multidisciplinary evaluation and management. Pediatrics. 1990;86(2):294–301.
31. Meyer AC, Lidsky ME, Sampson DE, Lander TA, Liu M, Sidman JD. Airway interventions in children with Pierre Robin Sequence. Otolaryngol Head Neck Surg. 2008;138(6):782–7.
32. Abel F, Bajaj Y, Wyatt M, Wallis C. The successful use of the nasopharyngeal airway in Pierre Robin sequence: an 11-year experience. Arch Dis Child. 2012;97(4):331–4.
33. Douglas B. The treatment of micrognathia associated with obstruction by a plastic procedure. Plast Reconstr Surg. 1946;1(3):300–8.
34. Kirschner RE, Low DW, Randall P, Bartlett SP, McDonald-McGinn DM, Schultz PJ, et al. Surgical airway management in Pierre Robin sequence: is there a role for tongue-lip adhesion? Cleft Palate Craniofac J. 2003;40(1):13–8.
35. Evans AK, Rahbar R, Rogers GF, Mulliken JB, Volk MS. Robin sequence: a retrospective review of 115 patients. Int J Pediatr Otorhinolaryngol. 2006;70(6):973–80.
36. Bijnen CL, Don Griot PJ, Mulder WJ, Haumann TJ, Van Hagen AJ. Tongue-lip adhesion in the treatment of Pierre Robin sequence. J Craniofac Surg. 2009;20(2):315–20.
37. Denny A, Kalantarian B. Mandibular distraction in neonates: a strategy to avoid tracheostomy. Plast Reconstr Surg. 2002;109(3):896–904; discussion 905–6.
38. Marcellus L. The infant with Pierre Robin sequence: review and implications for nursing practice. J Pediatr Nurs. 2001;16(1):23–34.
39. Figueroa AA. Commentary on "Craniofacial morphology in Treacher Collins syndrome", by Arvystas, M., Shprintzen, R.J. Cleft Palate Craniofac J. 1991;28:230–1.
40. Figueroa AA, Glupker TJ, Fitz MG, Begole EA. The mandible, tongue and airway in Pierre Robin sequence (PRS): a longitudinal cephalometric study. Cleft Palate Craniofac J. 1991;28:425–34.

Congenital Laryngomalacia: Disease Spectrum and Management

April Landry and Dana M. Thompson

Etiology

The precise etiology of the decreased laryngeal tone resulting in prolapse of the supraglottic tissues into the airway causing obstruction seen in laryngomalacia is unknown and continues to be an area of research. Theories of etiology include anatomic, cartilaginous, and neurologic origins. The anatomic theory suggests that the native laryngeal tissues are abnormal. The classic findings of shortened aryepiglottic folds, an omega-shaped or retroflexed epiglottis, and redundant arytenoid tissues seen in laryngomalacia (Figs. 1 and 2) may also present in infants without symptoms of laryngomalacia. Moreover, not all patients with laryngomalacia have these "abnormal" findings, challenging the validity of this theory.

The cartilaginous theory proposes that the cartilages of the infantile larynx are immature and have increased pliability. This theory has been refuted by histopathologic studies showing normal cartilage microanatomy in infants with severe laryngomalacia [1].

Published studies best support the neurologic theory of laryngomalacia which theorizes that neurosensorimotor dysfunction leads to decreased neuromuscular tone and coordination of the laryngeal structures leading to loss of laryngeal tone. An inference of a neurologic cause can be deduced from other conditions that affect the central nervous system leading to laryngomalacia or laryngomalacia-like clinical findings and symptoms. For example, central nervous system sedation can cause supraglottic obstruction in infants without laryngomalacia [2]. Moreover, late onset or acquired laryngomalacia has been seen to occur in children and adults who suffer a central nervous system insult such as a stroke, hypoxic brain injury, seizure, or trauma. Compression of the brainstem, like that of a Chiari malformation, has resulted in laryngomalacia with disease resolution following neurosurgical decompression [3]. It also is interesting to note that up to 20 % of infants with laryngomalacia have an associated neurologic abnormality [1, 3, 4].

Pathogenesis

Laryngeal tone and function is coordinated and modulated by a vagal nerve pathway called the laryngeal adductor reflex (LAR). Sensory information is gathered by superior laryngeal nerve fibers located in the aryepiglottic fold. Afferent signals pass through the nodose ganglion and are transmitted to the brainstem to synapses in the nucleus solitarius and nucleus ambiguous. These nuclei regulate breathing and swallowing. The efferent pathway is activated with signals propagating via the vagus nerve to the laryngeal muscles. In normal conditions, an involuntary motor response results in glottic closure and inhibition of respiration and swallowing, protecting the airway from the perceived laryngeal stimulus. This reflex also modulates baseline laryngeal tone. Abnormal sensorimotor integration of the LAR anywhere along the pathway results in decreased laryngeal tone, choking, aspiration, apnea, swallowing difficulty, and inability to clear secretions [1], all of which are within the spectrum of symptoms and clinical examination findings that may be seen in infants with laryngomalacia.

Laryngopharyngeal sensory testing in infants with laryngomalacia has demonstrated that the sensory stimulus threshold needed to begin the laryngeal adductor reflex is elevated in those with moderate and severe laryngomalacia. This finding suggests that peripheral afferent function and/or brainstem function are altered and lead to decreased laryngeal

A. Landry, M.D.
Department of Pediatric Otolaryngology Head and Neck Surgery, Cincinnati Children's Hospital Medical Center, The University of Cincinnati College of Medicine, Cincinnati, OH, USA

D.M. Thompson, M.D., M.S. (✉)
Department of Pediatric Otolaryngology Head and Neck Surgery, Ann & Robert H. Lurie Children's Hospital of Chicago, Northwestern University Feinberg School of Medicine, Chicago, IL, USA
e-mail: dmthompson@luriechildrens.org

J. Lioy and S.E. Sobol (eds.), *Disorders of the Neonatal Airway: Fundamentals for Practice*,
DOI 10.1007/978-1-4939-1610-8_6, © Springer Science+Business Media New York 2015

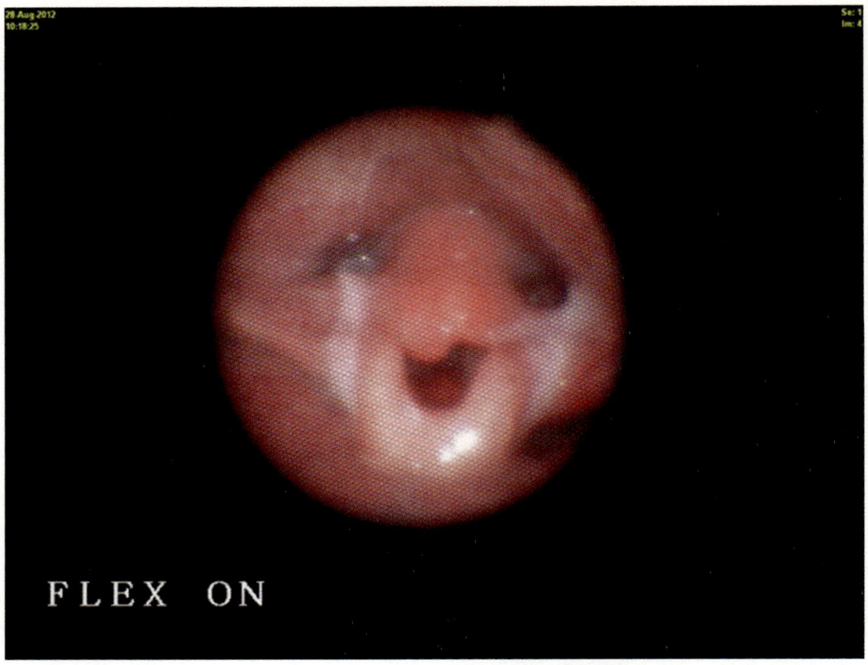

Fig. 1 Fiberoptic flexible laryngoscopy with endoscopic evaluation of swallowing in a 2-month infant with laryngomalacia. Typical anatomic features including shortened aryepiglottic folds, bilateral supraarytenoid prolapse, posterior glottic edema, and posterior pharyngeal wall cobblestoning effect. Laryngeal penetration of formula seen over the aryepiglottic fold

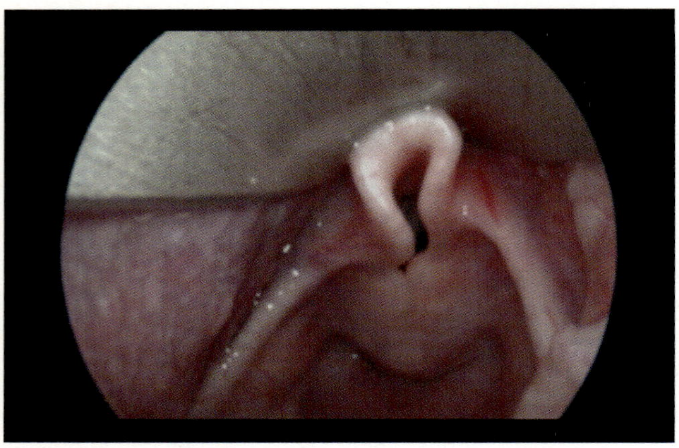

Fig. 2 Two-month child with severe laryngomalacia requiring supraglottoplasty. Typical features including omega-shaped epiglottis, short aryepiglottic folds, and arytenoid prolapse are seen

tone in patients with laryngomalacia. This theory is further supported by the finding of submucosal nerve hypertrophy in histological specimens of the supraarytenoid tissue in infants with severe laryngomalacia. It is unclear, however, if the noted nerve hypertrophy is the primary pathology or if it occurs secondary to inflammation from gastroesophageal reflux disease [4].

Alteration of brainstem responses may also contribute to the pathogenesis of laryngomalacia as they are often altered by states of hypoxia and hypercarbia, both of which may be seen in affected infants. The effect of brainstem modulation is further supported by case reports demonstrating reversal of laryngomalacia symptoms and findings after surgical decompression of the brainstem due to Chiari malformation or correction of a vertebral anomaly causing compression of the brainstem [3].

Gastroesophageal reflux likely plays an important role in the dysfunction of this neurological pathway by altering laryngeal sensation and causing tissue edema. Chronic acid exposure on the chemo- and mechanoreceptors of the larynx results in a functional denervation of the afferent response of the LAR. With decreased sensation the infant has difficulty handling secretions and initiating a swallow. Acid exposure also causes tissue edema, which can further exacerbate inspiratory prolapse of the supraglottic structures into the airway. Obstruction during inspiration can in turn increase negative intrathoracic pressure promoting further reflux and creating a vicious cycle. Until the airway obstruction/ reflux cycle is broken, the infant will continue to have symptoms.

Epidemiology

Laryngomalacia is the most common congenital laryngeal anomaly, and is implicated in 45–75 % of infants with stridor. The exact demographic data of laryngomalacia is not known. There is a reported male predominance of an average 1.6:1 male to female ratio [1, 5–10]. The clinical significance of this is unknown. No racial differences have been reported, but the majority of published literature has reported on Caucasian infants [11].

Congenital laryngomalacia can occur in newborns of any gestational age. The condition is seen in premature infants but has not been shown to have an increased incidence in this population. There may be a trend toward an association of prematurity and severity of disease, but larger populations with documented gestational age data are lacking [1, 12]. When comparing the specific sites of supraglottic collapse, preterm infants were found to have more of the classic features of laryngomalacia compared to term infants [13].

Clinical Presentation

Laryngomalacia is characterized by inspiratory stridor secondary to supraglottic tissue prolapse. The disease typically presents with stridor within 2 weeks of birth. The symptoms gradually increase until a peak is reached at 6–8 months of age. The majority of cases are self-limited and resolve by 18–24 months of age, but up to 20 % of infants will have significant airway obstruction and/or feeding issues requiring medical and surgical treatment [1, 14, 15].

Stridor is the primary symptom of laryngomalacia. On inspiration a high pitched, fluttering stridor is heard as the supraglottic tissues collapse over the glottis and vibrate against each other. Laryngomalacia increases with crying, agitation, and feeding due to the increase of negative intrathoracic airway pressures during these times. Supine positioning increases symptoms secondary to the posterior displacement of the base of tongue and laryngeal structures.

Feeding difficulties including regurgitation, emesis, cough, choking, and slow feeding are the most common associated symptoms of the disease. Airway obstruction interferes with the infant's ability to coordinate the suck-swallow-breathe sequence needed for feeding. Weight loss and failure to thrive can occur when there is a high metabolic demand of feeding and breathing against an obstruction.

In severe disease, infants may also present with suprasternal and subcostal retractions, tachypnea, apneic pauses, cyanosis, pectrus excavatum, pulmonary hypertension, and cor pulmonale.

Disease Spectrum

Laryngomalacia is a spectrum categorized into mild, moderate, and severe forms. Upon presentation to a health care provider, 40 % of infants have mild, 40 % moderate, and 20 % have severe disease [15].

Infants with mild disease have stridor without respiratory compromise and occasional cough, choking, and regurgitation with feeding. Despite this, these infants have normal coordination of the suck-swallow-breathe sequence and have an average resting oxygen saturation of 98–100 % [15]. The majority (70 %) of infants with mild disease have an uncomplicated course and resolution but 30 % will have worsening of feeding associated symptoms and progression to moderate laryngomalacia [15].

Forty percent of infants present with moderate laryngomalacia, which is characterized by stridor and frequent feeding-associated symptoms. Coughing, choking, regurgitation, fussiness, and cyanosis frequently occur during feeds (Fig. 1). Aspiration and weight loss may ensue if feeding modifications and acid reflux therapies are not initiated. Infants with moderate laryngomalacia are not hypoxic, but they may have a lower resting SAO_2 (96 %) [1, 15]. Even with feeding modifications and acid suppression, 28 % develop severe disease [15].

Those with severe disease have stridor along with associated symptoms of recurrent cyanosis, apneic pauses, suprasternal and subcostal retractions, aspiration, and failure to thrive. These infants also have a lower resting SAO_2 of 88–92 %. If not appropriately managed these infants may develop pectus excavatum, pulmonary hypertension and/or cor pulmonale. Up to 30 % of infants will have severe laryngomalacia with an additional medical comorbidity such as neurologic disease, congenital heart disease. or a genetic or syndromic condition.

Diagnosis

Diagnosis of laryngomalacia is primarily made by history and confirmed by an awake flexible nasopharyngoscopy. Caregivers often give a classic history of high pitched inspiratory stridor beginning within weeks of birth. The stridor is exacerbated with crying, agitation, supine positioning, and feeding. It is important to ask about feeding symptoms including cough, choking, regurgitation, and slow/fussy feeds. History of suprasternal and/or subcostal retractions, cyanosis, apnea, aspiration, and failure to thrive are worrisome and indicate severe disease. Cardiac, pulmonary, neurologic, gastrointestinal disease and the presence of a genetic disorder or syndrome history are important to note for treatment planning and prognostication.

The infant's birth, intubation, and surgical history are important in determining congenital versus acquired causes of stridor. The differential diagnosis of congenital stridor in an infant includes subglottic stenosis, vocal cord paralysis, tracheomalacia, and tracheal stenosis. Conditions that cause inspiratory stridor in infants and can mimic laryngomalacia include unilateral vocal fold paralysis, vallecular cyst, or a saccular cyst of the larynx. These entities can be differentiated by flexible laryngoscopy. In contrast to the inspiratory stridor of laryngomalacia, infants with bilateral vocal fold paralysis or subglottic stenosis have biphasic stridor with both inspiratory and expiratory components. The stridor of tracheomalacia and tracheal stenosis has a characteristic expiratory phase.

As noted above, confirmation of laryngomalacia is made by an awake flexible nasopharyngoscopy (Fig. 1). The infant is gently retrained on the caregivers lap in an upright or semi-reclined position. Sedation is not necessary, and may lead to false positive findings due to the resultant decrease in neuromuscular tone. A flexible scope is passed and the nasopharyngeal, oropharyngeal, hypopharyngeal, and laryngeal structures are inspected.

During the procedure, arytenoid mucosa and cartilage prolapse, shortened aryepiglottic folds and an omega or tubular epiglottis may be visualized. A retroflexed epiglottis with posterior pharyngeal contact can also be seen in more severe cases. One must visualize dynamic collapse of the supraglottic structures on inspiration and obtain a consistent history to diagnosis laryngomalacia. The presence of an omega-shaped epiglottis is not pathognomonic for laryngomalacia as up to 50 % of normal infants have this shape to the epiglottis [16]. Inspiratory stridor is heard during a positive exam. In severe disease the infant may also exhibit retractions and/or brief cyanosis.

The larynx may prolapse at one or multiple supraglottic locations. Multiple anatomic classification systems have been described based on the supraglottic location and direction of collapse [13, 17–19]. When redundant arytenoid mucosa and accessory cartilages prolapse, this is recognized as posterior prolapse. Foreshortened aryepiglottic folds obstruct the airway in the lateral plane, and anterior collapse occurs with posterior displace of the epiglottis. The pattern of collapse may help to guide surgical treatment.

After confirmation of the diagnosis, other adjuvant studies may be indicated depending on symptomatology and severity of disease. Videofluoroscopic swallow study or functional endoscopic evaluation of swallow (FEES) can be used to assess feeding symptoms and aspiration. In infants with known chronic aspiration, a chest X-ray should be obtained to determine the amount of pulmonary injury present. Concomitant gastroesophageal disease such as malrotation or pyloric stenosis should be ruled out with an esophagram in those with severe recurrent emesis.

Secondary Airway Lesions

Infants with laryngomalacia have a 7.5–64 % chance of having a secondary or synchronous airway lesion [20–24]. The wide range of incidence is likely due to the technique used to identify a secondary lesion and indication for screening. The most frequently identified lesions are tracheomalacia, subglottic stenosis, and vocal cord paralysis. The incidence of secondary lesions increases in congenital syndromic disorders such a Down syndrome.

Secondary lesions are associated with increased laryngomalacia severity and progression of disease which leads to a higher likelihood of requiring a surgical intervention. Secondary lesions add an additional level of obstruction thereby changing airflow dynamics. Increased resistance in the distal airway can exacerbate the degree of obstruction to the glottic level by means of the Venturi principle.

Secondary anomalies can also potentiate gastroesophageal reflux disease [14, 15, 21, 22]. Infants with mild to moderate disease that have a secondary lesion are 4.8 times more likely to need a surgical intervention [21]. Eliminating supraglottic obstruction with a supraglottoplasty allows the airflow at the secondary lesion to be more favorable. By performing a supraglottoplasty, the clinical significance of secondary lesions may decrease and eliminate the need for surgical treatment.

As lesions distal to the vocal folds are difficult to accurately diagnosis by flexible laryngoscopy alone, further studies may be indicated in certain infants. High-kilovoltage airway radiographs can be used in screening for a fixed obstruction such as subglottic stenosis; whereas, airway fluoroscopy are appropriate if there is a suspicion of dynamic tracheomalacia. Although awake flexible laryngoscopy with tracheoscopy in the office has been described in the literature, we do not routinely advocate this technique in infants [25]. The gold standard of secondary lesion diagnosis is rigid laryngoscopy and bronchoscopy. This evaluation can be used in conjunction to a planned supraglottoplasty or performed before a supraglottoplasty if the diagnosis is in question.

Management

Most infants with laryngomalacia have mild to moderate symptoms (80–90 %) and do not require surgical intervention [1, 14, 26]. Infants with mild disease can be expectantly managed by their pediatricians, and parents should be reassured.

Treatment should be initiated for those with frequent feeding symptoms. Feeding modifications and acid suppression therapy are the primary means of treatment. Strategies to improve feeding symptoms include pacing with frequent burping, texture modification by thickening formula/breast milk, and upright positioning for feeding. Bottle feeding is sometimes preferred over breast feeding because the amount of milk released is more controlled.

Acid suppression treatment often decreases the feeding symptoms and may shorten the natural course of the disease [1]. Gastroesophageal reflux treatment decreases supraglottic edema and the resultant increase in upper airway obstruction. The dose and duration of therapy has not been studied prospectively. Treatments regimens that have been proposed are proton pump inhibitor therapy, H2 receptor antagonist therapy, and combination of the two. An average of 9 months of acid suppression therapy is typically given. The response to medical therapy can be assessed by history and repeat physical exam. Up to 72 % of infants with moderate disease will have resolution of their symptoms within 12 months of using these management strategies [1, 15].

Those with severe laryngomalacia or worsening of moderate disease warrant surgical intervention [1, 14]. Surgical management is indicated in those who present with recurrent cyanosis, apneic pauses, severe suprasternal and subcostal retractions, aspiration, failure to thrive, pectus excavatum, pulmonary hypertension, and/or cor pulmonale. Infants who have worsening of their disease severity over time despite feeding modifications and acid suppression therapy are also candidates for surgical management. The primary operation use to manage laryngomalacia is a supraglottoplasty. Tracheostomy can be performed to definitively bypass the obstruction, but is reserved for those that have failed supraglottoplasty or have multiple other medical comorbidities that necessitate tracheostomy placement.

Multiple tools can be used to perform a supraglottoplasty, but the basic surgical principles remain the same regardless of instruments used. Briefly, the child is placed under mask ventilation with inhalational anesthetics. The otolaryngology and anesthesia team should be prepared for worsening obstruction during sedation. The airway should be fully evaluated for a secondary airway lesion with rigid laryngoscopy and bronchoscopy. The larynx is then visualized using a laryngoscope and laryngeal suspension system. The Benjamin-Lindholm or Parson's laryngoscopes are preferred by the authors as they give a wide view of the supraglottic structures. Insufflation of anesthetic gases and oxygen can be given via the side port of most laryngoscopes. The operative microscope is then brought into the field to allow for bimanual instrumentation and magnification during the procedure.

The aryepiglottic fold is incised at the base of the epiglottic cartilage. Prolapsed supraarytenoid mucosa is then removed bilaterally with a wedge resection. A cuff of mucosa should be maintained between the aryepiglottic fold incision and the arytenoid resection. Corniculate and cuneiform cartilages can also be removed with the wedge of supraarytenoid mucosa. Care must be taken to preserve the intra-arytenoid tissue and not violate the pharyngoepiglottic fold. In cases of shortened aryepiglottic folds and redundant arytenoid tissue, these procedures should result in a widened supraglottic airway.

These surgical maneuvers can be performed with cold steel microlaryngeal instruments or CO_2 laser depending on surgeon preference. Statically there is no difference between the outcomes of cold steel or CO_2 laser. CO_2 laser may give the surgeon better precision and hemostasis, but hemostasis does not tend to be significant risk during cold steel supraglottoplasty [14, 27, 28]. The risk of using the CO_2 laser includes airway fire, thermal injury, and theoretical risk of damage to the neural receptors of the supraglottic tissues which may lead to decreased laryngeal sensation.

Postoperative airway control depends on the age of the child, severity of disease, and extent of surgery performed. The patient may be extubated on the operating room table or remain intubated for a period of observation with planned extubation the following day. In infants younger than 1 year of age, overnight intubation with administration of a steroid dose before extubation is the recommended preference of the authors. Other experienced pediatric otolaryngologists extubate at the time of the procedure when safe, regardless of age. Racemic epinephrine may also be required at extubation.

When patients are tolerating room air and eating appropriately, they can be discharged to home. The authors recommend follow-up in appropriately 2 weeks. At that time, an assessment of weight gain and airway symptoms is important. A flexible laryngoscopy may be considered to assess surgical results and to assure the site is healing without granulation tissue. Postoperatively patients are continued on acid suppression medications for a minimum of 1 month. As symptoms and edema improve the reflux medications can be weaned. Functional endoscopic swallow evaluation and videofluoroscopy swallow studies are indicated for continued feeding difficulties or aspiration following surgery.

Complications following supraglottoplasty are rare; an 8 % complication rate is quoted in the literature [29]. Possible surgical site issues involve the development of granulation tissue, abnormal mucosal healing with webbing, bleeding, and infection. Supraglottic stenosis is a possible complication of supraglottoplasty which is difficult to manage. It reportedly occurs in 4 % of patients and is thought to be related to violation of the intra-arytenoid area or pharyngeo-epiglottic fold [29]. Systemic events that may complicate the procedure include aspiration, bronchiectasis, bronchiolitis, and pneumonia.

The success rate of supraglottoplasty is as high, and up to 94 % of infants have resolution of their symptoms [14]. Revision may be required in 19–45 % of infants. Infants with neurologic disease, cardiac disease, congenital syndromes, and secondary airway lesion are more likely to need revision supraglottoplasty and possible tracheostomy. These specific considerations are discussed later in this chapter [1].

Multidisciplinary Considerations

Gastrointestinal Disease

Gastroesophageal reflux is noted in 65–100 % of infants who have laryngomalacia [1, 12, 15]. Infants with moderate and severe disease should be started on empiric reflux therapy with a proton pump inhibitor, H2 receptor antagonist, or a combination of the two therapies. Feeding modifications to reduce reflux such as upright positioning and frequent burping are recommended. When these measures are not effective, gastroenterology consultation should be sought. In severe cases, pediatric surgery may consider fundoplication for those with continued refractory symptoms despite supraglottoplasty and maximum dose of acid suppression therapy [14].

Neurologic Disease

Neurologic disease is present in 20–45 % infants with laryngomalacia and when present may benefit from neurologic consultation [15]. Common neurologic comorbidities include hypotonia, developmental delay, cerebral palsy, mental retardation, microcephaly, and Chiari malformation. The association of neurologic disorders and laryngomalacia is not fully understood but is likely due to decrease of vagal-mediated laryngeal tone at the level of the brainstem. Infants with neurologic disease have increased severity of disease and a higher rate of surgical intervention. Revision supraglottoplasty is required in up to 70 % and tracheostomy in 60 % of those with neurologic comorbidities [30]. Those with persistent aspiration and severe symptoms after supraglottplasty should undergo MRI of the head to evaluate for brainstem or other CNS disease contributing to etiology.

Cardiac Disease

Congenital cardiac disease can be seen in up to 10 % of those with laryngomalacia and may exacerbate cyanosis, apnea, and respiratory distress when present [1, 15, 31]. Coordination of care with the patient's cardiologist and cardiac anesthesiologist may be necessary. Up to 34 % of infants with coexisting severe laryngomalacia and cardiac disease may require surgical treatment [1, 32]. Supraglottoplasty failure and subsequent tracheostomy is higher in this group of patients.

Congenital Anomalies/Syndromes/Genetic Disorders

Congenital anomalies and genetic disorders occur in 8–20 % of those with laryngomalacia [17, 31]. Down syndrome is the most commonly reportedly genetic disorder associated with the disease with 50 % of Down syndrome infants with respiratory symptoms having laryngomalacia [33, 34]. CHARGE association (coloboma, heart defect, chonal atresia, retardation, genital and ear abnormalities) and Pierre Robin sequence have also been associated with laryngomalacia. These syndromes are manifest with micrognathia which worsens laryngomalacia due to tongue base collapse into the hypopharynx. A supraglottoplasty in the setting of micrognathia is usually unsuccessful. Tracheostomy may be needed in these infants until their mandible grows or an advancement procedure is performed. Variants of 22q11.2 microdeletion syndrome are known to have upper airway obstruction which can be managed with a supraglottoplasty [3, 34, 35]. Cervical vertebral anomalies are common in this patient population and compression of the brainstem should be investigated as a possible cause of laryngomalacia.

Future Directions

Although laryngomalacia is a common anomaly, the exact neurologic etiology is still unknown. Research continues to focus on the role of the central nervous system, the peripheral nervous system, and the coordination of the two systems. The relationship between gastroesophageal reflux disease and laryngomalacia has been well proven, but standardized medical therapy and length of treatment has yet to be studied prospectively. Ongoing research to classify and describe the nature and anatomic pattern of collapse may better categorize patients by severity of disease. In the future, supraglottoplasty may be tailored to the type of collapse.

References

1. Thompson DM. Abnormal sensorimotor integrative function of the larynx in congenital laryngomalacia: a new theory of etiology. Laryngoscope. 2007;117:1–33.
2. Amin MR, Isaacson G. State-dependent laryngomalacia. Ann Otol Rhinol Laryngol. 1997;106:887–90.
3. Petersson RS, Wetjen NM, Thompson DM. Neurologic variant laryngomalacia associated with Chiari malformation and cervicomedullary compression: case reports. Ann Otol Rhinol Laryngol. 2011;120(2):99–103.
4. Munson PD, Saad AG, El-Jamal SM, Dai Y, Bower CM, Richter GT. Submucosal nerve hypertrophy in congenital laryngomalacia. Laryngoscope. 2011;121:627–9.
5. Holinger PH, Johnson KC, Schiller F. Congenital anomalies of the larynx. Ann Otol Rhinol Laryngol. 1954;63:581–606.
6. Holinger PH, Brown W. Congenital webs, cyst, laryngoceles and other anomalies of the larynx. Ann Otol Rhinol Laryngol. 1967;76: 744–52.
7. Ferguson CF. Congenital abnormalities of the infant larynx. Otolaryngol Clin North Am. 1970;3:185–200.
8. Friedman EM, Vastola AP, McGill TJ, Healy GB. Chronic pediatric stridor: etiology and outcome. Laryngoscope. 1990;100:277–80.
9. Zoulmalan R, Maddalozzo J, Holinger LD. Etiology of stridor in infants. Ann Otol Rhinol Laryngol. 2007;116(5):329–34.
10. Ayari S, Aubertin G, Girschig H, Van Den Abbeele T, Mondain M. Pathophysiology and diagnostic approach to laryngomalacia in infants. Eur Ann Otorhinolaryngol Head Neck Dis. 2012;129: 257–63.
11. Giannoni C, Sulek M, Friedman EM, Duncan III NO. Gastroesophageal reflux association with laryngomalacia: a prospective study. Int J Pediatr Otorhinolaryngol. 1998;43:11–20.

12. Adil E, Rager T, Carr M. Location of airway obstruction in term and preterm infants with laryngomalacia. Am J Otolaryngol. 2012;33:437–40.
13. Richter GT, Thompson DM. The surgical management of laryngomalacia. Otolaryngol Clin North Am. 2008;41:837–64.
14. Thompson DM. Laryngomalacia: factors that influence disease severity and outcomes of management. Curr Opin Otolaryngol Head Neck Surg. 2010;18:564–70.
15. Solomons NB, Prescott CA. Laryngomalacia: a review and the surgical management of severe cases. Int J Pediatr Otorhinolaryngol. 1987;13:31–9.
16. Olney DR, Greinwald Jr JH, Smith RJ, Bauman NM. Laryngomalacia and its treatment. Laryngoscope. 1999;109:1770–5.
17. Cotton RT. Congenital anomalies of the larynx. In: Cotton RT, Myer CM, editors. Practical pediatric otolaryngology. Philadelphia: Lippincott Williams & Wilkins-Raven Press; 1999. p. 497–514.
18. Kay DJ, Goldsmith AJ. Laryngomalacia: a classification system and surgical treatment strategy. Ear Nose Throat J. 2006;85: 328–31. 336.
19. Cohen S, Eavey R, Desmond M, May B. Endoscopy and tracheotomy in the neonatal period. A 10- year review. Ann Otol Rhinol Laryngol. 1977;86(5):577–83.
20. Dickson JM, Richter GT, Meinzen-Derr J, Rutter MJ, Thompson DM. Secondary airway lesions in infants with laryngomalacia. Ann Otol Rhinol Laryngol. 2009;118:37–43.
21. Schroeder JW, Bhandarkar ND, Holinger LD. Synchronous airway lesions and outcomes in infants with severe laryngomalacia requiring supraglottoplasty. Arch Otolaryngol Head Neck Surg. 2009;135(7):647–51.
22. Krashin E, Ben-Ari J, Springer C, DeRowe A, Avital A, Sivan Y. Synchronous airway lesions in laryngomalacia. Int J Pediatr Otorhinolaryngol. 2008;72(4):501–7.
23. Yuen HW, Tan HK, Balakrishnan A. Synchronous airway lesions and associated anomalies in children with laryngomalacia evaluated with rigid endoscopy. Int J Pediatr Otorhinolaryngol. 2006;70(10):1779–84.
24. Hartzell LD, Richter GT, Glade RS, Bower CM. Accuracy and safety of tracheoscopy or infants in a tertiary care clinic. Arch Otolaryngol Head Neck Surg. 2010;136:66–9.
25. Roger G, Denoyelle F, Triglia JM, et al. Severe laryngomalacia: surgical indications and results in 115 patients. Laryngoscope. 1995;105:1111–7.
26. Seid AB, Park SM, Kearns MJ, et al. Laser division of the aryepiglottic folds for severe laryngomalacia. Int J Pediatr Otorhinolaryngol. 1985;10:153–8.
27. Lee KS, Chen BN, Yang CC, et al. Co_2 laser supraglottoplasty for severe laryngomalacia: a study of symptomatic improvement. Int J Pediatr Otorhinolaryngol. 2007;71:889–95.
28. Denoyelle F, Mondain M, Gresillon N, et al. Faiures and complications of supraglottoplasty in children. Arch Otolaryngol Head Neck Surg. 2003;129:1077–80.
29. Hoff SR, Schroeder JW, Rastatter JC, Holinger LD. Supraglottoplasty outcomes in relation to age and comorbid conditions. Int J Pediatr Otorhinolaryngol. 2010;74:245–9.
30. Masters IB, Chang AB, Patterson L, et al. Series of laryngomalacia, tracheomalacia, and brnchomalacia disorders and their associations with the other conditions in children. Pediatr Pulmonol. 2002;34:189–95.
31. Reddy DK, Matt BH. Unilateral vs. bilateral supraglottoplasty for severe laryngomalacia in children. Arch Otolaryngol Head Neck Surg. 2001;127:694–9.
32. Bertrand P, Navarro H, Caussade S, et al. Airway anomalies in children with Down syndrome: endoscopic findings. Pediatr Pulmonol. 2003;36:137–41.
33. Mitchell RB, Call E, Kelly J. Diagnosis and therapy for airway obstruction in children with Down syndrome. Arch Otolaryngol Head Neck Surg. 2003;129:642–5.
34. Digilio MC, Mcdonald-McGinn DM, Heike C, et al. Three patients with oculo-auriculo-vertebral spectrum and microdeletion 22q11.2. Am J Med Genet A. 2009;149(12):2860–4.
35. Yu S, Cox K, Friend K, et al. Familial 22q11.2 duplication: a three-generation family with a 3-Mb duplication and a familial 1.5-Mb duplication. Clin Genet. 2008;73(2):160–4.

Neonatal Subglottic Stenosis

Kara K. Prickett and Ian N. Jacobs

Subglottic stenosis is classified as congenital or acquired based on a history of prior airway instrumentation. Milder cases can often be managed with medical support and endoscopic procedures, while patients with more pronounced narrowing may require open surgical repair. The most severe form of stenosis—laryngeal atresia—requires immediate recognition and management in the delivery room. Patients with subglottic stenosis can benefit from multidisciplinary evaluation and management coincident pathology in the upper aerodigestive tract.

Acquired Subglottic Stenosis

Epidemiology

The advent of neonatal resuscitation and ventilation in the late 1950s and 1960s lead to the emergence of acquired subglottic stenosis (SGS) as a disease entity in infants and small children. Reported incidence rates have ranged from 0.0 to 8.3 %, with declining incidence over the past several decades [1]. A 2001 review by Walner et al. concluded that less than 2 % of babies admitted to neonatal intensive care units (NICUs) develop SGS, and there is general agreement that this number drops to <1 % when very low birth weight infants are excluded [1]. A small number of children—on the order of 0.005 %—fail medical and endoscopic therapies and go on to require open surgical intervention to address their SGS [2].

K.K. Prickett, M.D.
Division of Otolaryngology, The Children's Hospital of Philadelphia, Philadelphia, PA, USA
e-mail: kara.prickett@emory.edu

I.N. Jacobs, M.D. (✉)
Division of Otolaryngology, The Children's Hospital of Philadelphia, Department of Otorhinolaryngology—Head and Neck Surgery, University of Pennsylvania, Perelman School of Medicine, Philadelphia, PA, USA
e-mail: jacobsi@email.chop.edu

Pathogenesis

Acquired subglottic stenosis is thought to represent the end result of cartilaginous remodeling in the airway due to underlying infection and chondritis. The process begins with a breach of the mucosal barrier caused by trauma or pressure from long-standing endotracheal intubation. Bacteria seed the underlying cartilage resulting in chronic chondritis. This leads to remodeling and distortion of the subglottic airway, as well as interarytenoid scarring (Fig. 1) [3, 4]. Autopsy studies have found inflammatory infiltrates in the tracheal perichondrium after as little as 24 h of intubation [5].

Since not all intubated neonates develop SGS, theorized risk factors for subsequent scarring include long-term intubation, traumatic intubation, excessive tube movement, intubation with an inappropriately large tube, multiple intubations, and systemic factors such as reflux and sepsis. However, the relative risk attributable to each of these factors has never been proven in a large, multicenter study. A 1996 review by da Silva found prematurity to be the only factor consistently associated with development of subglottic stenosis, while Manica et al. found length of intubation and need for rescue doses of sedation to be associated with development of SGS [6, 7].

Clinical Presentation

In the neonatal period, less severe forms of SGS may manifest as intermittent stridor or rapid fatigue with feeding. Infants under 6 months of age diagnosed with "croup," or children under 1 year of age who have been diagnosed with multiple episodes of croup should arouse suspicion for underlying structural narrowing of the airway.

Among premature and critically ill children, SGS often presents as failure to wean from ventilatory support once associated pulmonary pathology has been effectively managed. Inability to intubate an infant with an age-appropriate endotracheal tube may also be the first sign of subglottic narrowing.

J. Lioy and S.E. Sobol (eds.), *Disorders of the Neonatal Airway: Fundamentals for Practice*,
DOI 10.1007/978-1-4939-1610-8_7, © Springer Science+Business Media New York 2015

Diagnosis and Management

Initial evaluation of patients suspected of having SGS begins with a detailed history of birth, growth, development, and comorbid conditions. Patterns of exacerbation of stridor or respiratory effort should be noted. A detailed, but directed physical exam should assess the infant for signs of increased respiratory effort. The respiratory cycle creates alternating compressing and dilating forces on the intrathoracic and extrathoracic airways, and therefore the phase of respiration during which stridor is heard can help to localize the site of narrowing. Generally, supraglottic or glottic narrowing leads to inspiratory stridor, while tracheal and bronchial pathology cause expiratory stridor. SGS often presents with biphasic stridor.

Bedside flexible laryngoscopy can provide useful information about vocal fold mobility and supraglottic pathology in extubated patients, and may allow for limited examination of the subglottis. Simple neck X-rays can also detect SGS, and are often used to diagnose the acute subglottic narrowing seen in croup. Airway fluoroscopy provides a dynamic assessment of the larger airways and can aid in the diagnosis of tracheobronchomalacia or vascular compression.

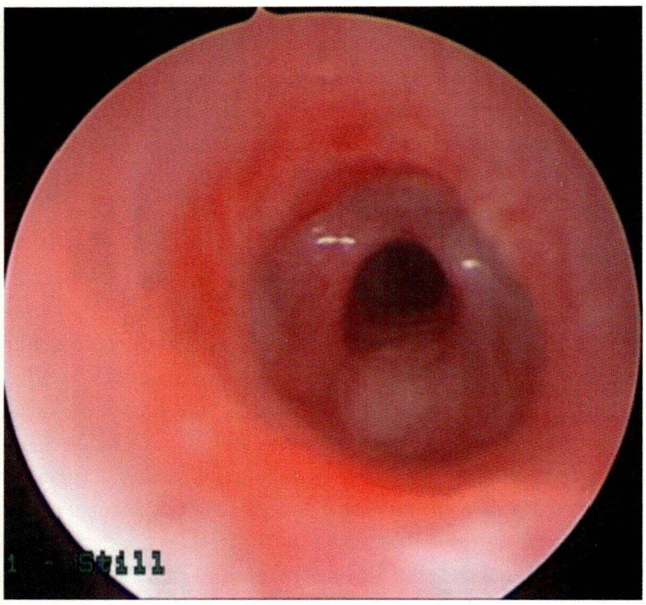

Fig. 1 Multi-level acquired subglottic stenosis in a 4-month-old child intubated during infection with respiratory syncytial virus

The gold standard for diagnosing SGS is rigid microlaryngoscopy and bronchoscopy (MLB). Assessment during spontaneous ventilation is preferred so that laryngotracheal dynamics may also be observed. The Cotton-Myer grading system (Fig. 2) is the most widely used classification scheme for SGS, and is easily adapted to standard endotracheal tube sizes [8]. "Sizing" of the subglottic airway is typically done with uncuffed endotracheal tubes under endoscopic visualization. The patient is intubated with serially larger tubes and assessed for an air leak around the tube at normal ventilatory pressures (10–25 cm H_2O). The outer diameter of the largest tube that permits a leak at appropriate pressures is considered to be the size of the airway. If a smaller-than-age-appropriate tube is needed, simple calculation can determine the percent of luminal obstruction.

Medical Management

Children with grade I SGS can often be managed conservatively with observation as long as the child is able to grow and effectively participate in normal daily activities. Intermittent medical treatment with inhaled or systemic steroids with or without racemic epinephrine may be required during periods of inflammatory upper airway obstruction. A strong working relationship between the caregivers and patient is essential, and open lines of communication must be in place so that small setbacks during periods of illness do not spiral into the need for intubation. These children often benefit from thorough aerodigestive evaluation to ensure that all potentially contributing factors are appropriately managed.

Although there continues to be debate in the literature surrounding the significance of acid reflux management in SGS, animal studies have shown that acid application to the injured subglottis causes fibrosis and scar proliferation, and adult studies have shown that idiopathic SGS refractory dilation may resolve with appropriate reflux management [9–11].

Percent airway obstruction based on endotracheal tube size									
Age	ETT	2	2.5	3	3.5	4	4.5	5	5.5
Pre-term		40%							
Pre-term		58%	30%			No obstruction			
0-3mo.		68%	48%	26%					
3-9mo.	No detectable lumen	75%	59%	41%	22%				
9mo-2yr		80%	67%	53%	38%	20%			
2yr		84%	74%	62%	50%	35%	19%		
4yr		86%	78%	68%	57%	45%	32%	17%	
6yr		98%	81%	73%	64%	54%	43%	30%	16%
	Grade IV		Grade III		Grade II		Grade I		

Fig. 2 Redrawn with modification from: Myer CM 3rd, O'Connor DM, Cotton RT. Proposed grading system for subglottic stenosis based on endotracheal tube sizes. Ann Otol Rhinol Laryngol. 1994 Apr;103(4 Pt 1):319–23

Endoscopic Balloon Dilation

Dilation has been a long-standing therapeutic option for subglottic stenosis. Beginning in the 1970s, balloon dilation gradually gained favor over the use of rigid, metal dilators due to the minimization of shearing forces, and the increased precision associated with endoscopic placement of the balloons. Typically, the area of stenosis is exposed with a suspension laryngoscope and the balloon is centered at the narrowest part of the airway, often with endoscopic guidance. The balloon is then inflated to just under burst pressure either for a pre-defined time period (such as 60 s) or until the patient exhibits evidence of oxygen desaturation. Depending on the response, dilation may be repeated with the same size balloon or with one of larger diameter. Topical or injected therapies, including triamcinolone or mitomycin, may be used to augment the effects of dilation and prevent further scar formation [12].

Initial evidence that thin or evolving stenoses responded better than firm, mature scars has been borne out with wider adoption of the technique. [13] Hebra et al. reported that patients who show no initial response are unlikely to benefit from further dilations [14]. In our experience, patients with very inflammatory stenoses or stenoses extending beyond the subglottis respond poorly to dilation. The need for repeat dilation is the rule rather than the exception, although there is limited evidence to show benefit beyond three repeated procedures for an acute symptomatic exacerbation.

Adjuvant Endoscopic Therapies

Focal obstruction of the subglottis by cysts or masses may also be managed endoscopically. Microlaryngeal instruments are often appropriately sized for use in the neonatal and infant subglottis. Simple scars and webs may be sharply divided prior to dilation, and small masses may be removed with microlaryngeal biopsy forceps. A powered tissue shaver (with an appropriately sized, laryngeal blade) can also be used for management of obstructing masses, subglottic cysts, or small hemangiomas [14].

Anterior Cricoid Split

Anterior cricoid split (ACS) was introduced in the 1980s as an alternative to tracheotomy in infants with SGS, with variable success rates. Reported extubation rates range from 58 to 100 %, although rates as low as 27–35 % have been noted among extremely premature infants (gestational age less than 28 weeks) [2, 15]. The procedure can be performed in open or endoscopic fashion, and involves complete transection of the anterior cricoid ring with or without associated balloon dilation of the airway. The lower portion of the thyroid cartilage is often divided in the midline as well, although the surgeon must take care to avoid the anterior commissure. A nasotracheal tube is left in the airway to serve as a stent during the preliminary healing phase—approximately 1 week—and soft tissue fibrosis is expected to fill the gap between the cut ends of the cricoid. The posterior cricoid may also be split to provide greater expansion of the subglottic airway.

Laryngotracheal Reconstruction

The addition of autologous cartilage grafts to augment the airway expansion achieved with cricoid split alone defines procedures classified as laryngotracheal *reconstructions* (LTR). In infants and neonates, reconstruction with a thyroid alar cartilage graft is the most commonly performed procedure. Pathologic study has shown that the thyroid alar graft can be effectively used from the glottis to the second tracheal ring, and is best for patients with grade II and select grade III stenoses [16]. Advantages of using the thyroid ala as a graft source include use of a single incision, elimination of potential for pulmonary complications related to the rib harvest and post-operative pain/splinting, and the excellent size match between the thyroid ala and the anterior cricoid ring in infants. Several retrospective studies have found increased operation-specific extubation rates when comparing primary LTR (81–89 %) with ACS alone (27–83 %) [15, 17, 18].

Reconstruction with costal cartilage grafting is typically done outside of the neonatal/infant period, after a bridging tracheotomy has been performed (Fig. 3). Techniques have been well-described in prior literature, and involve vertical incisions in the anterior or posterior midline of the cricoid plate with interposition of autologous cartilage grafts to stent open the airway. Anterior and posterior grafts may be placed together or in isolation, depending on the pathology present. Advantages of deferring LTR until around age 2 (or later) include growth of the airway leading to more working room and better tolerance of post-operative edema, maturation of the pulmonary system so that patients are better able to tolerate the surgery and post-operative recovery, and growth of the actual rib cage so that adequate grafts can be harvested with minimal morbidity. Recent studies, however, have focused on younger patients as earlier decannulation has been associated with better speech and language development outcomes [19].

Cricotracheal Resection

For children with high-grade III to grade IV lesions, cricotracheal resection (CTR) is an alternate surgical option. The anterior portion of the cricoid ring is removed with the associated stenotic segment of airway, and the distal trachea is anastomosed to the remaining cricoid posteriorly and to the inferior thyroid cartilage anteriorly. The procedure requires significantly more dissection around the airway, and therefore carries a greater risk to the recurrent laryngeal nerves than does LTR, but may offer better odds of operation-specific decannulation in selected patients [20, 21].

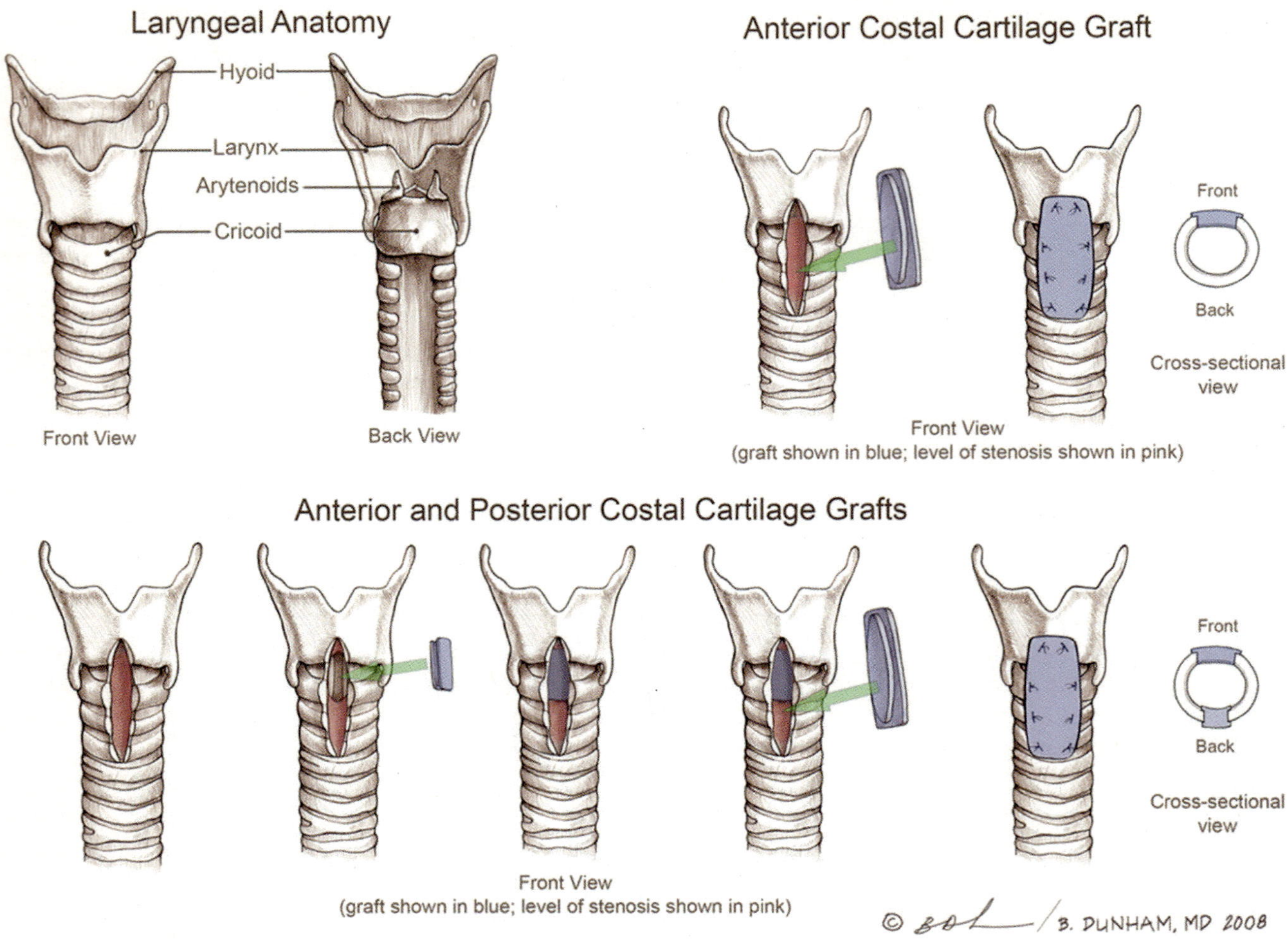

Fig. 3 Diagram of placement of anterior and posterior cartilage grafts during LTR, with resultant effect on cross-sectional airway diameter. (Permission granted for use of illustration by Brian Dunham, M.D © 2008)

Ikonomidis et al. have shown CTR to be safe and effective in children weighing less than 10 kg, but did find a high rate of post-op dysphonia (71 %) [20].

Tracheostomy

In patients with high-grade stenosis, inflammatory subglottic obstruction, or severe concomitant cardiac or pulmonary disease, tracheostomy may be the best initial option. This allows time for growth and for other medical comorbidities to be brought under control. Airway expansion surgery and decannulation can then be pursued under less acute circumstances.

Tracheostomy in the neonatal period is not without risk, though. The risk of mortality directly attributable to pediatric tracheostomy status is 0.5–1 % in the United States, with as many as 43 % of patients experiencing serious complications such as tube occlusion and accidental decannulation [22, 23]. Recent research has also suggested that neurodevelopmental outcomes may be worse among preterm infants who require tracheostomies [24].

Congenital Subglottic Stenosis

Epidemiology

Congenital SGS the third most common cause of neonatal stridor, and is thought to represent between 5 and 15 % of airway malformations [25, 26]. Congenital SGS refers to abnormal development of the cricoid ring, often resulting in a thickened, irregular structure imparting an elliptical shape to the subglottic airway. The true incidence of congenital SGS is unknown, as most infants with significant levels of obstruction are intubated at birth, thus making it very difficult to differentiate between acquired and congenital pathology.

Pathogenesis

In early embryonic development, the respiratory tree and foregut freely communicate. As the embryonic trachea is separated from the esophagus by the esophago-tracheal membrane, the epithelium of the airway proliferates rapidly, resulting in complete occlusion of the larynx and trachea. Recanalization is typically complete by the 7th week of gestation. Varying degrees of pathology may result when recanalization is incomplete, ranging from laryngeal webs to mildly obstructive subglottic shelves to complete atresia.

Clinical Presentation

Presentation of congenital SGS has a bimodal distribution, with severe cases causing immediate symptoms in the delivery room, and mild cases often going undiagnosed until later in childhood when patients prove susceptible to recurrent, severe upper respiratory infections. Congenital SGS may only be noted at the time of an unrelated surgical procedure when the anesthesiologist is unable to easily pass an age-appropriate tube.

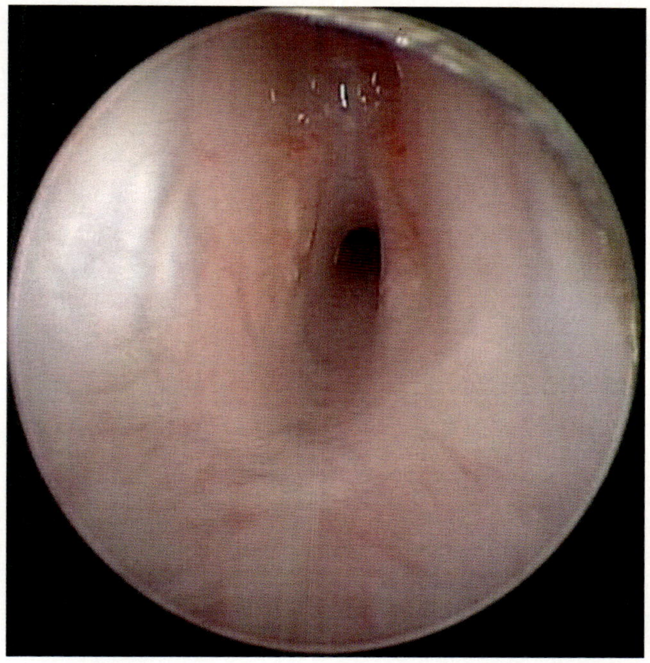

Fig. 4 Congenital subglottic stenosis in a 6-week-old neonate with a 1.5 mm airway lumen. The malformed cricoid manifests as firm, lateral subglottic shelves

Diagnosis and Management

Diagnosis of congenital SGS is made on rigid bronchoscopy, or can be made after failure to pass an age-appropriate endotracheal tube through the subglottis at the patient's first intubation. The normal diameter of the subglottic airway is 4.5–5.5 mm in a full-term infant, and 3.5 mm in a preterm infant, so most term infants should accommodate a 4.0 tube and most premature infants should accommodate a 3.0 endotracheal tube [26]. Extremely premature infants may require even smaller endotracheal tubes. On diagnostic bronchoscopy, the subglottic narrowing is typically firm due to the underlying abnormal cartilage, and lateral shelves or an elliptical opening are commonly seen (Fig. 4).

Grade I–II lesions

Many case of congenital SGS are mild and can be managed supportively. Medical management should be proactive and multidisciplinary with the goal of avoiding symptomatic exacerbations that might lead to airway instrumentation and scarring. Due to the cartilaginous nature of the narrowing in congenital SGS, patients rarely show a long-term response to balloon dilation.

Grade III–IV lesions

High-grade congenital SGS is best managed with surgical opening of the airway or tracheotomy. Patients without underlying lung disease or other comorbidities are often ideal candidates for primary LTR or CTR, as they lack the ongoing inflammatory pathology in the larynx and subglottis often seen in cases of acquired SGS. In children with other pathology present, tracheotomy with reconstruction at a later date may be the best option. Instrumentation of a congenitally narrowed airway carries the possibility of changing a stable stenosis into an unstable scar, with potential for worsening, rather than resolution, of the stenosis. Primary surgical candidates should be selected carefully.

Multidisciplinary Considerations in Subglottic Stenosis Management

Because many patients with acquired SGS carry an underlying diagnosis of prematurity, thorough evaluation and management of all associated medical issues is an important aspect of optimizing chances for successful airway surgery. Pulmonary health is often the limiting factor in determining candidacy for open airway reconstruction, and is even more critical in infants where many procedures are done in single-stage fashion (without a covering tracheotomy). Classic candidacy criteria for open airway reconstruction are shown in Fig. 5.

Patients with high-grade congenital stenosis should have a complete work-up for other congenital anomalies during the neonatal period. Patients requiring initial tracheotomy are followed by speech and swallowing therapists to ensure appropriate development of oromotor and communication skills while the tracheotomy is in place. Once patients become candidates for open airway reconstruction, we typically perform a "triple-scope" (laryngoscopy, bronchoscopy, and esophageal endoscopy) to ensure that all potential causes

Fig. 5 Guidelines for Airway Reconstruction

Guidelines for candidacy for open airway reconstruction
O_2 requirement ≤ 35%
No ventilatory support in preceding 1-2 months
No congestive heart failure in preceding 1 month
Absence of, or good control over, other aerodigestive pathology (gastro-esophageal reflux, reactive airway disease)
Weight ≥ 1500g
No evidence of active respiratory infection

*Adapted from Silver et. al[29]

of airway inflammation are well controlled. Impedance probes can be particularly useful in the assessment of reflux as a potential comorbidity due to their ability to measure both acid and non-acid refluxate.

A dedicated airway team, including representatives from otolaryngology, pulmonology, neonatology, gastroenterology, speech pathology, anesthesia, and social work provides an ideal level of support for these complex patients. Because these patients often require attention across the inpatient, outpatient, and home care spectrum, a dedicated midlevel provider (such as a nurse, nurse practitioner, or physician assistant) can be a valuable resource to families as they navigate the health system.

Future Directions

As neonatal intensive care outcomes have improved, more and more children are surviving extremely preterm birth, and are therefore at risk for acquired SGS. Research is ongoing to determine if better sedation management, optimal management of acid and non-acid reflux, and more aggressive use of noninvasive ventilatory support may help prevent acquired SGS. Endoscopic surgical options may expand as robotic surgery technology is adapted for smaller and smaller patients. Tissue engineering and biomaterials research may also yield new graft options that could decrease donor-site morbidity and minimize risk of cartilage graft resorption.

Laryngeal Atresia and Congenital High Airway Obstruction Syndrome

Epidemiology

Due to the high risk for fetal demise, the true incidence of Congenital High Airway Obstruction Syndrome (CHAOS) is unknown. It can occur in sporadic or syndromic fashion, with associated syndromes including Fraser's syndrome, Cri-du-Chat, short rib polydactaly syndrome, and velocardiofacial syndrome [27]. A single case of a father with two affected sons has been reported [28].

Pathogenesis

Fetal lungs produce fluid in utero, and obstruction of the trachea or larynx causes fluid to accumulate in the lungs and lower airways. This leads to expansion of the lungs with resultant compression of the heart and inversion of the diaphragm. Expansion of the lungs may impede fetal swallowing, contributing to polyhydramnios [29].

If tracheal atresia is accompanied by tracheo-esophageal fistula, classic signs may not be present, as the esophagus and pharynx provide an escape route for the lung fluid. Similarly, patients with oropharyngeal teratomas or other obstructing masses may not exhibit all the signs of CHAOS, as some fluid is typically able to pass around the mass and out of the lungs.

Clinical Presentation

Patients present in the neonatal period with ultrasound findings detailed in Fig. 6, or at birth with immediate cyanosis and inability to establish ventilation.

Diagnosis and Management

Diagnosis is typically made in the prenatal period when a specific constellation of ultrasound findings is noted (Fig. 6). If there is concern for CHAOS on ultrasound, confirmatory testing with 3D ultrasound or fetal MRI is frequently performed.

When diagnosis is made in the prenatal period, patients should be referred to a center capable of performing ex-utero intrapartum treatment (EXIT). During an EXIT procedure, the fetus is partially delivered by cesarean section while materno-fetal circulation is maintained by the placenta. Tracheotomy or a procedure to remove the obstructing lesion can then be performed in a controlled fashion. Should the patient present without prenatal diagnosis, rapid tracheotomy is the only treatment option. Even when appropriate prenatal diagnosis is made, risk of fetal demise remains high due to other coincident anomalies and risk for preterm birth due to polyhydramnios.

Ultrasound findings in CHAOS
Polyhydramnios
Increased echogenicity of lungs
Dilated trachea
Flattened or inverted diaphragm

Fig. 6 Ultrasound findings in CHOAS

Long-term management in CHAOS and laryngeal atresia typically requires CTR or segmental tracheal resection. This has not been reported in neonates or infants, likely due to coexisting pulmonary abnormalities.

Multidisciplinary Considerations in CHAOS Management

Effective management of patients with CHAOS requires coordination of multiple practitioners and treatment teams, including maternal-fetal medicine, surgery, otolaryngology, and neonatology. Dedicated surgical and anesthesia teams are often employed, so that all members of the treatment team are familiar with caring for simultaneous patients.

Once an initial airway has been established, surgical and medical teams must work closely with respiratory care providers and speech pathologists to ensure that a safe and stimulating environment is maintained while preparation for definitive airway reconstruction (if possible) is underway.

Future Directions

As prenatal diagnostics technologies improve, there is hope that more patients with CHAOS will be identified in utero. Timely diagnosis will allow for better characterization of the natural history of the disease during both the gestational and post-natal periods, with the ultimate goal of identifying early predictors of viability. Advances in fetal surgery may also allow for earlier intervention, thereby reducing the incidence of polyhydramnios and unexpected preterm delivery.

References

1. Walner DL, Loewen MS, Kimura RE. Neonatal subglottic stenosis—incidence and trends. Laryngoscope. 2001;111(1):48–51.
2. Leung R, Berkowitz RG. Incidence of severe acquired subglottic stenosis in newborns. Int J Pediatr Otorhinolaryngol. 2007;71(5):763–8. Epub 2007 Feb 21.
3. Suzumura H, Nitta A, Tanaka G, Kuwashima S, Hirabayashi H. Role of infection in the development of acquired subglottic stenosis in neonates with prolonged intubation. Pediatr Int. 2000;42(5):508–13.
4. Duynstee ML, de Krijger RR, Monnier P, Verwoerd CD, Verwoerd-Verhoef HL. Subglottic stenosis after endolaryngeal intubation in infants and children: result of wound healing processes. Int J Pediatr Otorhinolaryngol. 2002;62(1):1–9.
5. Gould SJ, Howard S. The histopathology of the larynx in the neonate following endotracheal intubation. J Pathol. 1985;146:301–11.
6. Manica D, Schweiger C, Maróstica PJ, Kuhl G, Carvalho PR. Association between length of intubation and subglottic stenosis in children. Laryngoscope. 2013;123(4):1049–54. doi:10.1002/lary.23771.. Epub 2013 Feb 1.
7. da Silva OP. Factors influencing acquired upper airway obstruction in newborn infants receiving assisted ventilation because of respiratory failure: an overview. J Perinatol. 1996;16(4):272–5.
8. Myer 3rd CM, O'Connor DM, Cotton RT. Proposed grading system for subglottic stenosis based on endotracheal tube sizes. Ann Otol Rhinol Laryngol. 1994;103(4 Pt 1):319–23.
9. Zalzal GH, Choi SS, Patel KM. The effect of gastroesophageal reflux on laryngotracheal reconstruction. Arch Otolaryngol Head Neck Surg. 1996;122(3):297–300.
10. Roh JL, Lee YW, Park HT. Effect of acid, pepsin, and bile acid on the stenotic progression of traumatized subglottis. Am J Gastroenterol. 2006;101(6):1186–92.
11. Blumin JH, Johnston N. Evidence of extraesophageal reflux in idiopathic subglottic stenosis. Laryngoscope. 2011;121(6):1266–73. doi:10.1002/lary.21776. Epub 2011 May 6.
12. Edmondson NE, Bent 3rd J. Serial intralesional steroid injection combined with balloon dilation as an alternative to open repair of subglottic stenosis. Int J Pediatr Otorhinolaryngol. 2010;74(9):1078–81.
13. Hebra A, Powell DD, Smith CD, Othersen Jr HB. Balloon tracheoplasty in children: results of a 15-year experience. J Pediatr Surg. 1991;26(8):957–61.
14. Ransom ER, Antunes MB, Smith LP, Jacobs IN. Microdebrider resection of acquired subglottic cysts: case series and review of the literature. Int J Pediatr Otorhinolaryngol. 2009;73(12):1833–6.
15. White DR, Bravo M, Vijayasekaran S, Rutter MJ, Cotton RT, Elluru RG. Laryngotracheoplasty as an alternative to tracheotomy in infants younger than 6 months. Arch Otolaryngol Head Neck Surg. 2009;135(5):445–7. doi:10.1001/archoto.2009.21.
16. Fayoux P, Devisme L, Merrot O, Chevalier D. Thyroid alar cartilage graft in laryngoplasty: anatomical study in premature and newborn babies. Int J Pediatr Otorhinolaryngol. 2002;66(3):259–63.
17. Forte V, Chang MB, Papsin BC. Thyroid ala cartilage reconstruction in neonatal subglottic stenosis as a replacement for the anterior cricoid split. Int J Pediatr Otorhinolaryngol. 2001;59(3):181–6.
18. Richardson MA, Inglis Jr AF. A comparison of anterior cricoid split with and without costal cartilage graft for acquired subglottic stenosis. Int J Pediatr Otorhinolaryngol. 1991;22(2):187–93.
19. Jiang D, Morrison GA. The influence of long-term tracheostomy on speech and language development in children. Int J Pediatr Otorhinolaryngol. 2003;67 Suppl 1:S217–20.
20. Ikonomidis C, George M, Jaquet Y, Monnier P. Partial cricotracheal resection in children weighing less than 10 kilograms. Otolaryngol Head Neck Surg. 2010;142(1):41–7.
21. Hartley BE, Cotton RT. Paediatric airway stenosis: laryngotracheal reconstruction or cricotracheal resection? Clin Otolaryngol Allied Sci. 2000;25(5):342–9.
22. Wetmore RF, Marsh RR, Thompson ME, Tom LW. Pediatric tracheostomy: a changing procedure? Ann Otol Rhinol Laryngol. 1999;108(7 Pt 1):695–9.
23. Carr MM, Poje CP, Kingston L, Kielma D, Heard C. Complications in pediatric tracheostomies. Laryngoscope. 2001;111(11 Pt 1):1925–8.
24. Demauro SB, D'Agostino JA, Bann C, Bernbaum J, Gerdes M, Bell EF, Carlo WA, C'Angio CT, Das A, Higgins R, Hintz SR, Laptook AR, Natarajan G, Nelin L, Poindexter BB, Sanchez PJ, Shankaran S, Stoll BJ, Truog W, Van Meurs KP, Vohr B, Walsh MC, Kirpalani H, Eunice Kennedy Shriver National Institute of Child Health and Human Development Neonatal Research Network.

Developmental outcomes of very preterm infants with tracheostomies. J Pediatr. 2014;164(6):1303–10.
25. Lyons M, Vlastarakos PV, Nikolopoulos TP. Congenital and acquired developmental problems of the upper airway in newborns and infants. Early Hum Dev. 2012;88(12):951–5.
26. Schroeder Jr JW, Holinger LD. Congenital laryngeal stenosis. Otolaryngol Clin North Am. 2008;41(5):865–75.
27. Artunc Ulkumen B, Pala HG, Nese N, Tarhan S, Baytur Y. Prenatal diagnosis of congenital high airway obstruction syndrome: report of two cases and brief review of the literature. Case Rep Obstet Gynecol. 2013;2013:728974.
28. Vanhaesebrouck P, De Coen K, Defoort P, et al. Evidence for autosomal dominant inheritance in prenatally diagnosed CHAOS. Eur J Pediatr. 2006;165(10):706–8.
29. Hedrick MH, Ferro MM, Filly RA, Flake AW, Harrison MR, Adzick NS. Congenital high airway obstruction syndrome (CHAOS): a potential for perinatal intervention. J Pediatr Surg. 1994;29(2):271–4.

Congenital and Acquired Disorders of the Vocal Folds

Jeffrey Cheng and Karen B. Zur

Introduction

The neonatal glottic apparatus is responsible for three main functions: respiration, protection from aspiration, and sound vocalization. Complex and coordinated actions, along with specialized mechanical properties, govern normal glottic physiology. A complete understanding of the physiology of the neonatal glottis is far from being achieved, and relatively few investigations have been focused in this area. Because of the complexities and variability in the development of neuromuscular pathways and the maturation of laryngeal reflexes, we have relatively little knowledge concerning the etiology of neonatal glottic disorders and many of our diagnostic and treatment approaches are extrapolated from experiences in older children and adults. As the subspecialty area of pediatric laryngology matures, our understanding and ability to diagnose, prognosticate, and treat congenital and acquired neonatal airway disorders will continue to evolve.

Embryology and Anatomy

Understanding the structure and function of the vocal folds is essential in the evaluation and management of glottic pathology. At birth, many different organ systems including the neonatal larynx are immature and undergo significant histologic and morphologic changes. The classic model of the mature vocal fold includes a composition of three distinct layers: a non-keratinizing stratified squamous layer, lamina propria, and the vocalis muscle, from superficial to deep, respectively. The lamina propria is further composed of three histologically separate layers—superficial, middle, and deep—which are believed to play a significant role in the pathophysiology of the fibrovascular and viscoelastic properties of the vocal folds. The middle and deep layers of the lamina propria are intimately related and make up the vocal ligament, which in neonates comprises approximately half the length of the vocal cord, as opposed to in adults, where the vocal ligament is about one-third the length of the vocal fold [6].

The currently accepted fundamentals of microlaryngeal phonosurgery describe the importance of the relationship between the superficial lamina propria and the vocal ligament. The superficial lamina propria plays an important role in the normal viscoelastic properties and forms the interface that promotes the normal fluid movement between the superficial epithelial layer and the vocal ligament. During the immediate neonatal period, this normal adult composition of the vocal folds has not yet matured. Histologic examination of neonatal larynges reveals the appearance of vocal folds lacking apparent layers within the lamina propria. Immediately after birth the lamina propria consists of a relative hypercellular monolayer, and is thought to begin maturation by 27 weeks gestation [3]. Within this monolayer, there is a uniform, histologic appearance throughout, with an even distribution of hyaluronic acid, which is the primary determinant of vocal cord viscosity and water content [17]. Given this immature arrangement within the neonatal lamina propria, it is thought that the collagen fiber arrangement within the lamina propria in the developing fetus may be important for vocalization at birth [4]. The lamina propria transitions to a bilayer by 5 months, but the mature lamina propria is not yet present until around the time of adolescence [15].

Due to the immaturity of the neonatal vocal fold structure, the incidence and types of vocal fold pathology are significantly different in neonates compared to older children

J. Cheng, M.D.
Division of Pediatric Otolaryngology, The Children's Hospital of Philadelphia, Philadelphia, PA, USA

K.B. Zur, M.D. (✉)
Division of Otolaryngology, The Children's Hospital of Philadelphia, Department of Otorhinolaryngology—Head and Neck Surgery, University of Pennsylvania, Perelman School of Medicine, Philadelphia, PA, USA
e-mail: zur@email.chop.edu

J. Lioy and S.E. Sobol (eds.), *Disorders of the Neonatal Airway: Fundamentals for Practice*,
DOI 10.1007/978-1-4939-1610-8_8, © Springer Science+Business Media New York 2015

and adults. Therefore, traditional microlaryngeal surgical techniques and principles that are performed in adults may not apply in this age group. In this chapter, we aim to describe the clinical presentation, endoscopic findings, and management strategies of congenital and acquired disorders of the neonatal vocal folds.

Vocal Fold Immobility

Etiology

Abnormal mobility of the true vocal folds in a neonate may be complete or incomplete. The etiology for absent or abnormal vocal fold motion may be secondary to an underlying mechanical or neural pathology, which may be elucidated through the patient's clinical history, physical exam, radiographic studies, endoscopic, and/or electrodiagnostic evaluations. A differential diagnosis for vocal fold immobility can be found in Table 1. Acquired etiologies may be related to iatrogenic causes, such as cervical or thoracic surgical procedures or trauma. A history of an instrument-assisted delivery may raise the suspicion for intracranial or cervical trauma. In rare cases, intracranial hemorrhage may be associated with vocal fold motion impairment. Neonates should be evaluated and monitored for vocal fold mobility issues if they have respiratory difficulty after common cervical or thoracic procedures such as patent ductus arteriosus (PDA) ligation and esophageal atresia or tracheoesophageal atresia repair. Factors beyond the surgical procedure, such as anastomic leakage after esophageal reconstruction, may also contribute to the immediate or delayed onset in the diagnosis or recognition of vocal fold paralysis.

Mechanical etiologies for neonatal vocal fold immobility are rare and may result from posterior glottic stenosis, a mass or arytenoid dislocation [14].

Neurogenic causes of unilateral or bilateral vocal fold immobility in neonates can be due to pathology anywhere along the neural pathway from the nucleus ambiguus to the motor endplates of the intrinsic laryngeal musculature. The etiology may be congenital or acquired. Congenital causes of vocal fold immobility include central nervous system (CNS) or neuromuscular abnormalities, Chiari malformation, infectious, or idiopathic. One rare cause is congenital myasthenic syndrome (CMS) and has been attributed to mutations in the DOK7 gene [7]. In other rare cases, the cause may be familial, and a genetics consultation may be helpful if there is a family history of bilateral vocal fold paralysis. A locus on chromosome 6 has been implicated in the autosomal dominant transmission of bilateral vocal cord paralysis [8]. A few cases of X-linked mode of inheritance have also been described and may occur with or without associated mental disabilities, musculoskeletal abnormalities, or neurologic anomalies [11].

Table 1 Differential diagnosis for congenital or acquired vocal fold immobility

Congenital	Acquired
Chiari malformation, intraventricular hemorrhage (IVH), or other CNS pathology	Iatrogenic (patent ductus arteriosus ligation, cervical or cardiothoracic surgery, traumatic delivery)
Congenital myasthenic syndrome (CMS)	Arytenoid dislocation
Familial inheritance	Posterior glottic stenosis
Infectious	
Congenital heart disease with cardiomegaly	

Epidemiology

Vocal fold immobility in neonates is the second most common cause of congenital stridor; it can be congenital or acquired, unilateral or bilateral. Premature and extremely low-birth weight neonates have a higher risk of left vocal cord paralysis after PDA ligation (up to 40 %), and in these children the associated morbidity is significantly higher with increased risks for bronchopulmonary dysplasia, reactive airway disease, and need for gastrostomy tube placement [2]. Neonates undergoing a PDA ligation may not present with respiratory symptoms despite the presence of a vocal fold paralysis, and up to 14 % of neonates may have this diagnosis missed without a scheduled post-extubation fiberoptic laryngoscopy [17]. Prospective efforts to assess vocal fold mobility after this procedure are being studied in high-risk, extremely low-birth weight/premature neonates. For all other cardiac surgery in neonates via a median sternotomy, the reported incidence for vocal fold paresis is between 1.7 and 67 %, depending on the type of surgery and the weight of the patient at the time of surgery [5]. On average, one in five neonates undergoing cardiac surgery may encounter vocal fold mobility issues postoperatively. Neonatal cardiac surgery that involves manipulation of the aortic arch may result in a higher incidence of immobility and longer hospitalizations.

Clinical Presentation

Vocal fold mobility disorders may have a greater negative impact on the neonate compared to older children or adults. While older patients may be asymptomatic due to compensation from the contralateral vocal fold, or present with dysphonia and a breathy voice, neonates with unilateral or bilateral vocal fold immobility often present with a weak cry, stridor, respiratory distress, and/or feeding difficulties. Neonates with bilateral vocal fold immobility present with more significant respiratory difficulties and may require endotracheal intubation or eventual tracheotomy placement in about 50 % of cases.

Diagnosis

Diagnostic consultation is often requested in neonates who present with dysphonia, stridor, and/or respiratory distress. A complete and thorough history and physical examination can often elucidate the etiology. In neonates with complex coexisting and comorbid medical and neurologic pathology, input from neonatal intensivists and pediatric neurologists may aid in the diagnostic considerations and workup, providing valuable information relating to the patient's overall prognosis.

Bedside fiberoptic laryngoscopy has become more readily available and is the primary diagnostic tool to assess vocal fold mobility. This nonsedated, awake endoscopic examination of the neonatal larynx will give the examiner the best opportunity to evaluate vocal fold mobility and dynamics. This evaluation may be more technically challenging than in the older patients as these infants have poorer pulmonary reserve and may have complicating, comorbid conditions. Inability to tolerate secretions, lack of patient cooperation, crowding of the nasopharyngeal, oropharyngeal, and supraglottic tissues, and enteric feeding tubes may interfere with introducing the equipment and visualization of the neonatal larynx. Recent extubation or significant laryngopharyngeal reflux can cause edema and erythema, which makes the examination even more challenging. Laryngomalacia, or floppiness of the supraglottic structures, may prohibit adequate visualization of the true vocal folds. Caution should be advised when performing bedside fiberoptic laryngoscopy, especially in the cardiac population, and advanced resuscitation equipment should be readily available when indicated in the unstable patient.

Given these limitations, an assessment of neonates vocal fold mobility can often be difficult, and careful attention should be placed on examining for adduction and abduction of the arytenoid cartilages which often serve as surrogate markers for vocal fold mobility. If there is a history of cardiothoracic surgery and symptoms of a hoarse cry and/or stridor, vocal cord immobility is often discovered. It is also important to rule out a subglottic pathology, as these patients have a history of intubation, which may lead to similar symptoms. Additionally, an initial assessment of pooling of secretions or the neonate's ability to handle secretions is important to help determine the patient's risk for aspiration and potential for oral feeding. Assessment for obvious masses or lesions in the supraglottic larynx should be undertaken. A detailed endoscopic view of the neonatal vocal folds, however, with current fiberoptic technology is limited. Large cysts or nodules should be readily visualized, but subtle nodules or submucosal lesions/scars will not be obvious in this age group. Accurate assessment of the subglottis is also not feasible with the bedside flexible laryngoscope.

Congenital infectious causes for vocal fold paralysis include varicella, for which the diagnosis may be confirmed by retinal imaging by the ophthalmologists [13].

The modified barium swallow (MBS) may be needed to be performed in order to assess the safety of oral feeding and the appropriateness of a particular diet under the guidance and supervision of a speech-language pathologist (SLP) and radiologist. The primary drawback to pursuing this study is the exposure of the neonate to ionizing radiation. The study, however, does provide some additional clinical information that may be useful in management and decision-making, as the managing team is also provided diagnostic radiographic images that may help to further delineate airway pathology and help protect the child from pulmonary soiling in cases of silent aspiration.

Cross-sectional imaging may be useful to help elucidate the etiology of vocal fold immobility. The choice is often between magnetic resonance imaging (MRI) and computed tomography (CT). The use of CT is often reserved for cases in which MRI cannot be performed or if there is a specific clinical indication. There is a growing body of literature cautioning the use of CT because of the potential effects of ionizing radiation, especially in young children [1]. MRI provides excellent, high resolution and high fidelity images evaluating for causes of vocal fold mobility disorders in neonates—Arnold Chiari malformation, central nervous system (CNS) abnormalities or malformations, intracranial hemorrhage, and neck or chest soft tissue lesions or vascular malformations. CT is often helpful in older patients to help detect arytenoid dislocation but is limited in neonates because of the lack of calcification of the maturing, laryngeal framework, which may make the pathology difficult to identify. MRI, when available, is probably the best choice for cross-sectional imaging in evaluating neonatal vocal fold paralysis. Small intracranial hemorrhages may be missed on CT. Evaluation and diagnosis of Chiari malformation almost always includes imaging with MRI. Detection of a Chiari malformation significantly impacts the clinical management of the child and necessitates neurosurgical consultation.

Management

The treatment of vocal fold immobility in neonates is primarily guided by the clinical severity of the affected patient. Often this is related to whether the vocal fold immobility is unilateral or bilateral. Unilateral vocal fold immobility in neonates is often managed conservatively, rarely causing significant enough respiratory symptoms to warrant tracheostomy placement. In these cases, medical management for feeding and reflux is often all that is required until further assessments can be made when the patient is older, and their needs can be better evaluated.

The most important aspects of the triage of unilateral vocal fold immobility are the respiratory status and the aspiration risk. Often, affected neonates demonstrate a hoarse cry but rarely any significant respiratory distress. Speech-language pathology consultation should be requested and assessment of the safety for oral intake made. Potential recovery may occur, and therefore, it is prudent to try to delay any permanent intervention for at least 12 months and often longer. If swallowing issues fail to be controlled, or handling of saliva and feeds is not remedied, then a sooner intervention may be needed to protect the lungs.

In rare cases of neonatal arytenoid dislocation there will be a history of stridor after extubation. Laryngoscopy will reveal unilateral immobility of the vocal fold, mimicking paralysis with an anterior and medial displacement of the ipsilateral arytenoid. Neonatal arytenoid dislocation may cause edema and mass effect, making intubation more challenging. In the neonate, management of the airway in such cases must be judicious and is rarely needed. The surgical approach would most likely involve a closed reduction with splinting of the cricoarytenoid joint with an endotracheal tube.

Bilateral vocal fold immobility usually presents with significantly more pronounced respiratory compromise necessitating early intervention. The primary management hinges upon the degree of respiratory symptoms, with 50 % of patients requiring tracheostomy placement. The goal is often to provide a safe temporary airway to bypass the glottic obstruction, and provide time for diagnostic evaluations, treatment options to be attempted, or to await spontaneous recovery.

When a neurologic etiology for bilateral vocal fold paralysis is established, such as in the case of a Chiari malformation, intraventricular hemorrhage, and/or neuraxial malformation, neurology and neurosurgical consultations are recommended. If the lesion is surgically correctable, repair of a central nervous system anomaly has the potential to reverse the paralysis.

Other surgical options include endoscopic or open airway procedures. These types of procedures are more established in infants and children with limited reports of outcomes in neonates. Partial cordotomy has been described to be safe and successful in avoiding tracheostomy placement or aiding in decannulation in a limited number of infants. The technique has not been reported to be associated with a significant risk for functional respiratory or feeding complications but may contribute to more dysphonia as the child grows, and often does not lead to a long-term benefit. This is anecdotal and not currently supported by substantial literature.

Laryngotracheal augmentation with placement of a posterior cricoid costal cartilage graft has been utilized for decannulating children with a tracheostomy in place or in management of airway compromise secondary to bilateral fold paralysis in older patients who have managed to avoid a tracheostomy tube placement at a younger age. This procedure is not well established in neonates as an alternative to placement of a tracheostomy placement in the acute situation.

A recent report of several patients who have undergone an endoscopic anterior–posterior cricoid split with balloon dilation and stenting with an indwelling endotracheal tube shows some promise in neonates who are symptomatic from bilateral vocal fold immobility [15]. Long-term results (>2 years) are not well known, but those patients were able to avoid placement of a tracheostomy tube in the critical period when one would be considered.

The neonate who presents with stridor, hoarseness, and/or feeding difficulties and is found to have a vocal fold mobility issue should undergo a clinical assessment for feeding. Performing a functional endoscopic evaluation of swallowing (FEES) in the infant is feasible, but may provide limited information in this age group. Clinical assessment by a speech-language pathologist is often more appropriate. Safety and prevention of aspiration are of the utmost importance. Often, when there is vocal fold immobility, the ability of the neonatal larynx to compensate and provide protection from aspiration is impaired, especially when compared to adults. The degree to which neonates are affected by vocal fold immobility can vary, but in very low-birth weight patients who develop left vocal cord paralysis after PDA ligation have been shown to have significant feeding difficulties and high rates of gastrostomy tube placement.

Multidisciplinary Considerations

The diagnosis and management of vocal fold immobility in neonates requires a multidisciplinary approach. The team of specialists may include otolaryngologists, speech-language pathologists, neurologists, neurosurgeons, ophthalmologists, and geneticists. The neonatal intensivist is vital in coordinating the appropriate services that need to be involved based on clinical assessment and the needs of the patient.

Future Considerations

One of the potentially promising future management options for bilateral vocal fold motion impairment is bilateral selective recurrent laryngeal nerve reinnervation. The champion of this procedure, Dr. Jean Paul Marie from Rouen, France, has been diligently studying this intricate procedure in adults and has performed a few cases in young children. The long-term effects are yet to be known, however a sizeable group of adult patients have done well following this intervention. This procedure requires a temporary tracheostomy tube due to the predicted synkinetic motion that occurs early during the reinnervation period. This leads to paradoxical vocal fold motion and respiratory distress. The appropriateness in children is yet to be determined.

Laryngeal electromyography (LEMG) is a useful diagnostic technology in adults for unilateral and bilateral vocal fold immobility. It can be used to aid in diagnosis, management, and prognosis for recovery of vocal fold motion impairment. In children, LEMG is used in a limited fashion since it requires a general anesthetic to allow for electrode placement in the larynx. Little data exists in the literature regarding the benefit of utilizing this tool in the infant, as it is rarely done in this age group. Treatment options may be guided by information obtained from the LEMG, as this study can provide prognostic data for recovery of vocal fold function. This should be an area for further study.

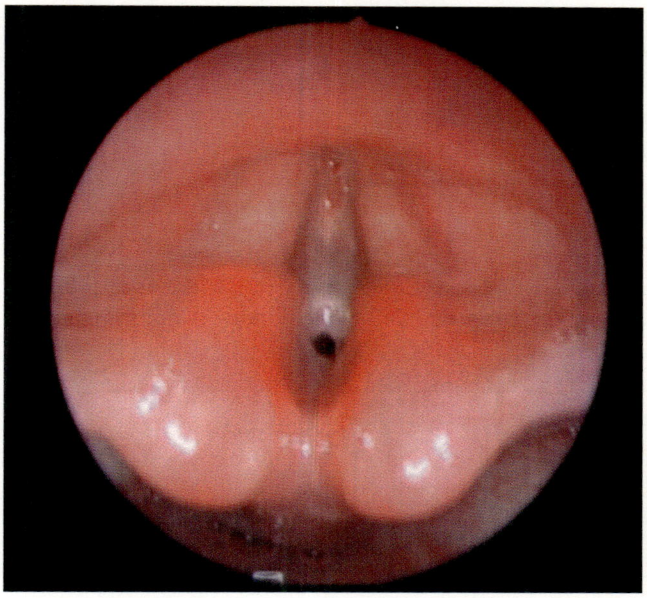

Fig. 1 Congenital laryngeal atresia with near-total fusion of the true vocal folds. Note the small glottis airway posteriorly

Glottic Webs

Etiology

Congenital glottic webs occur along the spectrum of laryngeal atresias. These are partial laryngeal atresias located in the area of the anterior commissure, across the anterior one-third of the true vocal folds, and may have a subglottic component that extends to the level of the cricoid. Rarely, a very thin glottic web may be present only at the level of the true vocal folds in the anterior commissure. These are the result of an embryologic failure of recanalization of the primitive larynx during the 10th week of embryogenesis.

Acquired glottic webs or synechiae can also be found after prolonged intubation or traumatic intubation. In these cases, opposing demucosalized and exposed deep layers of the true vocal folds may form scar bands, which limit abduction or mechanically restrict full vocal fold mobility. Infectious causes may also result in web formation, such as *Corynebacterium diphtheriae* or *Bacillus cereus*.

Epidemiology

In general, these are uncommon lesions of the neonatal vocal folds. However, 65 % of patients who have yet to be diagnosed with a 22q11 microdeletion syndrome may test positive for this genetic defect if an anterior glottic web is discovered. Nearly half of these patients may only present with a subtle clinical manifestation of velo-cardio-facial syndrome (VCFS), so a high-index of suspicion must be maintained [10].

Clinical Presentation

Older children may present with dysphonia more so than respiratory distress. However, due to the limited reserve in neonates, they may present with an abnormally weak, soft, husky, or absent cry. Stridor, usually biphasic, or respiratory distress may also be found.

Diagnosis

Bedside flexible laryngoscopy may allow identification of this pathology, but rigid microlaryngoscopy and bronchoscopy (MLB) should be pursued in order to make a definitive diagnosis. The initial diagnostic evaluation should have several primary objectives: (1) confirm the presence of a glottic web and attempt to determine if it is congenital or acquired; (2) initiate consultation and genetics evaluation for other associated anomalies; (3) accurately stage and define the extent of the web in order to guide optimal surgical and anesthetic options for reconstruction (Fig. 1).

During the general physical examination, special attention should be paid to the soft palate, looking for a submucous or open cleft; medialization of the internal carotid arteries with prominent pulsations along the posterior pharyngeal wall should also be noted. These are stigmata that can be seen in patients with Deletion 22Q. An abnormally shaped antihelix may also be seen in these patients.

Patients diagnosed with a laryngeal web should undergo fluorescent in situ hybridization (FISH) evaluation for the 22q11 microdeletion and other associated syndromes. A genetics evaluation is also recommended, as basic FISH testing may not rule out VCF syndrome. Depending on the clinical findings and genetics assessment, cardiology workup may be indicated in order to rule out or manage associated cardiac pathology.

Management

The treatment of glottic webs is challenging. The primary concern is for recurrence of anterior glottis scarring, and early intervention may result in persistent dysphonia or respiratory symptoms after treatment due to the small caliber of the infant larynx. Further evaluation may uncover other congenital defects and chromosomal abnormalities as previously discussed.

It may be advised to await and defer definitive management until beyond the neonatal period. However, in some cases, intervention may be warranted depending on the clinical severity of the patient's symptoms. Tracheostomy may also be an option for complex lesions with associated medical comorbidities that may make endoscopic or limited open procedures less likely to be successful in the neonatal period. Delayed, definitive treatment can be planned after tracheostomy placement.

When surgical intervention is entertained, the type of procedure will be guided by the severity of the lesion. With advancing surgical technologies, the goals of surgical intervention are to (1) resolve the airway obstruction and (2) preserve function while maintaining a serviceable voice. For simple thin anterior webs with normal respiration and voice, observation is recommended. In infants who are symptomatic, division with cold instrumentation and a short period of endotracheal intubation may resolve the problem. If the lesion is thicker, endoscopic or open division of the web and placement of a keel may be utilized to stent the anterior commissure in an attempt to prevent reformation. When an obstructing stent or keel is used, tracheostomy is required at least for the duration of stent placement. Realistically, infants who require a tracheostomy tube will likely not get decannulated in the first year of life. For the most involved lesions with subglottic extension, open laryngotracheal reconstruction with anterior cartilage grafting may be required at a later age.

Multidisciplinary Considerations

If a laryngeal abnormality, such as a glottic web, is encountered in a neonate and facial dysmorphism or cardiac anomalies are present, a genetics consultation is warranted to evaluate for a deletion 22Q. If present, patients with VCF will require multiple specialists and may be better served with referral to a center or institution with an established program or services to manage them. At the minimum, pediatric specialty services from pulmonary, cardiology, speech pathology, and genetics should be involved in the initial comprehensive evaluation of the patient.

Patients with 22Q deletion may have velopharyngeal insufficiency (VPI), which affects articulation and occasionally impacts vocal quality due to straining. The vocal quality may be independent of a history of laryngeal web and can occur without a history of one. A laryngeal evaluation of the velopharynx and the larynx should be performed to assess the cause of hoarseness in such patients. Depending on the institution, correction of VPI is addressed by the plastic surgery or otolaryngology service(s) in conjunction with a speech therapist.

Future Considerations

As airway reconstructive techniques advance, potentially more cases will be treatable endoscopically. Further study is required to investigate short and long-term voice outcomes and voice rehabilitative options for these patients. The type of stent/keel used to prevent re-webbing during the reconstructive procedure may impact the voice outcome postoperatively. Hopefully, advances in technology can assist in more customized stenting of the neonatal airway to improve the results of this procedure.

Granulomas

Etiology

The vocal process refers to the base of the arytenoid cartilage where the vocal ligament attaches. Granulomas of the vocal folds are found in this location and are referred to as vocal process granulomas. This pathology is commonly encountered in adults, usually as a result of trauma or related to endotracheal intubation for general anesthesia. As discussed earlier, the structure and composition of the neonatal vocal fold is different than in adults, with a higher portion of the vocal fold taken up by the vocal ligament. However, we do not have an understanding of how this relationship affects the susceptibility or protects neonates from vocal process granulomas.

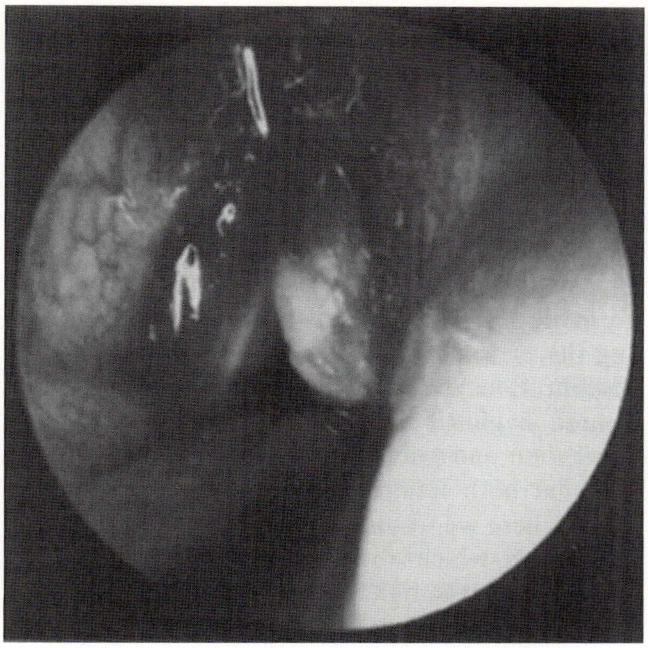

Fig. 2 Right sided vocal cord granuloma in a neonate (Reprinted from [8], copyright © 1996, Reprint by Permission of SAGE Publications)

Epidemiology

Even though prolonged or multiple episodes of endotracheal intubation commonly occur in neonates, vocal process granulomas are relatively rare in this age group. Little has been published on the management of this pathology for this age cohort. Only several cases have ever been reported in the literature [7, 8].

Clinical Presentation

Vocal process granulomas in neonates are associated with a history of endotracheal intubation with post-extubation stridor, dysphonia, or multiple failed extubation attempts.

Diagnosis

The diagnosis can be made with flexible, fiberoptic bedside laryngoscopy and/or rigid laryngoscopy. These lesions are exophytic, usually unilateral, affecting the posterior portion of the vocal cord, just anterior to the arytenoid on the vocal process (Fig. 2).

Management

The treatment recommendation for granulomas is a conservative approach. Management of potential insults such as gastroesophageal reflux, voice abuse, and removing a source of irritation such as an endotracheal tube are advocated. Systemic steroids may be helpful in reducing inflammation. For small nonobstructing lesions, it is recommended to avoid a surgical intervention, as surgical excision of a granuloma will likely result in regrowth of the lesion. Medical management is advised, and use of oral antibiotics is often employed as well, as an infectious process is often involved in the generation of a granuloma. For obstructing lesions, conservative observation may not be feasible. In these cases, microlaryngeal surgery is indicated for removal of the granuloma in conjunction with an intralesional steroid injection. This is done in order to avoid regrowth of the lesion. Avoidance of further laryngeal intubation and control of gastroesophageal reflux are recommended when possible.

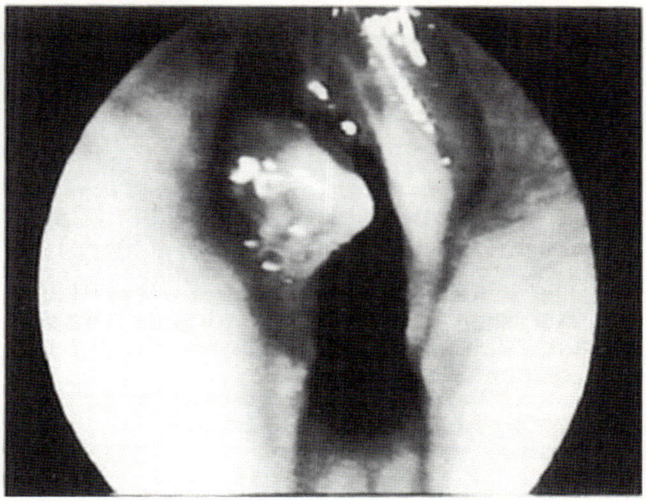

Fig. 3 Traumatic left vocal fold avulsion injury (Reprinted from [19], copyright © 1996, with permission from Elsevier, Ltd.)

Trauma

Etiology

Trauma of the larynx, albeit extremely rare in the neonatal group, is commonly the result of an injury related to airway management. Other modes of injury have not been described or reported in the literature. Traumatic intubation in neonates can be encountered with potentially devastating consequences. This may result in vocal fold avulsion injuries or disruption of the normal glottic architecture and passage into a false lumen (Fig. 3) [19].

Styletted endotracheal tubes, if not carefully placed, may predispose the neonatal vocal folds to injury because of the delicate nature of this structure. Caution should be exercised when using a stylette to aid in placement of an endotracheal tube.

Epidemiology

This is a rarely encountered complication in the neonatal age group with only sporadic case reports in the literature.

Clinical Presentation

During evaluation of post-extubation stridor, traumatic vocal cord avulsion should be considered in the differential diagnosis.

Diagnosis

The history will reveal the nature of the glottic injury. Endoscopic visualization can be utilized to assess the extent.

Management

The choice of therapy is dependent on the extent of the injury and the health of the neonate. Some traumatic events involving the neonatal vocal folds are unrepairable and have resulted in irreversibly poor outcomes. If the airway is impacted, a tracheostomy tube may be necessary to bypass the area of injury and to allow for healing or reconstruction. However, if the injury is mild, then conservative management strategies should be entertained, including observation with or without medical management of reflux. If an avulsion injury is encountered, anatomic realignment of the injured vocal musculature and mucosal covering may be pursued. This is followed by a short period of intubation, with the endotracheal tube serving as a stent. Reparative granulomas can occur, and may need to be addressed if large and impacting the airway (see previous section on Granulomas).

Conclusion

The vocal needs and abilities of neonates are unique and significantly different than at any other period of time in their life. The impact of the voice on the child's development is impossible to predict at such a young age. Therefore, conservative management and assurance of airway safety are the most important aspects of the management of the neonatal larynx. Awareness of associated dysphagia and aspiration is imperative in order to avoid soiling of the lungs. A multidisciplinary approach to the evaluation and management of these disorders is important, as the larynx is the gateway to respiration, phonation, and swallowing.

References

1. Andreassi MG, Picano E. Reduction of radiation to children: our responsibility to change. Circulation. 2014;130(2):135–7.
2. Benjamin JR, Smith PB, Cotten CM, Jaggers J, Goldstein RF, Malcolm WF. Long-term morbidities associated with vocal cord paralysis after surgical closure of a patent ductus arteriosus in extremely low birth weight infants. J Perinatol. 2010;30(6):408–13.
3. Boseley ME, Hartnick CJ. Development of the human true vocal fold: depth of cell layers and quantifying cell types within the lamina propria. Ann Otol Rhinol Laryngol. 2006;115(10):784–8.
4. Buhler RB, Sennes LU, Mauad T, Melo EC, Silva LF, Saldiva PH. Collagen fiber and versican distribution within the lamina propria of fetal vocal folds. Laryngoscope. 2008;118(2):371–4.
5. Dewan K, Cephus C, Owczarzak V, Ocampo E. Incidence and implication of vocal fold paresis following neonatal cardiac surgery. Laryngoscope. 2012;122(12):2781–5.
6. Hartnick CJ, Rehbar R, Prasad V. Development and maturation of the pediatric human vocal fold lamina propria. Laryngoscope. 2005;115(1):4–15.
7. Jephson CG, Mills NA, Pitt MC, et al. Congenital stridor with feeding difficulty as a presenting symptom of Dok7 congenital myasthenic syndrome. Int J Pediatr Otorhinolaryngol. 2010;74(9):991–4.
8. Kelly SM, April MM, Tunkel DE. Obstructing laryngeal granuloma after brief endotracheal intubation in neonates. Otolaryngol Head Neck Surg. 1996;115(1):138–40.
9. Lam DW, Abdullah V, van Hasselt CA. Intubation granuloma in a neonate. Otolaryngol Head Neck Surg. 1999;120(3):447–8.
10. Mace M, Williamson E, Worgan D. Autosomal dominantly inherited adductor laryngeal paralysis—a new syndrome with a suggestion of linkage to HLA. Clin Genet. 1978;14(5):265–70.
11. Miyamoto RC, Cotton RT, Rope AF, et al. Association of anterior glottic webs with velocardiofacial syndrome (chromosome 22q11.2 deletion). Otolaryngol Head Neck Surg. 2004;130(4):415–7.
12. Raza SA, Mahendran S, Rahman N, Williams RG. Familial vocal fold paralysis. J Laryngol Otol. 2002;116(12):1047–9.
13. Rizzardi E, Tagliaferro T, Snijders D, et al. Unilateral laryngeal paralysis in a newborn with congenital varicella syndrome. Int J Pediatr Otorhinolaryngol. 2009;73(1):115–8.
14. Roberts D, McQuinn T, Beckerman RC. Neonatal arytenoid dislocation. Pediatrics. 1988;81(4):580–2.
15. Rosenberg TL, Schweinfurth JM. Cell density of the lamina propria of neonatal vocal folds. Ann Otol Rhinol Laryngol. 2009;118(2):87–90.
16. Rutter MJ. Endoscopic management of bilateral vocal fold immobility [oral presentation]. Las Vegas (NV): American Society of Pediatric Otolaryngology; 2014.
17. Schweinfurth JM, Thibeault SL. Does hyaluronic acid distribution in the larynx relate to the newborn's capacity for crying? Laryngoscope. 2008;118(9):1692–9.
18. Smith ME, King JD, Elsherif A, Muntz HR, Park AH, Kouretas PC. Should all newborns who undergo patent ductus arteriosus ligation be examined for vocal fold mobility? Laryngoscope. 2009;119(8):1606–9.
19. Wohl DL. Traumatic vocal fold avulsion injury in a newborn. J Voice. 1996;10(1):106–8.

Laryngeal and Tracheal Clefts

David A. Gudis and David R. White

Etiology

A laryngeal cleft is a rare congenital anomaly of the upper aerodigestive tract characterized by a slit defect of the wall separating the laryngotracheal complex and the pharyngoesophageal complex. A laryngeal cleft (LC) is a defect limited to the posterior larynx, including the interarytenoid region with or without extension into the posterior cricoid plate, allowing communication between the larynx anteriorly and the hypopharynx posteriorly. A laryngotracheoesophageal cleft (LTEC) is a defect extending into the cervical or thoracic trachea, allowing communication between the larynx and trachea anteriorly and the hypopharynx and esophagus posteriorly. Although the anomaly has been described as far as back as 1792, its diagnosis was not definitively confirmed and published until an autopsy report in 1949 [1, 2]. While the diagnosis and treatment of LCs has developed substantially since then, the understanding and management of clefts continue to evolve today.

Epidemiology

Laryngeal clefts are very uncommon, representing approximately 0.5–1.5 % of congenital laryngeal anomalies [3]. The reported incidence varies widely by series from 1 in 2,000 to 1 in 20,000 live births [4–7]. However, many investigators believe that LCs are more common than previously thought, and in recent years the reported incidence has increased. Minor cases that may have been overlooked in the past appear to be diagnosed with increasing frequency, most likely due to an improved understanding of the pathology among practitioners, improved diagnostic methods, and the development of tertiary airway centers with experienced clinicians. Among patients evaluated operatively for related symptoms, the incidence is as high as 6–8 % with a slight male predominance [8–10]. Most cases are sporadic, though various inheritance patterns have been described [11].

D.A. Gudis, M.D. • D.R. White, M.D. (✉)
Department of Otolaryngology—Head and Neck Surgery, Medical University of South Carolina, Charleston, SC, USA
e-mail: whitedr@musc.edu

Pathogenesis

The embryology of LCs is controversial and incompletely described. The trachea and esophagus share a common lumen until they are separated by a septum in the fifth to sixth week of gestation. The abnormal development of the septum may result in a spectrum of congenital aerodigestive anomalies including esophageal atresia, tracheoesophageal fistulae, and clefts [12]. Risk factors include prematurity, polyhydramnios, and intrauterine exposure to drugs and alcohol, although the exact pathogenesis remains unclear [11, 13, 14].

Various theories exist to explain the normal embryological development of the aerodigestive system. The endoderm of the foregut develops from the fourth and sixth branchial arches, and the cricoid cartilage from the mesenchyme of the sixth arch [15]. Some investigators have suggested that, as the bilateral branchial complexes form the aerodigestive structures, lateral ridges arise into the common lumen and fuse in the midline to form a septum in a caudal to cranial direction between the ventral laryngotracheal complex and the dorsal pharyngoesophageal complex [16]. Therefore, an earlier arrest of septum development results in a longer defect and subsequently more severe congenital cleft [17]. However, some authors question the existence of lateral ridges as they have not been identified in animal studies, and suggest that the respiratory diverticulum develops from a stalk from the ventral aspect of the foregut and elongates to form the definitive airway, while the ventral foregut mesenchyme develops into the tracheoesophageal septum [18]. Still others have posited that apoptotic mechanisms may play a role in the developmental anatomy [19].

J. Lioy and S.E. Sobol (eds.), *Disorders of the Neonatal Airway: Fundamentals for Practice*,
DOI 10.1007/978-1-4939-1610-8_9, © Springer Science+Business Media New York 2015

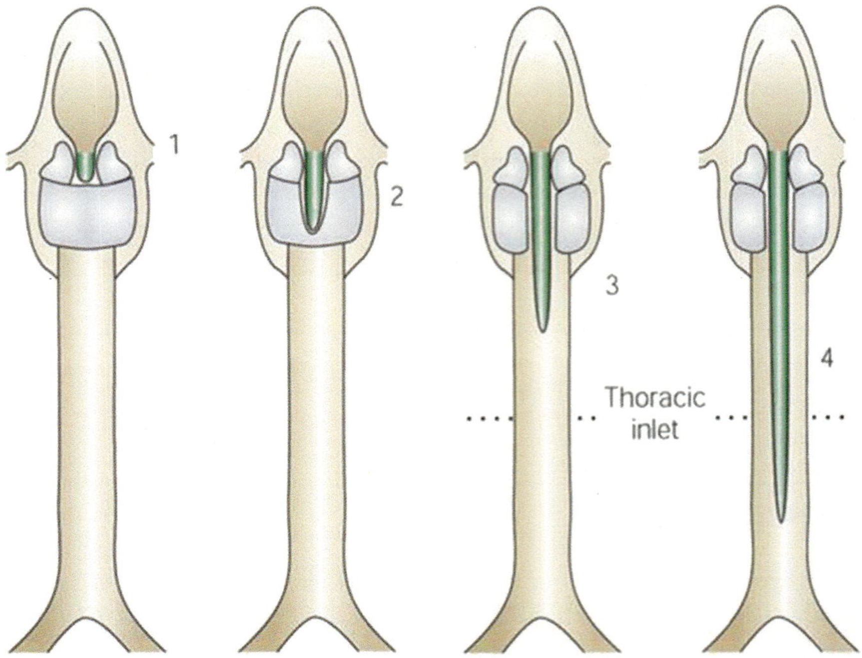

Fig. 1 The Benjamin and Inglis cleft classification

There are several structural and cellular models to explain the potential mechanisms for the failure of normal tracheoesophageal development. The intraembryonic pressure theory suggests that the development of the heart and the curvature of the cervical spine may lead to tension and distraction of the esophageal structures, resulting in failure of septum development. The epithelial occlusion theory states that the abnormal recanalization of the esophagus from its initial solid stage results in abnormal septum development. The vascular occlusion theory suggests that an aberrant vessel leads to vascular insufficiency and secondary failure of normal tissue development. Lastly, the differential cell growth theory suggests that the septum fails to develop due to abnormal cellular differentiation in that region [3, 18].

Various classification schemes have been published to distinguish laryngeal clefts based on their size and severity. The Benjamin and Inglis classification remains the most widely recognized (Fig. 1). The **Type I LC** is a supraglottic interarytenoid cleft, above the level of the vocal cords. The **Type II LC** extends into the cricoid cartilage beyond the level of the vocal cords. The **Type III LTEC** extends beyond the cricoid cartilage into the cervical trachea. And the **Type IV LTEC** extends beyond the thoracic inlet into the intrathoracic trachea and esophagus and occasionally into a mainstem bronchus [12]. Additional modifications have been made to the classification scheme for the purposes of reporting surgical technique, including description of a submucosal or occult laryngeal cleft, which may have functional consequences albeit without obvious anatomic abnormality [7, 20] In addition to the abnormal conduit between the respiratory and digestive tracts seen in LCs, there is frequently redundant mucosa along the cleft margin which contributes to airway obstruction [16].

Clinical Presentation

Respiratory and feeding difficulties are the hallmark symptoms of LCs, though they are generally nonspecific. The clinical presentation and severity of symptoms correlate to the extent of the cleft, and the acuity of presentation may range from incidental diagnosis of an asymptomatic cleft to neonatal life-threatening respiratory distress.

Type I and some Type II LCs can be asymptomatic or present with stridor, persistent coughing or choking with feeds, regurgitation, hoarseness, failure to thrive, stridor, shortness of breath, and recurrent aspiration pneumonia. Type II LCs and Type III LTECs tend to present with the same symptoms but worse in frequency and severity. Cyanosis with feeds, chronic aspiration pneumonia, and increased airway obstruction with stridor may be seen; noninvasive airway support with positive pressure or oxygen supplementation may be required. Type IV LTECs are marked by early respiratory distress and require emergent intervention.

Over 50 % of patients with LCs have an associated syndromic or nonsyndromic congenital abnormality, and the severity of the cleft may correspond with the incidence of concurrent anomalies [3, 6, 21, 22]. The most frequently identified concurrent pathologies are related to the aerodigestive system and include tracheomalacia, tracheoesophageal fistula, laryngomalacia, and gastroesophageal reflux. Other reported malformations include gastrointestinal (esophageal atresia, microgastria, imperforate anus), genitourinary (hypospadias, kidney anomalies), craniofacial (Pierre Robin sequence, cleft lip with or without cleft palate, choanal atresia), and cardiac and cardiovascular disorders (ventricular septal defect, aorta anomalies) [3, 15, 23].

Laryngeal clefts have been identified as part of several well-described syndromes, including Opitz-Frias Syndrome (cleft lip, cleft palate, hypospadias, external ear anomalies, and hypertelorism) and Pallister-Hall syndrome (central neurologic system anomalies, imperforate anus, cardiac, pulmonary, renal, and distal extremity abnormalities). LCs may also be seen with CHARGE syndrome (coloboma, heart defects, atresia of the nasal choanae, retardation of growth, genitourinary defects, and ear defects), Down Syndrome, and the spectrum of 22q11 deletion syndromes. Additionally, LCs have been identified as part of the congenital VACTERL association (vertebral anomalies, anal atresia, cardiac anomalies, tracheoesophageal fistulae, ear, renal, and limb anomalies).

Diagnosis

As the symptoms of a LC are nonspecific, the differential diagnosis is broad and includes laryngomalacia, tracheomalacia, tracheoesophageal fistula, gastroesophageal reflux, neuromuscular dysphagia, esophageal stricture, cricopharyngeal spasm, and unilateral or bilateral vocal cord paralysis. Even when the presentation is subtle, early definitive diagnosis is critical to an optimal outcome since chronic aspiration can lead to failure to thrive and chronic interstitial lung damage [22].

As with most pediatric airway pathology, endoscopic operative evaluation with microlaryngoscopy and rigid bronchoscopy is the mainstay of diagnosis and should be performed in any patient with persistent coughing, choking with feeds, stridor, respiratory distress, hoarseness, or recurrent aspiration pneumonia. The diagnosis of LC must be kept in mind during evaluation, as it can be easily missed when redundant mucosa prolapses into the cleft. The endoscopy is generally performed under general anesthesia with spontaneous ventilation, as endotracheal intubation would preclude an adequate exam. Several operative techniques have been described to examine the posterior laryngotracheal complex. Regardless of preferred technique, the interarytenoid space must be carefully examined and palpated to determine the presence and extent of a LC. Since flexible laryngoscopy and flexible bronchoscopy lack the required exposure and access for palpation, rigid endoscopy is the gold standard when evaluating for a LC (Fig. 2). Over one third of patients with a LC may also have a tracheoesophageal fistula; therefore, the initial identification of a cleft must not obviate the completion of a thorough bronchoscopic evaluation [6, 24]. The diagnosis of the Type I LC can be particularly challenging, as the symptoms are mild and the clefts subtle [8, 9, 21].

Several ancillary tests have proven useful in conjunction with endoscopy. Flexible fiberoptic laryngoscopy with the patient awake should be performed to determine vocal cord function and the presence and severity of potential concurrent laryngomalacia. A modified barium swallow and FEES (fiberoptic endoscopic examination of swallowing) examination are valuable for diagnosing and quantifying aspiration. It should be noted, however, that aspiration is a nonspecific finding for a LC and that normal swallow studies do not rule out the diagnosis of a cleft. Chest radiography can demonstrate findings of aspiration pneumonia and the development of interstitial lung disease. Finally, flexible bronchoscopy and bronchoalveolar lavage for lipid laden macrophages may quantify the severity of aspiration and help to predict which patients will benefit most from early surgical therapy [5]. When a LC is identified, a systemic evaluation is required to rule out concurrent congenital anomalies, including genetic, cardiothoracic, genitourinary, gastrointestinal, vertebral, and neurologic assessment.

Management

The treatment of LCs varies based on the extent of the cleft and the severity of the symptoms, but the underlying management principles are consistent. Airway protection is always the immediate concern and must be addressed first. When required, respiratory support should be delivered by noninvasive means if possible, such as nasal continuous or biphasic positive airway pressure, rather than prolonged endotracheal intubation. Intubation may lead to additional trauma and inflammation of the planned surgical site. When tracheotomy is required for severe clefts or due to associated tracheomalacia, it is ideally placed distal to the caudal end of the cleft to minimize contact of the tracheostomy tube with the surgical site. For severe Type IV LTECs, mainstem bronchus intubation may be emergently required to secure the airway.

Medical Management

Type I and some Type II LCs are often approached first with medical management, frequently initiated by a primary care physician, gastroenterologist, or pulmonologist prior to otolaryngology referral for endoscopic evaluation. Control of gastroesophageal reflux is the cornerstone of medical therapy. Proton-pump inhibitors, thickened feeds, upright positioning during feeds, and a speech and swallow evaluation may all be required for optimal reflux control, although it is not uncommon for patients with severe clefts to require ultimately gastrostomy tubes with or without Nissen fundoplication.

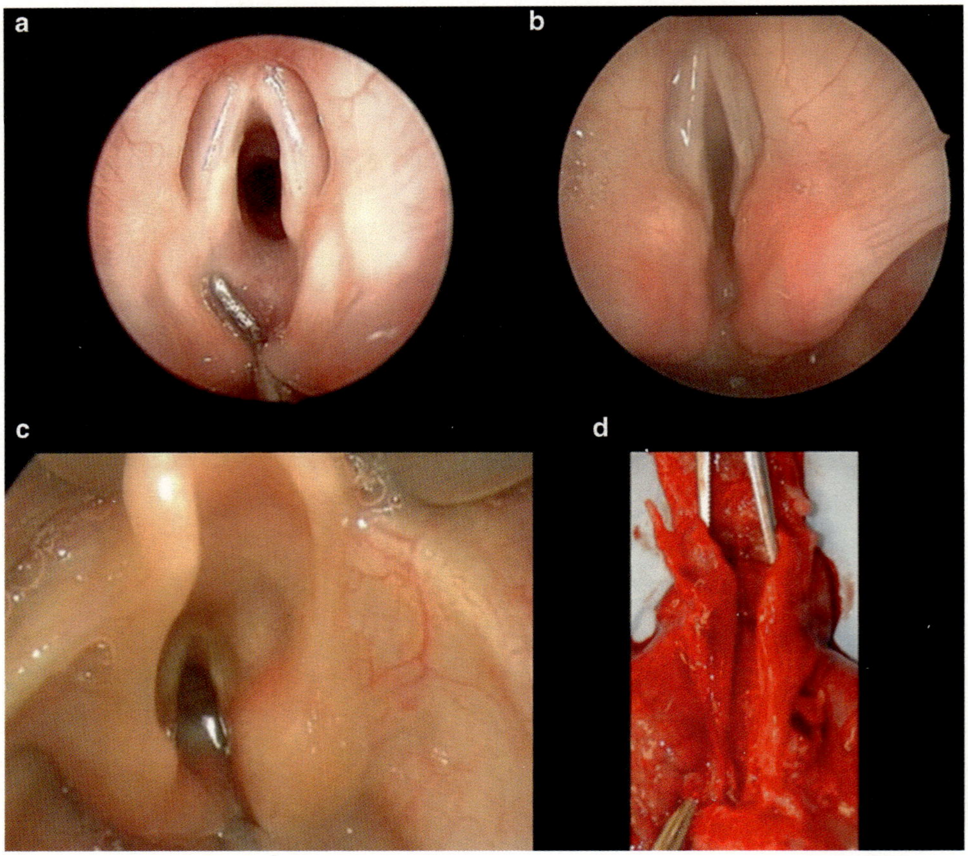

Fig. 2 (**a**) Type 1, (**b**) Type 2, (**c**) Type 3, (**d**) postmortem specimen of a Type 4 LTEC

Medical management alone may be sufficient for Type I and some Type II LCs. Furthermore, aggressive control of reflux has the added benefit of minimizing inflammatory changes to the cleft tissue and thus optimizing outcomes of surgery if required, as reflux is a risk factor for failure of cleft repair [25]. In patients whose symptoms persist despite medical therapy, early surgery has long been advocated [10]. Controversy remains regarding the regimen and time course of maximal medical therapy, and data conflict as to how many of such patients will ultimately require surgical intervention [8, 9, 21, 22].

Endoscopic Repair

With advances in endoscopic techniques in recent years, the endoscopic surgical approach has been widely applied to Type I LCs, Type II LCs, and some Type III LTECs. The endoscopic approach has several advantages: avoidance of an anterior cervical incision; reduced risk of laryngeal destabilization from an anterior laryngofissure in the setting of a known posterior cricoid deficiency; reduced need for postoperative intubation or tracheotomy; reduced risk of recurrent laryngeal nerve injury; and reduced risk of wound infection, breakdown, or fistula [7].

Prior to endoscopic or open surgery for laryngeal clefts, any other major congenital anomalies that might complicate surgery or anesthesia, such as cardiothoracic pathology, should be addressed first if possible. Laryngeal cleft surgery is ideally performed under general anesthesia with spontaneous ventilation. Inhalation anesthetic agent with judicious oxygen supplementation can be administered via an endotracheal tube placed in the hypopharyx above the larynx. The patient can then be intubated readily for desaturation or decompensation. Alternatively, the use of total intravenous anesthesia without an inhalation agent has also been described, with jet ventilation used intermittently when necessary [26]. The procedure can be performed with the patient intubated when necessary, but exposure is limited and the endotracheal tube can lead to excessive pressure on the surgical wound. In these settings, the smallest endotracheal tube to provide adequate ventilation should be used. The largest laryngoscope that can be accommodated is suspended to maximize surgical exposure.

Since the first report of laryngeal cleft surgery in 1955, the two-layer closure has been advocated and remains the fundamental principle of endoscopic or open surgical repair [27]. Using carbon dioxide laser or cold steel microlaryngeal instruments, two distinct mucosal planes are dissected into the cleft margin: an anterior laryngotracheal mucosal plane and a posterior pharyngoesophageal mucosal plane. Interrupted absorbable sutures are then placed in a caudal to cranial direction, usually posteriorly and then anteriorly for maximal access. Various methods of suturing and knot-tying have been described, and satisfactory results can be achieved using simple or mattress sutures, with either buried or extramucosal knots. Additionally, for Type I LCs, success has also been reported with endoscopic injection laryngoplasty with absorbable gelatin or calcium hydroxylapatite [23].

Open Repair

Open surgery is recommended for some Type III LTECs, Type IV LTECs, and some revision cleft surgery [28]. As these patients may have severe airway compromise, once the airway is secure the procedure may begin with a tracheostomy. Other practitioners have advocated using extracorporeal membrane oxygenation or intraoperative cardiopulmonary bypass to avoid the risks of the endotracheal or tracheostomy tube against the surgical site [17, 29]. Several surgical approaches to the cleft have been described, including an anterior cervical approach with laryngotracheal fissure, an anterior cervicothoracic approach, and a lateral pharyngotomy. The infant trachea is approximately 5 cm from subglottis to carina; therefore, even some Type IV LTECs with low intrathoracic extension can at times be repaired with an anterior cervical approach and no sternotomy or thoracotomy [17, 30]. A novel anterior cervical approach to the Type IV LTEC has recently been described, whereby a cricotracheal separation is performed to reflect the trachea anteriorly and expose the cleft [31].

Regardless of approach, the principle of a multilayer closure remains important. On one side of the cleft, a mucosal incision and submucosal dissection into the tracheal surface is performed 4–5 mm from the cleft margin. On the other side of the cleft, a mucosal incision and submucosal dissection into the esophageal mucosa is performed 4–5 mm from the cleft margin. Thus, with the creation of two distinct planes on either side of the cleft, the anterior mucosal planes and posterior mucosal planes can be opposed and repaired with longitudinal suture lines slightly offset rather than directly overlying one another. The posterior pharyngoesophageal closure is performed first with interrupted absorbable suture. A costal cartilage graft may be placed in the cleft of the posterior cricoid cartilage plate in a manner similar to laryngotracheal reconstructive surgery. Usually an autologous fascial graft is interposed between the two layers for added reinforcement. Various grafts have been described for this purpose, including tibial periosteum, sternal periosteum, pericardium, strap muscles, and temporalis fascia [15, 17, 28]. The anterior laryngotracheal mucosa is closed last.

Outcomes and Complications

With advances in diagnostic and therapeutic techniques, complications of LCs have fortunately reduced. The success of Type I LC and Type II LC management as measured by clinical cough, aspiration, and feeding difficulty may be as high as 80–90 %. The prognosis depends significantly on the extent of the cleft and presence of associated anomalies or comorbidities [14].

For more severe LCs, tracheobronchomalacia may remain a significant issue, sometimes resulting in the need for tracheostomy even after successful operation and perioperative period [32]. Persistent aspiration or dysphagia may also be seen, which likely reflects neuromuscular dysphagia, persistent structural pathology, or postoperative esophageal dysmotility. Breakdown of the repair may occur in up to 15 % of open approaches [28]. The presence of severe reflux and concurrent tracheoesophageal fistula both appear to be risk factors for wound breakdown [25, 33]. When breakdown of the repair occurs, revision surgery almost always requires an open approach with laryngotracheal fissure, as an intact closure at the cephalad end of the cleft would limit endoscopic access to the area of dehiscence.

Mortality of clefts overall has reduced substantially from approximately 46 % down to 6–25 % [4, 16]. A Type IV LTEC remains a life-threatening emergency with high mortality, although it too has reduced from 93 % or higher to approximately 50 % [4, 29, 32, 34, 35]. However, in over half of deaths in patients with LCs, the death is secondary to an associated anomaly and not the cleft itself [6, 28].

Multidisciplinary Considerations

Pediatric airway pathology is best served with a multidisciplinary approach. For LCs and LTECs, specialists to optimize patient care and outcomes include: otolaryngology, anesthesiology, neonatology, pediatric intensive care, pulmonology, gastroenterology, general surgery, cardiothoracic surgery, genetics, nutrition therapy, speech therapy, and intensive care level nursing.

Future Considerations

As the diagnosis becomes considered and identified more frequently, airway centers may be able to amass greater series of patients for better study of management considerations with the hope of reducing the rate of complications and mortality.

References

1. Richter CF. Dessertatio Medico de infanticide in artis obstetriciae [thesis for doctor of medicine]. Leipzig; 1792.
2. Finlay HV. Familial congenital stridor. Arch Dis Child. 1949;24:219.
3. Pezzettigotta SM, Leboulanger N, Roger G, Denoyelle F, Garabédian E-N. Laryngeal cleft. Otolaryngol Clin North Am. 2008;41:913–33.
4. Roth B, Rose KG, Benz-Bohm G, Günther H. Laryngo-tracheo-oesophageal cleft. Clinical features, diagnosis and therapy. Eur J Pediatr. 1983;140:41–6.
5. Kieran SM, et al. The lipid laden macrophage index as a marker of aspiration in patients with type I and II laryngeal clefts. Int J Pediatr Otorhinolaryngol. 2010;74:743–6.
6. Evans KL, Courteney-Harris R, Bailey CM, Evans JN, Parsons DS. Management of posterior laryngeal and laryngotracheoesophageal clefts. Arch Otolaryngol Head Neck Surg. 1995;121:1380–5.
7. Sandu K, Monnier P. Endoscopic laryngotracheal cleft repair without tracheotomy or intubation. Laryngoscope. 2006;116:630–4.
8. Parsons DS, Stivers FE, Giovanetto DR, Phillips SE. Type I posterior laryngeal clefts. Laryngoscope. 1998;108:403–10.
9. Chien W, et al. Type 1 laryngeal cleft: establishing a functional diagnostic and management algorithm. Int J Pediatr Otorhinolaryngol. 2006;70:2073–9.
10. Myer CM, Cotton RT, Holmes DK, Jackson RK. Laryngeal and laryngotracheoesophageal clefts: role of early surgical repair. Ann Otol Rhinol Laryngol. 1990;99:98–104.
11. Phelan PD, Stocks JG, Williams HE, Danks DM. Familial occurrence of congenital laryngeal clefts. Arch Dis Child. 1973;48:275–8.
12. Benjamin B, Inglis A. Minor congenital laryngeal clefts: diagnosis and classification. Ann Otol Rhinol Laryngol. 1989;98:417–20.
13. Mangat HS, El-Hakim H. Injection augmentation of Type 1 laryngeal clefts. Otolaryngol Head Neck Surg. 2012;146:764–8.
14. Rahbar R, et al. Endoscopic repair of laryngeal cleft type I and type II: when and why? Laryngoscope. 2009;119:1797–802.
15. Kubba H, Gibson D, Bailey M, Hartley B. Techniques and outcomes of laryngeal cleft repair: an update to the Great Ormond Street Hospital series. Ann Otol Rhinol Laryngol. 2005;114:309–13.
16. Leboulanger N, Garabédian E-N. Laryngo-tracheo-oesophageal clefts. Orphanet J Rare Dis. 2011;6:81.
17. Mathur NN, Peek GJ, Bailey CM, Elliott MJ. Strategies for managing Type IV laryngotracheoesophageal clefts at Great Ormond Street Hospital for Children. Int J Pediatr Otorhinolaryngol. 2006; 70:1901–10.
18. Merei J, Hutson J. Embryogenesis of tracheo esophageal anomalies: a review. Pediatr Surg Int. 2002;18:319–26.
19. Metzger R, Wachowiak R, Kluth D. Embryology of the early foregut. YSPSU. 2011;20:136–44.
20. Tucker GF, Maddalozzo J. 'Occult' posterior laryngeal cleft. Laryngoscope. 1987;97:701–4.
21. Watters K, Russell J. Diagnosis and management of type 1 laryngeal cleft. Int J Pediatr Otorhinolaryngol. 2003;67:591–6.
22. Thiel G, Clement WA, Kubba H. The management of laryngeal clefts. Int J Pediatr Otorhinolaryngol. 2011;75:1525–8.
23. Cohen MS, et al. Injection laryngoplasty for Type 1 laryngeal cleft in children. Otolaryngol Head Neck Surg. 2011;144:789–93.
24. Rahbar R, et al. The presentation and management of laryngeal cleft: a 10-year experience. Arch Otolaryngol Head Neck Surg. 2006;132:1335–41.
25. Hof E, Hirsig J, Giedion A, Pochon JP. Deleterious consequences of gastroesophageal reflux in cleft larynx surgery. J Pediatr Surg. 1987;22(3):197–9.
26. Ferrari LR, Zurakowski D, Solari J, Rahbar R. Laryngeal cleft repair: the anesthetic perspective. Paediatr Anaesth. 2013;23:334–41.
27. Pettersson G. Inhibited separation of larynx and the upper part of trachea from oesophagus in a newborn; report of a case successfully operated upon. Acta Chir Scand. 1955;110:250–4.
28. Monnier P. Pediatric airway surgery. Heidelberg: Springer; 2010.
29. Geller K, Kim Y, Koempel J, Anderson KD. Surgical management of type III and IV laryngotracheoesophageal clefts: the three-layered approach. Int J Pediatr Otorhinolaryngol. 2010;74:652–7.
30. Lee KS, Yang CC. Tracheal length of infants under three months old. Ann Otol Rhinol Laryngol. 2001;110:268–70.
31. Propst EJ, Ida JB, Rutter MJ. Repair of long type IV posterior laryngeal cleft through a cervical approach using cricotracheal separation. Laryngoscope. 2013;123:801–4.
32. Simpson BB, et al. Type IV laryngotracheoesophageal clefts: surgical management for long-term survival. J Pediatr Surg. 1996;31:1128–33.
33. Walner DL, Stern Y, Collins M, Cotton RT, Myer III CM. Does the presence of a tracheoesophageal fistula predict the outcome of laryngeal cleft repair? Arch Otolaryngol Head Neck Surg. 1999; 125:782.
34. Imbrie JD, Doyle PJ. Laryngotracheoesophageal cleft report of a case and review of the literature. Laryngoscope. 1969;79(7): 1252–72.
35. Kawaguchi AL, Donahoe PK, Ryan DP. Management and long-term follow-up of patients with types III and IV laryngotracheo-esophageal clefts. J Pediatr Surg. 2005;40:158–65.

Congenital Tracheal Stenosis

Michael J. Rutter, J. Drew Prosser,
and Alessandro deAlarcón

Overview

Compromised tracheal airflow in neonates is a rare but potentially life-threatening occurrence. Management of these infants is always subservient to the etiology of the tracheal compromise, and this compromise may be a consequence of any one of the following clinical scenarios: (1) extrinsic compression of the trachea (e.g., vascular compression); (2) a problem of the tracheal exoskeleton without the presence of stenosis (e.g., tracheomalacia); (3) a problem of the tracheal exoskeleton with stenosis (e.g., complete tracheal rings (CTRs), sleeve trachea, absent tracheal rings); and (4) an intraluminal obstruction with an adequate exoskeleton (e.g., congenital tracheal web). We will limit our discussion to an overview of the etiology, clinical presentation, and management of the three conditions that fall within the classification of problems of the tracheal exoskeleton with stenosis. We will also present a detailed description of the slide tracheoplasty procedure, which is now considered the operation of choice for the management of these conditions.

M.J. Rutter, M.B.Ch.B., F.R.A.C.S. (✉)
A. deAlarcón, M.D., M.P.H.
Division of Pediatric Otolaryngology—Head and Neck Surgery,
Cincinnati Children's Hospital Medical Center,
3333 Burnet Avenue, Cincinnati, OH 45229-3039, USA

Department of Otolaryngology—Head and Neck Surgery,
University of Cincinnati College of Medicine,
Cincinnati, OH, USA
e-mail: Mike.Rutter@cchmc.org

J.D. Prosser, M.D.
Division of Pediatric Otolaryngology—Head and Neck Surgery,
Cincinnati Children's Hospital Medical Center,
3333 Burnet Avenue, Cincinnati, OH 45229-3039, USA

Epidemiology, Etiology, and Pathogenesis

Congenital tracheal stenosis encompasses a wide range of anomalies resulting from aberrant embryogenesis of the respiratory system. It is infrequently seen and has an estimated incidence of 1 in 64,500 births [1]—representing only 0.3–1 % of all laryngotracheal stenoses [2]. A frequently cited article by Hoffer et al. [3] describes the associated embryologic processes and timing of the developmental aberrations that lead to the various manifestations of tracheal narrowing. As these authors point out, lung development begins during weeks 3 and 4 of gestation. The developing lung buds give rise to the trachea, infraglottis, and the glottic opening. By week 8 of gestation, the mesenchymal rudiments of the tracheal cartilages are present. During weeks 9 and 10, the cartilages form fibroelastic tissue, and smooth muscle is incorporated into the trachea. Hoffer and his colleagues postulate that (1) aberrant development in week 4 of gestation affects the developing respiratory and hepatic primordia and cause the more severe forms of the disease, which are associated with anomalies such as heart and skeletal malformations and that (2) aberrant development between gestational weeks 8 and 10 is confined to the developing cartilages and their supporting tissues. Abnormalities during this second critical time point likely result in less severe stenosis with fewer associated anomalies.

Clinical Presentation

Infants with compromised tracheal airflow classically present with biphasic stridor within the first weeks of life. Over the first few months of life, symptoms exacerbate, with retractions, dying spells, and severe deterioration occurring during intercurrent upper respiratory tract infections. Children with distal tracheal stenosis usually have a characteristic biphasic wet-sounding breathing pattern that transiently clears with coughing; this pattern is referred to as "washing machine breathing."

J. Lioy and S.E. Sobol (eds.), *Disorders of the Neonatal Airway: Fundamentals for Practice*,
DOI 10.1007/978-1-4939-1610-8_10, © Springer Science+Business Media New York 2015

Because the growth of the trachea is not commensurate with the growth of the infant over the first few months of life, decompensation frequently occurs around 4 months of age [4]. Important to note, however, even a neonate with a life-threatening tracheal stenosis may have surprisingly few symptoms.

Complete Tracheal Rings

CTRs are the most common etiology of congenital tracheal stenosis. In a normal trachea, luminal support is provided by C-shaped cartilaginous rings with a posterior sheet of muscle (the trachealis) completing the ring (Fig. 1a–c). In the infant with CTRs, the cartilaginous rings are circular and may affect varying lengths of the trachea. In addition, the trachealis muscle is absent. The diameter of the affected tracheal segment is always smaller than the trachea above that segment; however, the degree of stenosis may range from mild to severe. A classification system developed by Speggiorin et al. [5] delineates a number of recognizable morphological patterns. Of these patterns, the most frequently seen are: (1) CTRs that are of reasonable size proximally, but that cone down to a small distal ring close to the carina; (2) the "stovepipe" airway with a long segment of CTRs of similar diameter; (3) a short-segment stenosis, often in the mid-trachea; and (4) CTRs associated with a high tracheal (or pig) bronchus. More than 75 % of patients also have other congenital anomalies that may be severe. A relatively recent study conducted at Cincinnati Children's Hospital indicated that 60 % of patients with CTRs had cardiovascular abnormalities, particularly a pulmonary artery sling (21 %) [6].

Diagnostic Workup

The initial evaluation should include plain airway films, as these may indicate that congenital tracheal narrowing is present. Although imaging studies may be very useful, bronchoscopic evaluation remains the gold standard for definitive assessment. This should be performed with extreme care, as instrumentation in an area of stenosis may cause enough swelling to convert a narrow airway to a critical airway, necessitating abrupt intervention. If the smallest bronchoscope available (whether rigid or flexible), cannot be easily passed through the area of stenosis, it is better to identify the proximal extent of the stenosis without fully evaluating the distal airway. Good communication with anesthesia colleagues is essential, and to facilitate the bronchoscopy, the child should be spontaneously breathing. We recommend the use of sevoflurane and propofol; steroid administration is also advisable. The trachea is then suctioned with a soft 6 Fr catheter and the patient is preoxygenated. Next, a further propofol bolus is delivered to temporarily halt respiratory efforts during the bronchoscopy.

Ideally, the aims of endoscopic evaluation are: to confirm the diagnosis of tracheal stenosis; establish whether this is due to CTRs; estimate the size of the smallest ring; estimate the percentage of the airway involved with CTRs as well as the position of the rings within the trachea; and evaluate the bronchial anatomy.

In patients with distal tracheal stenosis, an adequate evaluation cannot be made with a ventilating bronchoscope, as even the smallest ventilating bronchoscope is too large for most complete rings. The Hopkins rod telescope (removed from the bronchoscope) should thus be introduced into the airway to assess the stenosis. The initial bronchoscopic view is often sufficient to establish the diagnosis, thereby avoiding the risk of airway edema.

Estimating the size of the airway is valuable. In a normal full-term neonate, the narrowest point of the airway is at the cricoid, and this should measure 4.5–5.5 mm. Subglottic stenosis is defined as an airway diameter of <4.0 mm (by comparison, a 2.5 mm endotracheal tube has an outer diameter of 3.6 mm). Although the trachea should be of greater capacity than the cricoid, the airway in patients with CTRs may be too small to easily permit safe passage of any form of instrumentation. For comparative purposes, the smallest Storz 2.5

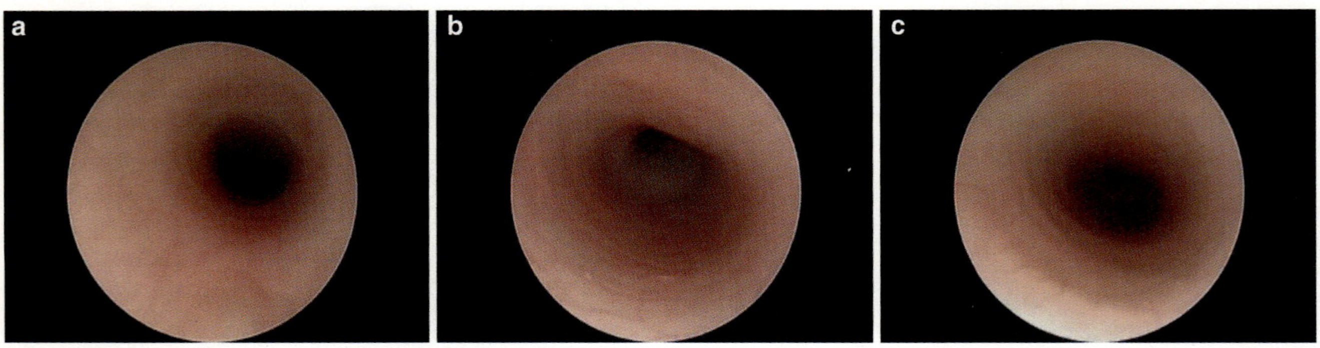

Fig. 1 Endoscopic views of a child with long-segment complete tracheal rings. (**a**) View showing beginning of rings; (**b**) view showing mid-section of rings; (**c**) view showing distal segment of rings

ventilating bronchoscope has an outer diameter (OD) of 3.7 mm. The smallest 20017 Hopkins rod telescope (as found in the Storz 2.5 ventilating bronchoscope) has an OD of 1.9 mm.

Because 50 % of children with CTRs have a tracheal inner diameter of approximately 2 mm at the time of diagnosis, the standard interventions for managing a compromised airway are not applicable. More specifically, the smallest endotracheal tube (2.0 mm inner diameter [ID]; 2.9 mm OD) and the smallest tracheotomy tube (2.5 mm ID; 3.9 mm OD) cannot pass through the stenotic segment without severe damage to mucosa or tracheal rupture. As the stenosis usually extends to the carina, bypassing the stenosis risks bronchial intubation. This may leave extracorporeal membrane oxygenation (ECMO) as the only viable alternative for stabilizing the child in the event of decompensation following bronchoscopy. In an effort to avoid ECMO in a child who is decompensating and poorly ventilating, intubation proximal to the complete rings is preferable. The endotracheal tube should be sized to the cricoid, with the Murphy eye just below vocal fold level. Given that it is unusual for the proximal two tracheal rings to be complete, shallow intubation is achievable in most children with CTRs. A nasal intubation to allow tube stabilization (as it is so shallow) is advisable. Ventilation requires a long inspiratory phase and an even longer expiratory phase to allow air to pass the stenosis. Higher than typical ventilator pressures may be tolerated, as the stenosis ensures that the lungs are not exposed to the same pressures as the subglottis. Maintenance of high humidity levels is crucial, as mucus accumulation may be lethal and is often heralded by rising CO_2 rather than low oxygen saturation. In a crisis, 1 mL of 1:10,000 epinephrine delivered down the endotracheal tube may assist ventilation. If possible, extubation is desirable, as most children with CTRs maintain ventilation more effectively themselves than on a ventilator. To prevent mucus accumulation, saline may be regularly nebulized if required.

In view of the high proportion of patients with other congenital anomalies, a thorough diagnostic investigation should include a contrast-enhanced computed tomography (CT) scan of the chest with three-dimensional reconstruction, and an echocardiogram. These tests will identify any coexisting cardiovascular pathology, which should be repaired concurrently with the tracheal repair. As mentioned earlier in this chapter, our clinical experience indicates that a pulmonary artery sling is the most common cardiovascular anomaly; intracardiac anomalies and the presence of a persistent left superior vena cava draining to the coronary sinus, with absence of the innominate vein are, however, also frequently seen. Other anomalies may be incidental (e.g., limb or central nervous system anomalies) or also affect the airway. Nearly one third of children with CTRs have a tracheal (or pig) bronchus, and subglottic stenosis is present in approximately 20 % [6]. Rarely, CTRs may coexist with a tracheoesophageal fistula or laryngeal cleft. Pulmonary anomalies may also occur, with subsegmental branching patterns almost universally aberrant, though of limited significance. Pulmonary hypoplasia or agenesis, more commonly affecting the right lung, is more significant, as it may cause mediastinal shift and aortic compression of the already stenotic trachea.

Although most children with CTRs require early tracheal reconstruction, some (10–15 %) have sufficient tracheal growth to avoid the need for reconstruction. A further 10–15 % eventually outgrows their trachea and requires late repair. The recommended surgical technique is the slide tracheoplasty (discussed later in this chapter). This approach yields significantly better results than any other tracheal reconstruction technique and is applicable to all anatomic variants of CTRs [6, 7].

Most children with CTRs have distal tracheal involvement. If the distal one-third of the trachea is involved or if there are coexistent cardiovascular anomalies that require repair, we recommend repair utilizing cardiopulmonary bypass. More than 90 % of children requiring slide tracheoplasty for CTRs fall into this category. If only the upper or mid-trachea is involved, repair may be performed with routine anesthesia through a cervical approach. Hyperextension of an infant's neck over a shoulder roll allows good access to the upper two thirds of the trachea through a cervical approach. Exposure can be further enhanced through a limited upper sternotomy if required.

Sleeve Trachea

Albeit extremely rare, tracheal sleeve is the second most common condition falling within the general classification of problems involving the tracheal exoskeleton with stenosis. In infants with this condition, the trachea consists of a single sheet of cartilage rather than 15–20 separate tracheal rings; this cartilaginous sheet may extend proximally into the cricoid and distally into the bronchi. Sleeve trachea is universally associated with a craniosynostosis syndrome, with Pfeiffer, Crouzon, and Apert syndromes, represented in that order [8]. Nonetheless, only a small number of patients with craniosynostoses have a sleeve trachea, and even fewer have associated tracheal obstruction with the posterior aspects of the tracheal cartilage overlapping, effacing the trachealis muscle (Fig. 2). In these cases, a slide tracheoplasty is still an effective reconstructive option, although technically more challenging than a straightforward repair of CTRs. Of note, most children with sleeve trachea have multiple levels of airway obstruction from the choana to the bronchi. Although a slide tracheoplasty may therefore not prevent the need for a tracheotomy, in some children, it does, however, allow for the safe placement of a tracheotomy.

Absent Tracheal Rings

Although compromised tracheal airflow in exoskeletal problems with stenosis usually results from abnormalities in cartilage structure, an infant may also present with stenosis or collapse resulting from an absence of cartilage [9]. This extremely rare condition generally presents in an otherwise normal child as an isolated segment of trachea (usually just proximal to the carina) that is missing cartilage in a two- to three-ring segment (Fig. 3a, b). Clinical presentation is similar to that in infants with complete tracheal rings; however, bronchoscopically the stenotic segment lacks cartilage and is therefore distensible. While most affected children are otherwise normal, we have seen associated congenital left vocal fold paralysis as well as esophageal atresia.

Management

Endoscopic techniques such as balloon dilation rarely have a role in the treatment of congenital tracheal stenosis. More specifically, they are contraindicated in the management of CTRs, as the risk of tracheal rupture is high. Balloon dilation may, however, have a role after reconstruction if restenosis occurs.

Although a number of approaches for repairing congenital tracheal stenosis have historically been used (i.e., pericardial patch, cartilage grafts, resection, and autografts), these approaches have been replaced by the slide tracheoplasty. This operation marks a clear turning point in the management of tracheal stenosis, as outcomes have dramatically improved since its inception. Although three decades ago the diagnosis of tracheal stenosis carried a mortality rate of 50–80 %, the survival rate currently exceeds 90 %. In essence, a patient's prognosis is now less about the compromised tracheal airway than about concomitant congenital anomalies.

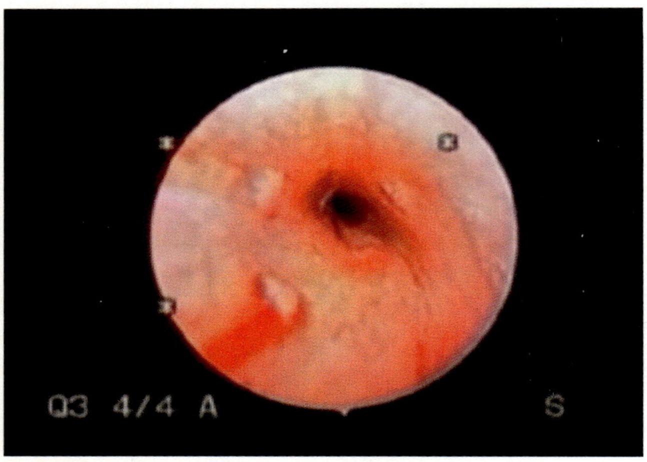

Fig. 2 Endoscopic view of sleeve trachea

Slide Tracheoplasty

Conceived by Goldstraw [10] in the 1980s and popularized by Grillo [11] in the 1990s, the slide tracheoplasty was originally designed as an operation to repair congenital tracheal stenosis caused by CTRs. Although this procedure may be performed using ECMO or jet ventilation, we prefer to use cardiopulmonary bypass to facilitate the repair [6, 7, 12]. Aside from the advantage of not requiring ventilation during the procedure, access is also enhanced, as the lungs and heart may be relatively "deflated." Typically, a sternotomy allows for exposure of the trachea, placement of atrial and aortic cannulae, and repair of any coexisting cardiovascular anomalies. Removal of the carinal lymph nodes facilitates tracheal exposure and mobilization. The extent of the tracheal stenosis is then assessed. The assessment usually requires bronchoscopic examination of the airway while a 30-gauge needle is placed into the trachea from the mediastinal side; this allows the proximal and distal extent of the stenosis to be precisely identified within the chest. The length of the stenosis is then measured and its midpoint is marked. Next, the trachea is transected at or just proximal to the midpoint of the stenosis, with the transection being slightly bevelled (anterior proximal to posterior distal). The transected trachea is

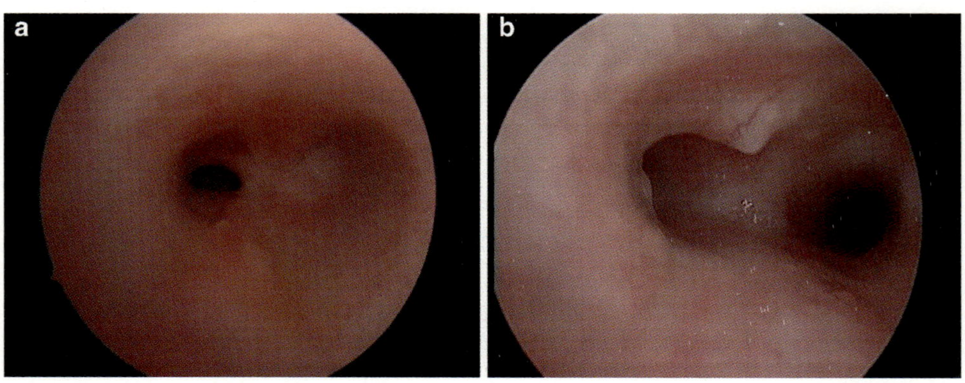

Fig. 3 Pre- and postoperative views of absent cartilage. (**a**) preoperative view; (**b**) postoperative view

mobilized by dissecting free the soft tissue attachments between the trachea and the esophagus of both the proximal and distal segments. Care is taken to preserve some lateral attachments to maintain a blood supply as well as to protect the vagus and recurrent laryngeal nerves. The distal segment is split posteriorly through all complete rings (to carina or down a bronchus if required) and the proximal segment is split anteriorly through the area of stenosis and into normal trachea. At the split, the trachea may be trimmed to round off either end at the transection margins to facilitate the closure. The anastomosis is commenced from distal posterior (carinal) in a running fashion using appropriately sized double-armed PDS sutures (usually 6–0 PDS in infants). Four to six throws of the suture are generally placed at the carina and tightened with a nerve hook. The anastomosis is then continued up the left and right sides of the trachea, with the sutures placed through cartilage and mucosa, therefore being exposed intraluminally. An effort is made to evert the lateral sides of the anastomosis to prevent internal bunching of the anastomotic lines (a "figure 8" trachea). Before the anastomotic suture lines rejoin in the midline at the proximal anterior aspect of the repair, the trachea is suctioned clear. The anastomosis is completed with a single proximal knot being thrown, leak tested (to 35 cm water pressure), and marked with Ligaclips applied to the proximal and distal ends of the anastomosis (for aid in radiographic positioning of the endotracheal tube). Fibrin glue is then applied to the anastomosis. The patient is reintubated and taken off cardiopulmonary bypass, and the chest is closed. At completion of the procedure, the airway is re-evaluated with a flexible bronchoscope to ensure that the repair is adequate and that blood and secretions are suctioned. A 2.8 mm flexible bronchoscope with a suction port can be placed into a 3.5 mm endotracheal tube and still allow for ventilation during the evaluation. If the patient's cardiovascular status permits, extubation is usually achieved within 24 h [12].

The slide tracheoplasty is an extremely versatile procedure [6]. If necessary, it is possible to slide: the entire length of the trachea; own a bronchus; into the anterior cricoid; or past a tracheal (pig) bronchus. The intrathoracic slide tracheoplasty may also be used to repair stenosis associated with absent tracheal rings, a sleeve trachea, or distal tracheoesophageal fistula repair. In addition, it may be used to repair an acquired tracheal stenosis.

The success of the intrathoracic slide tracheoplasty for long- or short-segment tracheal stenosis prompted us to use this technique to manage tracheal stenosis involving the more proximal trachea [13]. The upper half to two thirds of the trachea is accessible through a cervical approach, and the slide tracheoplasty is an effective method of repairing acquired upper tracheal stenosis, often in conjunction with partial resection of the most severely stenotic tracheal segment. The technique is similar to the intrathoracic slide, with the anastomosis commencing at the distal posterior aspect of the repair. In older children with a more proximal stenosis, the risk of developing a "figure 8" trachea is higher, and a temporary intrathoracic silicone stent may be placed for a week or more if required.

A child is typically extubated 24–96 h postoperatively. During this time we try to minimize positive pressure ventilation so as not to endanger the anastomosis. Chest drains are ideally left in place until after the extubation. Preoperatively, some children may present unstable and ventilated; rarely, some may be on ECMO support. In these circumstances, postoperative ECMO may be required. The aim is to establish endotracheal ventilation and remove the child from ECMO as rapidly as possible.

Most complications associated with the slide tracheoplasty have no long-term consequence. The "figure 8" trachea (lateral bunching of the anastomosis) seen in the majority of patients tends to spontaneously resolve over subsequent months and rarely causes obstruction or requires intervention. Although recurrent laryngeal nerve palsy occurs in less than 20 % of patients, it is usually unilateral and transient. Restenosis is rare, as is anastomotic dehiscence. Restenosis is more likely to occur at the proximal end of a slide tracheoplasty when a tracheal bronchus is present at this apex; it may be prevented by extending the slide two or three rings higher, proximal to the tracheal bronchus, into normal trachea.

Multidisciplinary Considerations

In view of the complexity of infants with the conditions described above and the likelihood that they may have serious coexisting conditions, syndromes, and/or anomalies (e.g., bronchial stenosis, lung agenesis or hypoplasia, craniosynostosis, cardiac disease), we cannot overemphasize the importance of a multidisciplinary team approach to management. The success rate at our own institution reflects the close collaborative efforts of a team comprising experienced pediatric subspecialists in otolaryngology, anesthesiology, pulmonology, critical care, and cardiothoracic surgery. The slide tracheoplasty is an operation with a steep learning curve, and research clearly shows that optimal outcomes are achieved through a team approach at a center of excellence [6, 14].

Future Considerations

Although slide tracheoplasty has markedly improved outcomes for children with congenital stenosis, there are circumstances in which this procedure does not provide a stable, viable, long-term solution. The two most common circumstances are (1) children with partial or total tracheal agenesis and (2) children in whom previous tracheal reconstruction has failed, with resultant damage to the tracheal exoskeleton that may be caused by infection. In these clinical scenarios, the ideal solution is to replace the trachea.

Historically, tracheal homografting was fraught with problems, frequently related to long-segment grafts with delayed reepithelialization. Tracheal homografting with pre-epithelialized or pre-vascularized segments of homograft trachea, zenograft trachea, or synthetic biologic scaffolds seeded with a patient's own respiratory epithelium does, however, offer promise. Pre-epithelialized homograft tracheal replacement remains an area of research that is being refined. Despite highly publicized cases, this is not yet a reality.

Acknowledgement The authors wish to thank Aliza P. Cohen for her assistance in writing this chapter.

References

1. Herrera P, Caldarone C, Forte V. The current state of congenital tracheal stenosis. Pediatr Surg Int. 2007;23:1033–44.
2. Ho AS, Koltai PJ. Pediatric tracheal stenosis. Otolaryngol Clin North Am. 2008;41:999–1021.
3. Hoffer ME, Tom LWC, Wetmore RF, et al. Congenital tracheal stenosis. The otolaryngologist's perspective. Arch Otolaryngol Head Neck Surg. 1994;120:449–53.
4. Rutter MJ, Cotton RT. Tracheal stenosis and reconstruction. In: Mattei P, editor. Surgical directives: pediatric surgery. Philadelphia: Lippincott Williams & Wilkins; 2003. Chap. 24.
5. Speggiorin S, Torre M, Roebuck DJ, et al. A new morphologic classification of congenital tracheobronchial stenosis. Ann Thorac Surg. 2012;93:958–61.
6. Manning PB, Rutter MJ, Lisec A, et al. One slide fits all: the versatility of slide tracheoplasty with cardiopulmonary bypass support for airway reconstruction in children. J Thorac Cardiovasc Surg. 2011;141:155–61.
7. Rutter MJ, Cotton R, Azizkhan R, et al. Slide tracheoplasty for the management of complete tracheal rings. J Pediatr Surg. 2003;38: 928–34.
8. Lertsburapa K, Schroeder Jr JW, Sullivan C. Tracheal cartilaginous sleeve in patients with craniosynostosis syndromes: a meta-analysis. J Pediatr Surg. 2010;45:1438–44.
9. Rutter MJ, Vijayasekaran S, Salamone FN, et al. Deficient tracheal rings. Int J Pediatr Otorhinolaryngol. 2006;70:1981–4.
10. Tsang V, Murday A, Gillbe C, Goldstraw P. Slide tracheoplasty for congenital funnel-shaped tracheal stenosis. Ann Thorac Surg. 1989;48:632–5.
11. Grillo HC, Wright CD, Vlahakes GJ, MacGillivray TE. Management of congenital tracheal stenosis by means of slide tracheoplasty or resection and reconstruction, with long-term follow-up of growth after slide tracheoplasty. J Thorac Cardiovasc Surg. 2002;123:145–52.
12. Manning PB, Rutter MJ, Border WL. Slide tracheoplasty in infants and children: risk factors for prolonged postoperative ventilatory support. Ann Thorac Surg. 2008;85:1187–91; discussion 1191–2.
13. de Alarcón A, Rutter MJ. Cervical slide tracheoplasty. Arch Otolaryngol Head Neck Surg. 2012;138:812–6.
14. Kocyildirim E, Kanani M, Roebuck D, et al. Long-segment tracheal stenosis: slide tracheoplasty and a multidisciplinary approach improve outcomes and reduce costs. J Thorac Cardiovasc Surg. 2004;128:876–82.

Tracheobronchomalacia

Eric E. Berg and John McClay

Etiology

Malacia is a term derived from the Greek word "malakia," meaning soft. Tracheomalacia and bronchomalacia, therefore, refer to softening of the trachea and bronchi, respectively. This anatomic softening of the cartilaginous airway elements, atrophy of the longitudinal elastic fibers of the posterior wall (pars membranacea), and/or decreased tone of myoelastic elements prevent the trachea from maintaining its shape through the stress of the respiratory cycle leading to collapse and intermittent airway obstruction [16, 39]. Tracheomalacia (TM) may be localized to a small portion of the trachea or may involve it entirely, and when the mainstem bronchi are involved the term tracheobronchomalacia (TBM) is used.

Epidemiology

Tracheomalacia is the most common congenital disorder of the trachea [28]. It was first described by Holinger et al. [29], and later defined by Baxter and Dunbar [5] as a condition in which the tracheal walls are weak from softening of cartilage and hypotonia of supporting myoelastic fibers [5, 29]. Tracheomalacia may be found in healthy infants, but is more commonly seen in premature infants [30]. Pediatric bronchoscopic series have noted observed rates of airway malacia between 15 and 57 % [17, 23, 30, 35, 43]. The incidence of primary malacia, that is airway malacia in otherwise normal infants without extrinsic vascular compression or other causative pathology, has been estimated to be at least 1 in 1,445–2,100 children [12, 15]. Masters et al. noted a higher incidence in males, with a male to female ratio of roughly 2:1 [35].

Tracheomalacia is often associated with additional malacic sites as well as other abnormalities. Masters et al. evaluated a series of 299 patients with airway malacia in order to determine the frequency of isolated versus multi-site involvement. The group noted isolated tracheomalacia in 26.7 % of patients, isolated bronchomalacia in 34.4 % of patients, and some combination of tracheobronchomalacia in 48 %. When present, bronchomalacia was most commonly left-sided, with a ratio of left- to right-sided lesions of 1.6:1 (Fig. 1).

Other abnormalities associated with tracheomalacia include a variety of syndromes and additional aerodigestive, cardiac, and neurologic anomalies (Table 1). In their series, Masters et al. found that tracheomalacia was associated with tracheoesophageal fistula (TEF) in 9.7 %. Eight percent of patients had defined syndromes [35]. Studies have found cardiovascular anomalies in 14–58 % of patients with TM, including patent ductus arteriosus, atrial or ventricular septal defects, vascular ring anomalies such as double aortic arch or pulmonary artery sling, hypoplastic left or right heart, Tetralogy of Fallot and other conotruncal cardiac disorders (affecting the cardiac outflow tract), dextrocardia, and valvular stenosis [10, 33, 35]. Bronchopulmonary dysplasia may be seen in up to 52 % of infants with TM, and gastroesophageal reflux disease is seen in about half of such patients. Subglottic stenosis, laryngomalacia, vocal cord paralysis, neurologic impairment, and overall developmental delay may also occur in association with TM [16]. Interestingly, 24 % of patients with laryngomalacia, a much more common condition, have also been found to have more distal airway malacia involving the trachea and/or mainstem bronchi [35].

E.E. Berg, M.D. (✉)
Division of Pediatric Otolaryngology,
Department of Otolaryngology—Head & Neck Surgery,
University of Texas Southwestern Medical Center,
5323 Harry Hines Boulevard, Dallas, TX 75390-9035, USA
e-mail: Eric.Berg@UTSouthwestern.edu

J. McClay, M.D.
Frisco ENT for Children, Dallas, TX USA
e-mail: JTMcClay@AOL.com

J. Lioy and S.E. Sobol (eds.), *Disorders of the Neonatal Airway: Fundamentals for Practice*,
DOI 10.1007/978-1-4939-1610-8_11,

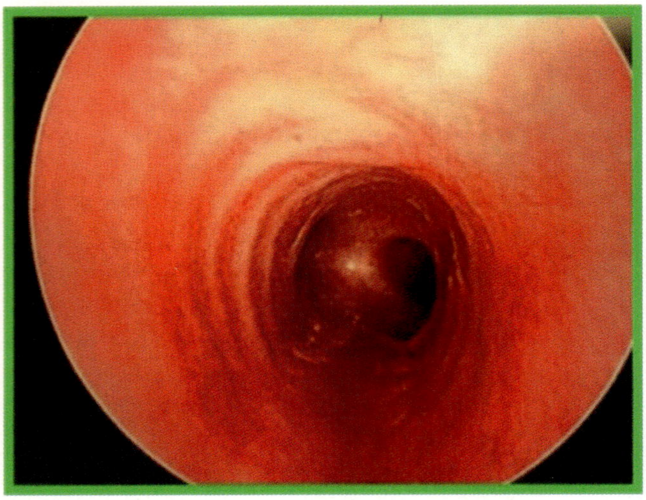

Fig. 1 Normal trachea with rigid cartilaginous support

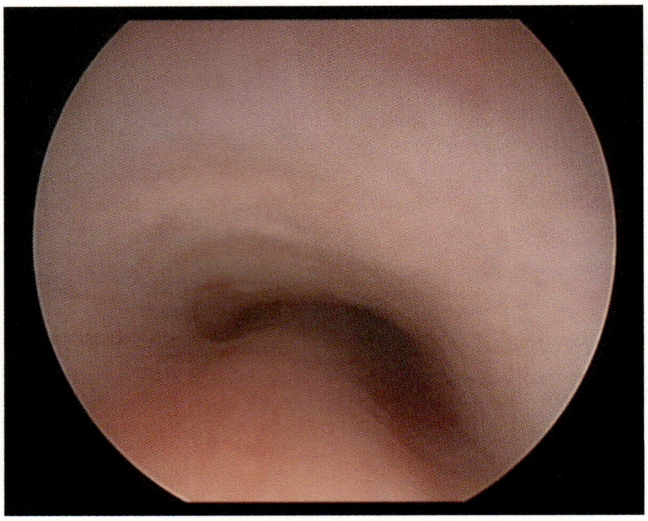

Fig. 2 Primary tracheomalacia with soft, collapsible cartilaginous support proximal to the carina

Table 1 Diseases associated with tracheobronchomalacia (adapted from [16])

Congenital (primary)	Acquired (secondary)
Normal infants (idiopathic)	*Prolonged intubation*
Prematurity	*Tracheotomy*
Pulsatile collapse with normal innominate artery	*Severe tracheobronchitis*
Congenital cartilage abnormalities	*Compressive*
Dyschondroplasia, chondromalacia, chondrodysplasia, polychondritis, Ehlers–Danlos syndrome	Vascular, cardiac, skeletal, tumors and cysts, infection, post-traumatic
Congenital syndromes associated with TBM	
Mucopolysaccharidosis (Hurler syndrome, Hunter syndrome), CHARGE syndrome, VATER anomaly, trisomy 9, trisomy 21, 22q11 deletion, DiGeorge syndrome, Pierre-Robin sequence, Pfieffer syndrome, Larsen syndrome	
Congenital anomalies associated with TBM	
Tracheoesophageal fistula, esophageal atresia with/without laryngeal cleft, bronchopulmonary dysplasia	

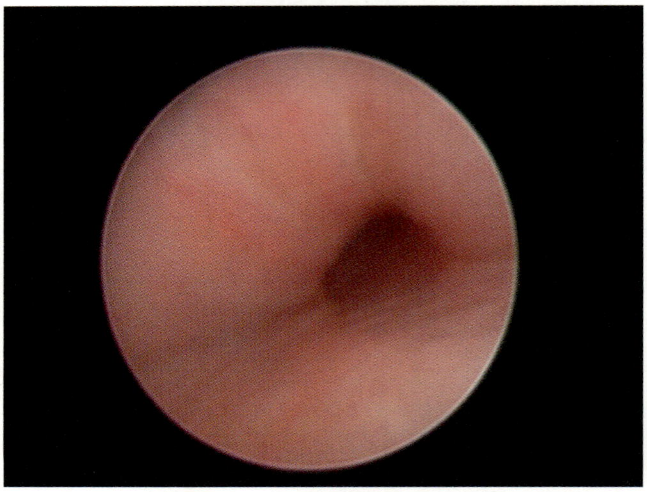

Fig. 3 Isolated left mainstem bronchomalacia

Pathogenesis

In order to fully understand the clinical presentation of a patient with tracheobronchomalacia, a brief review of the physical mechanics of the respiratory cycle is in order. In isolation, the natural tendency of the chest wall is to expand. Conversely, the natural tendency of the lungs is to collapse. In order to maintain inflation of the lungs, intrathoracic pressure must therefore be negative. With inspiration, the diaphragm contracts and descends and the chest wall expands, increasing thoracic volume and making intrathoracic pressure more negative. The lungs expand, and a gradient for airflow into the lungs is established. With expiration, the opposite occurs, and the lungs deflate until the gradient for airflow no longer exists.

Key to this model of normal pulmonary dynamics is that the trachea and bronchi maintain their shape in the face of fluctuating intrathoracic pressures. During inspiration, both intrathoracic pressure and intraluminal airway pressure are negative. During expiration, however, intrathoracic pressure becomes positive in relation to intraluminal airway pressure, and the cartilaginous rings of the normal trachea and bronchi serve to provide the necessary rigidity to resist the external force and prevent airway collapse (Fig. 2). If these cartilaginous elements fail to provide such support, as in tracheobronchomalacia, the airway collapses and obstruction occurs (Fig. 3).

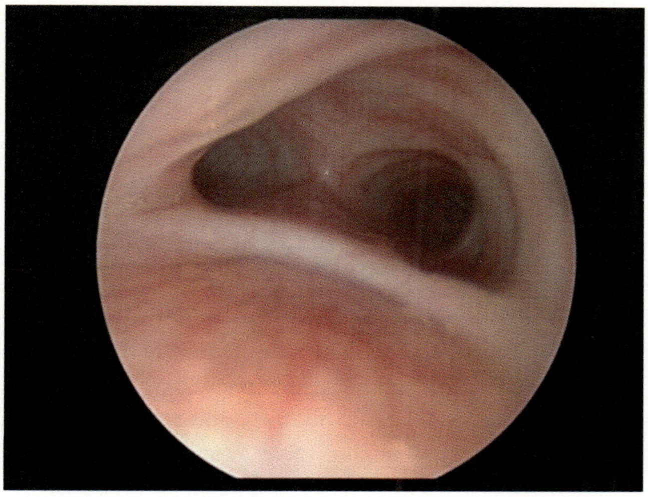

Fig. 4 Tracheomalacia in association with tracheoesophageal fistula

Baxter and Dunbar were the first to divide tracheomalacia into primary and secondary forms. Primary airway malacia was subsequently defined by Benjamin as isolated airway malacia in otherwise normal infants. Secondary airway malacia was defined as acquired malacia associated with TEF, esophageal atresia (EA), VATER/VACTERL association, vascular or external compression of the airways, or specific syndromes [6]. Disease processes that result in the formation of an abnormal cartilaginous matrix such as polychondritis and chondromalacia have since been included as primary forms, as have mucopolysaccharidoses such as Hunter syndrome and Hurler syndrome and other genetic syndromes [16].

Some controversy exists over the grouping of TM associated with TEF (Fig. 4) as an acquired rather than a congenital form of disease as there is inherent weakness of the involved portion of the trachea [16]. In 75 % of infants with TEF and EA, the trachea is more easily collapsible due to reduced circumference of tracheal cartilage and widening of the membranous trachea [50]. Blair and colleagues identified esophageal muscle in the histologic specimens taken from the posterior wall of the trachea in infants with TEF and/or EA. They subsequently proposed that idiopathic primary TM is actually the result of a defect in foregut division resulting in inherent tracheal weakness, just not severe enough to cause TEF or EA [10]. Others have supported the theory that congenital TM is due to faulty embryologic division of the foregut into the trachea and esophagus, suggesting that the trachea receives redundant tissue during separation with a subsequent decrease in structural integrity [33]. As a result of such findings, current classification schemes class TM associated with TEF under a primary, or congenital, form of disease (Table 1).

With such debate, Mair and Parsons were careful to reserve the term "tracheomalacia" for specific cases in which the posterior membranous wall of the trachea is widened. They noted a normal trachea to have a ratio of cartilage to posterior membrane of approximately 4–5:1, while in tracheomalacia this ratio approaches 2:1 [33]. In order to accommodate the entire spectrum of disease, they preferred to use the more encompassing term "major airway collapse" (MAC). They proposed a MAC classification system that includes three types. MAC Type I lesions represent congenital tracheal collapse due to abnormal cartilaginous development, including that seen in premature infants and those with EA, TEF, mucopolysaccharidoses, and Larsen syndrome. MAC type II lesions consist of tracheal collapse due to extrinsic compression alone. MAC type III lesions are acquired lesions, generally due to inflammatory stimuli such as severe or recurrent tracheobronchitis, gastroesophageal reflux disease, and intubation [33, 42].

Acquired TM is a result of the degeneration of normal cartilaginous support from a variety of causes and is slightly more common than congenital disease. MAC type III inflammatory lesions are the most common acquired lesion and are most often associated with prolonged endotracheal intubation with associated increases in airway pressure, oxygen toxicity, and recurrent infections [52]. Premature infants with respiratory distress syndrome are most commonly predisposed to the condition. One study of 50 infants with TM found that 52 % had "secondary" TM, and 96 % of these were premature infants with respiratory distress syndrome and a history of prolonged mechanical ventilation [30]. It should be noted, however, that it could be difficult to differentiate whether TM is truly a result of endotracheal intubation or a contributing factor in the need for endotracheal intubation from the outset [20, 30]. Tracheotomy also predisposes to TM, so a tracheotomy performed to help in management of primary TBM at one site may predispose to secondary tracheomalacia at the surgical site. Tracheotomy requires surgical interruption of the integrity of the tracheal rings, and over time the tube's presence may lead to cellular hypoxia and pressure necrosis due to impaired blood supply, tracheitis, and frictional mucosal damage [4, 22]. Finally, the role of gastroesophageal reflux as an inflammatory stimulus in the exacerbation and/or development of tracheomalacia may also be significant as it is more prevalent in children with large-airway malacia [9].

MAC type II lesions due to external tracheal compression present a less common form of acquired TM. Compression affects the integrity of the tracheal wall, at times severe enough to cause chronic obstruction but often only leading to transient collapse as intrathoracic pressure increases. Implicated structures and anomalies include double aortic arch (Fig. 5), abnormal branching of the innominate artery (Fig. 6), anomalous left pulmonary artery, right aortic arch with left ligamentum arteriosum, left atrial hypertrophy, and other vascular rings. Skeletal disorders such as scoliosis and

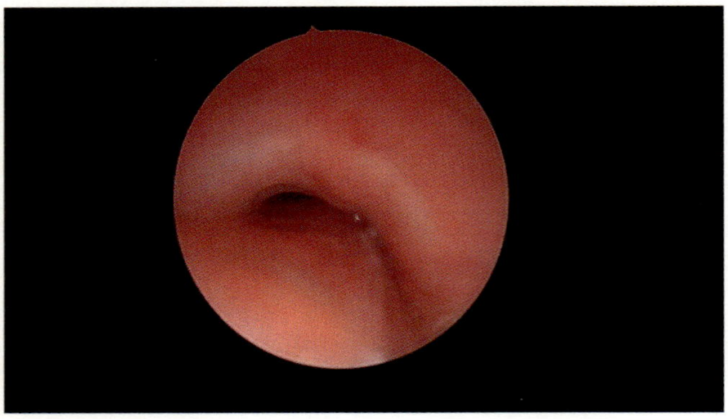

Fig. 5 Tracheomalacia in association with a double aortic arch

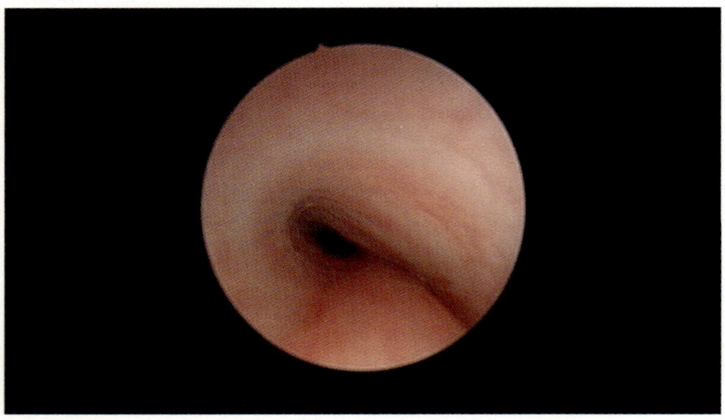

Fig. 6 Tracheomalacia in association with innominate artery compression and a large thymus

pectus excavatum may contribute as well. Mass lesions such as thymus enlargement, hemangiomas, lymphatic malformations, teratomas, other tumors, abscesses, cysts, and thyroid goiters are also implicated. Importantly, even after surgical relief of the compression, tracheal weakness and collapse may persist and require additional treatment [16].

Clinical Presentation

Since it was first defined in the 1950s and 1960s, the signs and symptoms of TBM have been classically described as appearing slowly over the first several weeks of life. A more recent study published in 1992, however, found that symptoms of primary TBM are apparent at birth in up to 95 % of infants [33]. Mild symptoms may include noisy breathing, intermittent stridor, and wheezing. More severe signs and symptoms include severe dyspnea, spontaneous hyperextension of the neck, increased work of breathing with retractions, cyanosis, and respiratory insufficiency or failure. Symptoms are often positionally dependent, better when prone and worse when supine. Generally, severe cases are detected in the neonatal period when patients present with acute episodes of severe obstruction, cyanosis, and desaturation and at times ventilator dependency. Recurrent lower airway infections and pneumonia may result from impaired mucociliary function as well as impaired clearance of secretions by the collapsed and obstructed airway lumen during cough [44].

The most common symptoms seen in isolated tracheobronchomalacia are expiratory stridor and a "brassy" or "barky" cough. Negative intraluminal pressure compared to intrathoracic pressure causes dynamic collapse of the insufficiently supportive cartilaginous elements of the airway. Airway obstruction can occur at any phase of respiration but is most pronounced with expiration, and resultant airway turbulence causes the high-pitched sound of stridor. The majority of the trachea and the entirety of the bronchi lie within the thoracic cavity and respond to changes in pressure accordingly.

While expiratory stridor is the most common presentation of tracheomalacia, it may be confused with the wheezing found in reactive airway disease or bronchiolitis. In all cases airway noise may worsen with activity or agitation as airflow increases. Similarly, it will generally worsen with upper respiratory tract infections as an already compromised airway becomes narrowed by edema and thicker, more abundant secretions. In contrast to the high-pitched and varied "squeaking" heard with the wheezing of reactive airway disease, the stridor associated with tracheomalacia is more centrally located and of a more uniform, slightly lower pitch. In addition, symptoms generally lessen when the patient is prone as the gravitational pressure of the intrathoracic structures on the collapsible airway present when supine is reversed. Symptoms that fail to improve when the patient is at rest or with positioning maneuvers should raise suspicion of fixed intraluminal airway obstruction or possible extrinsic airway compression.

Nevertheless, the classic presentation of tracheobronchomalacia as purely expiratory stridor may not always be so straightforward. A portion of the trachea is cervical and not subject to intrathoracic pressure. In addition, the underlying cartilaginous immaturity found in tracheomalacia is not uncommonly present in the larynx as well, causing laryngomalacia. Without the effect of negative intrathoracic pressure, these cervical structures are subject only to Bernoulli's principle. Briefly, an increase in airflow, i.e. during inspiration, causes a decrease in airway pressure. Intraluminal pressure becomes negative in relation to atmospheric pressure. Clinically insufficient airway support then allows collapse of the cervical airway and may cause *inspiratory* airway collapse and *inspiratory* stridor.

Though respiratory symptoms are generally the most alarming, feeding difficulties should not be overlooked. Dysphagia, regurgitation, cough, and cyanosis during feeding are not uncommon, particularly in association with vascular tracheal compression. During feeding, as the esophagus becomes engorged it may contribute to tracheal collapse and obstruction. Respiratory obstruction and desaturation may result, inhibiting the ability of the infant to feed normally and gain weight appropriately. Frequent interruption of feeding has been promoted as a means of preventing significant desaturation and cyanosis [10].

Finally, while the focus of this chapter is tracheobronchomalacia during the neonatal period, it should be noted that children with mild airway malacia may not present until after the neonatal period and will often have nonspecific symptoms such as rattling, wheeze, stridor, exercise intolerance, cough, and recurrent lower airway infections. In such patients it may be misdiagnosed as asthma, and due to its expected lack of response to standard asthma treatment may be further misdiagnosed as severe-persistent or therapy-resistant asthma [12].

Diagnosis

A thorough history and physical examination are critical as diagnosis is initially based upon the clinical presentation outlined above. As noted, TBM must be differentiated from asthma and other causes of intraluminal obstruction, and a high degree of suspicion is often necessary for accurate diagnosis. Reviews have demonstrated a mean delay from symptom onset to accurate diagnosis of 6–9 months [33, 47]. In mild cases with benign, intermittent noisy breathing that resolves at rest and with prone positioning and no evidence of clinically significant obstruction or increased work of breathing, clinical diagnosis may be sufficient. In cases where the diagnosis is in question, or when clinically apparent respiratory obstruction, increased work of breathing, and/or oxygen desaturation occurs, further diagnostic studies should be pursued.

The gold standard of diagnosis is operative bronchoscopy by an experienced airway endoscopist and anesthesia team. Communication between the surgeon and anesthesiologist is critical, as spontaneous ventilation is vital to achieving an accurate diagnosis. Only when the patient is breathing spontaneously, i.e. without positive-pressure support from the ventilator, can the dynamic airway collapse of tracheobronchomalacia be clearly seen. Therefore general inhalational anesthesia is necessary to avoid paralysis, heavy sedation, and positive-pressure ventilation that may impair recognition of dynamic airway collapse.

Based upon studies conducted in the 1960s by Wittenborg et al., a visualized decrease in airway diameter of >50 % is considered abnormal [54]. Most infants with TM will have >75 % collapse with complete collapse in up to 33 % of infants [54]. Collapse typically occurs in an anterior–posterior direction. Vascular compression may be appreciated with pulsatile collapse, and the level of collapse may help predict which vessel is likely to be the source of compression. A high riding innominate artery causes pulsatile compression of the anterior trachea a few centimeters above the carina, and compression of the mass with the bronchoscope will result in loss of the right upper extremity pulses. A double aortic arch, as the only complete vascular ring, will cause more pronounced pulsatile compression than other rings such as a right aortic arch with a left ligamentum arteriosum and aberrant left subclavian artery [46]. A pulmonary artery sling is classically associated with a "saber-shaped" tracheal stenosis and right middle segment bronchomalacia as the left pulmonary artery arises off of the right pulmonary artery and encircles the right mainstem bronchus and trachea as it courses between the trachea and esophagus towards the left lung [35].

Rigid bronchoscopy offers superior optics and, therefore better assessment of the tracheal mucosa and structure, with tracheal rings often distinct on visual inspection. It may be limited in its ability to assess past the level of the mainstem bronchi, however. Flexible bronchoscopy provides inferior image detail but may provide a more accurate picture of dynamic airway movement as less laryngeal manipulation is required to access the airway. Flexible bronchoscopy is also useful for assessing the distal bronchi for malacic change.

Tracheobronchomalacia's association with congenital heart lesions, especially conotruncal lesions, warrants consideration of a full cardiac evaluation when a diagnosis is made. Conotruncal heart defects as well as vascular rings have been described in association with 22q11 chromosomal defects such as DiGeorge syndrome and velocardiofacial syndrome, so providers should consider genetic and immunologic assessment for associated defects [35].

Nonoperative investigation is often invaluable in the evaluation and diagnosis of TBM and can be divided into static imaging, dynamic imaging, and spirometry. Static imaging includes plain films of the chest, chest CT, and chest MRI. Dynamic imaging generally includes airway fluoroscopy and esophagram, though development continues in using dynamic MRI and cine-CT as dynamic modalities. Diagnostic chest radiographs, as the most basic form of static imaging, include inspiratory and expiratory views. Tracheal narrowing may be seen on an expiratory film, and lung fields may demonstrate parenchymal abnormalities consistent with airway collapse and consolidation [35]. However, when compared to microlaryngoscopy and bronchoscopy, the sensitivity of plain films in diagnosing TM is only 62 % [51].

Airway fluoroscopy has been utilized in the evaluation of suspected TBM. Strauss et al. reported airway fluoroscopy to be as good as or even superior to bronchoscopy in the diagnosis of patients with combined stenosis and tracheomalacia [48]. A more recent study compared airway fluoroscopy to the gold standard of operative bronchoscopy and confirmed a specificity of 94 % for a diagnosis of tracheomalacia achieved by airway fluoroscopy. However, its sensitivity was only 20 % in detecting tracheomalacia, so its role as a screening study may be limited and further investigation is certainly warranted if clinical suspicion exists [7]. Barium esophagography may be useful when concern for associated TEF, EA, or reflux exists. It may also demonstrate esophageal compression due to a double aortic arch.

Computed tomography is a rapid and noninvasive diagnostic modality, often requiring no sedation that has demonstrated sensitivity of roughly 85 % in diagnosing airway lesions in children [24]. Advances in helical CT imaging have allowed images obtained at end-inspiration and during dynamic breathing to provide a noninvasive method for assessing tracheomalacia with studies demonstrating strong correlation between radiologic findings and bronchoscopy [11]. CT tracheobronchography gives three-dimensional airway renderings that depict the relationship of the external surface of the airway to adjacent structures, potentially valuable information in the assessment of complex airway abnormalities and specifically MAC type II compressive tracheomalacia [11]. Three-dimensional reconstruction also allows "virtual bronchoscopy," however, its utility in pediatric and especially neonatal populations has yet to be defined. The biggest limiting factor in the application of computed tomography in the evaluation of suspected TBM is exposure to ionizing radiation as well as iodinated contrast material when assessment of mediastinal vascular structures is desired. An increasing body of literature supports judicious use of CT and other studies involving ionizing radiation in children, even with pediatric dose reduction protocols, due to lifetime cancer risk [13, 25, 40].

Conversely, magnetic resonance imaging does not involve ionizing radiation. It is therefore the preferred modality for assessing paratracheal extrinsic airway abnormalities in children. Specifically, it is ideal for evaluating suspected MAC type II lesions such as vascular rings without the need for iodinated contrast agents. The primary disadvantage of MRI is that it requires either sedation, which may not be safe in patients prone to airway collapse, or intubation due to the length of the study. Dynamic MRI to avoid this has been evaluated in older populations [11]. From a practical standpoint, however, the inability of neonates and small infants to cooperate with breathing instructions will continue to limit the applicability of dynamic MRI and computed tomography techniques in this patient population.

Spirometry and flow-volume loops are noninvasive and repeatable methods to measure airflow and response to treatment. While other diagnostic modalities are useful for structural information, spirometry provides a functional assessment. In TBM the flow-volume loop may be flattened on expiration [19]. One can expect lower-than-expected values for mean peak expiratory flow, FEV1 and FEV1/FVC [12]. Unlike in asthma, these measures do not improve with bronchodilator therapy. Nevertheless, while its role in the evaluation and management of cooperative children is significant, pulmonary function testing is difficult and not routinely available for neonatal patients.

Management

Management is generally conservative, as the condition is benign and self-limiting in the majority of patients. Cartilaginous structures mature with age and provide better airway support. Conservative management may consist of simple observation with appropriate treatment of respiratory infections or may incorporate humidified air or oxygen and pulmonary physiotherapy as needed. Appropriate management of coexisting and possibly exacerbating conditions such as gastroesophageal reflux should be employed.

Historically, tracheotomy with long-term positive-pressure ventilation is the definitive treatment in those patients who fail to respond to conservative management. Jacobs et al reviewed 50 cases of TM in 1994 and found that 75 % of premature infants and 39 % of full-term infants required tracheotomy, with 71 % undergoing decannulation without further intervention at an average age of 30 months [30]. Other studies have reported the need for tracheotomy in infants with tracheomalacia to be anywhere from 12 to 62 % of infants [1, 2, 26, 33]. Even this "definitive" measure is not always sufficient, however, as custom tracheotomy tubes are often necessary to appropriately stent the diseased airway segment(s). Further complications include the risk of recurrent infections, as well as tracheal injury and scarring from the procedure and tube themselves. Frequent bronchoscopy and adjustment of tube length may be required as the child grows, and the presence of the tube may increase the risk of bronchospasm. Appropriate assessment of the ability to tolerate decannulation may also prove difficult. In a non-violated airway, positive intratracheal pressure that may help stent malacic segments can be generated against a closed glottis. With a tracheotomy present, the ability to generate this pressure is lost and true airway integrity becomes more difficult to evaluate. Assessment of the airway with a capped tracheotomy tube prior to decannulation is therefore essential [34].

Continuous positive airway pressure (CPAP), administered via nasal prongs, facemask, or tracheotomy is an effective treatment for TBM that prevents airway collapse by essentially creating a pneumatic stent [16]. Bronchoscopy [32, 36] and fluoroscopic evaluation [47] have confirmed the ability of CPAP to maintain airway patency during tidal respirations. The CPAP level can be adjusted based upon changing flow-volume measurements; however, more commonly it is adjusted based upon clinical response alone [16].

In their series, Jacobs et al. reported that CPAP was required for an average of 21.4 months in premature infants and 22.0 months in full-term infants [30]. In spite of its demonstrated efficacy, however, CPAP is not without its disadvantages, including delay in oral feeding, speech and language development, and the potential for overall developmental delay [30, 53].

Particularly within the first 6 months of life, airway smooth muscle plays a critical role in modulating the mechanical properties and dynamic behavior of the trachea [19]. Medical management with cholinergic agents (parasympathetic agonists) like bethanechol may help to support a malacic tracheobronchial tree by increasing smooth muscle tone. Panitch et al. demonstrated improvement in flow-volume curves following the administration of inhaled methacholine and oral bethanechol. Conversely, bronchodilation and relaxation of airway smooth muscle after albuterol administration had the opposite effect [39]. Ipratropium bromide has been utilized based on its similar mechanism of action. Neither has been widely studied in a prospective fashion.

In severe cases with recurrent infection, with dying spells, that do not respond to tracheotomy and positive pressure, or in whom tracheotomy and positive pressure ventilation somehow cannot be performed, more definitive surgical interventions such as stenting or thoracic surgery may be considered. It should first be noted, however, that patients with airway malacia deserve special consideration from an anesthetic standpoint. Like the intensive care team, the anesthesiologist must work to vigilantly minimize coughing and to prevent airway collapse and air trapping by judicious use of positive end-expiratory pressure [3].

Internal tracheal stenting is advantageous in that it is a less invasive approach, achieved endoscopically and with decreased surgical recovery time. Montgomery was the first to describe internal tracheal stent placement in 1965 [37]. He utilized a silicone stent, and since then a wide array of silicone and metal stents has been deployed. Metal stents are thinner with a wider intraluminal diameter and are more easily deployed overall. Silicone stents are more easily removed as the child outgrows the disease or requires larger stent placement. Both may cause significant complications, however, including airway obstruction from granulation tissue formation and stent migration. Granulation tissue is generally more problematic when metallic stents are utilized, so much so that endoscopic stent removal may be precluded and transthoracic approaches may be required. Currently, internal stents are only utilized for palliation and in situations in which more conventional therapies have failed. Resorbable biopolymer stents are in development and may have promise in overcoming current limitations [45].

Aortopexy has become a valuable procedure in the management of severe tracheomalacia and is considered the "gold standard" for surgical management, especially in cases caused by a vascular anomaly [49]. First described by Gross and Neuhauser in 1948, the procedure consists of a thoracotomy approach to the ascending aorta and placement of traction sutures from the adventitial layer of the aorta itself to the internal surface of the sternum [27]. By fixating the aorta anteriorly, the anterior–posterior dimension of the trachea is widened and the potential for clinically significant collapse is decreased. In a comparative study between intraluminal stents and aortopexy, Valerie et al. concluded that both treatment modalities are efficacious in severe cases. They did note, however, that although aortopexy has a higher perioperative complication rate, stents are more prone to long-term failure and morbidity and mortality [49]. Similarly, pexy of other compressive vessels may also be employed.

The flaccid trachea has been rigidly supported by external splinting using a variety of materials, including autologous costal cartilage along with a variety of prosthetic synthetics [16]. The supporting material is sutured directly to the trachea via a thoracotomy, cervical, or sternotomy approach depending upon the site of collapse. More recently the application of resorbable microplates to the lateral trachea has been described to support malacic segments [31]. Animal [14] and human studies [38], though limited, have not shown subsequent limitation of tracheal growth. While it may serve a valuable role in the care of patients with tracheomalacia, one must bear in mind that external tracheal stenting is not likely to adequately treat distal tracheal or bronchial malacia.

Additional surgical approaches have been reported with varied degrees of success, including tracheopexy, bronchopexy, segmental tracheal resection, and tracheal reconstruction [16]. Tracheal resection and primary anastomosis is efficacious in patients with short, focal malacic segments, however, this group represents only a small minority of affected patients overall [55]. Unfortunately, no perfect medical or surgical treatment exists for TBM and care must always be tailored to the individual patient.

Discussion of surgical interventions for TEF/EA and specific vascular anomalies associated with TM will be discussed elsewhere in this book.

Prognosis

In the majority of healthy and even premature infants, tracheobronchomalacia is generally a benign and self-limited condition associated with intermittent "noisy breathing" but without clinically significant obstruction or increased work of breathing. As a patient ages and airway structures mature, dynamic airway collapse no longer occurs. Conservative supportive care is generally all that is needed, including chest physiotherapy, humidified oxygen as needed, and treatment of infections. Symptomatic improvement is generally seen between 6 months and 1 year of age, and symptoms generally resolve by around 1–2 years of age [16]. As previously noted, there is a relatively higher incidence of respiratory illness due to poor mucociliary function and impaired ability to clear mucus and secretions past an obstructed tracheal lumen. When inflammatory or infectious respiratory illness occurs in patients with tracheomalacia, symptoms are often more pronounced and a more protracted course of illness can be expected.

A clinical severity scale has been described in which "mild" cases have respiratory difficulties only in association with infectious processes affecting the mucosa of the lower airway such as bronchitis or croup. "Moderate" cases present with stridor, wheezing, recurrent respiratory infections, and cyanosis with agitation, and other exacerbating factors. "Severe" cases are those in which children have stridor with normal respiration, significant difficulty with retained secretions, upper airway obstruction, reflex apnea, and in the most severe cases, cardiac arrest [18]. Reflex apnea, variably referred to as "death attacks," "dying spells," and "apneic spells," refers to reflexive respiratory arrest triggered by tracheal stimulation with secretions or compression by an engorged esophagus. It is felt to be the same mechanism by which infants may cease breathing during bronchoscopy, and may lead to cardiac arrest secondary to reflex apnea [33].

Patients with a more severe course of disease may also demonstrate increased work of breathing, oxygen desaturation, failure to thrive, and delayed development. Periodic episodes of apnea, cyanosis, and respiratory arrest ("death spells") may occur with ventilation-perfusion mismatch. Compression of the trachea by a full esophagus may cause periodic respiratory obstruction and oxygen desaturation. Failure to recognize or appropriately treat the condition may lead to significant morbidity and even mortality due to respiratory or cardiac arrest.

The mortality rate of patients with severe TM has been reported to be as high as 80 % [41]. Patients with connective tissue disorders and congenital syndromes are at even greater risk of more difficult disease course and poor outcomes. The prognosis of patients with TM secondary to a vascular ring should be considered distinct, however, with approximately 95 % long-term survival and nearly universal symptom relief after surgical correction. Further, while vocal cord paralysis is a known risk of surgery, the operation carries essentially no mortality in patients without coexisting cardiac defects [8].

Multidisciplinary Considerations

Tracheobronchomalacia may occur in isolation or in association with other anatomic abnormalities and syndromes. As noted, definitive diagnosis generally requires bronchoscopy by an appropriately trained endoscopist. Depending on the severity of disease, care may be managed by the pediatrician, neonatologist, or pediatric intensivist alone but will often require involvement of an otolaryngologist, pulmonologist, and cardiothoracic surgeon. When syndromes and associated anomalies are noted, a geneticist and additional services may be involved in care as appropriate.

Future Considerations

Management will continue to be patient-specific based upon observed symptomatology. In more severe cases requiring intervention, continued investigation into internal tracheal stenting and in particular stents composed of resorbable materials may provide a minimally invasive means of treatment without the problems of granulation and scar tissue previously noted with silicone and metallic stents. Research is ongoing [21, 45].

References

1. Altman KW, Wetmore RF, March RR. Congenital airway abnormalities requiring tracheotomy: a profile of 56 patients and their diagnoses over a 9 year period. Int J Pediatr Otorhinolaryngol. 1997;41:199–206.
2. Altman KW, Wetmore RF, March RR. Congenital airway abnormalities in patients requiring hospitalization. Arch Otolaryngol Head Neck Surg. 1999;125:525–8.
3. Austin J, Ali T. Tracheomalacia and bronchomalacia in children: pathophysiology, assessment, treatment, and anesthesia management. Paediatr Anaesth. 2003;13:3–11.
4. Azizkhan RG, Lacey SR, Wood RE. Anterior cricoid suspension and tracheal stomal closure for children with cricoid collapse and peristomal tracheomalacia following tracheostomy. J Pediatr Surg. 1993;28:169–71.
5. Baxter JD, Dunbar JS. Tracheomalacia. Ann Otol Rhinol Laryngol. 1963;72:1013–23.
6. Benjamin B. Tracheomalacia in infants and children. Ann Otol Rhinol Laryngol. 1984;93:438–42.
7. Berg E, Naseri I, Sobol SE. The role of airway fluoroscopy in the evaluation of children with stridor. Arch Otolaryngol Head Neck Surg. 2008;134(4):415–8.
8. Bhimji S. Vascular rings: treatment & management. Medscape Reference. WebMD LLC, New York. http://emedicine.medscape.com/article/426233-treatment#a25
9. Bibi H, Khvolis E, Shoseyov D, et al. The prevalence of gastroesophageal reflux in children with tracheomalacia and laryngomalacia. Chest. 2001;119:409–13.
10. Blair GK, Cohen R, Filler RM. Treatment of tracheomalacia: eight years' experience. J Pediatr Surg. 1986;21:781–5.
11. Boiselle PM, Ernst A. Recent advances in central airway imaging. Chest. 2002;121(5):1651–60.
12. Boogaard R, Huijsmans SH, Pijnenburg MWH, et al. Tracheomalacia and bronchomalacia in children: incidence and patient characteristics. Chest. 2005;128:3391–7.
13. Brody AS, Frush DP, Huda W, et al. Radiation risk to children from computed tomography. Pediatrics. 2007;120:677–82.
14. Cacciaguerra S, Bianchi A. Tracheal ring-graft reinforcement in lieu of tracheostomy for tracheomalacia. Pediatr Surg Int. 1998;13:556–9.

15. Callahan CW. Primary tracheomalacia and gastroesophageal reflux in infants with cough. Clin Pediatr. 1998;37:725–31.
16. Carden KA, Boiselle PM, Waltz DA, et al. Tracheomalacia and tracheobronchomalacia in children and adults: an in-depth review. Chest. 2005;127:984–1005.
17. Chang AB, Boyce NC, Masters IB, et al. Bronchoscopic findings in children with non-cystic fibrosis chronic suppurative lung disease. Thorax. 2002;57:935–8.
18. Davis S, Jones M, Kisling J, et al. Effect of continuous positive airway pressure on forced expiratory flows in infants with tracheomalacia. Am J Respir Crit Care Med. 1998;158:148–52.
19. Doshi J, Krawiec ME. Clinical manifestations of airway malacia in young children. J Allergy Clin Immunol. 2007;120:1276–8.
20. Duncan S, Eid N. Tracheomalacia and bronchopulmonary dysplasia. Ann Otol Rhinol Laryngol. 1991;100:856–8.
21. Eberhart RC, Su SH, Nguyen KT, et al. Bioresorbable polymeric stents: current status and future promise [Review]. J Biomater Sci Polym Ed. 2003;14(4):299–312.
22. Feist JH, Johnson TH, Wilson RJ. Acquired tracheomalacia: etiology and differential diagnosis. Chest. 1975;68:340–5.
23. Finder JD. Primary bronchomalacia in infants and children. J Pediatr. 1997;130:59–66.
24. Frey EE, Smith WL, Grandgeorge S, et al. Chronic airway obstruction in children: evaluation with cine-CT. Am J Roentgenol. 1987;148:347–52.
25. Frush DP, Donnelly LF, Rosen NS. Computed tomography and radiation risks: what pediatric health care providers should know. Pediatrics. 2003;112:951–7.
26. Greenholz SK, Karrer FM, Lilly JR. Contemporary surgery of tracheomalacia. J Pediatr Surg. 1986;21:511–4.
27. Gross RE, Neuhauser EBD. Compression of the trachea by an anomalous innominate artery: an operation for its relief. Am J Dis Child. 1948;75:570–7.
28. Holinger LD. Etiology of stridor in the neonate, infant, and child. Ann Otol Rhinol Laryngol. 1980;89:397–400.
29. Holinger PH, Johnston KC, Parchet VN, et al. Congenital malformations of the trachea, bronchi, and lung. Ann Otol Rhinol Laryngol. 1952;61:1159–80.
30. Jacobs IN, Wetmore RF, Tom LW, et al. Tracheobronchomalacia in children. Arch Otolaryngol Head Neck Surg. 1994;120:154–8.
31. Javia LR, Zur KB. How I do it: laryngotracheal reconstruction with resorbable microplate buttressing. Laryngoscope. 2012;122:920–4.
32. Kanter RK, Pollack MM, Wright WW, et al. Treatment of severe tracheobronchomalacia with continuous positive airway pressure (CPAP). Anesthesiology. 1982;57:54–6.
33. Mair EA, Parsons DS. Pediatric tracheobronchomalacia and major airway collapse. Ann Otol Rhinol Laryngol. 1992;101:300–9.
34. Mair EA, Parsons DS, Lally KP. Treatment of severe bronchomalacia with expanding endobronchial stents. Arch Otolaryngol Head Neck Surg. 1990;116:1087–90.
35. Masters IB, Chang AB, Patterson L, et al. Series of laryngomalacia, tracheomalacia, and bronchomalacia disorders and their associations with other conditions in children. Pediatr Pulmonol. 2002;34:189–95.
36. Miller RW, Pollack MM, Murphy TM, et al. Effectiveness of continuous positive airway pressure in the treatment of bronchomalacia in infants: a bronchoscopic documentation. Crit Care Med. 1986;14:125–7.
37. Montgomery WW. T-tube tracheal stent. Arch Otolaryngol. 1965;82:320–1.
38. Murphy JP, Filler RM, Muraji T, et al. Effect of prosthetic airway splint on the growing trachea. J Pediatr Surg. 1983;18:872–8.
39. Panitch HB, Keklikian EN, Motley RA, et al. Effect of altering smooth muscle tone on maximal expiratory flows in patients with tracheomalacia. Pediatr Pulmonol. 1990;9(3):170–6.
40. Pearce MS, Salotti JA, Little MP, et al. Radiation exposure from CT scans in childhood and subsequent risk of leukaemia and brain tumours: a retrospective cohort study. Lancet. 2012;380:499–505.
41. Picot C, Monnet P, Bethenod M, et al. Tracheomalacia in infants. Arch Fr Pediatr. 1969;26:493–506.
42. Poets CF. Gastroesophageal reflux: a critical review of its role in preterm infants. Pediatrics. 2004;113(2):e128–32.
43. Schellhase DE, Fawcett DD, Schutze GE, et al. Clinical utility of flexible bronchoscopy and bronchoalveolar lavage in young children with recurrent wheezing. J Pediatr. 1998;132:312–8.
44. Schwartz MZ, Filler RM. Tracheal compression as a cause of apnea following repair of tracheoesophageal fistula: treatment by aortopexy. J Pediatr Surg. 1980;15:842–8.
45. Sewall GK, Warner T, Connor NP, et al. Comparison of resorbable poly-L-lactic acid-polyglycolic acid and internal palmaz stents for the surgical correction of severe tracheomalacia. Ann Otol Rhinol Laryngol. 2003;112(6):515–21.
46. Shah RK, Mora BN, Bacha E, et al. The presentation and management of vascular rings: an otolaryngology perspective. Int J Pediatr Otorhinolaryngol. 2007;71:57–62.
47. Sotomayor JL, Godinez RI, Borden S, et al. Large-airway collapse due to acquired tracheobronchomalacia in infancy. Am J Dis Child. 1986;140:367–71.
48. Strauss HJ, Scheel W, Bartel M. Comparative cinematographic, endoscopic, and functional studies of the preoperative estimation of the severity of tracheal stenoses. Z Erkr Atmungsorgane. 1989;172:130–42.
49. Valerie EP, Durrant AC, Forte V, et al. A decade of using intraluminal tracheal/bronchial stents in the management of tracheomalacia and/or bronchomalacia: is it better than aortopexy? J Pediatr Surg. 2005;40:904–7.
50. Wailoo MP, Emery JL. The trachea in children with tracheaesophageal fistula. Histopathology. 1979;3:329–38.
51. Walner DL, Ouanounou S, Donnelly LF, et al. Utility of radiographs in the evaluation of pediatric upper airway obstruction. Ann Otol Rhinol Laryngol. 1999;108:378–83.
52. Windsor HM, Shanahan MX, Cherian K, et al. Tracheal injury following prolonged intubation. Aust N Z J Surg. 1976;46:18–25.
53. Wiseman NE, Duncan PG, Cameron CB. Management of tracheobronchomalacia with continuous positive airway pressure. J Pediatr Surg. 1985;20:489–93.
54. Wittenberg MH, Gyepes MT, Crocker D. Tracheal dynamics in infants with respiratory distress, stridor, and collapsing trachea. Radiology. 1967;88:653.
55. Wright CD, Graham BB, Grillo HC, et al. Pediatric tracheal surgery. Ann Thorac Surg. 2002;74:308–14.

Vascular Anomalies of the Neonatal Airway

David H. Darrow and Gresham T. Richter

Introduction

In 1982, Mulliken and Glowacki proposed a biological classification of vascular anomalies [1]. These authors described two major categories of vascular anomalies based on their clinical behavior, natural history, and cellular kinetics: *vascular tumors*, which are lesions characterized by endothelial proliferation, and *vascular malformations*, which result from errors in vascular morphogenesis while exhibiting normal endothelial turnover [1–3]. The modification of this classification accepted by the International Society for the Study of Vascular Anomalies (ISSVA) in 1996 [2] is shown in Table 1.

The most common vascular anomalies of the neonatal airway are infantile hemangiomas, lymphatic malformations, and venous malformations. Infantile hemangiomas, which are among the vascular tumors, have a predilection for the subglottic airway. In contrast, lymphatic and venous vascular malformations are typically pharyngeal and supraglottic and cause obstruction in higher regions of the airway [4].

Infantile Hemangioma of the Airway

Infantile hemangiomas (IHs) are benign tumors of the vascular endothelium. The most common tumors of infancy, IHs have the unique ability to involute after a period of rapid proliferation. Most IHs involve the skin, while only a small percentage involve the mucosa or the viscera.

IHs of the neonatal airway are relatively uncommon. Also known as "subglottic" hemangiomas, these lesions have a tendency to affect the narrowest portion of the pediatric airway, and therefore present with symptoms of stridor and cough. Growth of the tumor may result in airway compromise and severe respiratory distress.

Epidemiology

The incidence of IH in general has been estimated at 4–5 % based on retrospective and cross-sectional data [5], although other studies suggest rates of 1–3 % among newborns [6, 7], and 2.6–9.9 % among older children. [8, 9]. IHs occur more commonly among female infants at rate of about 3:1 [9, 10], and most studies report a significantly higher incidence in Caucasian infants [9–11]. The incidence of IH is increased among preterm infants, affecting 22–30 % of babies weighing less than 1 kg [10, 12]. Low birth weight has been implicated as the causal reason, with a 25 % increase in risk of IH development for every 500 g reduction in birth weight [13].

In a 1967 series, IHs of the airway accounted for 1.5 % of congenital laryngeal anomalies [14]. However, the actual incidence of IHs has not been determined in any formal study. An analysis of the 37-hospital Pediatric Health Information System (PHIS) database over the 5-year period from 2001 to 2005 found that of 2,890 admissions for a primary or secondary diagnosis of IH, 337 (12 %) underwent an airway procedure during at least one admission [15]. Thus, on average, pediatric hospitals in this cohort likely treated fewer than three symptomatic airway IHs each year. As with IH in general, airway IH of the subglottis have been reported more frequently in females, but with a 2:1 female to male preponderance [16–20]. It is unknown if the other risk factors associated with IH in general apply equally to the subset of IHs of the airway.

D.H. Darrow, M.D., D.D.S. (✉)
Department of Otolaryngology, Children's Hospital of The King's Daughters, Eastern Virginia Medical School, 600 Gresham Drive, Norfolk, VA 23507, USA
e-mail: David.Darrow@chkd.org

G.T. Richter, M.D.
Arkansas Children's Hospital, University of Arkansas Medical School, Little Rock, AR, USA

J. Lioy and S.E. Sobol (eds.), *Disorders of the Neonatal Airway: Fundamentals for Practice*,
DOI 10.1007/978-1-4939-1610-8_12, © Springer Science+Business Media New York 2015

Table 1 Classification of cutaneous vascular anomalies (Modified from issva.org/classification, updated 2014)

Vascular malformations
Venous
Lymphatic
Capillary
Arterial and arteriovenous
Mixed (combined)
Vascular neoplasms
Infantile hemangioma (IH)
Congenital hemangioma (CH)
Rapidly involuting (RICH)
Non-involuting (NICH)
Others
Kaposiform hemangioendothelioma (KHE)
Tufted angioma (TA)
Lobulated capillary hemangiomas (LCH) (pyogenic granuloma)[a]

Notes: [a]*considered cutaneous hyperplasia*

Etiology and Pathogenesis

The etiology and pathogenesis of IH remain theories that are incompletely proven. The endothelial progenitor cell theory suggests that IHs develop from clonal expansion of circulating endothelial progenitor cells (EPCs), resulting in vasculogenesis, or the de novo formation of new blood vessels. [21, 22]. The proposed stimulus for division of EPCs is a somatic mutation or abnormal signals from local tissues. The theory of placental origin suggests that fetal progenitor cells arise from disruption of the placenta during gestation or birth. This concept derived from research demonstrating that molecular markers unique to placental tissue were also present in IHs [23–25]. Clinical evidence for this theory is suggested by studies demonstrating an increased incidence of IH in association with chorionic villus sampling, placenta previa, and preeclampsia.

A unifying theory suggests that circulating EPCs find their way to certain locations that provide conditions favorable for growth into placenta-like tissues. In such tissues as the skin and liver, progenitor cells may encounter cellular signals and local tissue factors that stimulate their development. Such factors may include angiogenic and vasculogenic factors within the IH [26–28]. It is also theorized that disturbances causing placental hypoxia trigger a vascular response that increases the likelihood of IH [29–31]. Such disturbances include maternal chorionic villus sampling (CVS) or amniocentesis [[10, 32, 33], and placental anomalies such as retroplacental hematoma, infarction, and dilated vascular communications [29]. In utero hypoxia is also the most common cause of low birth weight and may explain the association seen with premature delivery.

Clinical Presentation

Although considered congenital lesions, airway IHs are not generally symptomatic at birth. However, like cutaneous IH, they typically exhibit a characteristic life cycle consisting of proliferation and involution. Proliferation occurs during early infancy, while gradual spontaneous involution or regression starts by 1 year of age [34–41]. Symptoms usually manifest during the early proliferative phase; accordingly, some airway IHs will become symptomatic during the neonatal period. 80–90 % of affected babies will present within the first 6 months with a mean age of 3.6 months at diagnosis [16, 42]. Symptoms are often present for several weeks before a definitive diagnosis is made. An intermediate period between proliferation and involution during mid-to-late infancy, often referred to as the "plateau" phase, more likely represents a period of temporary balance between individual cells that are proliferating and those undergoing involution and apoptosis [34–41]. The process of involution takes several years and varies in duration.

Most *symptomatic* airway IHs involve the subglottic larynx and, as a result, authors have traditionally referred to these lesions as "subglottic hemangiomas." In fact, many such IHs have been demonstrated to have transglottic or paratracheal extension [43]. Nevertheless, their associated symptom complex is consistent, including biphasic stridor and barky cough, usually in the absence of dysphonia. The symptoms are often mistaken for those of infectious or inflammatory croup, especially since the symptoms typically worsen in the presence of upper respiratory illness. Furthermore, IHs respond to many of the same treatments used for croup, including racemic epinephrine and nebulized and systemic steroids. As a result, recurrent croup-like symptoms and gradual worsening of stridor during early infancy are suggestive of airway IH and should be investigated further. Swallowing is usually normal; however feeding may be affected as the infant tries to coordinate sucking with breathing.

About one half of infants diagnosed with an airway IH also will have a cutaneous IH, although only 1–2 % of children with cutaneous IHs also have airway IHs [17, 44]. Even in asymptomatic children, the presence of cutaneous IH in the "beard distribution" (parotid area, lips, chin, neck) may be a predictor of IH in the airway (Fig. 1) [45]. Such cases likely represent "segmental" IHs [43, 46].

Once the proliferative phase is completed (9–12 months of age), respiratory symptoms tend to slowly resolve. Although the lesion itself may not involute completely or even significantly for many months, growth of the child over time allows the airway to better accommodate the IH, resulting in diminished stridor and cough.

Diagnosis

Diagnosis of airway IH begins with a high index of suspicion, since many congenital and inflammatory processes of the airway can mimic IH during the early months of infancy. The presence of cutaneous lesions and the persistence or recurrence of croup-like symptoms are important clues. When airway IH is suspected, the diagnosis may be confirmed by performing an imaging study or proceeding directly to laryngoscopy and bronchoscopy. In most cases, the uncertainty of the diagnosis or the severity of symptoms necessitates a trip to the operating room, where the pathology may be visualized directly and treated surgically if necessary. This approach avoids the risks associated with radiation exposure during infancy. Advocates of imaging, conversely, prefer to make a presumptive diagnosis based on flexible airway endoscopy, and confirm the diagnosis and assess the extent of the lesion by CT (computerized tomography) scan with angiography ("CT angio") [47]. This approach avoids the need for general anesthesia, especially given the recent trend to treat such lesions initially with medical therapy rather than surgery.

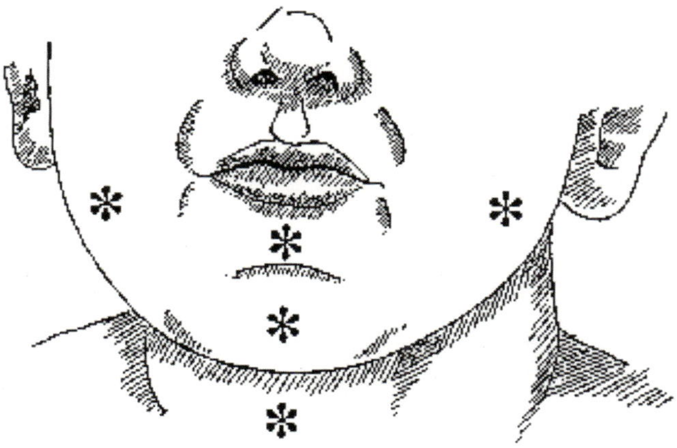

Fig. 1 Subsites of IHs in beard distribution, denoted by asterisks (Reprinted from [45], copyright © 1997, with permission from Elsevier, Ltd)

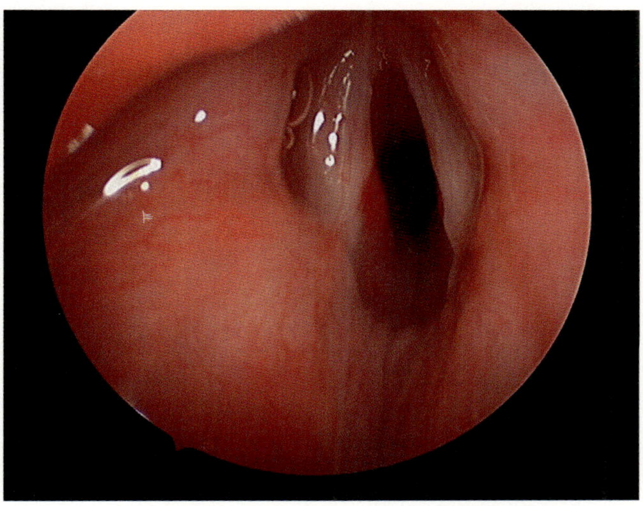

Fig. 2 Hemangioma on posterior wall of glottic and subglottis

When endoscopy is performed, symptomatic airway IHs are usually found to involve the subglottis, but bulk and blush may be present at adjacent and distant sites as well. The bulky lesion is smooth, submucosal, compressible, and pink or blue in color (Fig. 2). A left-sided predominance has been reported, but IHs may be bilateral, circumferential, or multiple. Biopsy is not usually necessary to establish the diagnosis; however when the diagnosis is in doubt, specimens from true IHs will stain positively for GLUT1 (glucose transporter protein isoform 1) [24, 48]. The most useful and widely used immunohistochemical marker for the diagnosis of IH, GLUT1 is strongly expressed by IH endothelial cells and not by other benign vascular anomalies, and has been validated for the identification of IHs of the airway [49].

On CT imaging, IHs will demonstrate an intensely staining, well-circumscribed mass with lobular architecture. MRI, although often diagnostic, is less advantageous since the duration of the study generally requires general anesthesia, often with endotracheal intubation. Fluoroscopy or anterior-posterior radiographs of the neck may demonstrate an asymmetric subglottic narrowing; however these studies do not definitively establish the diagnosis.

A staging system for airway IHs has been proposed by Perkins et al. [47]. IH stage is determined from CT angiography based on location, percentage of laryngeal airway obstruction, and estimated total volume of the IH (Table 2).

Table 2 Proposed airway IH staging system and treatment protocol

Stage[a]	Unilateral airway hemangioma	Circumferential or bilateral airway hemangioma	Percent laryngeal airway obstruction	CTA or MRI extralaryngeal hemangioma volume (mm^3)
1	Yes	No	≤50	<4,000
2	Yes	Yes	>50–90	4,001–10,000
3	No	Yes	>90	>10,000

CTA CT angiography, *IH* infantile hemangioma
[a]Stage based on lowest stage in a row with two or more positive findings
From Perkins et al. [47]

Management

Once the diagnosis of airway IH has been established, the need for and type of intervention is determined by several factors, including the degree of airway obstruction, the extent of extralaryngeal IH, the location of the patient at the time of diagnosis, the experience of the treating physician, and the preferences of the caretaker.

Since involution is the ultimate fate of nearly all infantile IHs, "watchful waiting" is reasonable in cases involving minimal symptomatology. For those patients with symptomatic IHs whose caretakers prefer no intervention for the lesion itself, tracheotomy with observation is highly successful [18]. This approach, however, requires a high level of maintenance to avoid tube occlusion, accidental decannulation, and exposure of the airway to water over a long period of time. As a result, in most cases, some sort of intervention for the IH itself is more desirable.

Pharmacotherapy

In a landmark 2008 publication by Léauté-Labrèze et al., the authors described their serendipitous observation that involution of IHs may be accelerated with the administration of propranolol [50]. At doses of 2–3 mg/kg/day used to treat cardiac complications of their IHs, two children experienced marked and rapid involution of their IHs. These results were replicated in a case series reported by the same authors [51] and in publications by a number of other investigators [52–62].

Several mechanisms have been proposed to explain the mechanism by which propranolol inhibits IH growth, including vasoconstriction due to decreased release of nitric oxide, blocking of proangiogenic signals (vascular endothelial growth factor, basic fibroblast growth factor, matrix metalloproteinases 2 and 9), and induction of apoptosis in proliferating endothelial cells [51, 62–64]. It has also been suggested that propranolol may prevent the differentiation of IH stem cells into endothelial cells or pericytes [65], or that it may hasten the differentiation of progenitor cells into adipocytes [51].

Several clinicians have reported success using propranolol in the management of airway IHs [66–76], but response is not universal [77]. The pretreatment assessment, optimal dose, and appropriate duration of therapy vary considerably in the literature. After considering contraindications such as cardiogenic shock, sinus bradycardia, hypotension, heart block greater than first-degree, heart failure, bronchial asthma, and known hypersensitivity to the drug, most clinicians will perform a cardiac evaluation, including at least an examination and a pretreatment electrocardiogram. In most series, the drug is started at a dose of 1 mg/kg/day divided two to three times a day, and then increased over several days to a week to 2–3 mg/kg/day. Heart rate and blood pressure are checked each hour for the first 2–3 h after the initial dose and with each dosage increase. The drug is administered throughout most of the first year of life. Although protocols for propranolol initiation do appear in the otolaryngology literature [78, 79], a consensus multidisciplinary protocol has also been published [62].

Propranolol has a well-established safety profile based on years of use at higher doses for control of high blood pressure and cardiac pathology. Potential side effects and complications include sinus bradycardia, hypotension, reactive airways, hypoglycemia with secondary seizures, diarrhea, and cool extremities. Patients should be monitored for evidence of bradycardia, hypotension and/or hypoglycemia [62, 65, 80]. However, such complications are reported rarely, and it has been suggested that propranolol should become the standard for initial management of all airway IHs [81].

Although propranolol has largely supplanted systemic corticosteroids as first line pharmacotherapy, the latter are occasionally useful in refractory cases. Steroid medications inhibit growth of the lesion during the proliferative phase, losing their effectiveness once involution begins [82]. Doses of prednisolone at 2–3 mg/kg/day are generally necessary to control growth of the mass and should be maintained for 1–2 weeks before starting a 2–4 week taper. Response rates reported in the literature vary between 30 and 93 %, although there is little consistency among dosing regimens [82, 83]. Long-term management on steroids carries a significant risk of complications, including gastroesophageal reflux, gastritis, immune suppression, cushingoid changes, hyperglycemia and glycosuria, hypertension, fluid and electrolyte disturbances, and growth retardation [82]. IH patients on maintenance steroids should concomitantly receive courses of H_2 receptor blockers and trimethoprim-sulfamethoxasole as prophylaxis against gastritis and pneumocystis carinii infection, respectively. Live vaccinations should also be avoided while a child is taking high-dose steroids.

Interferon α-2A has been used with success in treating IHs, but should only be considered when all other traditional modalities fail [84–87]. Potential side effects are associated with this therapy, including fever, myalgia, transient elevation of hepatic transaminase levels, transient neutropenia, anemia, and spastic diplegia [88, 89].

Surgical Intervention

Indications for surgical management of airway IH have become few since the efficacy of propranolol was established. Surgery is a reasonable consideration when (1) the obstruction found at operative endoscopy is severe and will likely require a lengthy intubation while medical therapy is initiated, and (2) the patient remains severely symptomatic despite an adequate trial of medical therapy.

Operative intervention may include intralesional injection of corticosteroids and/or partial ablation of the IH, or complete surgical excision the portion of the lesion within the airway. In most cases, the patients will remain on

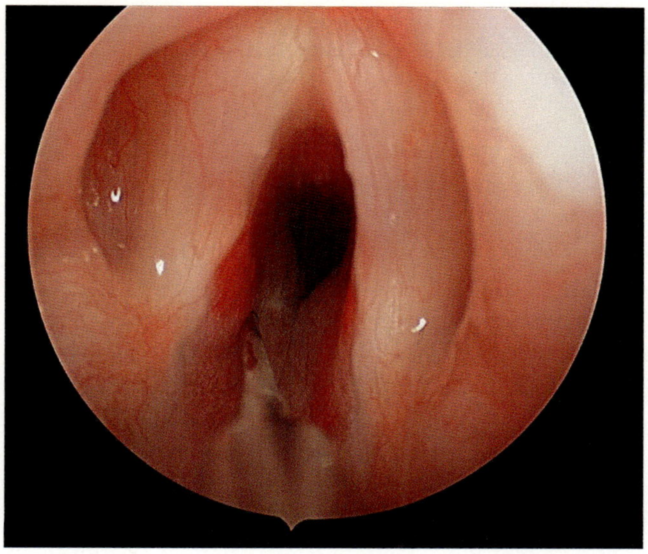

Fig. 3 Triamcinolone/betametasone steroid injection with needle in left side of subglottic hemangioma

medical therapy postoperatively to reduce the likelihood of recurrence. This is of particular importance in "segmental" airway lesions with known extension outside of the airway.

Intralesional steroids should be considered for patients whose IHs have necessitated a trip to the operating room for endoscopy or endoscopic resection. While repeated injections are usually necessary as single modality therapy [90], these medications may be effective adjuvant therapy for patients whose lesions are being observed, treated pharmacologically, or partially resected. In most cases, triamcinolone 40 mg/cm^3 is administered at a dose of 3–5 mg/kg either alone or supplemented by betamethasone 6 mg/cm^3 dosed at 0.5–1.0 mg/kg (Fig. 3) [82]. Total volume delivered may be limited by the size of the lesion, and care must be taken to avoid depositing the steroid medication deep enough to affect the underlying cartilage. Patients will usually require at least overnight intubation due to the increased volume of the lesion after injection. Cure rates of 77–87 % using intralesional steroids have been reported [42, 90].

Airway IHs causing focal obstruction may be addressed surgically by a subtotal endoscopic approach using a microscope or telescope, or by total excision through an open approach, dividing the thyroid and cricoid cartilages in the midline. Subtotal resection, more often than total excision, carries the risk of growth of the residual lesion during the proliferative phase, potentially resulting in additional surgical procedures unless combined with pharmacologic therapy. Endoscopic excision is usually performed using an apneic anesthesia technique, intermittently interrupting the surgery for reinsertion of the tube and ventilation of the patient. Alternatively, the procedure may be performed under spontaneous ventilation with anesthetic insufflation or Venturi jet ventilation.

The laser has been the most popular endoscopic surgical modality [42], with the carbon dioxide (CO_2) [17, 19, 44, 91, 92] potassium titanyl phosphate (KTP) [93, 94], and neodymium:yttrium-aluminum-garnet (Nd:YAG) [95, 96] lasers all demonstrating some effectiveness. All of these lasers are currently available for airway use through fiber delivery systems, however only CO_2 is used by direct beam. CO_2 lasers are preferentially absorbed by water, while KTP and Nd:YAG lasers take advantage of absorption peaks that approximate those of hemoglobin and are thought to penetrate more deeply. However, all of these lasers cause destruction by ablation rather than selective photothermolysis. As a result, in addition to the risk of recurrence, laser treatment carries a risk of subglottic stenosis of 5–25 % that is likely greatest with deeper resections and in cases of bilateral or circumferential disease [19, 44, 89, 97]. Debulking of the lesion using rotary powered instrumentation (microdebrider or "shaver") has also been reported [98, 99]. Postoperatively, patients are observed in an intensive care setting. Some clinicians recommend face tent humidification to prevent airway obstruction due to eschar formation.

Although the first open surgical excision of a focally obstructing airway IH was reported in 1949, the procedure did not gain popularity until the 1990s, after complications of laser therapy became increasingly apparent [100–105]. Over the 15 years prior to the discovery of effects of propranolol, open resection appeared to be emerging as the intervention of choice for airway IHs. The procedure is of greatest advantage in patients with bilateral or circumferential lesions that may otherwise been at risk for postoperative stenosis, recurrence, or tracheotomy. However, open surgical excision may be more difficult in cases involving significant extra-laryngeal extension, and the procedure may potentially result in some degree of dysphonia.

After initial intubation through the obstructed portion of the airway, the lesion is approached through the anterior neck via laryngofissure. After the tube has been relocated to the inferior aspect of the incision, the IH is removed submucosally under the operating microscope. At the conclusion of the dissection, the patient is intubated; in some cases a thyroid cartilage graft may be placed to enlarge the subglottic laryngeal framework. After the neck is closed, the patient is transported to the intensive care unit where intubation is maintained for 3–7 days.

Multidisciplinary Considerations

Management of airway IH requires good communication among pediatric specialists, both in terms of diagnosis of the lesion as well as management after the diagnosis has been made. It is estimated that some 50 % of patients with airway

IHs have cutaneous lesions as well, many with problematic segmental involvement in the "beard" distribution. In addition, there is an important association of airway IH with PHACE(S) syndrome, including *P*osterior fossa defects, *H*emangiomas, cerebrovascular *A*rterial anomalies, *C*ardiovascular anomalies including *C*oarctation of the aorta, *E*ye anomalies, and *S*ternal cleft and/or *S*upraumbilical raphe (OMIM 606519) [106]. In one study of 23 PHACE patients, 52 % were found to have airway IH, many of whom required treatment for stridor [107]. Another study found eight patients (42 %) meeting the criteria for PHACE among 17 with large "beard" distribution IHs and airway IHs [108]. In such cases, early consultations with pediatric dermatology and genetics are advisable.

During diagnostic endoscopy, as with all lesions of the airway, moment-to-moment communication between the otolaryngologist and the anesthesiologist is critical to successful management. Since in most cases a subglottic lesion is predictable based on symptoms, the two clinicians should have a game plan in place for intubation, management of the airway during any intervention, and emergency contingencies, and the two should agree on a plan for airway management in the immediate postoperative period.

Postoperatively, the otolaryngologist must continue to coordinate the airway management plan with the pediatric intensivists and hospitalists that will administer care to patients with airway IH while they recover from endoscopy and start on medical therapy. Such care includes the duration of intubation (if any), management of medical therapy for the IH and for reflux if indicated, and use of adjunctive racemic epinephrine and/or steroids to control exacerbations of stridor. In most cases, consultation with a pediatric cardiologist is advisable prior to starting propranolol therapy while the child is still hospitalized.

Future Considerations

There are still several important unanswered questions in the diagnosis and management of IH of the airway. One key issue in pathogenesis is the predilection of IH to involve the subglottis as opposed to other areas of the airway. As the etiology of IH in general becomes clearer, it may be possible to theorize plausible reasons for this clinical observation. It is also not yet clear if there is some subset of patients with a presentation of cutaneous IH that should undergo endoscopy prior to the development of symptomatic airway obstruction. Finally, in terms of therapeutic intervention, propranolol therapy is a relatively new tool in the management of airway IH, and additional research will be required to determine optimal administration, including dosage, frequency, and duration of therapy.

Vascular Malformations of the Neonatal Airway

Vascular malformations are congenital disorders of vasculogenesis with ectatic vascular networks and the propensity for relentless expansion and recruitment of new vessels. Unlike hemangiomas, vascular malformations do not experience a cycle of growth and involution. They are present at birth and grow commensurate with the child until periods of rapid expansion lead to functional and aesthetic compromise. Trauma, infection, and hormonal fluctuation have been associated with acute growth of these vascular anomalies [109, 110].

Vascular malformations may be composed of any blood vessel type and they are named accordingly, including capillary malformations (port wine stains), venous malformations, lymphatic malformations, and arteriovenous malformations. The most common vascular malformations affecting the neonatal airway are lymphatic and venous malformations [111–113]. Relative to subglottic hemangiomas and other disorders of the newborn airway, these malformations are rare. Although they may occur in isolation, neonatal vascular malformations of the airway are more commonly associated with diffuse cervicofacial lesions [114, 115]. Diffuse involvement of the head and neck will commonly affect the aerodigestive tract mucosa to include the oral cavity, tongue, hypopharynx and larynx (Fig. 4) [113]. Vascular malformations typically experience slow growth but airway involvement may necessitate urgent intervention, especially in the setting of acute or chronic obstruction.

Lymphatic Malformations

Epidemiology

Lymphatic malformations are believed to occur in 1 in 500 live births and comprise about 12 % of vascular cases referred to a vascular center [116]. Within the head and neck, lymphatic malformations occur at a rate of between 1 in 2,000 and 1 in 4,000 [117]. Fifty percent of cases present after birth and 80–90 % by 2 years of age. There does not appear to be a gender or race predilection for LMs.

Etiology and Pathogenesis

Lymphatic malformations (LMs) are slow flow vascular malformations composed of dilated ectatic lymphatic channels. They are thought to arise from disruptions in embryonic lymphangiogenesis but their etiology and pathogenesis remain unclear. Lymphatic malformations are present at

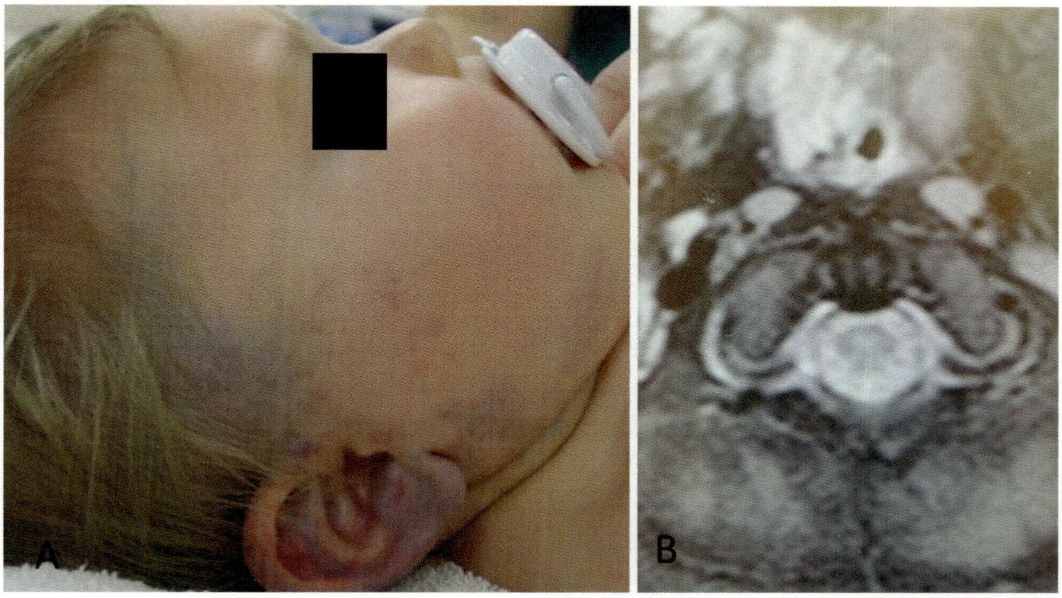

Fig. 4 Infant with venous malformation of facial soft tissue and larynx. The malformation is characterized by blue cutaneous staining (left) and enhancing lesion of supraglottis on MRI (right)

birth but may not be detectible until later in life. The majority of LMs occur in the head and neck, making them the second most common congenital mass found at these sites [118, 119]. Exacerbated by infection, cervicofacial LMs may expand in infancy or early childhood when the rate of ear and upper respiratory infections are at their peak. Diffuse lesions are more likely to progress than those that are localized. If left untreated, the likelihood of progression is significantly higher in adolescence than childhood [120]. The earlier intervention may thus be warranted in many cases.

Clinical Presentation

Based upon their response to treatment, LMs have been categorized by the size of the fluid filled lymphatic cysts present. In particular, cysts greater than 1–2 cm in diameter are considered macrocysts, while microcysts are those 1–2 cm in diameter or less [121]. While LMs may be predominantly macrocystic or microcystic, most LMs of the head and neck region are mixed lesions. Venous malformations may also be present within extensive cervicofacial LMs.

Macrocystic and microcystic LMs have different clinical courses. Macrocystic LMs grow by accumulated lymphatic fluid and expansion of the cysts into areas of least resistance. They have a tendency to encompass and compress surrounding architecture. In the neonate, they can affect the larynx and trachea by direct or indirect compression of these structures. Stridor, grunting, or symptoms consistent with obstructive sleep apnea may be present when the larynx, trachea, or pharynx are involved, respectively. With rapid expansion or internal bleeding, macrocystic LMs may cause acute compromise of vital structures. Chronic expansion in the head and neck frequently leads to upper aerodigestive symptoms such as dysphagia and gradual airway obstruction, especially during recumbence.

Unlike macrocystic LMs, microcystic LMs are infiltrative in nature. In this condition, small microcystic vesicles penetrate soft tissue including skin, muscle, and mucosa [122, 123]. Non-descript soft tissue swelling and the emergence of weeping vesicles in the skin or mucosa often note its presence. Isolated disease commonly occurs in the tongue, upper lip, and larynx (Fig. 5). When associated with mixed cervicofacial lesions, microcysts in the tongue and larynx can cause acute life-threatening airway obstruction upon delivery, shortly after birth, or during periods of acute infection and swelling (Fig. 6) [124].

Isolated microcystic LMs rarely cause respiratory obstruction in the newborn period. However, in the presence of massive cervicofacial disease of mixed or microcystic LM, rapid airway compromise may occur, especially during periods of acute edema [124]. Upper airway obstruction is exacerbated by infiltrating disease of the tongue and floor of mouth (Fig. 6) [123, 125–127]. Laryngeal involvement will exacerbate symptoms.

Diagnosis

Airway endoscopy with office-based flexible laryngoscopy, followed by rigid microlaryngoscopy and bronchoscopy, will provide best evidence of the extent of obstruction and its effect on the airway. Distinct margins of macrocystic LMs may also be detected on physical exam and on magnetic resonance imaging (MRI), the diagnostic study of choice for LMs. An MRI of the head and neck will demonstrate the depth of disease and differentiate macrocystic LM from more common conditions of the pediatric head and neck. Hyperintense lesion on T2 weighted images and air-fluid levels within the lesion are hallmark MRI findings for macrocystic LM [128]. Frequently mixed lesions are discovered. Microcystic and macrocystic lymphatic malformations may coexist with deep neck space venous malformations which will also be evident on MRI.

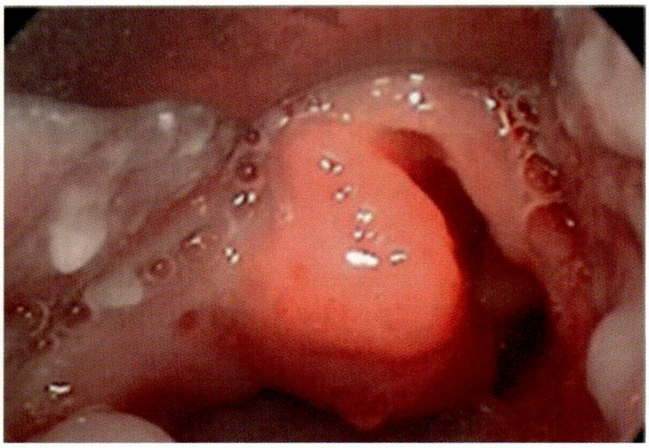

Fig. 5 Isolated lymphatic malformation of the supraglottic larynx. Lymphatic vesicles are seen on the left pharyngeal wall and vallecula

Management and Multidisciplinary Considerations

Except in rare cases, LMs ultimately need intervention to control symptoms associated with their accumulated lifetime growth. Timing of intervention for LMs in infants is dependent upon the acuity of symptoms and dictated by the presence, or risk of, acute and chronic upper aerodigestive dysfunction or pain due to inflammation. Acute airway obstruction, sleep apnea, and dysphagia are the most common reasons for intervention in these patients [113, 118, 126]. Sclerotherapy and surgery constitute the therapeutic approach to lymphatic malformations and is typically conducted in a multidisciplinary fashion. However, symptom control may be best achieved acutely with oral steroids and antibiotics that reduce the inflammation, lymph accumulation, and expansion of LMs.

Macrocystic Disease

A small percentage of isolated macrocystic LMs have been reported to spontaneously resolve [129, 130]. Because these isolated lesions usually occur in the neck, they rarely cause significant dysfunction in the newborn and can be observed into early childhood before treatment is considered.

Most macrocystic LMs compressing the neonatal airway require treatment. In acute situations, needle aspiration of the responsible cyst or cysts may alleviate the airway compromise until more definitive management with either surgical excision or sclerotherapy is possible. Sclerotherapy is the direct injection of agents that cause epithelial damage and

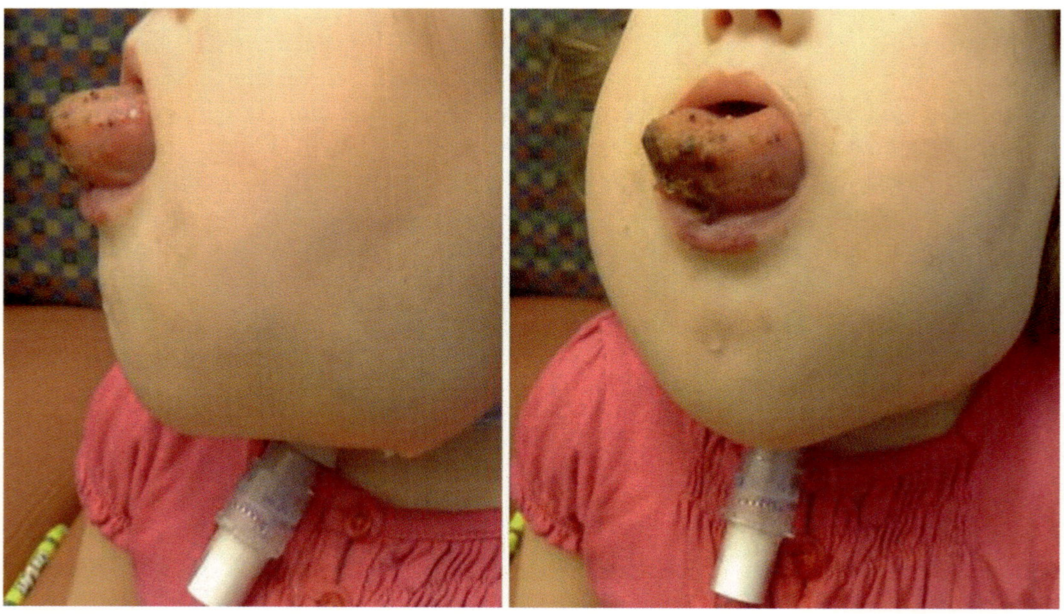

Fig. 6 Cervicofacial microcystic lymphatic malformation with multiple levels of airway obstruction leading to early tracheostomy

subsequent disruption of the LM channels. Various materials have been employed with equal success including doxycycline, ethanol, sodium tetradodecyl, and OK-432, an immunostimulant derived from Group A streptococci [131–135]. With these therapies, dissolution occurs as the result of intravascular injury and luminal absorption by the body. Multiple treatment sessions, under radiographic fluoroscopy, may be required for significant reduction in volume using this technique. Postoperative edema with potentially worsening compression may occur following sclerotherapy. Expectant airway management with intubation or intensive care observation is necessary when treating compressive lesions of the neonatal airway. Risk to adjacent nerves ranges from 5 to 10 % with temporary dysfunction being more common than complete injury [134].

Surgical excision can provide immediate relief of airway obstruction caused by macrocystic cervical LMs. The risk of injury to important neurovascular structures in the neck is real but fortunately rare in experienced hands. Coexistent venous malformations may be found during surgical excision of deep neck LMs. Recurrence, persistent lymphatic drainage, and postoperative scarring often occur following excision [136]. These risks are minimized by removing as much disease as possible, placing perioperative drains, and hiding incisions in natural creases of the neck.

Outcomes of surgical excision are not affected by age with successful management of head and neck macrocystic LMs in the newborn. Small recurrent LMs or seromas that occur following excision are best managed with symptom-directed sclerotherapy. Routine use of intraoperative intravenous dexamethasone and a short course of postoperative systemic steroids are recommended to prevent acute and dramatic lymphatic drainage and soft tissue edema that occurs following any intervention for LMs.

When venous malformations are found in mixed LMs, patients need to be screened for local intravascular coagulation. Elevated D-dimers and low fibrinogen levels indicate a coagulation disturbance and may be found in these patients prior to intervention. Perioperative management with low-molecular weight heparin can reduce the risk of intraoperative disseminated intravascular coagulation and perioperative thrombi in patients when these coagulation factors are abnormal.

Congenital high airway resistance syndrome (CHAOS) may occur in the presence of complex cervicofacial LMs at birth. If detected during ultrasonography and confirmed by fetal MRI, massive LMs that are expected to obstruct the newborn airway at delivery can be managed with ex utero intrapartum treatment, also known as the EXIT procedure [124]. This is a specialized surgical delivery of the newborn by a multidisciplinary team to manage potentially immediate life-threatening conditions at birth [137]. The newborn is delivered by cesarean section with the umbilical cord and placenta attached with the goal to deliver oxygen as urgent interventions are performed. The team has 1–1.5 h to stabilize the airway and establish adequate respiration to the baby. This may require intubation or tracheostomy. Fortunately, most infants with macrocystic LMs do not require an EXIT procedure as expansion of the lesion is primarily external and not towards the airway (Fig. 7). If necessary, intubation can be performed by an airway specialist. The larynges of such patients are typically easy to access. Bilateral mixed or microcystic LMs may be more difficult when other compressive components are present.

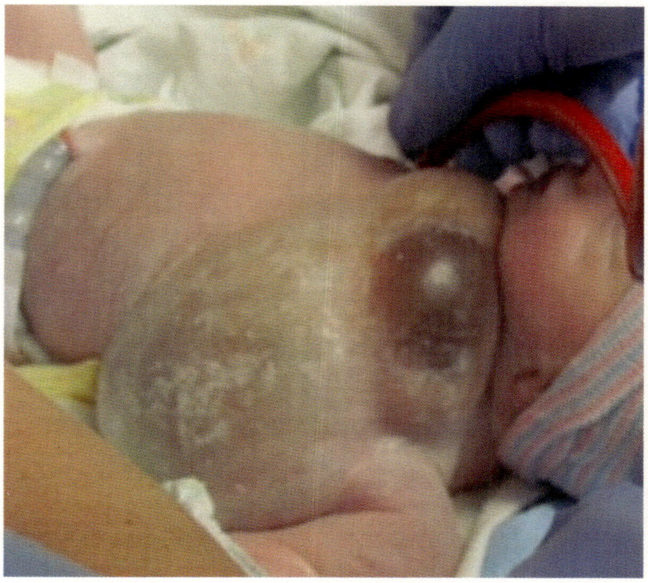

Fig. 7 Macrocystic lymphatic malformation of neck and chest in an infant. The malformation extends externally, but the airway is not compromised

Microcystic Disease

The infiltrative nature and protracted course of microcystic LM make them particularly difficult to manage, especially when the upper aerodigestive tract is involved. In these patients urgent tracheostomy may be required as an infant that is thereby followed by periodic and staged treatments. Management of the neck, tongue, pharynx, and larynx is often necessary to ultimately relieve chronic obstruction. Unfortunately, microcystic disease is poorly responsive to sclerotherapy, due to the limited retention of sclerosing agents in the small cysts. Excision requires desiccation of normal tissue since this condition integrates into surrounding structures. Unfortunately, high rates of recurrence (90–100 %) are also experienced following excision of microcystic LM [125, 138].

Nonetheless, the tongue may be addressed with local ablative therapy. Infiltrative disease of the deep musculature of the tongue is best controlled by excision or coblation, which can reduce significant bulk and relieve obstruction.

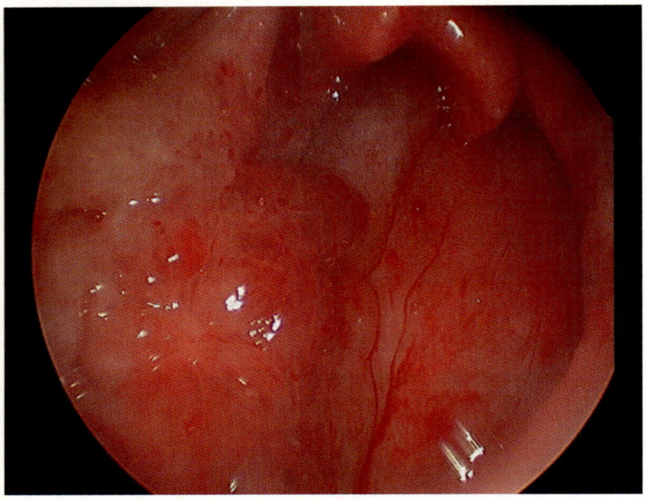

Fig. 8 Posterior and lateral pharyngeal involvement of microcystic lymphatic malformation

Early studies using intralesional bleomycin and doxycycline therapy in the management microcystic lymphatic disease have demonstrated promising results [138, 139]. Direct injections of bleomycin within the involved tissue have led to disease control and symptom improvement in some studies [139]. The risks of these agents are equivalent to those with other sclerotherapy tools, including nerve injury, pain, incomplete response, and the need for numerous treatments. There is theoretically an added risk of pulmonary fibrosis when using bleomycin, but this does not likely occur at the low doses typically used. The impact of these agents on laryngeal disease has not been closely examined.

Microcystic LM of the neonatal trachea is unlikely. However, early disease involving the larynx may be found [140–142]. This is often associated with adjacent pharyngeal or hypopharyngeal involvement (Fig. 8). Stabilization of life-threatening airway symptoms in this setting may be necessary as primary treatment with a tracheotomy [140]. A staging system for laryngeal disease demonstrates the frequent need of tracheotomy in these patients [143].

Surgical management of microcystic laryngeal disease must be performed in a staged fashion. The carbon dioxide (CO_2) laser may be used to ablate weeping or bleeding mucosal vesicles of the oral cavity, tongue, or pharynx. However, precise excision of involved laryngeal tissue is performed using the CO_2 laser in cutting mode [143, 144]. When employed, the laser is directed to the larynx to remove unwanted and obstructive microcystic disease. Unilateral treatment with management of the contralateral side at a later date will prevent unwanted scarring and worsening obstruction. This mucosa-sparing approach with partial excision of involved supraglottic disease is a complicated procedure and should be performed judiciously by experienced otolaryngologists. Temporary intubation may be required postoperatively. Again perioperative steroids will reduce significant edema associated with interventions directed at LMs.

Future Considerations

The management of microcystic lymphatic malformations is particularly difficult. The deep tissue penetration, small vesicular cysts, and high recurrence rates of microcystic LMs limit the therapeutic benefit of surgery and sclerotherapy. Pharmacologic interventions have recently been explored for these complicated lesions with limited benefit. Rapamycin, an mTOR inhibitor, and sildenafil, a phosphodiesterase inhibitor, in particular have been tried with some early reported success. Prospective studies are necessary to determine if these tools can be truly useful in the search for a cure of microcystic disease. Nonetheless, genetic and molecular profiling may help identify new pharmacologic targets in the future.

Venous Malformations

Epidemiology

Due to their rarity, the actual incidence of venous malformations is unclear. However, based upon the referral pattern to a prominent vascular anomalies center, slow-flow vascular malformations have an incidence of about 1 in 10,000 people (0.01 % of population) [144]. There exists no race predilection for venous malformation but recent publications suggest a female predominance over males of 1.5:1 [145]. They are sporadic in 93 % of affected patients and usually unifocal. Approximately 7 % of cases of venous malformations are multifocal and associated with inherited forms comprised of cutaneomucosal venous malformations (VMCM).

Etiology and Pathogenesis

Venous malformations (VMs) are rare, low flow, slowly progressive vascular malformations. They are primarily composed of small to medium sized ectatic venous channels that coalesce to form a vascular mass of poorly draining veins. With time, gradual accumulation of blood, loss of vascular elasticity, and vascular expansion lead to growth of involved soft tissue. The etiology of VMs remains unclear although familial patterns and genetic links have been reported in patients with multifocal disease. TIE 2 mutations causing autophosphorylation of an endothelial cell specific tyrosine kinase are believed to lead to cell proliferation and cause VM to intermittently develop throughout life [144]. A second type of inherited multifocal form is the glomovenous malformation (GVM) secondary to a glomulin gene mutation and resulting in abnormal differentiation of smooth muscle cells [144]. In familial cases of venous malformations, autosomal inheritance pattern has been observed and linked to the 9p locus [146].

Venous malformations frequently affect the head and neck. However, extremity involvement is most common (60.9 %) followed by head and neck (32.7 %) and trunk (9.8 %). The majority of venous malformations involve the integument (skin and subcutaneous tissue) but 50 % of lesions invade deeper structures including fat, muscle, bone and viscera. In the deep venous malformations, phlebectasia is the most common deep venous anomaly and is seen in about 40–50 % of patients [147, 148].

Sites commonly involved in the head and neck include the parotid gland, submandibular space, buccal space, and masseter muscle [114, 149]. Mucosal disease is the norm rather than the exception. Venous malformations of the tongue, lips, gingiva, cheek, palate, retromolar trigone, pharynx, hypopharynx, and larynx have been described and are frequently identified in early childhood [150–152]. Because of the slow expansion of VMs, they are rarely found in the newborn. When present in the airway, they may be asymptomatic in the neonatal period. Discovery during surveillance of disease elsewhere in the head and neck is common (Fig. 4).

Diagnosis and Clinical Presentation

Laryngeal involvement of VMs can lead to chronic upper airway resistance, especially during recumbence as the venous channels fill with dependency. Inspiratory stridor during eating, crying, and agitation may occur. Symptoms consistent with sleep apnea such as loud snoring, stertor, neck hyperextension, and restlessness are also common when supraglottic disease is present [149]. Acute airway obstruction is rare. Dysphagia may be present in infants with post-cricoid disease. Head and neck masses that worsen with Valsalva and dependency are consistent with deep cervical VMs. Skin involvement will appear as blue telangiectatic vessels (Fig. 4). The presence of extensive superficial or deep neck disease should prompt evaluation of the upper aerodigestive tract.

Endoscopic exam of the entire airway and MRI of the neck will provide the best evidence of mucosal involved VMs and their associated deep components. Pupuric to blue discoloration of the mucosa that expands with Valsalva or recumbence is consistent with venous malformations of the airway. Gadolinium enhancement on T1 weighted images is a common indicator of VMs on MRI. Focal hypolucencies on MRI suggest phleboliths, which are a hallmark sign of VMs compared to other vascular anomalies [128].

Management and Multidisciplinary Considerations

Early intervention for venous malformation of the airway includes raising the head of the bed to prevent progressive expansion of the venous channels during sleep. Like lymphatic malformations, both sclerotherapy and surgical excision can be employed for deep and superficial cervicofacial venous malformations with a high degree of success. However, management of upper aerodigestive and airway venous malformations requires a different approach. Sclerotherapy may injure or slough involved mucosa leading to profound edema, bleeding, and scarring. Excision of aerodigestive lesions requires the removal of involved normal tissue and can lead to functional deficits in breathing, voice, or swallowing. For these reasons surgery and sclerotherapy are secondary modalities in the management of neonatal airway venous malformations.

An alternative and effective treatment for mucosal and airway disease is Nd:YAG laser therapy [114, 151, 152]. This technique utilizes the process of selective photothermolysis to target and injure small to medium sized veins while preserving surrounding normal tissue. The Nd:YAG laser, with a wavelength of 1,064 nm, can heat and disrupt anomalous veins while preserving the overlying mucosa. The treatment is effective up to 7 mm below the mucosal surface. Immediate reduction in the size of involved aerodigestive lesions can be observed at the time of laser treatment. The reduction from a single treatment is often sustained for several months while multiple treatments spaced in 3–6 month intervals are often required for maximal benefit and control of symptoms [153]. This approach can be particularly effective for the tongue and larynx with preservation of function. Airway complications or injury following Nd:YAG therapy have not yet been reported. Interstitial laser therapy, by placing the laser deep into the tongue musculature has also proven effective. Thus the ND:YAG laser therapy of the aerodigestive tract is a healthy alternative to excision or sclerotherapy that are at higher risk of untoward functional deficits.

Cervicofacial venous malformations that compress the airway but do not directly extend into it can be addressed with sclerotherapy, surgical excision, or a combination of these modalities. Because of slow and gradual expansion, neck disease without mucosal involvement will lead to airway obstruction predominately with recumbence and sleep. Symptoms are rarely acute or life threatening in this situation and planned procedures can be performed at appropriately spaced intervals.

Future Considerations

Due to their infiltrative nature, rarely are VMs "cured." Management techniques of laser, surgery, and sclerotherapy reduce disease bulk, improve symptoms, and control disease progression. As novel mutations are identified in VMs, molecular targets for pharmacotherapy may become evident and exploited. Laser therapy and sclerotherapy may then selectively destroy VMs by targeted disease specific factors while reducing risk of injury to be involved and adjacent normal tissue.

References

1. Mulliken JB, Glowacki J. Hemangiomas and vascular malformations in infants and children: a classification based on endothelial characteristics. Plast Reconstr Surg. 1982;69:412–22.
2. Enjolras O, Mulliken JB. Vascular tumors and vascular malformations (new issues). Adv Dermatol. 1997;13:375–423.
3. Mulliken JB, Fishman SJ, Burrows PE. Vascular anomalies. Curr Probl Surg. 2000;37:517–84.
4. Rahbar R, McGill TJ, Mulliken JB. Vascular tumors and malformations of the head and neck. In: Cummings CW, Flint PW, editors. Otolaryngology head and neck surgery. 4th ed. Philadelphia: Mosby; 2005. p. 4013–20.
5. Kilcline C, Frieden IJ. Infantile hemangiomas: how common are they? A systematic review of the medical literature. Pediatr Dermatol. 2008;25:168–73.
6. Pratt AG. Birthmarks in infants. Arch Dermatol. 1953;67:302–5.
7. Jacobs AH, Walton RG. The incidence of birthmarks in the neonate. Pediatrics. 1976;58:218–22.
8. Dickison P, Christou E, Wargon O. A prospective study of infantile hemangiomas with a focus on incidence and risk factors. Pediatr Dermatol. 2011;28:663–9.
9. Hoornweg MJ, Smeulders MJ, Ubbink DT, van der Horst CM. The prevalence and risk factors of infantile haemangiomas: a case-control study in the Dutch population. Paediatr Perinat Epidemiol. 2012;26:156–62.
10. Haggstrom AN, Drolet BA, Baselga E, Chamlin SL, Garzon MC, Horii KA, et al. Prospective study of infantile hemangiomas: demographic, prenatal, and perinatal characteristics. J Pediatr. 2007;150:291–4.
11. Chiller KG, Passaro D, Frieden IJ. Hemangiomas of infancy: clinical characteristics, morphologic subtypes, and their relationship to race, ethnicity, and sex. Arch Dermatol. 2002;138:1567–76.
12. Amir J, Metzker A, Krikler R, Reisner SH. Strawberry hemangioma in preterm infants. Pediatr Dermatol. 1986;3:331–2.
13. Drolet BA, Swanson EA, Frieden IJ. Infantile hemangiomas: an emerging health issue linked to an increased rate of low birth weight infants. J Pediatr. 2008;153:712–5. e1.
14. Holinger PH, Brown WT. Congenital webs, cysts, laryngoceles and other anomalies of the larynx. Ann Otol Rhinol Laryngol. 1967;76:744–52.
15. Perkins JA, Oliaei S, Garrison MM, Manning SC, Christakis DA. Airway procedures and hemangiomas: treatment patterns and outcome in U.S. pediatric hospitals. Int J Pediatr Otorhinolaryngol. 2009;73:1302–7.
16. Shikhani AH, Marsh BR, Jones MM, et al. Infantile subglottic hemangiomas: an update. Ann Otol Rhinol Laryngol. 1986; 95:336–47.
17. Sherrington CA, Sim DK, Freezer NJ, Robertson CF. Subglottic haemangioma. Arch Dis Child. 1997;76:458–9.
18. Feuerstein SS. Subglottic hemangioma in infants. Laryngoscope. 1973;83:466–75.
19. Chatrath P, Black M, Jani P, et al. A review of the current management of infantile subglottic haemangioma, including a comparison of CO_2 laser therapy versus tracheostomy. Int J Pediatr Otorhinolaryngol. 2002;64:143–57.
20. Hughes CA, Rezaee A, Ludemann JP, Holinger LD. Management of congenital subglottic hemangioma. J Otolaryngol. 1999;28: 223–8.
21. Yu Y, Flint AF, Mulliken JB, Wu JK, Bischoff J. Endothelial progenitor cells in infantile hemangioma. Blood. 2004;103:1373–5.
22. Greenberger S, Boscolo E, Adini I, Mulliken JB, Bischoff J. Corticosteroid suppression of VEGF-A in infantile hemangioma-derived stem cells. N Engl J Med. 2010;362:1005–13.
23. North PC, Waner M, James CA, Mizeracki A, Frieden IJ, Mihm MC. Congenital nonprogressive hemangioma. A distinct clinicopathologic entity unlike infantile hemangioma. Arch Dermatol. 2001;137:1607–20.
24. North PE, Waner M, Mizeracki A, Mihm Jr MC. GLUT1: a newly discovered immunohistochemical marker for juvenile hemangiomas. Hum Pathol. 2000;31:11–22.
25. Leon-Villapalos J, Wolfe K, Kangesu L. GLUT1: an extra diagnostic tool to differentiate between haemangiomas and vascular malformations. Br J Plast Surg. 2005;58:348–52.
26. Greenberger S, Adini I, Biscolo E, Mulliken JB, Bischoff J. Targeting NF-kB in infantile hemangioma-derived stem cells reduces VEGF-A expression. Angiogenesis. 2010;13:327–35.
27. Chang J, Most D, Bresnick S, Mehrara B, Steinbrech DS, Reinisch J, et al. Proliferative hemangiomas: analysis of cytokine gene expression and angiogenesis. Plast Reconstr Surg. 1999;103:1–9. discussion 10.
28. Razon MJ, Kräling BM, Mulliken JB, Bischoff J. Increased apoptosis coincides with onset of involution in infantile hemangioma. Microcirculation. 1998;5:189–95.
29. Colonna V, Resta L, Napoli A, Bonifazi E, et al. Placental hypoxia and neonatal haemangioma: clinical and histological observations. Br J Dermatol. 2010;162:208–9.
30. Drolet BA, Frieden IJ. Characteristics of infantile hemangiomas as clues to pathogenesis: does hypoxia connect the dots? Arch Dermatol. 2010;146:1295–9.
31. Kleinman ME, Blei F, Gurtner GC. Circulating endothelial progenitor cells and vascular anomalies. Lymphat Res Biol. 2005;3: 234–9.
32. Bauland CG, Smit JM, Bartelink LR, Zondervan HA, Spauwen PH. Hemangioma in the newborn: increased incidence after chorionic villus sampling. Prenat Diagn. 2010;30:913–7.
33. Bauland CG, Smit JM, Scheffers SM, Bartels RH, van den Berg P, Zeebregts CJ, et al. Similar risk for hemangiomas after amniocentesis and transabdominal chorionic villus sampling. J Obstet Gynaecol Res. 2012;38:371–5.
34. Lister WA. Natural history of strawberry nevi. Lancet. 1938; 231(5991):1429–30.
35. Bivings L. Spontaneous regression of angiomas in children: twenty-two years' observation covering 236 cases. J Pediatr. 1954;45:643–7.
36. Margileth AM, Museles M. Current concepts in diagnosis and management of congenital cutaneous hemangiomas. Pediatrics. 1965;36:410–6.
37. Moroz B. Long-term follow-up of hemangiomas in children. In: Williams HB, editor. Symposium on vascular malformations and melanotic lesions. St Louis: CV Mosby; 1982. p. 27–35.
38. Mulliken JB. Diagnosis and natural history of hemangiomas. In: Mulliken JB, Young AE, editors. Vascular birthmarks: hemangiomas and malformations. Philadelphia: WB Saunders; 1988. p. 41–62.
39. Esterly NB. Cutaneous hemangiomas, vascular stains and malformations, and associated syndromes. Curr Probl Pediatr. 1996; 26:3–39.
40. Bowers RE, Graham EA, Tominson KM. The natural history of the strawberry nevus. Arch Dermatol. 1960;82:667–70.

41. Chang LC, Haggstrom AN, Drolet BA, Baselga E, Chamlin SL, Garzon MC, et al. Growth characteristics of infantile hemangiomas: implications for management. Pediatrics. 2008;122:360–7.
42. Bitar MA, Moukarbel RV, Zalzal GH. Management of congenital subglottic hemangioma: trends and success over the past 17 years. Otolaryngol Head Neck Surg. 2005;132:226–31.
43. Perkins JA, Duke W, Chen E, Manning S. Emerging concepts in airway infantile hemangioma assessment and management. Otolaryngol Head Neck Surg. 2009;141:207–12.
44. Sie KC, McGill T, Healy GB. Subglottic hemangiomas: 10 years experience with the carbon dioxide laser. Ann Otol Rhinol Laryngol. 1994;103:167–72.
45. Orlow S, Isakoff M, Blei F. Increased risk of symptomatic hemangiomas of the airway in association with cutaneous hemangiomas in a "beard" distribution. J Pediatr. 1997;131:643–6.
46. O TM, Alexander RE, Lando T, et al. Segmental hemangiomas of the upper airway. Laryngoscope. 2009;119:2242–7.
47. Perkins JA, Chen EY, Hoffer FA, Manning SC. Proposal for staging airway hemangiomas. Otolaryngol Head Neck Surg. 2009; 141:516–21.
48. North PE, Waner M, Mizeracki A, Mrak RE, Nicholas R, Kincannon J, et al. A unique microvascular phenotype shared by juvenile hemangiomas and human placenta. Arch Dermatol. 2001;137:559–70.
49. Badi AN, Kerschner JE, North PE, Drolet BA, Messner A, Perkins JA. Histopathologic and immunophenotypic profile of subglottic hemangioma: multicenter study. Int J Pediatr Otorhinolaryngol. 2009;73:1187–91.
50. Léauté-Labrèze C, Dumas de la Roque E, Hubiche T, Boralevi F, Thambo JB, Taïeb A. Propranolol for severe hemangiomas of infancy. N Engl J Med. 2008;358:2649–51.
51. Sans V, Dumas de la Roque E, Berge J, et al. Propranolol for severe infantile hemangiomas: follow-up report. Pediatrics. 2009;124:e423–31.
52. Tan ST, Itinteang T, Leadbitter P. Low-dose propranolol for multiple hepatic and cutaneous hemangiomas with deranged liver function. Pediatrics. 2011;127:e772–6.
53. Mousa W, Kues K, Haas E, et al. Successful treatment of a large hemangioma with propranolol. J Dtsch Dermatol Ges. 2010;8: 184–6.
54. Marsciani A, Pericoli R, Alaggio R, Brisigotti M, Vergine G. Massive response of severe infantile hepatic hemangioma to propanolol. Pediatr Blood Cancer. 2010;54:176.
55. Saint-Jean M, Léauté-Labrèze C, Mazereeuw-Hautier J, Bodak N, Hamel-Teillac D, Kupfer-Bessaguet I, et al. Propranolol for treatment of ulcerated infantile hemangiomas. J Am Acad Dermatol. 2011;64:827–32.
56. Cheng JF, Gole GA, Sullivan TJ. Propranolol in the management of periorbital infantile haemangioma. Clin Experiment Ophthalmol. 2010;38:547–53.
57. Li YC, McCahon E, Rowe NA, Martin PA, Wilcsek GA, Martin FJ. Successful treatment of infantile haemangiomas of the orbit with propranolol. Clin Experiment Ophthalmol. 2010;38:554–9.
58. Fulkerson DH, Agim NG, Al-Shamy G, Metry DW, Izaddoost SA, Jea A. Emergent medical and surgical management of mediastinal infantile hemangioma with symptomatic spinal cord compression: case report and literature review. Childs Nerv Syst. 2010;26: 1799–805.
59. Vanlander A, Decaluwe W, Vandelanotte M, Van Geet C, Cornette L. Propranolol as a novel treatment for congenital visceral haemangioma. Neonatology. 2010;98:229–31.
60. Theletsane T, Redfern A, Raynham O, Harris T, Prose NS, Khumalo NP. Life threatening infantile haemangioma: a dramatic response to propranolol. J Eur Acad Dermatol Venereol. 2009;23:1465–6.
61. Hogeling M, Adams S, Wargon O. A randomized controlled trial of propranolol for infantile hemangiomas. Pediatrics. 2011;128: e259–66.
62. Drolet BA, Frommelt PC, Chamlin SL, Haggstrom A, Bauman NM, Chiu YE, et al. Initiation and use of propranolol for infantile hemangioma: report of a consensus conference. Pediatrics. 2013; 131:128–40.
63. Greenberger S, Bischoff J. Infantile hemangioma-Mechanism(s) of drug action on a vascular tumor. Cold Spring Harb Perspect Med. 2011;1(1):a006460.
64. Dai Y, Hou F, Buckmiller L, et al. Decreased eNOS protein expression in involuting and propranolol-treated hemangiomas. Arch Otolaryngol Head Neck Surg. 2012;138:177–82.
65. Frieden IJ, Drolet BA. Propranolol for infantile hemangiomas: promise, peril, pathogenesis. Pediatr Dermatol. 2009;26:642–4.
66. Mistry N, Tzifa K. Use of propranolol to treat multicentric airway haemangioma. J Laryngol Otol. 2010;7:1–4.
67. Truong MT, Chang KW, Berk DR, Heerema-McKenney A, Bruckner AL. Propranolol for the treatment of a life-threatening subglottic and mediastinal infantile hemangioma. J Pediatr. 2010;156:335–8.
68. Maturo S, Hartnick C. Initial experience using propranolol as the sole treatment for infantile airway hemangiomas. Int J Pediatr Otorhinolaryngol. 2010;74:323–5.
69. Buckmiller LM, Munson PD, Dyamenahalli U, Dai Y, Richter GT. Propranolol for infantile hemangiomas: early experience at a tertiary vascular anomalies center. Laryngoscope. 2010;120:676–81.
70. Manunza F, Syed S, Laguda B, et al. Propranolol for complicated infantile haemangiomas: a case series of 30 infants. Br J Dermatol. 2010;162:466–8.
71. Jephson CG, Manunza F, Syed S, Mills NA, Harper J, Hartley BE. Successful treatment of isolated subglottic haemangioma with propranolol alone. Int J Pediatr Otorhinolaryngol. 2009;73:1821–3.
72. Buckmiller L, Dyamenahalli U, Richter GT. Propranolol for airway hemangiomas: case report of novel treatment. Laryngoscope. 2009;119:2051–4.
73. Leboulanger N, Fayoux P, Teissier N, Cox A, Van Den Abbeele T, Carrabin L, et al. Propranolol in the therapeutic strategy of infantile laryngotracheal hemangioma: A preliminary retrospective study of French experience. Int J Pediatr Otorhinolaryngol. 2010;74:1254–7.
74. Anderson de Moreno LC, Matt BH, Montgomery G, Kim YJ. Propranolol in the treatment of upper airway hemangiomas. Ear Nose Throat J. 2013;92:209–14.
75. Mahadevan M, Cheng A, Barber C. Treatment of subglottic hemangiomas with propranolol: initial experience in 10 infants. ANZ J Surg. 2011;81:456–61.
76. Rosbe KW, Suh KY, Meyer AK, Maguiness SM, Frieden IJ. Propranolol in the management of airway infantile hemangiomas. Arch Otolaryngol Head Neck Surg. 2010;136:658–65.
77. Raol N, Metry D, Edmonds J, Chandy B, Sulek M, Larrier D. Propranolol for the treatment of subglottic hemangiomas. Int J Pediatr Otorhinolaryngol. 2011;75:1510–4.
78. Bajaj Y, Kapoor K, Ifeacho S, Jephson CG, Albert DM, Harper JI, et al. Great Ormond Street Hospital treatment guidelines for use of propranolol in infantile isolated subglottic haemangioma. J Laryngol Otol. 2013;127:295–8.
79. Parikh SR, Darrow DH, Grimmer JF, Manning SC, Richter GT, Perkins JA. Propranolol use for infantile hemangiomas: American Society of Pediatric Otolaryngology Vascular Anomalies Task Force practice patterns. JAMA Otolaryngol Head Neck Surg. 2013;139:153–6.
80. Lawley LP, Siegfried E, Todd JL. Propranolol treatment for hemangioma of infancy: risks and recommendations. Pediatr Dermatol. 2009;26:610–4.
81. Denoyelle F, Garabédian EN. Propranolol may become first-line treatment in obstructive subglottic infantile hemangiomas. Otolaryngol Head Neck Surg. 2010;142:463–4.
82. Waner M, Suen JY. Treatment options for the management of hemangiomas. In: Waner M, Suen JY, editors. Hemangiomas and

vascular malformations of the head and neck. New York: Wiley-Liss, Inc.; 1999. p. 233–62.
83. Waner M, Suen JY. Advances in the management of congenital vascular lesions of the head and neck. Adv Otorhinolaryngol. 1996;10:31–54.
84. Ezekowitz RAB, Mulliken JB, Folkman J. Interferon alfa-2A therapy for life-threatening hemangiomas of infancy. N Engl J Med. 1992;326:1456–63.
85. Ohlms LA, Jones DT, McGill TJ, Healy GB. Interferon alfa2A therapy for airway hemangiomas. Ann Otol Rhinol Laryngol. 1994;103:1–8.
86. Bauman MN, Burke DK, Smith RJH. Treatment of massive or life-threatening hemangiomas with recombinant α 2a-interferon. Otolaryngol Head Neck Surg. 1997;117:99–110.
87. MacArthur CJ, Senders CW, Katz J. The use of interferon Alfa-2A for life-threatening hemangiomas. Arch Otolaryngol Head Neck Surg. 1995;121:690–3.
88. Barlow CF, Priebe CJ, Mulliken JB, et al. Spastic diplegia as a complication of interferon Alpha-2a treatment of hemangiomas of infancy. J Pediatr. 1998;132:527–30.
89. Michaud AP, Bauman NM, Burke DK, Manaligod JM, Smith RJ. Spastic diplegia and other motor disturbances in infants receiving interferon-alpha. Laryngoscope. 2004;114:1231–6.
90. Hoeve LJ, Kuppers GLE, Verwoerd CDA. Management of infantile subglottic hemangioma: laser vaporization, submucous resection, intubation or intralesional steroids? Int J Pediatr Otorhinolaryngol. 1997;42:179–86.
91. Walker P, Cooper D, MacDonald D. Subglottic haemangioma: controversies in management. J Paediatr Child Health. 1999;35:392–5.
92. Re M, Forte V, Berardi C, Mallardi V. Role of endoscopic CO_2 laser surgery in the treatment of congenital infantile subglottic hemangioma. Experience in the Department of Otolaryngology, "Sick Children Hospital", Toronto, Canada. Acta Otorhinolaryngol Ital. 2003;23:175–9.
93. Madgy D, Ahsan SF, Kest D, Stein I. The application of the Potassium-Titanyl-Phosphate (KTP) laser in the management of subglottic hemangioma. Arch Otolaryngol Head Neck Surg. 2001;127:47–50.
94. Kacker A, April M, Ward RF. Use of potassium titanyl phosphate (KTP) laser in management of subglottic hemangiomas. Int J Pediatr Otorhinolaryngol. 2001;59:15–21.
95. Fu CH, Lee LA, Fang TJ, Wong KS, Li HY. Endoscopic Nd:YAG laser therapy of infantile subglottic hemangioma. Pediatr Pulmonol. 2007;42:89–92.
96. Azizkhan RG. Laser surgery: new applications for pediatric skin and airway lesions. Curr Opin Pediatr. 2003;15:243–7.
97. Cotton RT, Tewfik T. Laryngeal stenosis following carbon dioxide laser in subglottic hemangioma. Ann Otol Rhinol Laryngol. 1985;94:494–7.
98. Pransky SM, Canto C. Management of subglottic hemangioma. Curr Opin Otolaryngol Head Neck Surg. 2004;12:509–12.
99. Jai H, Huang Q, Lü J, Li J, Zhang Z, Wang Z, et al. Microdebrider removal under suspension laryngoscopy: an alternative surgical technique for subglottic hemangioma. Int J Pediatr Otorhinolaryngol. 2013;77:1424–9.
100. Froehlich P, Stamm D, Floret D, Morgon A. Management of subglottic hemangioma. Clin Otolaryngol. 1995;4:336–9.
101. Wiatrak BJ, Reilly JS, Seid AD, Pransky SM, Castillo JV. Open surgical excision of subglottic hemangioma in children. Int J Pediatr Otorhinolaryngol. 1996;34:191–206.
102. Van Den Abbeele T, Triglia J-M, Lescanne E, et al. Surgical removal of subglottic hemangiomas in children. Laryngoscope. 1999;109:1281–6.
103. Vijayasekaran S, White D, Hartley BEJ, Rutter MJ, Elluru RG, Cotton RT. Open excision of subglottic hemangiomas to avoid tracheostomy. Arch Otolaryngol Head Neck Surg. 2006;132:159–63.
104. Bajaj Y, Hartley BEJ, Wyatt ME, Albert DM, Bailey CM. Subglottic haemangioma in children: experience with open surgical excision. J Laryngol Otol. 2006;120:1033–7.
105. O-Lee TJ, Messner A. Open excision of subglottic hemangioma with microscopic dissection. Int J Pediatr Otorhinolaryngol. 2007;71:1371–6.
106. Frieden IJ, Reese V, Cohen D. PHACE syndrome: the association of posterior fossa brain malformations, hemangiomas, arterial anomalies, coarctation of the aorta and cardiac defects, and eye abnormalities. Arch Dermatol. 1996;132:307–11.
107. Durr ML, Meyer AK, Huoh KC, Frieden IJ, Rosbe KW. Airway hemangiomas in PHACE syndrome. Laryngoscope. 2012;122:2323–9.
108. Haggstrom AN, Skillman S, Garzon MC, Drolet BA, Holland K, Matt B, et al. Clinical spectrum and risk of PHACE syndrome in cutaneous and airway hemangiomas. Arch Otolaryngol Head Neck Surg. 2011;137:680–7.
109. Duyka LJ, Fan CY, Coviello-Malle JM, Buckmiller L, Suen JY. Progesterone receptors identified in vascular malformations of the head and neck. Otolaryngol Head Neck Surg. 2009;141:491–5.
110. Rahbar R, Rowley H, Perez-Atayde AR, McGill TJ, Healy GB. Delayed presentation of lymphatic malformation of the cervicofacial region: role of trauma. Ann Otol Rhinol Laryngol. 2002;111:828–31.
111. Ohlms LA, Forsen J, Burrows PE. Venous malformation of the pediatric airway. Int J Pediatr Otorhinolaryngol. 1996;37:99–114.
112. Thompson DM, Kasperbauer JL. Congenital cystic hygroma involving the larynx presenting as an airway emergency. J Natl Med Assoc. 1994;86:629–32.
113. O TM, Rickert SM, Diallo AM, et al. Lymphatic malformations of the airway. Otolaryngol Head Neck Surg. 2013;149:156–60.
114. Richter GT, Braswell L. Management of venous malformations. Facial Plast Surg. 2012;28:603–10.
115. Konez O, Burrows PE, Mulliken JB. Cervicofacial venous malformations. MRI features and interventional strategies. Interv Neuroradiol. 2002;8:227–34.
116. Manning SC, Perkins J. Lymphatic malformations. Curr Opin Otolaryngol Head Neck Surg. 2013;21:571–5.
117. Kennedy TL, Whitaker M, Pellitteri P, Wood WE. Cystic hygroma/lymphangioma: a rational approach to management. Laryngoscope. 2001;111:1929–37.
118. Padwa BL, Hayward PG, Ferraro NF, Mulliken JB. Cervicofacial lymphatic malformation: clinical course, surgical intervention, and pathogenesis of skeletal hypertrophy. Plast Reconstr Surg. 1995;95:951–60.
119. Harsha WJ, Perkins JA, Lewis CW, Manning SC. Pediatric admissions and procedures for lymphatic malformations in the United States: 1997 and 2000. Lymphat Res Biol. 2005;3:58–65.
120. Hassanein AH, Mulliken JB, Fishman SJ, Quatrano NA, Zurakowski D, Greene AK. Lymphatic malformation: risk of progression during childhood and adolescence. J Craniofac Surg. 2012;23:149–52.
121. Smith RJ, Burke DK, Sato Y, Poust RI, Kimura K, Bauman NM. OK-432 therapy for lymphangiomas. Arch Otolaryngol Head Neck Surg. 1996;122:1195–9.
122. Edwards PD, Rahbar R, Ferraro NF, Burrows PE, Mulliken JB. Lymphatic malformation of the lingual base and oral floor. Plast Reconstr Surg. 2005;115:1906–15.
123. Wiegand S, Eivazi B, Zimmermann AP, et al. Microcystic lymphatic malformations of the tongue: diagnosis, classification, and treatment. Arch Otolaryngol Head Neck Surg. 2009;135:976–83.
124. Stefini S, Bazzana T, Smussi C, et al. EXIT (Ex utero Intrapartum Treatment) in lymphatic malformations of the head and neck:

discussion of three cases and proposal of an EXIT-TTP (Team Time Procedure) list. Int J Pediatr Otorhinolaryngol. 2012;76:20–7.
125. Lei ZM, Huang XX, Sun ZJ, Zhang WF, Zhao YF. Surgery of lymphatic malformations in oral and cervicofacial regions in children. Oral Surg Oral Med Oral Pathol Oral Radiol Endod. 2007; 104:338–44.
126. Perkins JA, Manning SC, Tempero RM, Cunningham MJ, Edmonds Jr JL, Hoffer FA, et al. Lymphatic malformations: review of current treatment. Otolaryngol Head Neck Surg. 2010;142:795–803. 803 e791.
127. Renton JP, Smith RJ. Current treatment paradigms in the management of lymphatic malformations. Laryngoscope. 2011;121:56–9.
128. Dubois J, Alison M. Vascular anomalies: what a radiologist needs to know. Pediatr Radiol. 2010;40:895–905.
129. Dasgupta R, Adams D, Elluru R, Wentzel MS, Azizkhan RG. Noninterventional treatment of selected head and neck lymphatic malformations. J Pediatr Surg. 2008;43:869–73.
130. Perkins JA, Maniglia C, Magit A, Sidhu M, Manning SC, Chen EY. Clinical and radiographic findings in children with spontaneous lymphatic malformation regression. Otolaryngol Head Neck Surg. 2008;138:772–7.
131. Boardman SJ, Cochrane LA, Roebuck D, Elliott MJ, Hartley BE. Multimodality treatment of pediatric lymphatic malformations of the head and neck using surgery and sclerotherapy. Arch Otolaryngol Head Neck Surg. 2010;136:270–6.
132. Nehra D, Jacobson L, Barnes P, Mallory B, Albanese CT, Sylvester KG. Doxycycline sclerotherapy as primary treatment of head and neck lymphatic malformations in children. J Pediatr Surg. 2008;43:451–60.
133. Smith MC, Zimmerman MB, Burke DK, Bauman NM, Sato Y, Smith RJ. Efficacy and safety of OK-432 immunotherapy of lymphatic malformations. Laryngoscope. 2009;119:107–15.
134. Cahill AM, Nijs E, Ballah D, et al. Percutaneous sclerotherapy in neonatal and infant head and neck lymphatic malformations: a single center experience. J Pediatr Surg. 2011;46:2083–95.
135. Shiels 2nd WE, Kang DR, Murakami JW, Hogan MJ, Wiet GJ. Percutaneous treatment of lymphatic malformations. Otolaryngol Head Neck Surg. 2009;141:219–24.
136. Chen WL, Zhang B, Wang JG, Ye HS, Zhang DM, Huang ZQ. Surgical excision of cervicofacial giant macrocystic lymphatic malformations in infants and children. Int J Pediatr Otorhinolaryngol. 2009;73:833–7.
137. Otteson TD, Hackam DJ, Mandell DL. The Ex Utero Intrapartum Treatment (EXIT) procedure: new challenges. Arch Otolaryngol Head Neck Surg. 2006;132:686–9.
138. Burrows PE, Mitri RK, Alomari A, et al. Percutaneous sclerotherapy of lymphatic malformations with doxycycline. Lymphat Res Biol. 2008;6:209–16.
139. Bai Y, Jia J, Huang XX, Alsharif MJ, Zhao JH, Zhao YF. Sclerotherapy of microcystic lymphatic malformations in oral and facial regions. J Oral Maxillofac Surg. 2009;67:251–6.
140. Sobol SE, Manoukian JJ. Acute airway obstruction from a laryngeal lymphangioma in a child. Int J Pediatr Otorhinolaryngol. 2001;58:255–7.
141. Kenton A, Duncan N, Bhakta K, Fernandes CJ. Laryngeal lymphatic malformation in a newborn. J Perinatol. 2003;23:567–71.
142. Chan J, Younes A, Koltai PJ. Occult supraglottic lymphatic malformation presenting as obstructive sleep apnea. Int J Pediatr Otorhinolaryngol. 2003;67:293–6.
143. Berg EE, Sobol SE, Jacobs I. Laryngeal obstruction by cervical and endolaryngeal lymphatic malformations in children: proposed staging system and review of treatment. Ann Otol Rhinol Laryngol. 2013;122:575–81.
144. Brouillard P, Vikkula M. Genetic causes of vascular malformations. Hum Mol Genet. 2007;16(Spec No. 2):R140–9.
145. Hassanein AH, Mulliken JB, Fishman SJ, Alomari AI, Zurakowski D, Greene AK. Venous malformation: risk of progression during childhood and adolescence. Ann Plast Surg. 2012;68:198–201.
146. Gallione CJ, Pasyk KA, Boon LM, et al. A gene for familial venous malformations maps to chromosome 9p in a second large kindred. J Med Genet. 1995;32:197. e9.
147. Eifert S, Villavicencio JL, Kao TC, Taute BM, Rich NM. Prevalence of deep venous anomalies in congenital vascular malformations of venous predominance. J Vasc Surg. 2000;31(3):462–71.
148. Gloviczki P, Stanson AW, Stickler GB, Johnson CM, Toomey BJ, Meland NB, Rooke TW, Cherry Jr KJ. Klippel-Trenaunay syndrome: the risks and benefits of vascular interventions. Surgery. 1991;110(3):469–79.
149. Glade RS, Richter GT, James CA, Suen JY, Buckmiller LM. Diagnosis and management of pediatric cervicofacial venous malformations: retrospective review from a vascular anomalies center. Laryngoscope. 2010;120:229–35.
150. Dompmartin A, Vikkula M, Boon LM. Venous malformation: update on aetiopathogenesis, diagnosis and management. Phlebology. 2010;25:224–35.
151. Eivazi B, Wiegand S, Teymoortash A, Neff A, Werner JA. Laser treatment of mucosal venous malformations of the upper aerodigestive tract in 50 patients. Lasers Med Sci. 2010;25:571–6.
152. Scherer K, Waner M. Nd:YAG lasers (1,064 nm) in the treatment of venous malformations of the face and neck: challenges and benefits. Lasers Med Sci. 2007;22:119–26.
153. Glade R, Vinson K, Richter G, Suen JY, Buckmiller LM. Endoscopic management of airway venous malformations with Nd:YAG laser. Ann Otol Rhinol Laryngol. 2010;119:289–93.

Vascular Rings and Pulmonary Artery Slings

Aseem Srivastava, Matt Harrison, and Stephanie Fuller

The term vascular ring describes a group of congenital intrathoracic vascular anomalies caused by abnormal regression and differentiation of the aortic arches during fetal development that result in compression of the trachea, esophagus, or both. Albeit rare, these vascular rings can lead to serious and at times life threatening respiratory compromise. Surgical treatment is therefore indicated in all symptomatic patients.

Classification

Vascular rings have previously been classified as complete or incomplete based upon whether the vascular encirclement around the trachea and esophagus is complete or partial. More recently, the International Congenital Heart Surgery Nomenclature and Database Committee has proposed a classification system based on the anatomic configuration of the ring [1] (Table 1).

Double aortic arches are further subgrouped based upon arch dominance (right dominant, left dominant, or balanced). Those vascular rings associated with a right arch are classified as right arch with mirror image branching, right arch with retro esophageal left subclavian artery, or circumflex aorta which denotes a right arch but a left-sided descending thoracic aorta. This can be associated with aortic arch hypoplasia.

A. Srivastava, M.D. • S. Fuller, M.D. (✉)
The Division of Cardiothoracic Surgery, The Children's Hospital of Philadelphia, Philadelphia, PA, USA

University of Pennsylvania, Perelman School of Medicine, Philadelphia, PA, USA
e-mail: fullers@email.chop.edu

M. Harrison, M.D.
Division of Cardiology, The Children's Hospital of Philadelphia, Philadelphia, PA, USA

Embryology

In a human embryo, there are six paired pharyngeal (aortic) arches. They arise from the aortic sac and course posteriorly to connect to the right and left dorsal aorta, respectively. After a series of regression and differentiation events, this embryonic arch system ultimately gives rise to the adult aortic arch, its branches, and the pulmonary arteries. A brief understanding of this embryonic process is helpful to appreciate the anatomy of these vascular rings and for the interpretation of radiological images.

Arches 1 and 2 regress and give rise to maxillary and stapedial arteries. In humans, the fifth arch does not form to any significant degree. The third arch forms the common carotid arteries bilaterally. The sixth arch forms the left and right pulmonary arteries respectively along with the patent ductus arteriosus. Normally, the left fourth pharyngeal arch will form a portion of the adult aortic arch (between the left carotid and left subclavian arteries) whereas the right fourth arch will regress and form the right subclavian artery. A right aortic arch results when this pattern of normal regression is reversed. Similarly, persistence of both right and left fourth arches will form a double aortic arch.

Clinical Presentation and Diagnosis

Depending on the severity of compression of both the esophagus and trachea due to a vascular ring, patients may have symptoms within the first few months of life. However, it is not unusual to see patients that present with significant symptoms at a much later date, even in adulthood. Presentation is generally dependent upon the severity of obstruction based upon the "tightness" of the ring itself. Tighter lesions, like the double aortic arch and pulmonary artery slings, usually present earlier (within 3 months of age) relative to those that are loose such as aberrant right subclavian artery that typically present at greater than 6 months of age [2].

J. Lioy and S.E. Sobol (eds.), *Disorders of the Neonatal Airway: Fundamentals for Practice*,
DOI 10.1007/978-1-4939-1610-8_13, © Springer Science+Business Media New York 2015

Table 1 Classification of vascular rings

Double aortic arch
Right arch dominant
Left arch dominant
Balanced double arch
Right aortic arch
Mirror image branching
Retroesophageal left subclavian artery
Circumflex aorta
Pulmonary artery sling
Innominate artery compression

The most common symptoms from these vascular anomalies arise from the external compression of trachea and esophagus. These symptoms include inspiratory stridor, dyspnea, cough, wheezing, and dysphagia. In addition to obstruction of airflow, tracheal compression also impedes mucociliary clearance and, as a result, many patients will also suffer with recurrent respiratory tract infections [3]. Since these symptoms are shared with many other and more prevalent childhood illnesses, these patients can have a significant delay in diagnosis. Often they will receive long-term bronchodilators in an attempt to treat asthma and multiple courses of antibiotics to treat upper respiratory infections before the actual disease is accurately diagnosed. Persistence of these symptoms, especially when they do not respond to routine treatment, should alert the pediatrician of the possibility of a vascular ring. Only a high index of suspicion will ensure these patients receive early diagnosis and appropriate therapy.

Diagnosis

With the availability of more sophisticated imaging techniques, many recent publications give only historical value to the chest radiograph findings in these patients [4]. The chest X-ray is usually the first imaging study performed in a child with airway obstruction and can frequently point toward the presence of a vascular ring. Films should be assessed for the laterality of the aortic arch and for evidence of tracheal compression at the level of the arch, often better visualized on lateral films.

Absence of an aortic knuckle on the left side suggests a right arch, and when present in a child with symptoms of airway obstruction, a vascular ring should be strongly suspected. A right aortic arch may be suspected if the distal trachea is seen slightly deviated to the left instead of the right, because of the aortic arch bowing over the right main stem bronchus instead of the left. Similarly, a double aortic arch is likely if the sidedness of the arch cannot be determined on chest X-ray. Hyperinflation of the left lung with the left hilum lower than the right may suggest a pulmonary artery sling. The location of the descending aorta can usually be determined by inspecting the paraspinal line and the azygoesophageal recess.

A barium esophagogram used to be the most extensively used imaging study for the diagnosis of a vascular ring. Contrast swallow will show a posterior indentation of the esophagus in all vascular anomalies except in the presence of a pulmonary artery sling, which will produce an anterior indentation on the esophagus and an increase in the space between the esophagus and trachea at the same level.

Upon bronchoscopy, vascular rings appear as an external compression of the trachea just above the carina. Routine bronchoscopy is not necessary in a symptomatic patient with a radiologically proven vascular ring. However, it plays an essential role in the diagnostic workup of an infant with airway obstruction and an unclear cause. Bronchoscopy may also reveal additional associated airway lesions, such as tracheomalacia, complete tracheal rings, and tracheal stenosis, which may be commonly associated with vascular anomalies. In fact, vascular rings and innominate artery compression are the most common congenital cause for secondary tracheomalacia [5]. The diagnosis of innominate artery compression is almost always based on its classical findings on bronchoscopy of anterior pulsatile compression of lower trachea.

Both computed tomography (CT) and magnetic resonance imaging (MRI) are extremely useful techniques in the diagnosis of a vascular compression of the airway. The greatest advantage of these imaging modalities is their capability to completely delineate the anomaly along with their relationship to the adjacent structures. Both provide post-processed 3D images that can be very helpful in planning a surgical intervention. However, a limitation common to both these techniques is their inability to directly visualize obliterated structures. Even so, based on branching patterns, the laterality of the arch, and compression of the airway, a diagnosis of vascular ring can usually be reached. There are advantages as well as disadvantages to both modalities. We feel that CT provides excellent tracheal images at a minimal risk of ionizing radiation. MRI, on the other hand, provides a superior assessment of cardiac anatomy and function in the case that additional information is helpful. Yet, scan times are much longer thus requiring sedation and anesthesia in most infants and toddlers.

Echocardiogram can easily identify branching patterns and sidedness of the arch. It can also identify a double aortic arch when both the arches are patent. However, it is not useful to identify an obliterated lumen. It is helpful in the identification of congenital heart disease commonly associated with vascular rings such as the association between right aortic arch and tetralogy of Fallot, the incidence of which can be as high as 30 %.

Before CT and MRI were widely available, angiography was very frequently used to diagnose vascular rings. Since MRI and CT can provide essentially the same information noninvasively, a cardiac catheterization is now very infrequently utilized, unless needed for an associated cardiac disease.

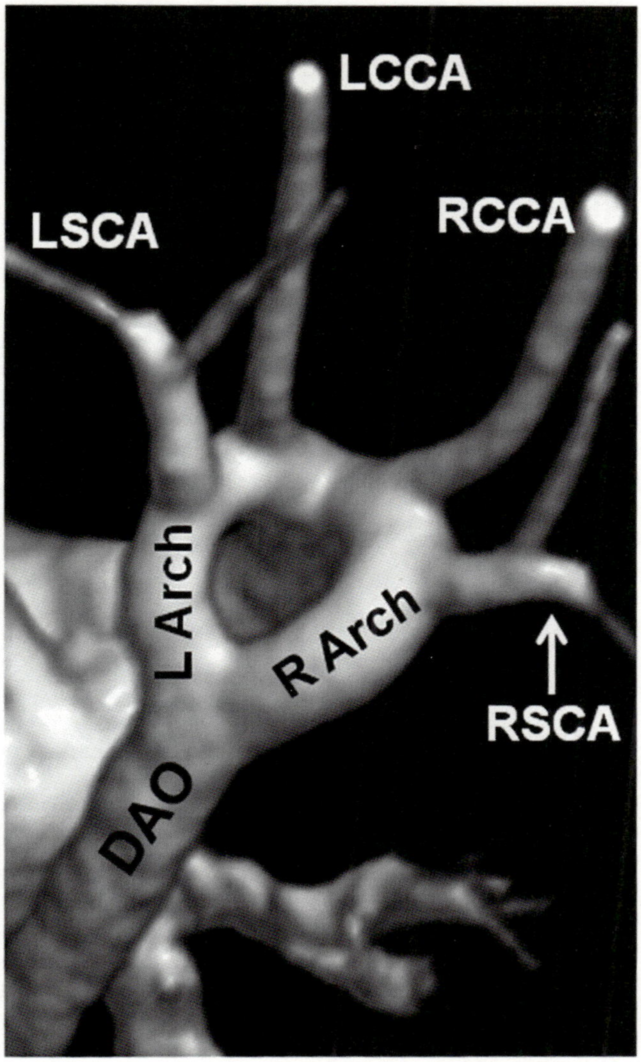

Fig. 1 Magnetic resonance angiogram of an unobstructed double aortic arch viewed from right posterior oblique with cranial angulation. Note that the right aortic arch is slightly larger. Descending Aorta (DAO), Left-Sided Arch (L Arch), Left Common Carotid Artery (LCCA), Left Subclavian Artery (LSCA), Right-Sided Arch (R Arch), Right Common Carotid Artery (RCCA), Right Subclavian Artery (RSCA)

Double Aortic Arch

This is the most common symptomatic vascular ring present in 0.05–0.3 % of the population and results from the persistence of both right and left fourth primordial arches. Two aortic arches arise from the ascending aorta and pass on either sides of trachea and esophagus to meet the descending aorta posteriorly, forming a complete ring. The right and left carotid and subclavian arteries arise from their respective arch. In almost 70 % patients, the right arch is larger (dominant), posterior, and more cephalad than the left, in about 25 % the left arch is dominant and in about 5 % patients both arches are balanced (Fig. 1).

A double aortic arch will usually cause significant narrowing and anterior bowing of thoracic trachea, and this can occasionally be seen on a lateral chest radiograph.

The surgical treatment of a double aortic arch consists of division of the lesser of the two arches.

For most patients, the approach is through a left posterolateral thoracotomy. In rare circumstances, a right thoracotomy is utilized in patients with a dominant left arch. After adequate exposure via thoracotomy, the ligamentum arteriosum, both arches, neck vessels, and descending aorta are clearly identified and both the ligamentum as well as the lesser of the two aortic arches are divided between vascular clamps, usually where the arch joins the descending aorta posteriorly. The divided ends are then oversewn using polypropylene sutures. Frequently, there will be an atretic segment in the lesser aortic arch in which case this site is then ideally suited for division.

Intraoperatively, it is useful to have pulse oximetry and/or pressure monitoring available for both upper and lower limbs. With balanced arches, blood pressure is checked in the lower limbs, while the clamps are alternately applied to each arch. The arch associated with a lesser fall in blood pressure in the lower limbs is then divided. If no appreciable difference is noted, it is preferable to divide the right arch, as its anatomical location poses a higher risk of continued compression of the trachea.

Right Arch

As previously mentioned, a right aortic arch will form if the left fourth arch regresses. Different configurations of vascular rings result depending upon the site of regression.

Right arch and retroesophageal left subclavian artery. This is the most common (65 %) type of right arch seen [10] and results from the involution of the left fourth arch between the left common carotid and left subclavian arteries. As a result, the left subclavian now arises from the descending aorta and passes behind the esophagus to reach the left arm. The ligamentum connects the descending aorta to the left pulmonary artery and, in doing so, completes the ring.

Occasionally, the origin of the aberrant left subclavian will have a bulb like dilation, known as Kommerell's diverticulum (Fig. 2).

This represents the remnant of fourth embryonic arch. When present, it implies a left ligamentum arteriosum and denotes the presence of a ring. Additionally, Kommerell's diverticulum may dilate over time and can compress the trachea and/or esophagus, leading to a recurrence of symptoms.

Surgical approach to these patients is again through a left posterolateral thoracotomy. With careful dissection, the ligamentum, aortic arch, brachiocephalic vessels, and descend-

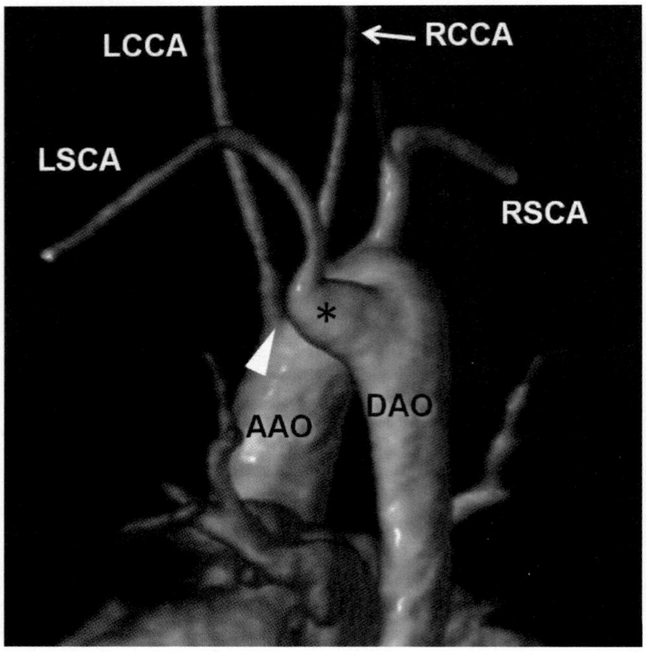

Fig. 2 Magnetic resonance angiogram viewed from left posterior oblique demonstrates a right aortic arch with an aberrant left subclavian artery originating from a retroesophageal diverticulum (diverticulum of Kommerell). The location of the left-sided ligamentum arteriosum (*arrowhead*), though not directly observed, is implied by the regionally dilated proximal left subclavian artery (*) completing the vascular ring. Aberrant Left Subclavian Artery (ALSCA), Aberrant Right Subclavian Artery (ARSCA), Descending Aorta (DAO), Left Common Carotid Artery (LCCA), Right Common Carotid Artery (RCCA)

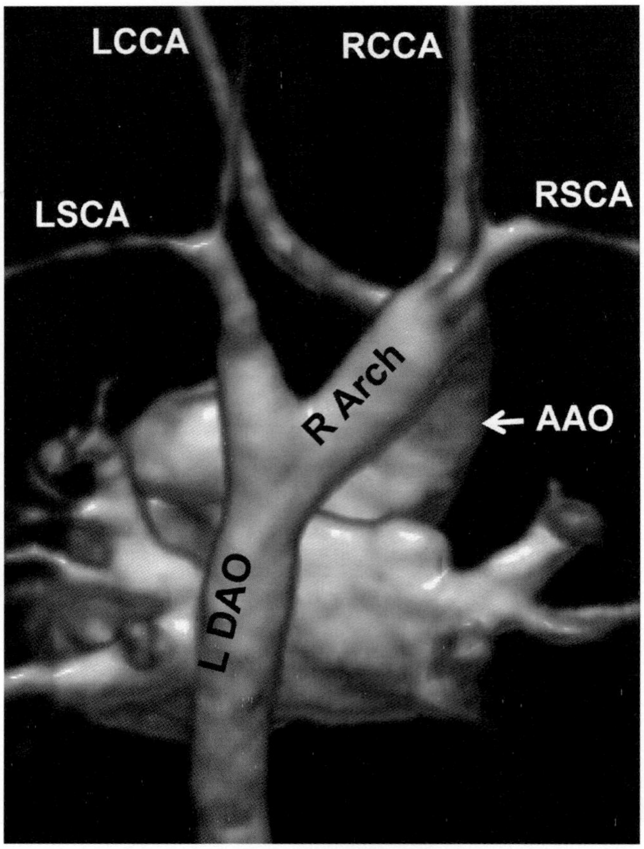

Fig. 3 Magnetic resonance angiogram from a direct posterior view demonstrates a right aortic arch with left-sided descending aorta (circumflex aortic arch). The combination of right arch and left-sided thoracic descending aorta implies a left ligamentum which completes the ring. Left-Sided Descending Aorta (L DAO), Left Common Carotid Artery (LCCA), Left Subclavian Artery (LSCA), Right-Sided Arch (R Arch), Right Common Carotid Artery (RCCA), Right Subclavian Artery (RSCA)

ing aorta are clearly identified. The ligamentum is then divided and its stumps are oversewn.

When a Kommerell's diverticulum is present, controversy exists whether or not it should be resected, or whether the left subclavian artery should be transferred to the left carotid artery. Division of the ligamentum and pexy of the diverticulum may be associated with late dilation of the diverticulum and recurrence of symptoms [6–8].

Right arch mirror image branching. A right aortic arch with mirror image branching occurs when the left fourth arch regresses between the subclavian artery and the descending aorta. As a result, the branching pattern resembles a "mirror image" of the normal left arch. A vascular ring may form if the ligamentum arises from the descending thoracic aorta. However, it most commonly originates from the innominate artery and therefore does not form a compressive vascular ring.

Right aortic arch with left descending aorta (circumflex aorta). This is a rare variant of right aortic arch, where the transverse arch courses posterior to the esophagus and continues as a left descending aorta. A vascular ring is formed in the setting of a left ligamentum (Figs. 3 and 4).

Optimal surgical treatment for this anomaly is known as an "Aortic Uncrossing" and is a more complicated operation, requiring a median sternotomy, the use of cardiopulmonary bypass and deep hypothermic circulatory arrest. The arch along with its branches is extensively mobilized and then divided at a point where it hooks around the esophagus. The proximal end of the arch may be oversewn while the distal retro esophageal segment is brought anteriorly and anastomosed to a counter-incision on the left lateral side of the ascending aorta. Alternatively, both sides of the arch are mobilized anterior to the trachea with great care not to injure both recurrent laryngeal nerves. This lesion may occur in conjunction with severe long segment coarctation of the retro esophageal and descending aorta. In these rare cases, the coarctation requires augmentation using a patch material.

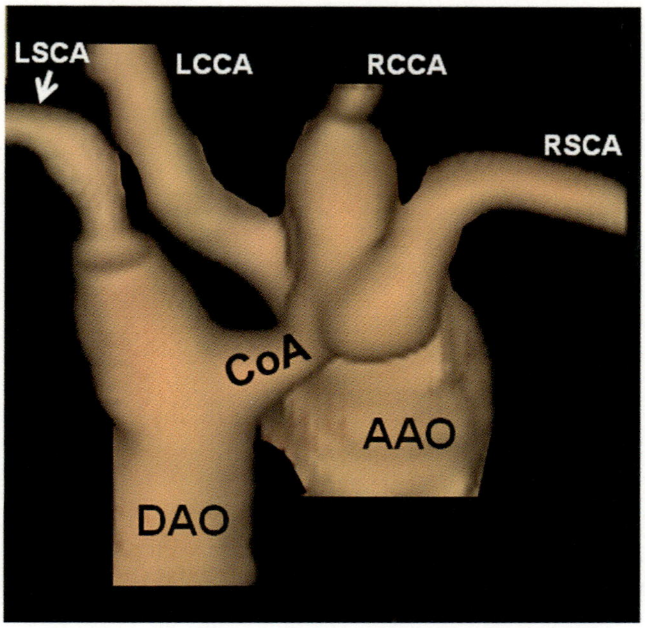

Fig. 4 Magnetic resonance angiogram from a direct posterior view demonstrates a right aortic arch with left-sided descending aorta. The combination of right arch and left-sided thoracic descending aorta implies a left ligamentum which completes the ring. In this particular patient there is also the rare presence of coarctation of the right-sided aortic arch

Pulmonary Artery Sling

This is a relatively uncommon vascular anomaly in which the left pulmonary artery arises extra-pericardially, from the posterior aspect of the right pulmonary artery. It then hooks over the right bronchus and passes between the trachea and esophagus to reach the left pulmonary hilum (Fig. 5).

With this configuration, the left pulmonary artery compresses the lower trachea leading to severe stenosis [9]. Additionally, this anomaly is also strongly associated with tracheal stenosis, due to the presence of complete tracheal rings, in almost 50–65 % patients (known as the ring-sling complex). The tracheal cartilage forms a complete circle with an absence of membranous trachea.

Repair of a pulmonary artery sling requires a median sternotomy and cardiopulmonary bypass [10]. The ductus or the ligamentum is divided. The left pulmonary artery is dissected circumferentially from its origin on the right pulmonary artery to its left hilar branches. It is then divided between clamps at its origin from the right pulmonary artery. It is then brought anterior to the bronchus, and anastomosed to a counter-incision on the main pulmonary artery with great care not to kink the vessel at its neo-origin.

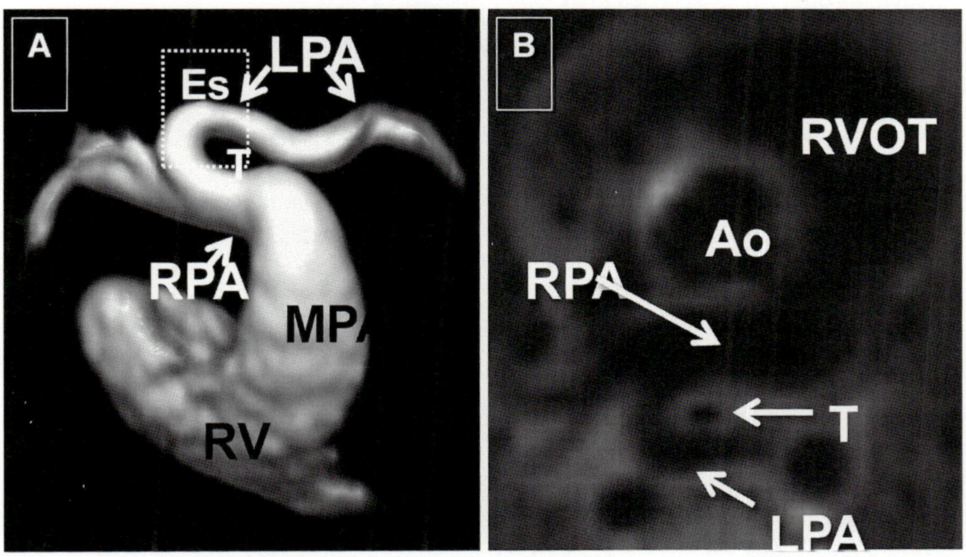

Fig. 5 (**a**) Magnetic resonance angiogram demonstrating a Pulmonary Sling. In this disease, the left pulmonary artery originates from the proximal right pulmonary artery and then passes between the relatively anterior trachea and the relatively posterior esophagus as it heads back toward the left lung. This creates a sling around the trachea with a leftward pull typically producing severe tracheal symptoms. In contrast, vascular rings encompass both the trachea and the esophagus and therefore may cause both stridor and dysphagia. (**b**) Spin Echo Dark Blood Image demonstrating tracheal narrowing at the level where the left pulmonary artery creates a sling around the trachea. Aorta (Ao), Esophagus (Es), Left Pulmonary Artery (LPA), Right Pulmonary Artery (RPA), Right Ventricle Outflow Tract (RV), Trachea (T)

In the presence of complete tracheal rings, a concomitant repair of the trachea (slide tracheoplasty) must be performed.

Innominate Artery Compression

This results from an innominate artery that arises a more distal on the aortic arch than normal and compresses the lower end of trachea as it crosses it anteriorly from left to right (Fig. 6).

The incidence of this anomaly seems to be relatively high. However, only a fraction of these patients are symptomatic, leading to a lot of debate on the optimal management of these patients.

For those symptomatic patients with respiratory distress, persistent stridor and reflex apnea should have an aggressive diagnostic workup followed by aortopexy [11].

The diagnosis is usually made on bronchoscopy by the presence of a pulsatile anterior narrowing of the lower trachea on a child with symptoms of airway obstruction. Additional radiological imaging (CT, MRI) may further support the diagnosis.

Aortopexy, in which the innominate artery and proximal arch are suspended with sutures, to the posterior surface of the sternum, is a simple and effective procedure for the treatment of this malformation. Surgical approach is typically through a small right anterior thoracotomy in the second intercostal space. The right lobe of thymus is resected, taking care to avoid injury to the phrenic nerve. The proximal innominate artery and arch adjacent to its origin are suspended to the posterior sternal periosteum using 3–4 pledgeted mattress sutures that are tied down, at times under direct bronchoscopic guidance. If needed, these sutures can also be passed trans-sternally, and tied on the anterior surface of the sternum. It is important, not to dissect the space between innominate artery and the trachea, as this fibrous tissue will necessary to effectively pexy the anterior wall of trachea.

Left Aortic Arch and Aberrant Right Subclavian

When the right fourth pharyngeal arch regresses between the subclavian and the carotid arteries, the right subclavian artery will arise "aberrantly" from the descending aorta. The incidence of this anomaly ranges between 0.5 and 1.8 %. The majority of these individuals will remain asymptomatic, and only rarely when the ligamentum is right sided will a vascular ring form.

Postoperative Care

Most patients have a relatively straightforward postoperative course after surgical repair. Early extubation is recommended except in those with a concomitant procedure of the trachea or tracheomalacia. Therapies that may prove useful in the early postoperative period include oxygen, humidity, inhaled steroids, bronchodilators, and aggressive early chest physiotherapy. Vocal cord paresis and/or paralysis are a known complication of surgical repair and should be watched for in the post op. Persistent airway obstruction after surgical repair can be due to residual compression, tracheomalacia, or intrinsic lesions of the airway.

Results

Long-term results of surgical repair of vascular rings are generally good, with no reported operative mortality and a very low risk of recurrence as highlighted in many recent publications [11]. Of note, complete resolution of symptoms may not always be evident immediately after surgery, and this is commonly due to an associated tracheal lesion (malacia), and

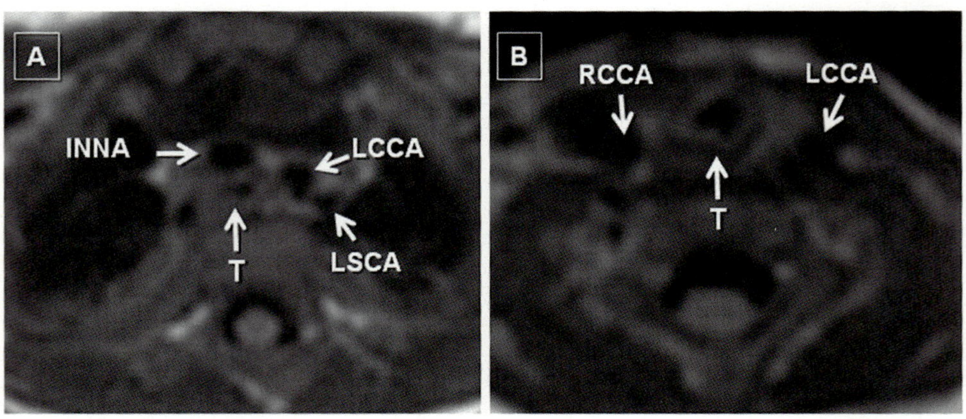

Fig. 6 (**a**) Turbo spin echo dark blood image in transverse view demonstrates severe tracheal flattening at the point where the innominate artery crosses anterior to the trachea. Bronchoscopy demonstrated tracheomalacia of the proximal trachea associated with an anterior pulsating mass. These findings are consistent with innominate artery compression of the trachea. (**b**) More superiorly above the thoracic inlet, the trachea appears round and patent

improves over time. By 1 year, almost 70 % of all patients are expected to be symptom free [7, 12], and most of the remaining patients will have experienced a substantial improvement in symptoms.

Multidisciplinary Considerations

While surgical repair is performed by the cardiothoracic surgeon, management of vascular anomalies often involves multidisciplinary input from neonatology, otolaryngology, pulmonology, and cardiology.

Future Considerations

Over the past few years, there has been a push to expand the role of minimally invasive cardiac surgery in pediatric patients. In 1995, based on an experience with video-assisted interruption of the patent ductus arteriosus, Burke et al. [13] reported their initial results with video-assisted vascular ring division, and recently, robotically assisted vascular ring division represents a further step in this direction [14]. By avoiding muscle division and rib spreading, these minimally invasive operations decrease post-thoracotomy pain, tearing of intercostal ligaments, and may also improve early postoperative respiratory function, in addition to better cosmetic results. However, operative times are longer, conversion rates are still significant, along with a much higher procedural cost.

Importantly, the use of these minimally invasive procedures is limited to relatively bigger kids, and for non-patent (atretic) vascular rings. Recent advances in thoracoscopic and robotic instruments have undoubtedly contributed to an increasing use of these techniques. In the present, however, the use of this technology for surgical correction of vascular rings is very limited and its future application will depend largely on follow-up studies, further advances, and improved cost-effectiveness.

References

1. Backer CL, Mavroudis C. Congenital Heart Surgery Nomenclature and Database Project: vascular rings, tracheal stenosis, pectus excavatum. Ann Thorac Surg. 2000;69:S308–18.
2. Smith RJ, Smith MC, Glossop LP, Bailey CM, Evans JN. Congenital vascular anomalies causing tracheoesophageal compression. Arch Otolaryngol. 1984;110:82–7.
3. McLaughlin Jr RB, Wetmore RF, Tavill MA, Gaynor JW, Spray TL. Vascular anomalies causing symptomatic tracheobronchial compression. Laryngoscope. 1999;109:312–9.
4. McLaren CA, Elliott MJ, Roebuck DJ. Vascular compression of the airway in children. Paediatr Respir Rev. 2008;9:85–94.
5. Thompson DM, Willging JP, Cotton RT. Lesions of the larynx, trachea and upper airway. In: Coran AG, editor. Pediatric surgery, vol. 2. New York: Elsevier; 2012. p. 837–54.
6. Ruzmetov M, Vijay P, Rodefeld MD, Turrentine MW, Brown JW. Follow-up of surgical correction of aortic arch anomalies causing tracheoesophageal compression: a 38-year single institution experience. J Pediatr Surg. 2009;44:1328–32.
7. Backer CL, Russell HM, Wurlitzer KC, Rastatter JC, Rigsby CK. Primary resection of Kommerell diverticulum adn left subclavian artery transfer. Ann Thorac Surg. 2012;94:1612–7.
8. Ota T, Okada K, Takanashi S, Yamamoto S, Okita Y. Surgical strategy for Kommerell's diverticulum. J Thorac Cardiovasc Surg. 2013;131:574–8.
9. Sailer R, et al. Pulmonary artery sling associated with tracheobronchial malformations. Arch Otolaryngol Head Neck Surg. 1992;118:864–7.
10. Fiore AC, Brown JW, Weber TR, Turrentine MW. Surgical treatment of pulmonary artery sling and tracheal stenosis. Ann Thorac Surg. 2005;79:38–46.
11. Gardella C, et al. Tracheal compression by aberrant innominate artery: clinical presentations in infants and children, indications for surgical correction by aortopexy, and short- and long-term outcome. J Pediatr Surg. 2010;45:564–73.
12. Woods RK, Sharp RJ, Holcomb III GW, Snyder CL, Lofland GK, Ashcraft KW, Holder TM. Vascular anomalies and tracheoesophageal compression: a single institution's 25-year experience. Ann Thorac Surg. 2001;72(2):434–8.
13. Burke RP, Rosenfeld HM, Wernovsky G, Jonas RA. Video-assisted thoracoscopic vascular ring division in infants and children. J Am Coll Cardiol. 1995;25(4):943–7.
14. Suematsu Y, Mora BN, Mihaljevic T, del Nido PJ. Totally endoscopic robotic-assisted repair of patent ductus arteriosus and vascular ring in children. Ann Thorac Surg. 2005;80(6):2309–13.

Malformations, Deformations, and Disorders of the Neonatal Airway: A Bullet Point Review

Pamela Mudd, Steven Andreoli, and Steven E. Sobol

The Nose

Nasal obstruction in the neonate is often symptomatic as infants are preferential nasal breathers. Immediate presentation may be cyclical cyanosis relieved by crying, airway distress, and feeding difficulties. The differential diagnosis for nasal obstruction includes: rhinitis/inflammation, arhinia, piriform aperture stenosis, nasal septal deviation, nasolacrimal duct cyst (bilateral or unilateral), nasal hemangioma, and other rare tumors, encephalocele/glioma, choanal stenosis/atresia.

- Piriform aperture and nasal stenosis
  - Etiology
    - The nasal inlet is narrowed by overgrowth or medial position of the nasal process of the maxilla at the level of the piriform aperture bilaterally.
    - Partial obstruction of the nasal inlet, which may be associated with craniofacial or skull base anomalies.
  - Epidemiology
    - Rare
    - May be associated with a single central incisor or anterior pituitary abnormalities.
  - Pathogenesis
    - The narrowed aperture or nasal cavity leads to increased nasal resistance.
  - Clinical presentation
    - Difficulty is with breathing and/or feeding.
    - Anterior rhinoscopy identifies a narrowed nasal inlet, may be unable to pass 6 French catheter or 2.2 mm scope into the nasal aperture.
  - Diagnosis
    - Clinical evaluation is complemented by non-contrasted CT scan of the skull and sinuses inclusive of the pituitary and maxillary dentition.
    - Diagnosis is made when the nasal aperture is less than 11 mm on axial CT scan.
  - Medical management
    - Observation if minimally symptomatic.
    - Conservative management with nasal saline or steroids if moderate symptomatology.
    - Oral breathing appliance such as McGovern nipple or intubation for acute respiratory distress.
  - Surgical management
    - Most often required when piriform aperture width is <5 mm. Most common approach is sublabial with drill out of the piriform aperture, nasal dilation, with or without stent placement.
  - Multidisciplinary considerations
    - Endocrinology/Neurology: Association with anterior pituitary abnormalities, holoprosencephaly spectrum.
    - Dentistry/OMFS: Often associated with median central incisor.
    - Genetics: When syndrome suspected.
- Choanal atresia and stenosis (bilateral and unilateral)
  - Etiology
    - Failure of recanalization of the buccal pharyngeal membrane during 4th–12th week of gestation leads to atresia (complete obstruction) or stenosis (narrowing) of the posterior choanae.
    - May be unilateral or bilateral.
    - Most common abnormality is bony/membranous obstruction; the vomer (posterior septum) is often bowed.
    - May be associated with skull base or midline defects, especially when presenting as part of a syndrome.

P. Mudd, M.D. • S. Andreoli, M.D.
Division of Otolaryngology, The Children's Hospital of Philadelphia, Philadelphia, PA, USA

S.E. Sobol, M.D., M.Sc., FRCS(C) (✉)
Pediatric Otolaryngology, The Center for Pediatric Airway Disorders, The Children's Hospital of Philadelphia, Philadelphia, PA, USA

Department of Otorhinolaryngology-Head and Neck Surgery, University of Pennsylvania Perelman School of Medicine, Philadelphia, PA, USA
e-mail: sobols@email.chop.edu

J. Lioy and S.E. Sobol (eds.), *Disorders of the Neonatal Airway: Fundamentals for Practice*, DOI 10.1007/978-1-4939-1610-8_14, © Springer Science+Business Media New York 2015

- Epidemiology
  - 1: 7,000 live births, female to males equal in the recent literature.
  - 50 % associated with syndrome or additional anomalies.
- Pathogenesis
  - Atresia occludes passage of air or drainage of nasal secretions. Stenosis increases airway resistance.
- Clinical presentation
  - Neonate with bilateral atresia/stenosis will present with labored breathing, desaturations, cyclical cyanosis, and feeding difficulties.
  - Unilateral stenosis often presents with unilateral rhinorrhea/sinusitis, rarely with respiratory distress.
- Diagnosis
  - Failure to pass a 5/6 french catheter.
  - Nasal endoscopy revealing the atretic plate.
  - Non-contrast fine cut CT scan of the skull base/sinuses.
- Medical management
  - Conservative management: Oral airway or McGovern nipple and side or prone positioning may help initially. Intubation often necessary with bilateral atresia.
- Surgical management
  - Endoscopic approach is most common. Serves to dilate and or repair the membranous and bony narrowing often with a posterior septectomy.
  - Bilateral atresia should be repaired once work-up is complete.
  - Unilateral atresia/stenosis repair can be delayed until childhood to allow for skull and patient.
- Multidisciplinary considerations
  - Genetics: Associated syndromes: CHARGE.

The Oropharynx

The oropharyngeal airway may be obstructed by a prolapsing tongue base or a space-occupying mass. When the oropharynx is obstructed, air cannot pass fluidly from the nasal cavity or mouth into the larynx. The differential diagnosis for oropharyngeal obstruction includes: macroglossia, glossoptosis, nasopharyngeal mass extension, oropharyngeal mass, vallecular cyst, an undescended thyroid, or thyroglossal duct cyst.

- Glossoptosis
  - Etiology
    - Most commonly associated with Pierre Robin Sequence: Congenital micrognathia which leads to glossoptosis (tongue base obstruction of the posterior pharynx) and airway distress of the neonate.
    - Most cases associated with a secondary cleft palate: U shaped, involving the soft palate.
  - Epidemiology
    - 1 in 8,500–14,000 births.
  - Pathogenesis
    - Airway obstruction secondary to displacement of the tongue into the hypopharynx occluding the airway at the level of the epiglottis.
  - Clinical presentation
    - Airway distress in the neonate with apparent obstruction, which may be positional (worse on back), feeding difficulties, including airway distress or desaturation during feeding.
  - Diagnosis
    - Clinical diagnosis is complemented by a modified polysomnogram to quantify the severity of obstruction.
    - Awake flexible nasopharyngolaryngoscopy can aid in assessment of the tongue base position relative to the posterior pharyngeal wall.
    - Imaging with plain film or more commonly CT scan with 3D reconstructions of the face is obtained if considering surgical management.
  - Medical management
    - Prone or side lying positioning.
    - Nasal trumpet/nasopharyngeal airway.
    - Airway support with high flow nasal catheter or positive pressure ventilation.
  - Surgical management
    - Tongue–lip adhesion: Tongue musculature is sutured to that lower lip musculature to prevent ptosis of tongue base; the adhesion is later released.
    - Mandibular distraction: The mandible is advanced forward using distraction osteogenesis technique—internal and external devices.
    - Tracheostomy: Definitive management in refractory or complicated cases.
  - Multidisciplinary considerations
    - Plastic surgery: May consider mandibular distraction osteogenesis (MDO) for cases associated with micrognathia.
    - Genetics: More than 40 associated syndromes. Most common: Stickler and 22q11.2 deletion syndrome.
- Vallecular cyst
  - Etiology
    - Etiology related to either a trapped minor salivary gland or a variant of a thyroglossal duct cyst present solely in the tongue base.
  - Epidemiology
    - Congenital airway cysts occur in 1.87–3.49 cases per 100,000 live births.
      - Vallecular cysts account for ~10.5 %.
  - Pathogenesis
    - Cyst may grow slowly or rapidly leading to a spectrum of airway symptoms. Most commonly presents within the first 2 weeks of life.
    - Secondary laryngomalacia may occur secondary to the Bernoulli Effect.

- Clinical presentation
  - Most commonly presents with inspiratory stridor similar to laryngomalacia. Depending on the size may lead to complete airway obstruction with distress.
  - Large cysts also associated with feeding difficulties.
- Diagnosis
  - Awake flexible fiberoptic pharyngolaryngoscopy.
  - Microlaryngoscopy demonstrates a mucous-filled cyst in the vallecula between the tongue base and laryngeal surface of the epiglottis.
- Management
  - Surgical management is the mainstay of treatment.
  - Microlaryngoscopy and bronchoscopy with endoscopic marsupialization or excision with microlaryngeal instruments, microdebrider, or laser.
  - Preservation of lingual surface of the epiglottis is important to prevent vallecular scarring.
  - Cyst recurrence is rare.
- Multidisciplinary considerations
  - Speech therapy: For evaluation and management of aspiration, if indicated.

The Larynx

The larynx consists of the supraglottic, glottic, and subglottic structures. Difficulties at the level of the larynx are commonly associated with stridor or noisy breathing. Some congenital anomalies present immediately with airway distress while others are asymptomatic or discovered later in infancy or childhood as feeding and growing difficulties arise.

Supraglottic Airway

Supraglottic anomalies affect the airway at the level of the epiglottis through the ventricle, which sits immediately superior to the vocal cords. Anomalies discussed below include laryngomalacia, bifid epiglottis, saccular cyst, and laryngeal cleft.

- Laryngomalacia
  - Etiology
    - Most common cause of stridor in infants, resulting from dynamic collapse of the supraglottic structures into the laryngeal inlet during inspiration.
  - Epidemiology
    - Incidence is unknown but accounts for 70–95 % of all neonatal stridor.
    - Incidence of synchronous airway lesions is ~15 % (more frequent in severe cases).
  - Pathogenesis
    - Collapse related to: Omega-shaped epiglottis, short aryepiglottic folds, and/or redundant supra-arytenoid tissue and cuneiform cartilages.
  - Clinical presentation
    - Fluttering inspiratory stridor most pronounced while supine, crying, sleeping, or with feeding.
    - Obstructive sleep apnea may be present.
    - Severe cases may present with failure to thrive or respiratory distress.
    - High concomitant incidence of gastroesophageal reflux.
  - Diagnosis
    - Awake fiberoptic laryngoscopy demonstrates an omega-shaped epiglottis, short aryepiglottic folds, and/or redundant and prolapsing soft tissue over the arytenoid cartilages.
    - Microlaryngoscopy and bronchoscopy may be necessary to rule out significant synchronous airway lesions.
    - Reflux evaluation may be indicated when feeding or swallowing symptoms are present.
  - Medical management
    - Most cases self-resolve over 12–18 months and require no medical treatment.
    - Reflux management should be considered in patients with feeding or respiratory concerns.
  - Surgical management
    - Consider microlaryngoscopy and bronchoscopy in recalcitrant cases to identify secondary airway lesions.
    - Supraglottoplasty is performed with microlaryngeal instruments or laser for children with failure to thrive, cyanotic spells, severe OSA, or recurrent respiratory admissions.
  - Multidisciplinary considerations
    - Pulmonary: May consider PSG to evaluate for central and obstructive sleep apnea.
    - Speech therapy: Preoperative and postoperative aspiration risk.
    - Gastroenterology: If significant reflux is present and recalcitrant to therapy.
- Bifid epiglottis
  - Etiology
    - Clefted epiglottis involving at least 2/3 of the height of the epiglottis. The embryology is not clear though the epiglottis is derived from the hypobranchial eminence with likely involvement of the 4th branchial pouch.
    - Teratogen theory as hand, hypothalamus, and oral cavity development occurs during the same time period and may have associated anomalies.
  - Epidemiology
    - Usually does not present as an isolated anomaly, incidence not well reported.
    - Associated with Pallister–Hall syndrome.
  - Pathogenesis
    - Midline cleft within the epiglottis rendering it incompetent.

- Clinical presentation
  - Inspiratory stridor, worse with feeding.
  - Choking or gagging with feeds if aspiration.
- Diagnosis
  - Awake flexible laryngoscopy.
  - Consider rigid laryngoscopy and bronchoscopy to assess for additional anomalies.
  - Modified barium swallow to assess epiglottic competency and aspiration risk.
- Management
  - Medical and genetic work-up for associated conditions including: Pallister–Hall, polydactyly, congenital hypothyroidism, and hypothalamic dysfunction.
  - Surgical management is not well described.
- Multidisciplinary considerations
  - Genetics: Commonly associated with anomalies of the hands/feet (most commonly syndactyly), oral cavity, and hypothalamus/pituitary axis.
  - Endocrine: Hypothalamus and pituitary axis abnormalities.
  - Speech therapy: If aspiration or feeding issues.

- Saccular cyst
  - Etiology
    - Cystic blockage at the opening of the saccule of the laryngeal ventricle, which extends between the false and true vocal folds.
    - Originate from an obstruction of the excretory duct of laryngeal epithelial mucous glands.
  - Epidemiology
    - Congenital airway cysts occur in 1.87–3.49 cases per 100,000 live births.
      - Saccular cysts account for ~25 %.
  - Pathogenesis
    - Cystic accumulation of fluid within the laryngeal saccule. May partially or complete block the laryngeal inlet.
  - Clinical presentation
    - May present with the spectrum of airway obstruction depending on the size and location.
    - Most commonly presents with stridor similar to laryngomalacia but may also be associated with hoarse cry or cyanotic spells and may progress to complete airway obstruction as the cyst enlarges.
  - Diagnosis
    - Fiberoptic laryngoscopy.
    - Anterior cysts project medially into the laryngeal ventricle. Lateral cysts project into the false cord, aryepiglottic fold, and may extend extralaryngeal.
    - MRI or CT complementary to determine origin and extent of cyst once identified.
  - Management
    - Surgical management is the mainstay of treatment.
    - Microlaryngoscopy and bronchoscopy with endoscopic excision may be used for medially projecting lesions using cold instrumentation or laser excision/marsupialization.
    - Lesions with extralaryngeal extent may be approached from an external thyrotomy.
  - Multidisciplinary considerations
    - Speech therapy: For evaluation and management of aspiration, if indicated.
- Laryngeal/interarytenoid cleft
  - Etiology
    - Type I cleft defined as supraglottic cleft—depth of the interarytenoid notch extends to the level of the vocal cords—diastasis of the interarytenoid musculature.
    - Type II cleft involves the superior posterior cricoid cartilage—incomplete fusion of the posterior cricoid ring.
  - Epidemiology
    - Historical incidence is 0.1–0.47 % with type I clefts being most common.
  - Pathogenesis
    - Branchial anomaly: Failure of the cricoid (6th arch) to fuse posteriorly.
  - Clinical presentation
    - Aspiration and/or chronic cough.
    - Recurrent pneumonia.
  - Diagnosis
    - Videofluoroscopic swallow study.
    - Microlaryngoscopy with suspension laryngoscopy and palpation of the interarytenoid space.
  - Medical management
    - Trial of conservative management involves antireflux therapy, a thickened liquid feeding regimen, and maneuvers during feeding to prevent aspiration.
  - Surgical management
    - Surgery is recommended if persistent symptoms despite medical management or if symptom severity warrants immediate treatment. Surgical intervention includes interarytenoid bulking procedure with injection, endoscopic laryngeal cleft repair, and open laryngeal cleft repair through a laryngofissure.
  - Multidisciplinary considerations
    - Speech therapy: For evaluation and management of aspiration risk once cleft identified.

Glottic Airway

Glottic anomalies affect the airway involving the vocal cords. Glottic anomalies lead to a dysphonic or aphonic cry and may also present with stridor. In the most extreme case of laryngeal agenesis the laryngeal structures fail to form and present prenatally requiring an EXIT procedure in order to secure the airway. Other anomalies discussed below include vocal cord paralysis and laryngeal/glottic web.

- Bilateral vocal cord paralysis
  - Etiology
    - Most common etiology is idiopathic. Other causes secondary to medical conditions include: Arnold–Chiari malformation, intracranial hemorrhage, hydrocephalus, meningocele, and myasthenia gravis.
  - Epidemiology
    - The second most common cause of neonatal stridor.
    - Incidence of 0.75 cases per million births per year.
  - Pathogenesis
    - Bilateral abductor paralysis leads to medial position of the vocal cords which limits glottic opening leading to stridor and increased airway resistance.
  - Clinical presentation
    - High-pitched inspiratory or biphasic stridor is the most common manifestation, but may also include dyspnea, chronic aspiration, and cyanosis. Voice may range from weak to normal depending on the site of the lesion.
  - Diagnosis
    - Fiberoptic laryngoscopy with patient awake.
    - Microlaryngoscopy and bronchoscopy with palpation of the arytenoid to rule out cricoarytenoid joint fixation and posterior glottis stenosis.
    - MRI (including imaging of the posterior fossa and course of recurrent laryngeal nerves) to investigate intracranial and compressive causes is paralysis.
    - Laryngeal EMG may be used to monitor motor function and recovery.
    - Videofluoroscopic swallow study (VFSS) or fiberoptic endoscopic evaluation of swallow (FEES) may be used to detect aspiration.
  - Medical management
    - Spontaneous resolution of idiopathic paralysis occurs in up to 70 % of patients up to 11 years later.
    - Treatment for underlying condition with VP shunt or posterior fossa decompression may result in recovery of function in secondary cases.
  - Surgical management
    - Tracheotomy is traditionally recommended for persistent paralysis with respiratory distress or failure to thrive (up to 50 % of patients).
    - Endoscopic transverse cordotomy, arytenoidectomy, arytenoid lateralization, open or endoscopic laryngotracheoplasty with posterior costochondral grafting, and laryngeal reinnervation procedures are options for treatment.
    - Reinnervation uses superior branch of phrenic anastomosed to the posterior cricoarytenoid muscle and ansa-hypoglossal to laryngeal adductors.
  - Multidisciplinary considerations
    - Neurology and/or neurosurgery: Evaluate central causes of paralysis.
    - Speech therapy: Evaluation and management for aspiration risk.
- Laryngeal/glottic web
  - Etiology
    - Partial failure of laryngeal recanalization during gestation.
  - Epidemiology
    - Rare
  - Pathogenesis
    - Anterior glottic involvement is most common leading to voice alteration.
    - Respiratory distress can occur if there is posterior or inferior extension leading to increased airway resistance.
  - Clinical presentation
    - Hoarseness if thin, aphonia in thicker lesions.
    - Depending on length of involvement and subglottic extent may result in respiratory distress.
    - Rare interarytenoid webs present with stridor secondary to inability to abduct the vocal cords.
  - Diagnosis
    - Fiberoptic laryngoscopy for identification, microlaryngoscopy and bronchoscopy to assess character and inferior extent of web.
    - Described according to the Cohen classification:
      - Type I: Thin glottic web without subglottic extension, <35 % airway obstruction
      - Type II: Thicker web with minimal subglottic extension, 35–50 % airway obstruction
      - Type III: Solid web with subglottic involvement, 50–75 % airway obstruction
      - Type IV: Solid web with subglottic involvement and stenosis, 75–90 % airway obstruction
  - Management
    - Surgical management is the mainstay of treatment.
    - Thin webs may be managed endoscopically with lysis and dilation.
    - More complex webs may be treated with endoscopic unilateral local flap reconstruction.
    - Large webs with cartilaginous subglottic involvement most commonly require laryngotracheoplasty with anterior grafting. Persistent webs can be managed with endoscopic or open keel insertion and tracheostomy.
  - Multidisciplinary considerations
    - Genetics: Evaluation for 22q11.2 deletion.

- Laryngeal agenesis/CHAOS (Complete High Airway Obstruction Syndrome)
  - Etiology
    - Complete failure of laryngeal recanalization at approximately 10 weeks gestation.
  - Epidemiology
    - Rare
  - Pathogenesis
    - Congenital laryngeal atresia results in a lack of connection between the upper and lower airway. The defect may be isolated or occur in association with other congenital abnormalities, notably the presence of a tracheoesophageal fistula, esophageal atresia, and encephalocele.
  - Clinical presentation
    - Acute respiratory distress at birth.
    - Presence of polyhydramnios during gestation may lead to fetal diagnosis.
  - Diagnosis
    - Fetal diagnosis made using ultrasound and complemented with fetal MRI. In addition to polyhydraminos, fetal findings include: flat diaphragms, distal airway dilation, and echogenic lungs. Synchronous tracheoesophageal fistula allows egress of fetal lung fluid and may prevent prenatal diagnosis. Postnatal diagnosis results in acute respiratory failure with inability to ventilate.
  - Management
    - Primary management is surgical with tracheostomy.
    - Prenatal diagnosis warrants delivery by EXIT (Ex-utero Intrapartum Treatment) procedure. Uterotomy is performed with preservation of placental blood flow and recirculation of amniotic fluid. The head and neck of the neonate are delivered and the airway is secured via tracheostomy.
    - Postnatally diagnosed cases are managed by emergent tracheostomy.
    - May consider laryngotracheoplasty in select cases for definitive management.
  - Multidisciplinary considerations
    - Special delivery unit for planned EXIT procedure.

Subglottic Airway

The subglottic airway is the area immediately below the vocal cords, extending to the level of the inferior edge of the cricoid cartilage. Narrowing of the subglottis is typically from a fixed lesion and typically presents with biphasic stridor. Anomalies discussed below include subglottic cysts, subglottic stenosis, and hemangioma.

- Subglottic cyst
  - Etiology
    - Most commonly associated with prematurity and a history of intubation.
    - Results from obstruction of subglottic mucous glands secondary to subepithelial fibrosis.
  - Epidemiology
    - Unknown.
  - Pathogenesis
    - Single or multiple cysts may occur as fixed lesions in the immediate subglottis increasing airway resistance.
  - Clinical presentation
    - Infant with a history of prematurity and prior intubation who presents with biphasic stridor should raise clinical suspicion. May also be associated with apnea, recurrent croup, or feeding problems.
  - Diagnosis
    - Microlaryngoscopy and bronchoscopy demonstrate obvious cysts or asymmetric subglottic narrowing.
  - Medical management
    - Asymptomatic cysts may be managed with observation with consideration of medical management of acid reflux.
  - Surgical management
    - Endoscopic marsupialization: Technique is surgeon dependent, most commonly performed using microlaryngeal instrumentation or the CO_2 laser.
    - High recurrence rates range from 12 to 70 %.
  - Multidisciplinary considerations
    - Pulmonary: Often associated with lower airway pathology.
    - Gastroenterology: Acid reflux may potentiate or worsen subglottic inflammation.
- Subglottic stenosis
  - Etiology
    - Membranous subglottic stenosis due to embryologic failure of laryngeal recanalization.
    - Cartilaginous subglottic stenosis secondary to either cricoid cartilage deformity or entrapment of the first tracheal ring within the cricoid cartilage.
    - Acquired in 95 % of cases, most commonly secondary to intubation trauma.
  - Epidemiology
    - Congenital in 5 % of cases.
    - Acquired in 95 % of cases.
  - Pathogenesis
    - Subglottic narrowing leading to increased airway resistance.
  - Clinical presentation
    - Biphasic stridor is most common. Depending on severity children may be asymptomatic, have episodes

of recurrent croup in mild cases, or respiratory distress in severe cases.

- Diagnosis
  - Fiberoptic laryngoscopy may reveal evidence of subglottic narrowing, but gold standard diagnosis and classification via microlaryngoscopy and bronchoscopy.
  - Airway films may demonstrate subglottic narrowing.
  - Degree of stenosis identified using Cotton-Myer classification (see chapter on Subglottic Stenosis).
- Management
  - Grade I stenosis most commonly managed conservatively and often outgrown with time.
  - Endoscopic procedures including lysis and dilation for symptomatic grade I and II membranous stenoses.
  - Grade III membranous stenosis may be treated with endoscopic techniques, but often requires open laryngotracheal reconstruction.
  - Symptomatic cartilaginous stenoses require airway expansion via laryngotracheoplasty with or without tracheostomy depending on degree of stenosis and health of the patient.
  - Grade IV stenosis requires tracheostomy and laryngotracheoplasty or cricotracheal resection.
- Multidisciplinary considerations
  - Pulmonary: Often associated with lower airway pathology.
  - Gastroenterology: Acid reflux may potentiate or worsen stenosis.

- Hemangioma
  - Etiology
    - Hemangiomas occur secondary to an abnormal proliferation of small blood vessels.
  - Epidemiology
    - Hemangioma is the most common tumor of infancy.
    - Incidence of 1–2.6 % at birth and ~10 % by 1 year of age.
    - Female to male ratio 3:1. 60 % occur in the head and neck.
  - Pathogenesis
    - Benign vascular tumor involving the subglottis, glottis, and/or supraglottis with a natural history similar to cutaneous hemangiomas, including proliferation and involution phases.
  - Clinical presentation
    - Inspiratory or biphasic stridor: Approximately 30 % of cases present at birth, with nearly all cases symptomatic by 6 months. Symptoms worsen during the proliferative phase.
    - Natural history: Proliferative phase (first 8–12 months of life), quiescence, slow involution (begins at about 12 months of age and involute at variable rates typically over 5–8 years).
  - Diagnosis
    - 80 % are noted within the first month of life, typically presenting at 2–4 weeks of age.
    - Cutaneous hemangiomas are present in 50 % of children with subglottic hemangiomas.
    - Beard distribution facial hemangioma is more likely to have a synchronous airway hemangioma.
    - Airway X-ray show asymmetric subglottic narrowing.
    - Microlaryngoscopy and bronchoscopy reveals a compressible soft tissue mass with vascular congestion.
  - Medical management
    - Small subglottic hemangiomas with resulting low-grade obstruction are managed with propranolol. Dosing escalates to a maximum of 3 mg/kg. Propranolol carries a risk of hypoglycemia and is contraindicated in children with severe asthma.
    - Moderate to large hemangiomas with respiratory distress can be acutely managed with intralesional or systemic steroids.
  - Surgical management
    - Mass is routinely soft and compressible allowing for intubation even in severe stenoses.
    - Hemangiomas refractory to propranolol are managed with laryngotracheoplasty with open submucosal resection of the lesion.
  - Multidisciplinary considerations
    - Dermatology: Evaluate patient for systemic medical therapy.

The Trachea

The trachea begins immediately below the cricoid and extends distally to the cricoid where the mainstem bronchi diverge. Tracheal anomalies often require multidisciplinary intervention with pediatric surgery and/or cardiothoracic surgery. The timing and clinical presentation of tracheal anomalies is more variable as the pathology is more heterogeneous. Anomalies discussed below include complete tracheal rings, vascular extrinsic rings, tracheal cleft, tracheoesophageal fistula, and tracheomalacia.

- Complete tracheal rings
  - Etiology
    - Abnormal development of the tracheal rings, likely after the 8th week of gestation.
    - The typical C-shaped cartilage is fused posteriorly and there is a lack of the posterior membranous trachea.
  - Epidemiology
    - Incidence estimated to be 1 in 64,500.

- Pathogenesis
  - The posterior membranous portion of the trachea is absent leading to fixed, narrowed dimension of the trachea. May involve a few tracheal rings or the entire length of the trachea (sleeve trachea).
- Clinical presentation
  - "Washing machine" breathing; stridor may be inspiratory (cervical trachea) expiratory (thoracic trachea) or biphasic.
  - Symptoms may not be apparent until >50 % stenosis and may be uncovered in a setting of respiratory illness which exacerbates the narrowing.
- Diagnosis
  - Plain chest films may provide indication of stenosis by demonstrating a narrowed air column.
  - Airway fluoroscopy can be utilized to assess narrowing and associated pulmonary tree anomalies, which are present in up to 20 % of cases.
  - CT or MRI along with vascular studies may be used to further evaluate the stenosis as well as evaluate for vascular malformations/anomalies and extrinsic compression.
  - Rigid bronchoscopy remains the gold standard for diagnosis to assess the length of involvement.
- Medical management
  - In select cases patients with mild symptoms may be monitored and respiratory illness mass require steroids and close monitoring.
- Surgical management
  - Slide tracheoplasty performed through a sternal or cervical approach is the current surgical modality of choice.
  - Augmentation using cartilage or perichondrium has been used for repair with variable results.
- Multidisciplinary considerations
  - Cardiothoracic surgery: For thoracic tracheal involvement, may require ECMO or temporary cardiac bypass for surgical management. Vascular malformations present in up to 50 % of cases.

- Vascular extrinsic rings
  - Etiology
    - Abnormal development of branchial arch system.
  - Epidemiology
    - Rare, frequently associated with other cardiac abnormalities.
  - Pathogenesis
    - Anomalous branching pattern of the vessels originating from the aortic arch or pulmonary trunk.
  - Clinical presentation
    - Degree of respiratory problems and/or feeding difficulties varies depending on degree and site of compression at the trachea, the bronchi, and/or the esophagus.
    - Range from asymptomatic to severe respiratory distress.
    - May present as recurrent pulmonary infection, cough, stridor, and /or dysphagia.
  - Diagnosis
    - Barium esophagogram, echocardiography, computed tomography (CT), magnetic resonance imaging (MRI), and angiography aid in diagnosis.
    - Rigid bronchoscopy and esophagoscopy for definitive evaluation and to identify synchronous tracheobronchial anomalies including complete rings and abnormal bronchial take off.
  - Medical management
    - None
  - Surgical management
    - Heterogeneous anomalies, therefore no single surgical operation defined.
    - Cardiothoracic surgery most common service to address surgical needs.
    - Most frequently managed with vessel pexy or division with or without re-implantation.
  - Multidisciplinary considerations
    - Cardiology: Cardiac evaluation and identification of secondary cardiac anomalies.
    - Cardiothoracic surgery: Definitive surgical management.
    - Pediatric surgery: May be involved with esophageal management.
- Tracheal cleft
  - Etiology
    - Incomplete development of the tracheoesophageal septum.
  - Epidemiology
    - Associated syndromes include: Pallister–Hall, Opitz–Frias, and VACTERL.
    - Clefts are present in 6 % of patients with tracheoesophageal fistulas.
  - Pathogenesis
    - Most commonly present with aspiration. As a result, may have respiratory distress or cyanosis with feeding. Severe aspiration leads to failure to thrive or recurrent pneumonia.
    - Excessive redundant mucosa may also cause stridor and airway obstruction.
  - Clinical presentation
    - High index of suspicion for this anomaly in children with aspiration.
    - Additionally may present with difficult intubation or difficulty ventilating secondary to a large air leak.
  - Diagnosis
    - Modified barium swallow or FEES exam may show a posterior to anterior aspiration pattern.

    - Fiberoptic laryngoscopy demonstrates the" Ram sign" in large clefts with redundant soft tissue adjacent to the arytenoids which prolapses into the cleft margin.
    - Formal diagnosis requires microlaryngoscopy and bronchoscopy with palpation of the posterior commissure.
    - Suspension with use of vocal cord spreaders may aid in diagnosis.
    - Clefts are commonly described according to the Benjamin–Inglis classification.
      - Type I: Involves the interarytenoid region down to and including the vocal cords
      - Type II: Extension into the cricoid cartilage
      - Type III: Extension through the cricoid into the cervical trachea
      - Type IV: Extension into the intrathoracic trachea
  - Management
    - Endoscopic management with suture approximation may be feasible with smaller clefts.
    - Open repair via a transtracheal or lateral pharyngotomy approach is often indicated for deeper clefts.
    - Often require ECMO or cardiopulmonary bypass (CPB) for repair of type IV cleft.
    - Despite repair, mortality >90 % for patients with a type IV cleft.
  - Multidisciplinary considerations
    - General surgery for management of esophagus and often gastric exclusion.
      - Microgastria is a common associated finding
    - Pulmonology: Severe often recalcitrant tracheobronchomalacia which may lead to prolonged tracheostomy dependence.
- Tracheoesophageal fistula and pouches
  - Etiology
    - No unifying theory proposed to address this heterogeneous group of anomalies.
    - Likely multifactorial, 50 % associated with other malformations.
  - Epidemiology
    - Incidence of 1 in 2,500–4,500 live births.
    - Associated with VACTERL, CHARGE, Fanconi anemia, Opitz G, and Goldenhar.
  - Pathogenesis
    - Various degree of esophageal atresia with or without associated fistula.
    - Connection to the trachea prevents egress of saliva and feeds into stomach and provides direct connection for gastric contents to pass into the tracheobronchial tree.
    - Respiratory symptoms are often exacerbated by associated tracheobronchomalacia.
  - Clinical presentation
    - Most patients are symptomatic within first few hours of life.
    - Excessive saliva, pooling of secretions are often the first noted symptoms.
    - Feeding difficulties with coughing, regurgitation, cyanosis with feeds, and potentially respiratory distress.
  - Diagnosis
    - AP/Lateral X-ray with air or contrast to aid in delineation of the pouch, coiled catheter/feeding tube may be seen.
    - Fluoroscopy for more detailed evaluation of the anomaly.
    - Microlaryngoscopy and bronchoscopy for evaluation of the tracheal pouch and endoscopic evaluation with rubber catheter pull through.
    - Ladd and Gross classification
      - Type A: Esophageal atresia (EA) without fistula (6 %)
      - Type B: EA with proximal fistula (5 %)
      - Type C: EA with distal fistula (84 %)
      - Type D: EA with double fistula (1 %)
      - Type E: Tracheoesophageal fistula without atresia—H-type (4 %)
  - Medical management
    - Sump catheter for salivary and gastric diversion to prevent pneumonitis prior to surgical management.
    - Positioning to minimize secretion burden on lungs.
    - Antibiotics may be indicated.
  - Surgical management
    - Surgical management for repair once medically able.
    - The operative approach to an infant with EA depends greatly on the specific type of anomaly present and the occurrence of associated anomalies.
  - Multidisciplinary considerations
    - Pediatric surgery: Often primary team for management.
    - Genetics: 50 % of patients have associated malformations.
- Tracheomalacia
  - Etiology
    - Primary tracheomalacia is described isolated weakness of the tracheal wall which leads to airway symptoms.
    - Secondary tracheomalacia is weakness of the tracheal wall that occurs as a result of extrinsic compression by a vascular anomaly or in association with a tracheoesophageal fistula or tracheal cleft. Secondary tracheomalacia commonly persists

after surgical repair of the associated tracheal anomalies.

- Epidemiology
  - Rare
  - May be associated with syndromic conditions and other anomalies of the tracheobronchial tree.
- Pathogenesis
  - Weakness of the cartilaginous trachea leads to varying degrees of dynamic collapse of the tracheal wall during expiration, which increases airway resistance.
- Clinical presentation
  - Most common presentation is expiratory stridor/wheeze.
  - Wide spectrum of respiratory symptoms ranging from chronic cough to life-threatening recurrent apnea.
- Diagnosis
  - Gold standard for diagnosis is bronchoscopy.
  - Radiological airway screening/fluoroscopy, chest CT, MRI, or tracheobronchogram may also be utilized for diagnosis.
- Medical management
  - Mild cases should be observed.
  - Symptom management with inhaled agents, chest physiotherapy, positive pressure ventilation with CPAP or BiPAP may be indicated for more severe cases.
- Surgical management
  - May require short- or long-term tracheostomy for positive pressure.
  - Internal airway stenting, endoscopic interventions are rarely indicated and controversial.
  - Management of extrinsic compression with vessel pexy or diversion.
  - Management of tracheoesophageal fistula.
- Multidisciplinary considerations
  - Pulmonology: Flexible bronchoscopy, medial management, noninvasive ventilation.
  - Cardiothoracic of pediatric surgery: Surgical management of associated conditions.

References

Wine TM, Dedhia K, Chi DH. Congenital nasal pyriform aperture stenosis: is there a role for nasal dilation? JAMA Otolaryngol Head Neck Surg. 2014;140(4):352–6.

Belden CJ, Mancuso AA, Schmalfuss IM. CT features of congenital nasal piriform aperture stenosis: initial experience. Radiology. 1999;213(2):495–501.

Evans KN, Sie KC, Hopper RA, Glass RP, Hing AV, Cunningham ML. Robin sequence: from diagnosis to development of an effective management plan. Pediatrics. 2011;127(5):936–48.

Tsai YT, Lee LA, Fang TJ, Li HY. Treatment of vallecular cysts in infants with and without coexisting laryngomalacia using endoscopic laser marsupialization:fifteen-year experience at a single-center. Int J Pediatr Otorhinolaryngol. 2013;77(3):424–8.

Dobbie AM, White DR. Laryngomalacia. Pediatr Clin North Am. 2013;60(4):893–902.

Ayari S, Aubertin G, Girschig H, Van Den Abbeele T, Mondain M. Pathophysiology and diagnostic approach to laryngomalacia in infants. Eur Ann Otorhinolaryngol Head Neck Dis. 2012;129(5):257–63.

Tsurumi H, Ito M, Ishikura K, Hataya H, Ikeda M, Honda M, Nishimura G. Bifid epiglottis: syndromic constituent rather than isolated anomaly. Pediatr Int. 2010;52(5):723–8.

Ho AS, Koltai PJ. Pediatric tracheal stenosis. Otolaryngol Clin North Am. 2008;41(5):999–1021.

Kir M, Saylam GS, Karadas U, Yilmaz N, Çakmakçi H, Uzuner N, Güzeloğlu M, Ugurlu B, Oto Ö. Vascular rings: presentation, imaging strategies, treatment, and outcome. Pediatr Cardiol. 2012;33(4):607–17.

Sharma N, Srinivas M. Laryngotracheobronchoscopy prior to esophageal atresia and tracheoesophageal fistula repair—its use and importance. J Pediatr Surg. 2014;49(2):367–9.

Harmon CM, Coran AG. Congenital anomalies of esophagus. In: Coran AG, Adzick NS, Krummel TM, et al., editors. Pediatric surgery. 7th ed. Philadelphia: Elsevier Saunders; 2012. p. 893–918.

Part II

Assessment, Evaluation and Treatment

Challenges of the Neonatal Airway

Janet Lioy, Hitesh Deshmuhk, and J. Thomas Paliga

Overview

It has been well known in pediatric medicine that children are not just small adults—whether it is in response to stress, disease presentation, or overall anatomic and physiologic adaptation. It is also true that neonates are not just small children with respect to exactly the same set of differences. The neonatal airway is especially different from larger children's due mostly to the small size of all tubular structures, a proportionally large head and occiput, and the position of all these structures relative to the entire airway. These factors generally differentiate the neonate from the older child and adult, however, more specific differences exist as well.

The Neonate vs. the Adult

Anatomical Differences: Overview

Non-airway anatomical differences relate to head size, tongue size, jaw angle, the palatal arch, overall position, and muscle tone. One major difference is that the narrowest point of the neonatal airway is at the cricoid ring not the vocal cords as in adults [45]. This fact may be very important in explaining why many neonatologists intubating small infants can pass an endotracheal tube past the vocal cords but not advance beyond. The glottis opening is higher at C-1 and more anterior than adults [27]. Often there is a perception that there is some sort of obstruction, when it is simply the level of the cricoid cartilage that is reached. This has been considered a factor in referrals to pediatric ENT in many neonatal and infant intensive care units. Microscopic laryngoscopy bronchoscopy after referrals usually is normal in these infants, which highlights the importance of having bronchoscopy done at a center experienced with operating room set-up and equipment. It is very common that an infant referred for an airway obstruction ultimately has a normal bronchoscopy, reflecting only the normally occurring narrowed cricoid cartilage (Fig. 1).

The Upper Airway

The airway of the younger child is very different from that of the older child or adult, and these pediatric features are usually present until about age 8 or 9. After this age, the airway becomes more adult-like in configuration, and the generalist emergency physician is on more familiar grounds. There are many levels of differences from the nose and mouth to the tracheal bifurcation and, generally, more malacia of structures due to a relatively greater amount of connective tissue and weak supraglottic tissue. In general, the segments of the upper airway include the nasopharynx, oropharynx, hypopharynx, and larynx.

Nasopharynx

One of the most important factors in the infant's anatomical differences is the nasal anatomy. It is long standing common knowledge amongst neonatal physicians and caregivers that the infant is an obligate nose breather until approximately 3–6 months of age [32]. The obvious consequence of this fact is that they are reliant upon patent nares for adequate ventilation. Even the smallest nasal congestion is thought to potentiate

J. Lioy, M.D. (✉)
Attending Neonatologist, Director Neonatal Outreach, Medical Director, Neonatal Airway Program, The Children's Hospital of Philadelphia, Associate Professor of Clinical Pediatrics, The University of Pennsylvania Perelman School of Medicine, 3400 Spruce Street, Philadelphia, PA 19104, USA
e-mail: Lioy@email.chop.edu

H. Deshmuhk, M.D., Ph.D.
Division of Neonatology, Pulmonary Biology, Cincinnati Children's Hospital Medical Center, University of Cincinnati School of Medicine, Cincinnati, OH, USA

J.T. Paliga, M.S.
Division of Plastic Surgery, Department of Surgery, The Children's Hospital of Philadelphia, Philadelphia, PA, USA

Duke University School of Medicine, Durham, NC, USA

J. Lioy and S.E. Sobol (eds.), *Disorders of the Neonatal Airway: Fundamentals for Practice*,
DOI 10.1007/978-1-4939-1610-8_15, © Springer Science+Business Media New York 2015

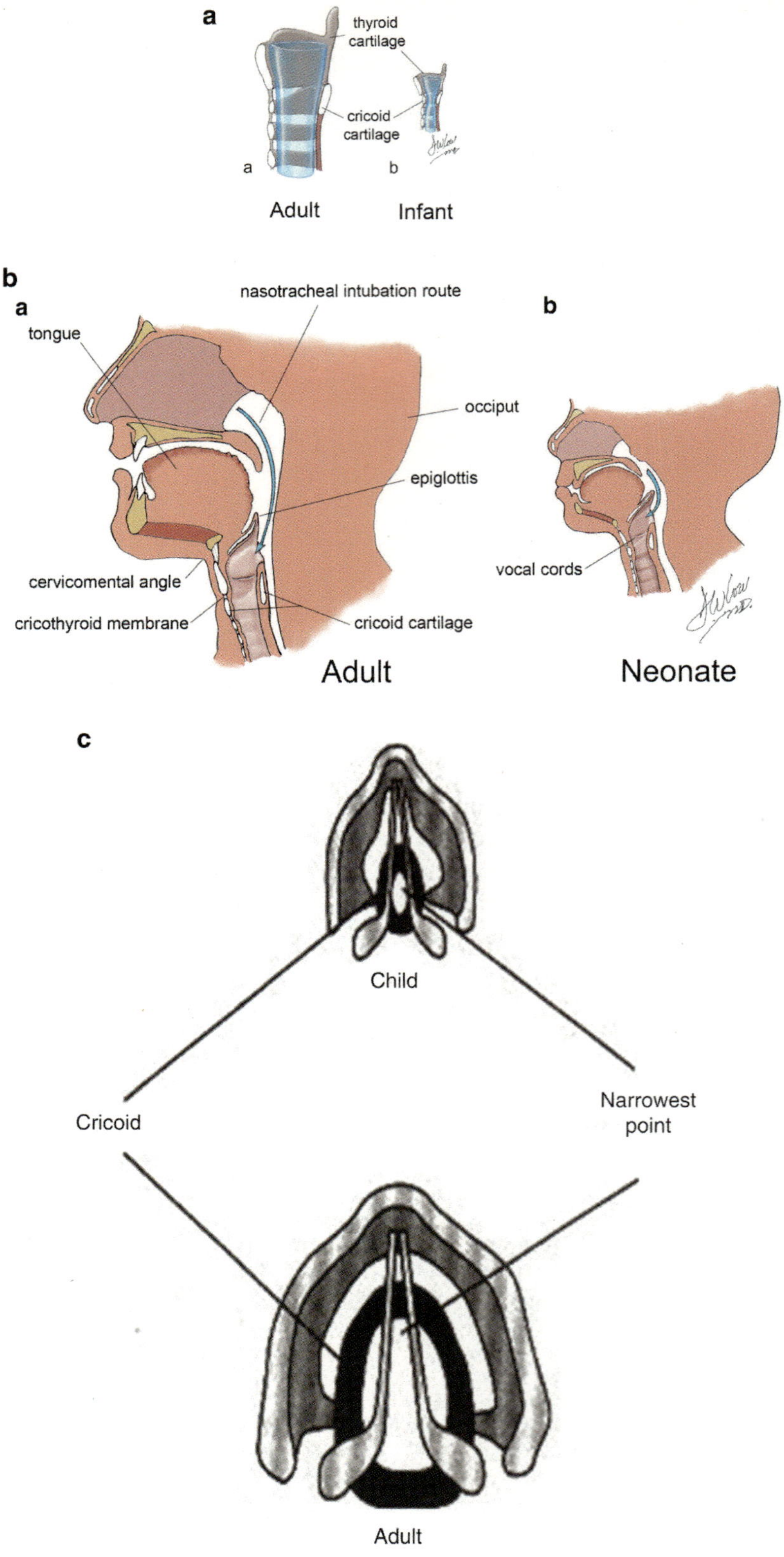

d

	Infant	Adult
Head	Large, prominent occiput	Flat occiput
Tongue	Relatively larger	Relatively smaller
Larynx	Cephalad position Opposite to C2–C3	Opposite to C4–C6
Epiglottis	Omega-shaped & soft	Flat and flexible
Vocal cords	Short & concave	Horizontal
Narrowest portion	Cricoid ring, below cords	Vocal cords
Cartilage	Soft	Firm
Lower airways	Smaller, less developed	Larger, more cartilage

Fig. 1 (**a**) Narrowest point of airway: Adult vs Neonate. Note the more superior position of cricoid ring in the neonatal airway vs adult. (Courtesy of David Low, CHOP). (**b**) Sagittal View of the Adult vs Neonatal Airway. Note the reduced nasopharyngeal space and larger occiput of the neonate contributing to the tendency for tongue based obstruction during airway emergency situations. (Courtesy of David Low, CHOP). (**c**) Cross section of the narrowest point of the airway: Neonates vs Adults, (adapted from Wheeler and Shanley, et al. eds. Resuscitation and Stabilization of the Critically Ill Child). Springer, 2009. (**d**) Major anatomic differences between infants and adults

obstructive apnea. Due to a high metabolism, small lung volumes, and reduced functional residual capacity, the oxygen reserve is relatively decreased, which can relate to rapid desaturations and cyanosis. Interestingly, however, recent studies have shown that infants can mouth breathe during both spontaneous breathing and nasal occlusion. [3]. The term preferential nose breathers may be a better term as, under normal circumstances, the infant does breathe through the nose. Subsequently, any decrease in airway diameter due to secretions or inflammation can significantly add to the infant's work of breathing. As such, rapid respiratory rate, grunting, and nasal flaring are key signs of respiratory distress in infants.

In considering the nasal anatomy, there are also some common conditions that obstruct the nasal cavity in neonates. *Choanal stenosis/atresia*, a posterior nasal obstruction, is seen approximately one in every 5,000–7,000 births and increasingly diagnosed with the utilization of high definition prenatal ultrasound. Rarely, nacrimal duct cyst or nasal mass can present as nasal obstruction and must also be ruled out by CT during the evaluation process. The surgical outcome for choanal stenosis/atresia is largely dependent upon the degree of bony atresia, size of the infant, and frequency of restenosis [25, 26, 42]. *Congenital pyriform sinus aperture stenosis*, also a rare condition, is a cause of nasal obstruction but a different entity than choanal atresia by virtue of location. In this case, obstruction occurs at the anterior nasal bony inlet, and the diagnosis carries genetic significance in that it is associated with holoprosencephaly, hypopituitarism and septo optic dysplasia [26, 42, 48]. Nonetheless, surgery is required for both conditions with stent placement and long hospitalization, giving rise to many potential airway obstructive episodes during the healing process. Other less common causes of nasal obstruction include nasal encephaloceles, nasal septal deviation, and tumor of the nasopharyngeal cavity (Fig. 2).

Oropharynx

The oropharynx consists mostly of the tongue and palatal structures. Macroglossia with tongue-based obstruction is frequently seen in neonates with certain genetic conditions such as trisomy 21 and Beckwith Weidmann syndrome, which can require tracheostomy in extreme cases. The palatal structures usually do not cause airway obstruction by themselves, unless congenital malformations of the palate occur causing complete oropharyngeal obstruction. In addition, tumors arising from the palate may be the source of oropharyngeal obstruction in rare cases (Fig. 3).

Mandible

Retrognathia and micrognathia cause life-threatening airway obstructions in neonates if either is present in a severe form. While retrognathia relates to a recessed position of the jaw, micrognathia relates to the actual size of the mandible with both causing tongue-based obstructions. Many genetic syndromes like Robin sequence and Stickler syndrome can be associated with these conditions and should be ruled out. Treatments such as tongue–lip adhesion and tracheostomy have long been the mainstay of treatment for tongue-based obstruction. Of particular interest, mandibular distraction osteogenesis has recently proven to be an effective technique in relieving the obstruction in a relatively short period of time (Fig. 4).

Tongue

In proportion to the adult, the infant tongue is larger and potentially more obstructive [45]. Although instrumental in the suck-and-swallow mechanism, the tongue can compromise the pulmonary status of the infant by falling to the back of the pharynx and causing an airway obstruction. Generalized neck muscle or pharyngeal muscle hypotonia can exist with other conditions and together create a tongue-based obstruction and airway emergency. It is well known and obvious to those caring

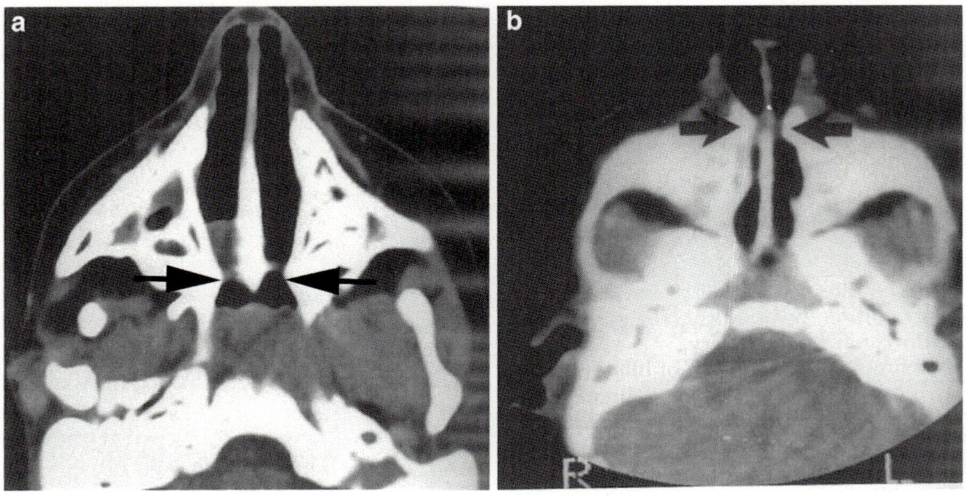

Fig. 2 (**a**, **b**) CT scan of head showing: (**a**) Choanal atresia and (**b**) pyriform aperture stenosis. Note the differences in location of these embryologically different but similar clinical nasal obstructions. (Courtesy of Steve Sobol, CHOP Neonatal Airway Program)

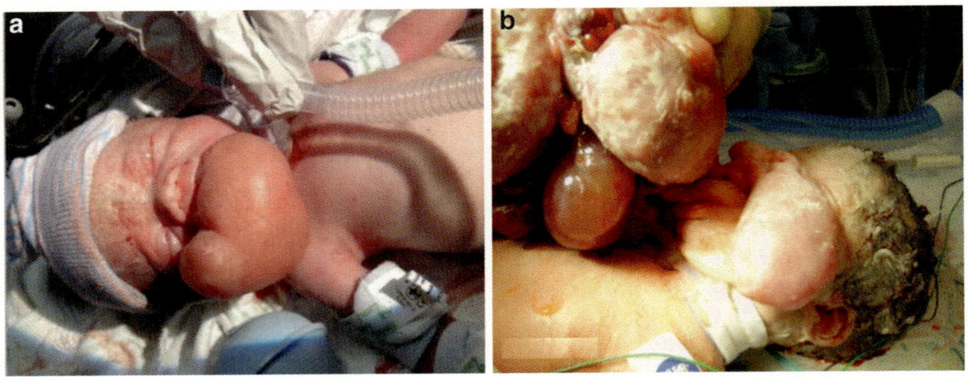

Fig. 3 (**a**, **b**) Photographs of infants with complete oropharyngeal airway obstruction: (**a**) oropharyngeal teratoma and (**b**) Epignathus (Courtesy of Alan Flake MD, Children's Hospital of Philadelphia)

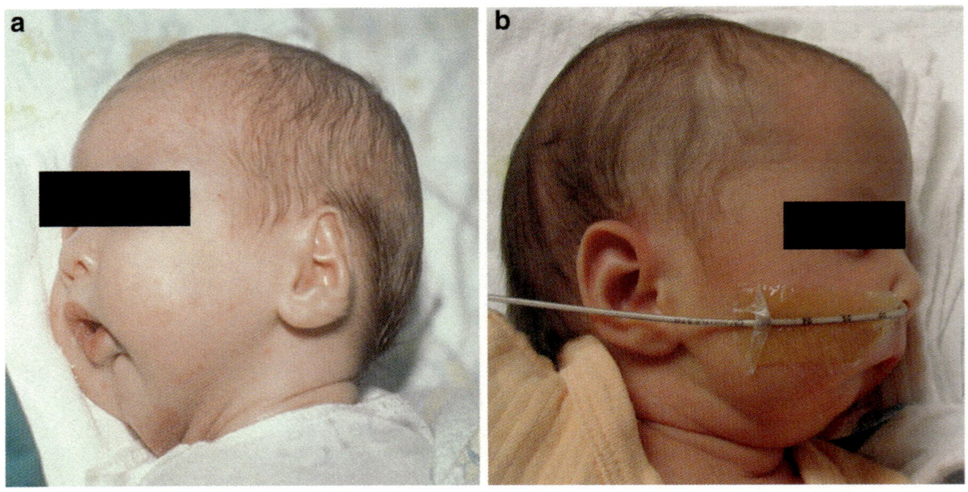

Fig. 4 (**a**, **b**) Photographs of infants with severe Micrognathia (**a** and **b**), (Courtesy of Jesse Taylor MD, Children's Hospital of Philadelphia)

for sick neonates that the tongue always seems too large for the mouth. As such, the tongue frequently impedes intubations and is one of the major causes of failure to maintain a stable airway. Conditions such as Trisomy 21 and Beckwith-Wiedemann syndrome are regularly associated with large tongues. Flexion may also provide a positional contribution to upper airway obstruction in these neonates. Many of these tongue-based obstruction syndromes are underappreciated and are often mistaken for central apnea, gastroesophageal reflux, or other cardiovascular episodes causing an unstable situation. During an emergency, insertion of an oral airway is important in maintaining a patent airway in these types of infants. In neonates, anything that is inserted into the nose or mouth can obstruct the airway further. However, in a spontaneously breathing infant a nasopharyngeal trumpet or a simple nasopharyngeal endotracheal tube is often underutilized and should be considered when intubation is impossible (Fig. 5).

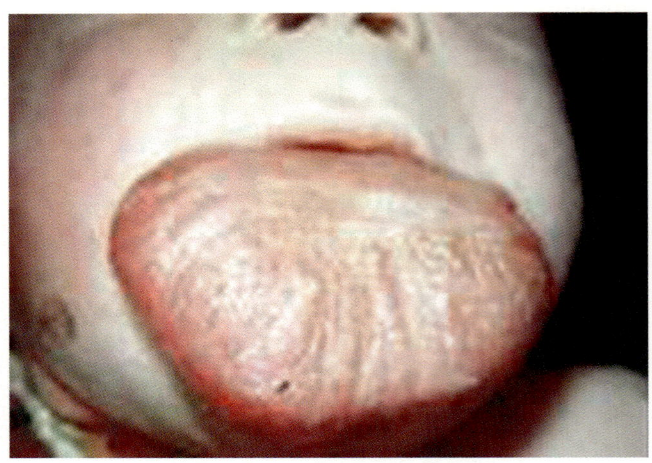

Fig. 5 Photograph of infant with Beckwith-Wiedemann syndrome showing extreme macroglosssia (Courtesy of Ian Jacobs MD, Children's Hospital of Philadelphia)

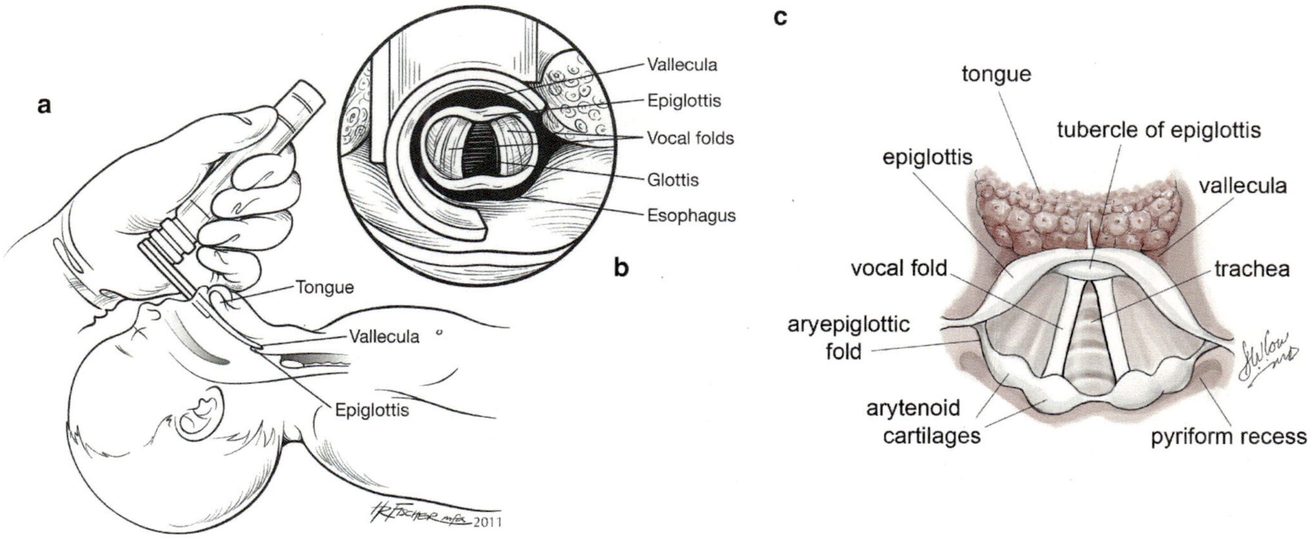

Fig. 6 (**a–b**) Proper view during laryngoscopy of the neonate. Note the correct position of the blade in relation to the glottis opening. Compare with the detailed anatomic drawing of the neonatal airway showing all structures in relation to one another. (adapted from Weissman and Donn. Steve Donn, et al. Manual of Neonatal Respiratory Care, 3rd ed. Springer 2012. (**c**) (Courtesy of David Low, CHOP)

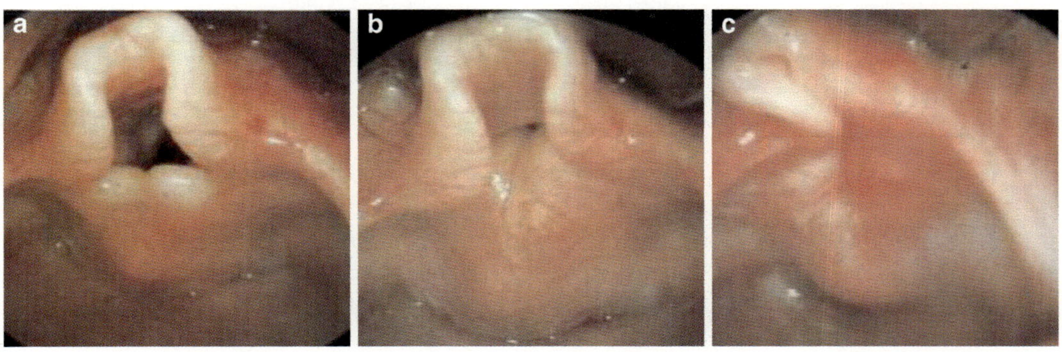

Fig. 7 (**a–c**) Photographs showing severe laryngomalacia. (Courtesy of Steve Sobol, Neonatal Airway Program, CHOP)

Hypopharynx and Larynx

The hypopharynx includes the structures seen during intubation such as the epiglottis and vallecula, and the larynx is the entrance to the airway including both the true and false vocal cords.

Typically described as being cone-shaped with the narrowest segment at the level of the cricoid cartilage the infant larynx lies higher in the neck in relation to the cervical spine [27, 28] (Fig. 8). The larynx is also proportionally smaller, while the surrounding arytenoids and folds are larger relative to the surrounding larynx [26, 42]. The larynx descends as the infant grows into a child and is similar to an adult airway by the age of six. The most important structure, the epiglottis differs in infants from adults in three ways: it is proportionally longer, narrower, larger, less flexible, and often Omega-shaped. These factors may lend to airway obstruction under certain conditions and also make it extremely susceptible to trauma during intubating, suctioning, or examining the infant upper airway.

The supraglottic and glottic anatomy in the neonate is more compact and difficult to visualize for the inexperienced. The aryepiglottic folds, arytenoid cartilages, and epiglottis can all look like one structure when secretions and edema obscure a clear view. Critical landmarks for exposure include the base of the tongue, tip of epiglottis, and vallecula. When intubating with a rigid blade, knowledge of these landmarks is essential to successful intubation (Fig. 6).

Laryngomalacia is a major and common problem in certain neonates resulting from a combination of the aforementioned anatomic characteristics and the physics of airflow through a tube (Bernoulli's effect of less pressure on tubular walls with fast flow and Venturi effect of collapse of these low pressure walls with inspiration) [26, 42]. Recent use of supraglottoplasty surgery with release of tight aryepiglottic folds early in neonates with severe laryngomalacia has allowed earlier feeding and discharge. Previously many of these neonates experienced repeated bouts of airway obstruction, some even going on to tracheostomy (Fig. 7).

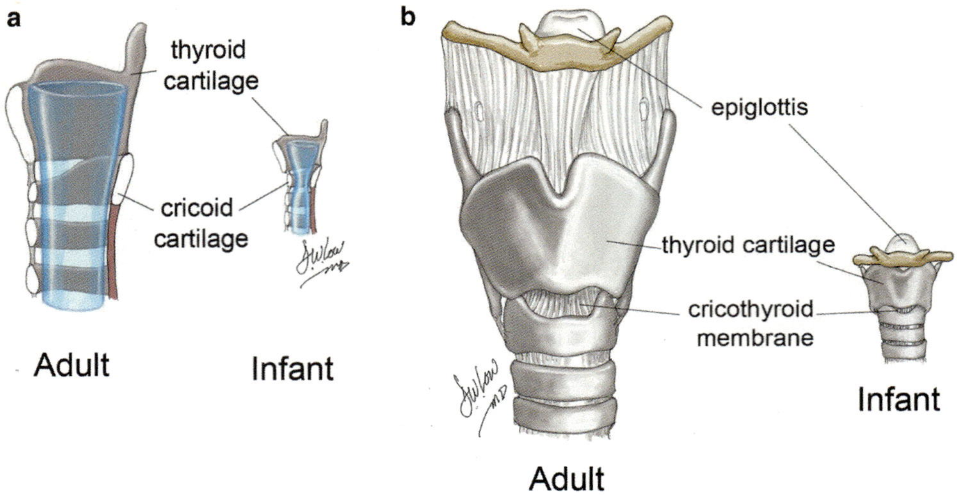

Fig. 8 (**a**, **b**) Differences in the size and location of cricothyoid membrane, cricoid and thyroid cartilage in infants and adult. (Courtesy of David Low, CHOP)

	Tracheal length	Tracheal diameter
Neonate	3 cm	6.5 mm
Toddler	5-7 cm	6 mm
Adult	9-15 cm	14-16.5 mm

Fig. 9 Table of tracheal dimensions: neonates vs adults (Adapted from Chap. 25, Ian Jacobs, MD Fundamentals of Pediatric Surgery, in Peter Mattei editor: Springer

The larynx is separated from the trachea by the cricoid cartilage which is and is entirely composed of cartilage [26, 42].

The narrowest point in the infant airway is the cricoid cartilage ring (in contrast to adults—which is the epiglottis). Due to the narrowing of the airway of this cricoid ring, many people refer to the infant airway as funnel shaped. A 3-D image of the neonatal trachea looks more like an "hourglass" than a tube. Again, it is the cartilaginous cricoid cartilage making up the narrowest part of neonatal airway with a point of resistance at the cricoid ring, often a common area of difficulty in a preterm infant during intubation of a difficult/critical airway by most neonatologists (Fig. 8a, b). This natural narrowing is the reason that uncuffed endotracheal tubes are used almost exclusively in neonates. Anatomically, this area forms a complete cartilaginous ring approximately 2 cm in length starting below the vocal cords. Knowledge of these airway differences is the most important factor in determining the skill and ease of airway visualization and access and ultimate success in intubation [27, 28].

The Lower Airway

The cricoid cartilage marks the true beginning of the lower airway.

The first structure encountered is the trachea, which ends at the carina. The tracheal size and length vary with age (Fig. 9).

The neonatal trachea is much shorter, narrower, and more compact than the adult trachea proportionally, and a high tracheal position at C1-2 can result in anteroposterior differences. There are major differences in the length and diameter of the trachea at different age groups (Fig. 9). The trachea is "C" shaped with soft trachealis muscle posteriorly and a 3:1 ratio of rings/muscle circumference. The soft muscle provides flexibility during breathing but can be the source of severe collapse in cases of significant tracheomalacia [45]. At the level of the cricoid ring any mucosal edema will encroach on the lumen, resulting in exponential increases in resistance to airflow per Poiseuille's law (that is, air flow is proportional to the fourth power of the airway radius) [27, 28].

Neck

The neck of the infant compared to the adult is much shorter, composed of more subcutaneous fat, and often requires different maneuvers while intubating when compared to a child or an adult. Cricoid pressure is often necessary during intubation to overcome the limited space and lack of anatomical landmarks easily seen in adults or children.

Airway Resistance

The diameter of the pediatric airway is much smaller than the adult airway, making it far more vulnerable to obstruction by either foreign objects or edema. Minor narrowing from respiratory infections or bronchospasm may result in

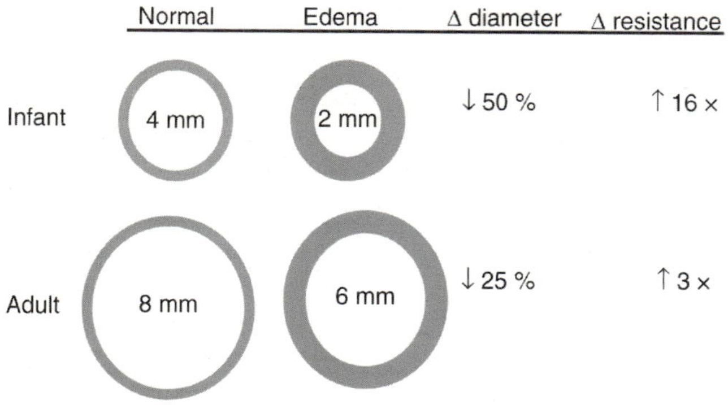

Fig. 10 Differences in luminal size and airway resistance with 1 mm circumferencial edema: Adult vs Infant. (Adapted from Wheeler et al., [56]. In Wheeler et al., Resuscitation and Stabilization of the Critically Ill Child). Springer, 2009

profound airway difficulties in the pediatric patient. Airflow through a pipe like the bronchi is described by Poiseuille's equation. Airflow in the narrowed airway meets resistance that is described by an inverse proportion to the fourth power of the radius of the airway for laminar airflow, and to the fifth power for turbulent airflow (Fig. 10).

$$R=1/r^4$$

(R is resistance and r is the radius)

Illustrating that a mere 1 mm of circumferential edema in an infant's airway will increase the airflow resistance 16-fold. With turbulent airflow, such as in a crying child, the work of breathing increases 32-fold.

Soft Tissue

Developmental changes in the soft-tissue structures of the upper airway occur with age. Radiographic studies show that bony structures remain proportionately the same size. Adenoidal tissue disproportionately increases in the size between 3 and 5 years of age, resulting in a narrowing of the nasopharyngeal airway. Subsequently, bony growth outstrips soft tissue growth, and the airway dimensions increase [34]. Therefore, due to these anatomic differences when muscle tone is reduced, for example, in the setting of a reduced level of consciousness, the head will flex and pharyngeal tone will diminish, resulting in reduced oropharyngeal volume and occlusion of the oropharynx by the tongue. Accordingly, airway-opening maneuvers are required to maintain airway patency. Here, the application of basic adult principles is usually sufficient to provide airway support until additional pediatric help is available. Simple airway-opening techniques, such as head tilt and jaw thrust, are usually sufficient to open the child's airway [9, 10].

Physiological Differences

First, it is well known that lung function in neonates is like no other time in life. There are notable differences with chest wall compliance, functional residual capacity, oxygen metabolism, and muscle fiber type and function. Term healthy infants have reduced functional lung capacity due to more compliant rib cages, a challenging diaphragm angle with unfavorable insertion anatomy for minimal work of breathing. However, by the age of 8, the overall lung function, alveolar growth, and airway properties are very similar to that of an adult [45]. The child's chest wall is more compliant than an adult's because it is more cartilage than bone. The diaphragm is higher due to the relatively larger size of the abdominal contents and the smaller lung volumes of the child. Additionally, the child's lungs are also small in relation to the child's metabolic needs, so there is a smaller margin than in the adult. Infants and children have basal oxygen consumption twice that of adults [27, 28]. Overall, infants and small children are at high risk of respiratory problems because of their immature physiologic responses. The infant will become apneic and bradycardic in response to a hypoxic challenge, instead of increasing the respiratory effort and heart rate.

Differences in pulmonary physiology also affect airway management. Infants have higher oxygen consumption rates (6–8 mL/kg/min vs. 4–6 mL/kg/min) than adults. Infants also have a higher ratio of minute ventilation to functional residual capacity. This results in steep declines in arterial oxygen partial pressures if the airway becomes occluded and subsequently requires more rapid resolution of airway compromise if hypoxic injury is to be avoided [46]. The child's diaphragmatic muscles can be fatigued by increased work of respiration, and the mechanics of the child's inspiration can suffer. Likewise, a distended stomach can compress the diaphragm, even after intubation.

Identifying Potential Airway Emergencies

Overview

An airway emergency in a neonatal intensive care unit can be disastrous without the right training, the right equipment, and the right people capable of responding within minutes. Additionally, knowledge about the differences between preterm and term neonates compared with the pediatric patient and even the adult is necessary to ensure rapid adaptation during an emergency. Practical guidelines for extreme airway emergencies in neonates do not exist as they do for pediatric or adult patients, and neonatal resuscitation program (NRP) guidelines are often used for resuscitation in community delivery room settings [63].

Neonatal and infant airway emergencies are often chaotic and there needs to be an organized team effort. Babies are

Fig. 11 Common diagnosis posing potential airway emergencies in neonate

Level of Obstruction	Conditions
Nasal	Choanal Stenosis Choanal Atresia Nasal Encephalocele Nasal Dermoid Pyriform Aperture Stenosis Nasal Cyst Nasal Septal Deviation Tumor/Teratoma Nasal Polyps
Pharyngeal	Vallecular Cyst Cleft Palate Tumor/Teratoma Micro/Retrognathia Macroglossia Hypotonia/Reduced Pharyngeal tone
Cervical	Lymphatic Malformations (Cystic Hygroma) Teratoma
Laryngeal	Laryngomalacia Laryngeal Cleft Ventricular or Other Laryngeal Cysts Subglottic Stenosis Vocal Cord Paralysis
Tracheal	Congenital Tracheal Stenosis Complex Tracheomalacia (esophageal atresia) Vascular Ring Tracheal Cyst
Bronchial	Bronchial Tumors
Pulmonary	Bronchopulmonary Dysplasia Congenital Cystadenomatoid Malformation
Chest wall (Mechanical/ Neuromuscular)	Asphyxiating Thoracic Dystrophy Muscular Dystrophies
Multiple Craniofacial/ Airway Anomalies	Pierre Robin Sequence Treacher Collins syndrome Crouzon syndrome Apert syndrome Trisomy 21 Beckwith-Wiedemann syndrome

often admitted to neonatal units with unrecognized problems, which can quickly become emergencies during accidental extubations or onset of acute illness. Thus, having a well-thought-out approach to identifying potential airway emergencies is imminently important. The following table lists common disorders associated with neonatal airway emergencies (Fig. 11).

Airway Emergency Profiles

Non-Intubated (Unanticipated Emergencies)

A surprisingly common group of patients that develop airway emergencies are non-intubated. Thus, these cases represent unanticipated emergencies. The origin of the emergency often relates to comorbidities and the onset of acute illness (i.e. sepsis). Additionally, an emergency may develop during attempts at anesthesia. These patients are not labeled as airway risks, but the potential for emergency is realized as additional problems arise. For example, a neonate will get sick and require an airway, but the airway is surprisingly difficult to establish. In these attempts, the airway problem is revealed. Perhaps unsurprisingly, these are the most shocking cases because you can never predict which patients will fall into this category.

Unplanned Extubation (Unanticipated Emergencies)

This group of patients presents with an endotracheal tube already in place. However, they have no previously identified

Fig. 12 Difficult vs. critical airway

Difficult Airway	***Critical Airway***
Non-life threatening History of difficult intubation	Life threatening Impossible visualization
BMV-LMA possible	BMV-LMA impossible
Experienced intubator necessary	ENT required
Mild craniofacial micrognathia Midface hypoplasia Macroglossia Anterior larynx Subglottic narrowing Small mouth	Fresh tracheostomy < 1week Laryngeal web Severe subglottic stenosis Tracheal clefts Severe craniofacial defect Severe micrognathia Severe macroglossia Oropharyngeal tumor Lymphangioma Obstructing Neck mass

airway issues. It is often in the case of an inadvertent extubation that the problem is uncovered. Upon replacing the endotracheal tube, the patient becomes classified as a difficult airway. The key in this subset of patients is that they would never be realized as a potential airway emergency until the need to reestablish the airway.

Tracheostomy Patients

Classically high-risk patients with tracheostomies are especially high-risk in the first week of placement when the stoma is not well formed. Essentially, an open wound still exists, in other words a "fresh tracheostomy." As such, stay sutures are necessary because of the high potential for a problem.

Fresh Tracheostomy with Accidental Decannulation in the First Week

The most obviously high-risk patients that exist in the neonatal ICU are those who had a tracheostomy placed in the last week due to the lack of maturity of the stoma and the nature of the fresh wound. In these cases, it is extremely easy to false track a tracheostomy tube while reinserting. Often, unsuccessful attempts at replacement can lead to false passage into the mediastinum, resulting in pneumothorax/pneumomediastinum and potentially death.

Mature Tracheostomy Reinsertion Difficulty with Distress

Occasionally, an infant with a mature tracheostomy can still have difficulty with insertion of a tube upon changing. Since routine cleaning (approximately every 7 days) and upsizing make reinsertion of tube relatively frequent events, there is a high potential for complications. Even with a mature stoma, there is still a risk of false tracking. Additionally, during upsizing of tracheostomy tubes, accidental false passage can occur if the procedure is not correctly followed or the wrong size tube is applied. An over- or undersized tube inherently leads to poor fitting and placement, substantially increasing risk of emergency. Sadly, neonatal patients can go home with mature tracheostomies and die at home because reestablishment of the tracheostomy becomes unexpectedly difficult during routine maintenance.

Labeling Patients

As noted previously, the neonate that represents a challenge in establishing an airway is classified as either a difficult airway or a critical airway. Labeling patients with regards to airway risk severity is an important aspect of avoiding and responding to emergencies (Fig. 12).

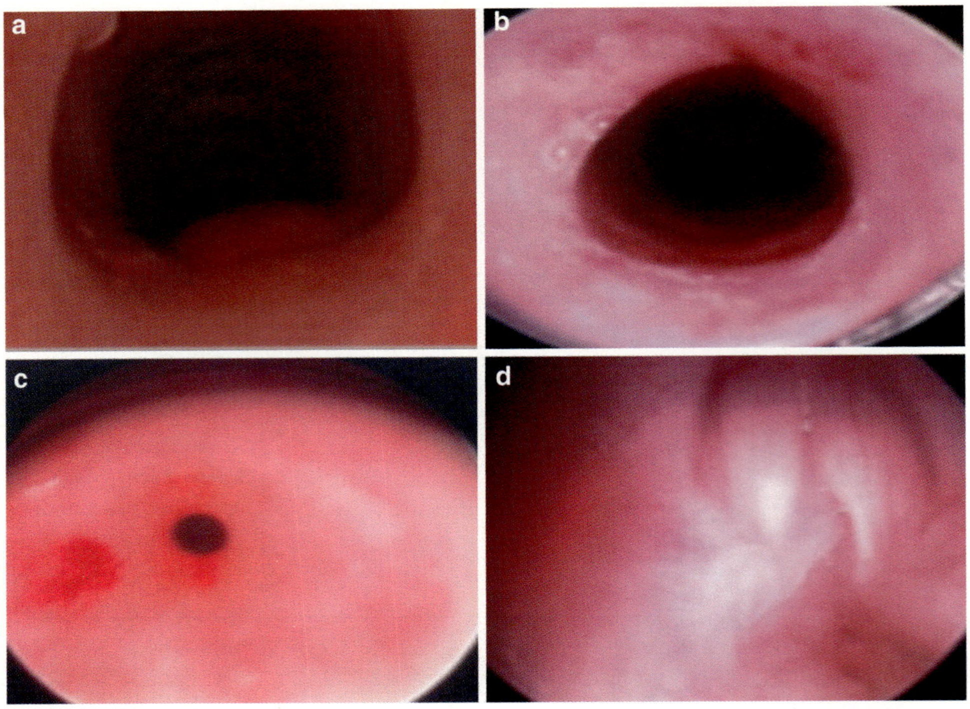

Fig. 13 (**a–d**) Myer-Cotton staging for subglottic stenosis. (**a**) Grade 1–50 % obstruction. (**b**) Grade 2: 51–70 % obstruction. (**c**) Grade 3 >70 % obstruction. (**d**): Grade 4—No detectable lumen. (Courtesy of Steve Sobol MD, Children's Hospital of Philadelphia)

Difficult Airway

The American Society of Anesthesiologists Task Force on Difficult Airway Management defined use of the term *difficult airway* to represent a clinical situation where an experienced, conventionally trained anesthesiologist encounters difficulty with bag mask ventilating or intubation or both [24, 39, 43]. This definition also includes but is not limited to difficulties with visualization on laryngoscopy. A difficult airway is usually when bag mask ventilation is ultimately successful, but intubation can only be accomplished by a skilled, high-level clinician, and the risk of death is low. Although these guidelines are now 10 years old, they still hold true today. While defined by anesthesiologists, this classification is important for the neonatologist as airway management skills in the neonate falls within their scope of practice.

Critical Airway

As an extension of the difficult airway, the critical airway is defined by a situation where bag mask ventilation is unsuccessful and fiber optic intubation by high-level ENT clinician is required to establish an airway. Neonates with a critical airway are at serious risk of cardiopulmonary decompensation and would ultimately die without the airway. Also included in this category are patients with a fresh tracheostomy in the first week of placement. While still a particularly stressful clinical scenario, "the critical airway can be safely and effectively managed when a composed surgeon follows a sensible thought process and conducts a directed work up as part of a multidisciplinary care team" [63].

A common example of patients with a critical airway is witnessed in cases of acquired subglottic stenosis. The Myer-Cotton staging system is useful for mature, firm, circumferential stenosis confined to the subglottis. It describes the stenosis based on the percent relative reduction in cross-sectional area of the subglottis as determined by differing sized endotracheal tubes. Four grades of stenosis are described with this system: [35] (Figs. 13 and 14).

Summary

Knowledge of the differences between adult and neonatal airway size, structure and function is essential in understanding the specific conditions both congenital and acquired that affect neonates. Awareness and familiarity of different levels of anatomic and physiologic distress will be vital in responding to airway obstruction requiring different emergent treatment solutions. Finally, understanding the differences between "difficult" and "critical" airways is necessary for proper preparation and anticipation for airway emergencies that cannot be predicted beforehand.

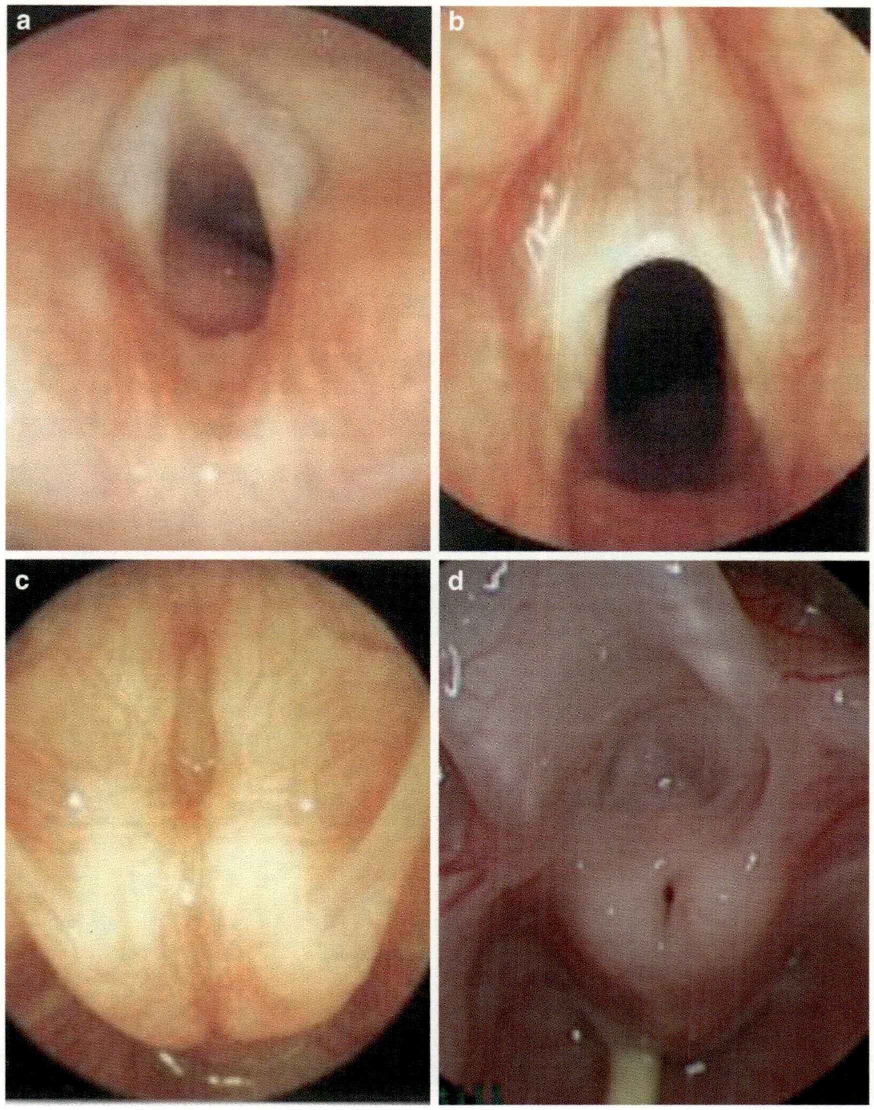

Fig. 14 (**a**–**d**) MLB pictures of congenital laryngeal anomalies causing airway obstruction. (**a**) Glottic lymphangioma; (**b**) Laryngeal Web; (**c**) Tracheal Atresia; (**d**) Vocal Cord Atresia. (Courtesy of Ian Jacobs, Children's Hospital of Philadelphia)

References

1. Altman KW, Wetmore RF, Marsh RR. Congenital airway abnormalities in patients requiring hospitalization. Arch Otolaryngol Head Neck Surg. 1999;125(5):525–8. PubMed PMID: 10326809.
2. Arensman R. Surgical intervention for respiratory distress and airway management. In: Goldsmith J, Karotkin E, editors. Assisted ventilation of the neonate. 5th ed. Philadelphia: Elsevier Saunders; 2011.
3. Bergeson PS, Shaw JC. Are infants really obligatory nasal breathers? Clin Pediatr (Phila). 2001;40(10):567–9. PubMed PMID: 11681824.
4. Bull P. Evaluation of the pediatric airway by rigid endoscopy. In: Mayer C, Cotton R, editors. Practical pediatric otolaryngology. Philadelphia: Lippincott Williams & Wilkins; 1996.
5. Carrelton S, Brown C. Bag mask ventilation. In: Walls R, Murphy M, editors. Manual of emergency airway management. Philadelphia: Lippincott Williams & Wilkins; 2012.
6. Cotton R, Prescott CA. Congenital anomalies of the larynx. In: Cotton R, Mayer C. ed. Philadelphia: Lippincott Williams & Wilkins; 1996.
7. Desai B, Beattie L, Ryan MF, Falgiani M. Visual diagnosis: pediatric airway emergency. Case Rep Emerg Med. 2012;2012:495363. PubMed PMID: 23326717. Pubmed Central PMCID: 3542885.
8. Dickison AE. The normal and abnormal pediatric upper airway. Recognition and management of obstruction. Clin Chest Med. 1987;8(4):583–96. PubMed PMID: 3322644.
9. Dieckmann R. Pediatric assessment. In: Gausche-Hill M, Fuchs S, Yamamoto L, editors. APLS: the pediatric emergency medicine. 4th ed. Sudbury: Jones and Bartlett; 2004.
10. Drummond GB. Keep a clear airway. Br J Anaesth. 1991;66(2):153–6. PubMed PMID: 1817613.
11. Fearon B, Whalen JS. Tracheal dimensions in the living infant (preliminary report). Ann Otol Rhinol Laryngol. 1967;76(5):965–74. PubMed PMID: 6074243.
12. Fiascone J, Vreel P. Neonatal lung disease and respiratory care. In: Burton G, Hodgkin JE, Ward J, editors. Respiratory care: a guide to clinical practice. 4th ed. Philadelphia: Lippincott Williams & Wilkins; 1997.
13. Finer NN, Rich W, Wang C, Leone T. Airway obstruction during mask ventilation of very low birth weight infants during neonatal resuscitation. Pediatrics. 2009;123(3):865–9. PubMed PMID: 19255015.
14. Gerber M, Dunham ME, Holinger LD. Stridor, aspiration and cough. In: Byron J, editor. Bailey's head & neck surgery—otolaryngology. Philadelphia: Lippincott Williams & Wilkins; 2001.
15. Gibson S. Aerodigestive tract foreign bodies. In: Cotton R, Mayer C, editors. Practical pediatric otolaryngology. Philadelphia: Lippincott Williams & Wilkins; 1996.

16. Hess D, Susan P. Neonatal lung disease and respiratory care. In: Burton J, Hodgkin M, Ward J. (eds.) 4th ed. Lippincott Williams & Wilkins; 1997.
17. Hobolth N, Buchmann G, Sandberg LE. Congenital choanal atresia. Acta Paediatr Scand. 1967;56(3):286–94. PubMed PMID: 5340416.
18. Hudgel DW, Hendricks C. Palate and hypopharynx–sites of inspiratory narrowing of the upper airway during sleep. Am Rev Respir Dis. 1988;138(6):1542–7. PubMed PMID: 3202504.
19. Jacobs I. Bronchoscopy. In: Mattei P, editor. Fundamentals of pediatric surgery. New York: Springer; 2011.
20. John S, Swischuk LE. Airway imaging in children. In: Johnson J, Newlands S, Bailey BJ, editors. Bailey's head & neck surgery—otolaryngology. Philadelphia: Lippincott Williams & Wilkins; 2001.
21. Karlovich G, Goldsmith J, Karotkin E. Resusication. In: Goldsmith J, Karotkin K, editors. Assisted ventilation of the neonate. 5th ed. New York: Elsevier Saunders; 2011.
22. Keller JL, Kacker A. Choanal atresia, CHARGE association, and congenital nasal stenosis. Otolaryngol Clin North Am. 2000;33(6):1343–51. viii. PubMed PMID: 11449791.
23. Keller R, Farmer D. Surgical disorders of chest and airways. In: Tauesch E, Gleason M, Devaskar S, editors. Avery's diseases of the newborn. New York: Elsevier Saunders; 2010.
24. Kurth CD, LeBard SE. Association of postoperative apnea, airway obstruction, and hypoxemia in former premature infants. Anesthesiology. 1991;75(1):22–6. PubMed PMID: 2064055.
25. Litman RS, Weissend EE, Shibata D, Westesson PL. Developmental changes of laryngeal dimensions in unparalyzed, sedated children. Anesthesiology. 2003;98(1):41–5. PubMed PMID: 12502977.
26. Lowinger D, Ohlms L. Otolaryngology: head and neck surgery. In: Hansen A, Pudler M, editors. Manual of neonatal surgical intensive care. 2nd ed. Shelton: People's Medical Publishing House; 2009. p. 70–118.
27. Luten R, Kissoon N. Approach to the pediatric airway. In: Walls R, Murphy MF, Luten RC, editors. Manual of emergency airway management. Philadelphia: Lippincott, Williams & Wilkins; 2004. p. 263–81.
28. Luten R, Mick N. Differentiating aspects of pediatric airway. In: Walls R, Murphy M, editors. Manual of emergency airway management. 4th ed. Philadelphia: Lippincott, Williams & Wilkins; 2012.
29. Mace SE, Khan N. Needle cricothyrotomy. Emerg Med Clin North Am. 2008;26(4):1085–101. xi. PubMed PMID: 19059102.
30. Maniglia AJ, Goodwin Jr WJ. Congenital choanal atresia. Otolaryngol Clin North Am. 1981;14(1):167–73. PubMed PMID: 7254838.
31. Mehta R, Hariprakash S, Cox P, Wheeler D. Diseases of upper respiratory tract. In: Wheeler D, Wong H, Shanley T, editors. The respiratory tract in pediatric critical illness and injury. New York: Springer; 2009.
32. Miller MJ, Carlo WA, Strohl KP, Fanaroff AA, Martin RJ. Effect of maturation on oral breathing in sleeping premature infants. J Pediatr. 1986;109(3):515–9. PubMed PMID: 3746545.
33. Morley C. Continuous distending pressure. Arch Dis Child Fetal Neonatal Ed. 1999;81(2):F152–6. PubMed PMID: 10448188. Pubmed Central PMCID: 1720991.
34. Moss I. Physiologic considerations. In: McMillian J, Feigin RD, DeAngelis CD, editors. Oski's pediatrics. Philadelphia: Lippencott Williams & Wilkins; 2006. p. 300–5.
35. Myer 3rd CM, O'Connor DM, Cotton RT. Proposed grading system for subglottic stenosis based on endotracheal tube sizes. Ann Otol Rhinol Laryngol. 1994;103(4 Pt 1):319–23. PubMed PMID: 8154776.
36. Myers C. Inflammatory diseases of the pediatric airway. In: Cotton R, Mayer C, editors. Practical pediatric otolaryngology. Philadelphia: Lippincott Williams & Wilkins; 1996.
37. Nandi PR, Charlesworth CH, Taylor SJ, Nunn JF, Dore CJ. Effect of general anaesthesia on the pharynx. Br J Anaesth. 1991;66(2): 157–62. PubMed PMID: 1817614.
38. Othetrsen H, Andre H. Choanal atresia, intraoral obstructions, laryngeal obstructions, laryngomalacia, webs, atresia, laryngoceles, lymphangiomas and hemangiomas papilloma. Ashcraft and holder: pediatric surgery. New York: W.B. Saunders; 1993.
39. Paterson SJ, Byrne PJ, Molesky MG, Seal RF, Finucane BT. Neonatal resuscitation using the laryngeal mask airway. Anesthesiology. 1994;80(6):1248–53; discussion 27A. PubMed PMID: 8010471.
40. Polgar G. Airway resistance in the newborn infant. Preliminary communication. J Pediatr. 1961;59:915–21. PubMed PMID: 14487521.
41. Polgar G, Kong GP. The nasal resistance of newborn infants. J Pediatr. 1965;67(4):557–67. PubMed PMID: 5833190.
42. Pudler M. Cleft Lip/Palate and Robin Sequence. In: Hansen A, Pudler M, editors. Otolaryngology: head and neck surgery. 2nd ed. Shelton: People's Medical Publishing House; 2009.
43. Rennie J. Neonatal resuscitation. In: Donn S, Sinha S, editors. Manual of neonatal respiratory care. New York: Springer; 2012.
44. Rutter M. Congenital airway and respiratory tract anomalies. In: Wheeler D, Wong H, Shanley T, editors. The respiratory tract in pediatric critical illness and injury. New York: Springer; 2009. p. 163–93.
45. Santillanes G, Gausche-Hill M. Pediatric airway management. Emerg Med Clin North Am. 2008;26(4):961–75. ix. PubMed PMID: 19059095.
46. Sarnaik A, Heidemann SM. Respiratory pathophysiology and regulation. In: Kleigman R, Rehrman RE, Jenson HB, editors. Nelson's textbook of pediatrics. 18th ed. Philadelphia: Saunders; 2007.
47. Scanlon C, Spearman C, Sheldon R. Neonatal and pediatric respiratory care. In: Kacmarek R, Stoller J, Heuer A, editors. Egan's fundamentals of respiratory care. 10th ed. New York: Springer; 1995.
48. Schaffer T, Wolfson M. Upper airway: structure, function and development. In: Abman S, Polin R, Fox W, editors. Fetal and neonatal physiology. 4th ed. Philadelphia: Elsevier Saunders; 2011.
49. Schmolzer GM, Dawson JA, Kamlin CO, O'Donnell CP, Morley CJ, Davis PG. Airway obstruction and gas leak during mask ventilation of preterm infants in the delivery room. Arch Dis Child Fetal Neonatal Ed. 2011;96(4):F254–7. PubMed PMID: 21081593.
50. Stern Y, Cotton RT. Evaluation of the noisy infant. In: Cotton R, Charles M, editors. Practical pediatric otolaryngology. Philadelphia: Lippincott Williams & Wilkins; 2001.
51. Vauthy P. Evaluation of the pediatric airway by flexible endoscopy. In: Cotton R, Mayer C, editors. Practical pediatric otolaryngology. Philadelphia: Lippincott, Williams & Wilkins; 1999.
52. Walner D, Cotton RT. Acquired anomalies of the larynx and trachea. In: Cotton R, Mayer C, editors. Practical pediatric otolaryngology. Philadelphia: Lippincott Williams & Wilkins; 1996.
53. Wetmore R. Management of acute airway obstruction. In: Wetmore R, Muntz HR, McGill TJ, editors. Pediatric otolaryngology: principles and practice pathways. New York: Thieme; 2000.
54. Wetmore R. Tracheotomy. In: Wetmore R, Muntz HR, McGill TJ, editors. Pediatric otolaryngology. Philadelphia: Springer; 2003.
55. Wetmore RF, Marsh RR, Thompson ME, Tom LW. Pediatric tracheostomy: a changing procedure? Ann Otol Rhinol Laryngol. 1999;108(7 Pt 1):695–9. PubMed PMID: 10435931.
56. Wheeler D, Spaeth J, Mehta R, Hariprakash S, Cox P. Assesment and management of pediatric airway. In: Wheeler D, Wong H, Shanley T. (eds.) New York: Springer; 2009.
57. Whitaker K. Assessment of the neonatal and pediatric patients. In: Whitaker K, editor. Comprehensive perinatal & pediatric respiratory care. 3rd ed. New York: Delmar; 2001.
58. Wilson TG. Stridor in infancy. J Laryngol Otol. 1952;66(9):437–51. PubMed PMID: 12990908.
59. Wiseman K, Donn S. Laryngoscopy and endotracheal intubation. In: Donn S, Sinha S, editors. Manual of neonatal respiratory care. 3rd ed. New York: Springer; 2012.
60. Wittenborg MH, Gyepes MT, Crocker D. Tracheal dynamics in infants with respiratory distress, stridor, and collapsing trachea. Radiology. 1967;88(4):653–62. PubMed PMID: 6020927.

61. Wood R. Bronchoscopy in pediatric intensive care unit. In: Wheeler D, Wong H, Shanley T, editors. The respiratory tract in pediatric critical illness and injury. New York: Springer; 2009.
62. Wycoff M, McGowan J, Coby C, Fairchild K, Henry L, Steven R. Textbook of neonatal resuscitation. In: McGowan J, ed. 6th ed. Elkgrove: American Academy of Pediatrics and American Heart Association; 2012.
63. Zur K. The critical airway. In: Mattei P, editor. Fundamentals of pediatric surgery. New York: Springer; 2011.

Genetics of Neonatal Airway Disorders

Sulagna C. Saitta and Daniel T. Swarr

Introduction

Genetic disorders can significantly influence airway development and a functioning respiratory system in the newborn infant. These differences are likely the culmination of numerous developmental processes, involving dozens of separate structures and thousands of genes guiding each step. The development of diverse structures, ranging from the nose and facial bones, to the trachea, esophagus, and distal lung tissue must be carefully coordinated. Disruption in the formation of any one of these structures may lead to a disorder of the neonatal airway. A vast array of developmental disruptions, single gene disorders, and chromosomal syndromes have been associated with congenital airway anomalies. This chapter reviews the genetic diagnostic approach to an infant who presents with an airway disorder and the types of genetic testing currently available. The genetics of specific airway malformations, and identifiable syndromes commonly associated with significant airway malformations, are discussed.

An Overview of the Etiology of Congenital Airway Disorders

As seen with other congenital anomalies, congenital airway disorders may result from any process that disrupts normal development: an environmental exposure, deformation from an external physical force, or an underlying genetic abnormality. Congenital anomalies are frequently classified as malformations, disruptions, or deformations. *Malformations* result from a primary abnormality in the formation of a tissue or structure during organogenesis. The etiology is often genetic or environmental. The abnormal craniofacial structures and complete cartilaginous tracheal sleeve that lead to airway complications in Crouzon (Fig. 1a, b), and Apert syndromes (Fig. 1c, d) are examples of malformations. In contrast, *disruptions* result from a process that alters normally forming structures during or after formation. Processes that result in disruptions can include external compressive forces, amniotic bands, hemorrhage, or other vascular abnormalities including thrombosis. If such an insult affects the developing facial structures, airway patency at birth may be significantly compromised. *Deformations* result from alteration in the normal shape of a structure by mechanical forces, which may be either intrinsic or extrinsic to the developing fetus [1].

A *syndrome* refers to a recurrent pattern of malformation arising from a single underlying etiology. A well-known example is Trisomy 21 or Down syndrome. The multiple associated features affect various organ systems ranging from the characteristic facies to major structural defects, including cardiac septal defects, Tetralogy of Fallot, duodenal atresia, and anal stenosis. The findings are collectively identified as a syndrome because of the single underlying cause, an extra 21st chromosome. In contrast, when a collection of anomalies is recognized to occur together more frequently than expected by chance, but when no unifying etiology can be established, it is referred to as an *association*. Many associations, such as VACTERL or OAVS (Oculo-Auriculo-Vertebral Spectrum), exhibit significant and even life-threatening airway anomalies. Finally, a pattern of anomalies that results from a single primary anomaly or mechanical force with secondary effects on other structures is referred to as a *sequence*. Pierre-Robin sequence, in which primary micrognathia results in glossoptosis and cleft palate, is an example of a sequence with important airway implications.

S.C. Saitta, M.D., Ph.D. (✉)
Clinical Genetics, Cedars-Sinai Medical Center,
Department of Pediatrics, David Geffen School of Medicine
at UCLA, Los Angeles, CA, USA
e-mail: Sulagna.Saitta@cshs.org

D.T. Swarr, M.D.
Divisions of Neonatology, Department of Human Genetics, The
Children's Hospital of Philadelphia, University of Pennsylvania,
Perelman School of Medicine, Philadelphia, PA, USA

J. Lioy and S.E. Sobol (eds.), *Disorders of the Neonatal Airway: Fundamentals for Practice*,
DOI 10.1007/978-1-4939-1610-8_16, © Springer Science+Business Media New York 2015

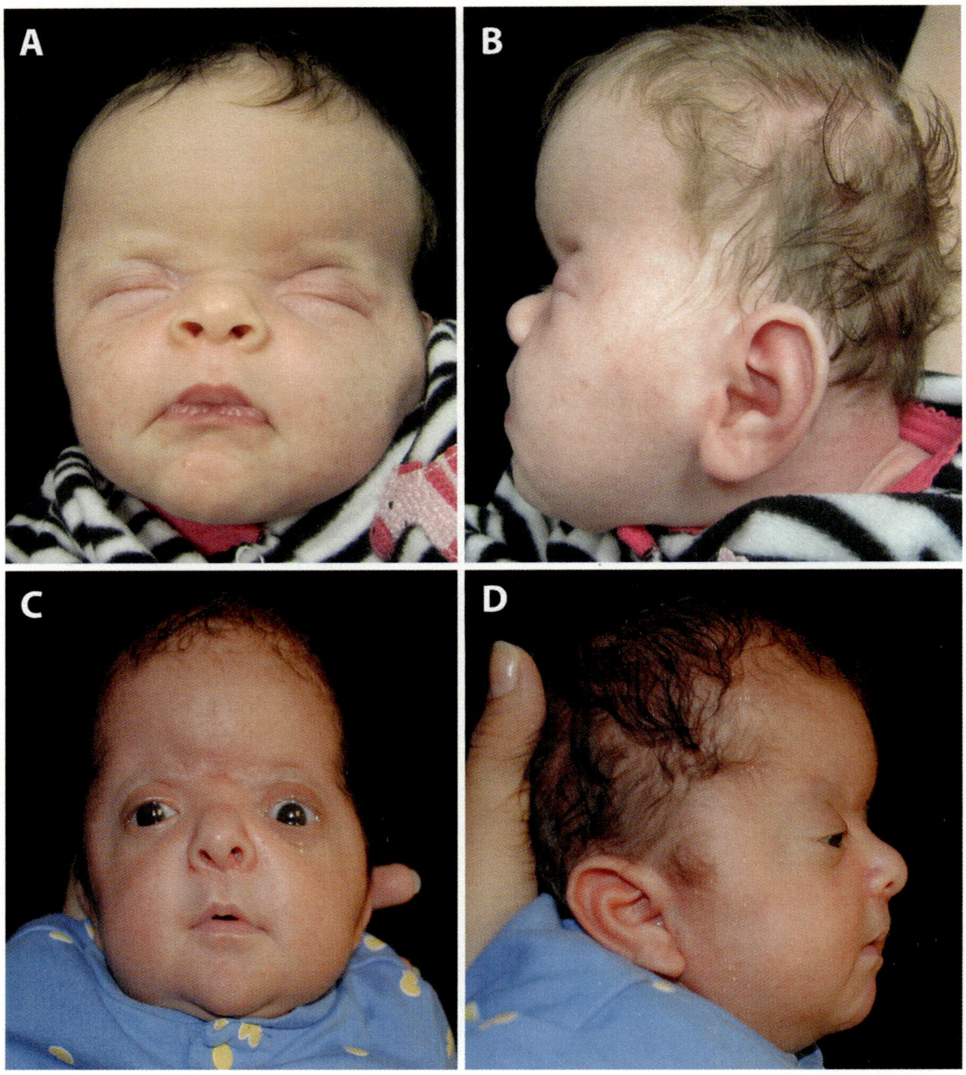

Fig. 1 Crouzon & Apert Syndromes. (**a**) Front, & (**b**) Side view of Crouzon Syndrome. Note brachycephaly (short skull in AP dimension, with flat occiput), frontal bossing, maxillary hypoplasia with mandibular prognathism, shallow orbits and hypertelorism. Similar features are seen in Apert syndrome (**c**—Front, **d** Side), although ptosis is more evident in this infant because his eyes are open. Syndactyly of all five fingers ("mitten hand" deformity; not shown here) in Apert syndrome would easily distinguish these otherwise very similar-appearing conditions. Courtesy of CHOP Craniofacial Program, Permission Obtained

Among the airway anomalies with an identifiable genetic etiology, the nature of the genetic lesions leading to these disorders is equally diverse, ranging from the involvement of an entire chromosome (e.g., Trisomy 18 or 21), to a single base pair change in a critical gene, as with the FGFR2 mutation in Crouzon syndrome. Overall, it is estimated that 10 % of all birth defects are due to a chromosomal abnormality [2]. *Aneuploidy* refers to the presence of an abnormal number of chromosomes and includes the important syndromes such as Trisomy 18 and 21, both of which have been associated with significant airway anomalies (Table 1). Deletions or duplication of genetic material can also affect just a portion of a chromosome and also cause significant life-threatening airway malformations.

For nearly half of all congenital malformations, a comprehensive diagnostic evaluation will fail to reveal an underlying genetic etiology [3]. This may be due to the limitations of available diagnostic techniques and also likely reflects our incomplete understanding of human genetics. The failure to identify an associated genetic change also highlights the fact that a variety of nongenetic factors can contribute to human birth defects. Environmental

Table 1 Airway anomalies associated with Trisomy 13, 18, and 21

Trisomy 18	Cleft lip/palate
	Tracheoesophageal fistula
	Pulmonary hypoplasia or aplasia
Trisomy 21	Laryngeal web
	Laryngeal cleft
	Subglottic stenosis
	Tracheal stenosis
	Tracheoesophageal fistula

Table 2 Syndromes associated with TEF/EA

Disorder	Key features	Etiology/Gene
22q11.2 microdeletion syndrome	Congenital heart defects, hypocalcemia, immune deficiency (thymic aplasia), characteristic facial features	Deletion of chromosome 22q11.2
Trisomy 18	Growth retardation, microcephaly, microphthalmia, malformed ears, microretrognathia, clenched fists, rocker-bottom feet, congenital heart disease	Trisomy 18
Trisomy 21	Characteristic facial features, infantile hypotonia, intellectual disability, congenital heart disease, duodenal atresia, hypothyroidism	Trisomy 21
CHARGE	*C*oloboma of the eye, *H*eart defects, choanal *A*tresia, *R*etardation of growth/development, *G*U anomalies, *E*ar anomalies	CHD7 gene (AD)
Feingold	Microcephaly, limb malformations, esophageal/duodenal atresia, hand/foot malformations, cardiac, renal, vertebral malformations, intellectual disability	MYCN gene (AD)
OAVS	Facial asymmetry with malar, maxillary, and mandibular hypoplasia, microtia, ear tags, ocular anomalies (e.g., epibulbar dermoids), and vertebral anomalies	Unknown
Optiz-G BBB	Hypertelorism, broad nasal bridge, anteverted nares, grooved nasal tip, cleft lip/palate, congenital heart disease, imperforate anus, hypospadias, widow's peak, agenesis of corpus callosum	MID1 (X-linked)
VACTERL	*V*ertebral anomalies, *A*nal atresia, *C*ardiac defects, *TE*F/*E*A, *R*enal, *L*imb anomalies	Unknown

AD autosomal dominant, *AR* autosomal recessive

factors, including infectious agents, maternal disease states, drugs, chemicals, and radiation, have all been linked to disrupted human development. While beyond the scope of this review, exposures to agents like diphenylhydantoin (Dilantin) or vitamin A (e.g., excessive supplemental vitamin intake, isotretinoin) can lead to altered craniofacial development and cleft lip/palate, while other drugs including warfarin can lead to choanal stenosis. Our understanding of how subtle environmental exposures, including dietary factors or common environmental contaminants interact with genetic factors to contribute to the formation of congenital malformations, is rudimentary, but future research in this area will likely greatly enhance our understanding of many complex congenital airway disorders.

Similarly, recent research has begun to elucidate how chemical modifications of DNA or its supporting structure (chromatin) that leaves the DNA sequence itself unchanged, can alter normal development and result in human disease. These *epigenetic* changes can even be passed on from one generation to the next and often reflect a response to environmental cues such as starvation and obesity. Examples exist of known human disorders in which the normal epigenetic marks are disrupted. These include Prader-Willi and Angelman syndromes in chromosome 15q11, and Beckwith-Wiedemann syndrome in chromosome 11p15. It is possible that epigenetic changes may contribute to complex and likely multifactorial airway malformations. For example, although laryngotracheal clefts and tracheosophageal fistulas have been associated with several syndromes (Tables 2 and 3), the precise etiology of these complex disorders remain almost completely unexplored, and such areas of investigation will also likely contribute greatly to our understanding of the etiology of these disorders over the coming years.

Table 3 Syndromes associated with laryngeal clefts/LET clefts

• Opitz-G BBB syndrome
• Pallister-Hall syndrome
• Rhizomelic chondrodysplasia punctata syndrome
• Trisomy 21

Comprehensive Diagnostic Approach to the Infant with An Airway Disorder

Physical Assessment

The genetics evaluation of a neonate with airway malformation is guided by the type and location of the malformation, a specific medical history and a detailed physical examination. *History*: A complete prenatal history should be obtained, including results of any prenatal testing. Maternal and paternal ages at conception are important to discern, since there is an increased risk of chromosomal nondisjunction and subsequent chromosomal anomalies that occurs with increasing maternal age at conception. Similarly, advanced paternal age is associated with increasing risk for single gene disorders, such as achondroplasia. The use of assisted reproductive techniques to achieve pregnancy and use of donor gametes should be identified. In addition, the results of any imaging studies such as ultrasound evaluation, fetal echocardiogram and fetal MRI in cases where such modalities have been utilized should be reviewed. For example, an ultrasound assessment of abnormal levels of amniotic fluid may provide a clue to an underlying malformation and potential diagnosis. *Oligohydramnios* or decreased amniotic fluid could indicate leakage of fluid or a malformation of the renal or urinary tract structures. Instead, excess fluid, or *polyhydramnios* may indicate poor fetal swallowing and relate to a neurologic condition in the fetus precluding normal movement or a gastrointestinal malformation such as tracheoesophageal fistula. Anatomic differences of the uterus can result in fetal constraint and a deformational effect on airway structures. Such underlying issues may have already been identified on imaging studies of the pregnancy.

A general maternal health history such as the presence of diabetes, hypertension, drug and alcohol exposures, infections, and use of medications is important to elicit. Teratogenic exposures, to ethanol for example, may cause structural effects on the exposed fetus. There are numerous known teratogens, many with specific associated structural anomalies and dysmorphisms. These include well-documented human teratogens such as thalidomide, warfarin, valproate, hydantoin, and trimethadione. Some can display a pronounced effect on airway structures. For example, fetal warfarin exposure can result in severe nasal hypoplasia, compromising the upper airway. Similarly, oral isotretinoin use, (a synthetic retinoic acid derivative used for dermatologic disorders), particularly early in pregnancy, can cause severe craniofacial malformations. The effect of a given teratogen may vary depending on the timing, dosage and duration of the exposure. In general, exposures early in gestation and at relatively higher doses have more pronounced effects on fetal development. Ascertainment of teratogen exposure is crucial, since many of these effects can mimic a chromosomal disorder; however the adjunct genetic testing and recurrence risk counseling would be quite different.

In evaluating the infant, documenting data on fetal activity, fetal size, position, evidence of fetal distress and gestational age is highly relevant to the differential diagnosis. For example, a case of a neonate with hypotonia at birth who has a history of poor fetal movement and breech presentation suggests a long-standing developmental issue rather than simply perinatal depression.

In many pregnancies, genetic studies including screening analyses such as standard maternal serum screening and more recently, noninvasive prenatal testing (NIPT) may have been performed. This latter screening test utilizes cell-free DNA circulating in the maternal peripheral blood and sequencing-based techniques to assess for commonly encountered aneuploidies such as Trisomy 21. Data from genetic diagnostic tests such as chorionic villus sampling (CVS) or amniocentesis where karyotyping and/or chromosomal microarray may have been performed should also be reviewed.

It is important to document a complete three-generation family history. Eliciting a history of consanguinity in a couple increases the likelihood of a recessive condition in the infant. Consideration of seemingly unrelated birth defects, such as cardiac or renal anomalies in other family members may provide a clue to an underlying diagnosis in the proband. Intellectual disability in close relatives is also important to document. In addition, a history of multiple (>2) unexplained miscarriages may be suggestive of an underlying chromosomal predisposition such as the presence of a balanced translocation carried by one of the parents, that may be related to the proband's condition. Data from a formal pedigree analysis can be quite helpful in ascertaining an underlying pattern of inheritance, such as an X-linked recessive disease with affected males, relatively unaffected females, and transmission on the maternal side of the family.

Dysmorphology Exam

This detailed physical exam assesses for defects in the structure or morphology of an organ or organ system that reflects an abnormal developmental process. In assessing for congenital defects and in order to develop an appropriate differential diagnosis, a detailed physical exam with emphasis on the craniofacial exam is performed and measurements are compared to published age-matched standards [4]. The initial assessment begins with the newborn growth parameters, adjusted for any prematurity. The height, weight, and head circumference will provide a snapshot view of fetal health and intrauterine environment. For example, head-sparing intrauterine growth retardation where HC >length >weight may reflect poor nutrition or placental insufficiency, while microcephaly might instead suggest underlying neurological malformation with a genetic etiology or infectious agent such as cytomegalovirus. The dysmorphology exam focuses on assessing the patient for anatomic features that diverge from normal standards with the understanding that some might be familial variants. The shape and size of the head and fontanelles and assessment of the cranial sutures should be obtained. The presence of craniosynostosis may significantly narrow down the diagnoses under consideration and an unusual head shape or size would prompt imaging studies that might reveal a brain malformation (Fig. 2a, b). In further assessing the head, notation of any scalp defects, differences in the shape of the forehead, eyebrows, and distribution of hair should be sought. The spacing of the eyes with measurements of the canthi and palpebral fissure lengths is performed. The presence of colobomata, cataracts, and the surrounding structures such as the presence of epicanthal folds or downward or upward slant of the palpebral fissures is also documented as these can be characteristic findings of some syndromes. Careful examination of the ears, assessing their placement, rotation and appropriate folding of the ear is important as is assessment for auricular pits and tags which can be specific for certain disorders. The nose is evaluated for proper formation of the bridge, alar nasi, nares, and nasal tip. Patency of the chonae is also assessed. The mouth and throat are evaluated for evidence of defects or clefts of the lip and/or palate. The shape of the palate and the uvula are examined, with direct implications for functional issues of

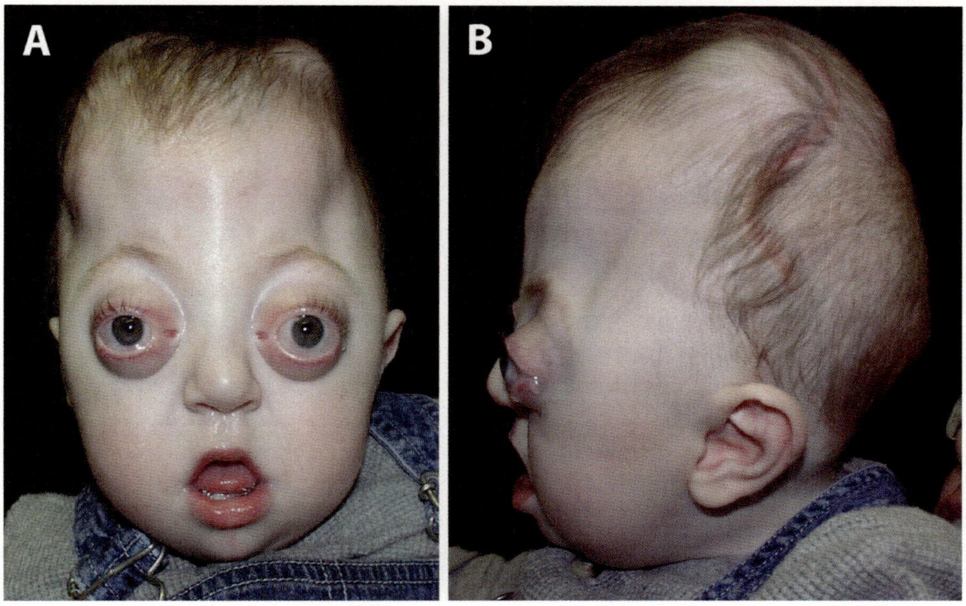

Fig. 2 (**a**, **b**)—Pfeiffer Syndrome. (**a**)—Front, (**b**)—Side. Note the short, tall skull (turribrachycephaly), maxillary hypoplasia with mandibular prognathism, shallow orbits with striking ocular proptosis, small nose, flat nasal bridge, and irregular skull shape due to the presence of craniosynostosis. The presence of broad thumbs and toes (not shown) is also characteristic of this disorder. Courtesy of CHOP Craniofacial Program, Permission Obtained

the airway. The mouth is carefully examined for findings such as natal teeth, gum abnormalities, lip pits, frenulae, and tongue malformations that might be suggestive of a diagnosis. Evaluation of the chin is critical in a patient with airway involvement and micrognathia and retrognathia can be part of distinct syndromic entities. They can also occur as isolated malformations. Finally, the neck is evaluated for webbing, excess nuchal skin, or bony cervical abnormalities, which would prompt a subsequent cervical spine stability evaluation, affecting airway management.

Examination of the chest and thorax notes any bony deformities such as pectus or narrow chest and internipple distances. Abnormalities should prompt imaging studies such as chest X-ray evaluating for bone malformations, while presence of a murmur would prompt cardiac evaluation. The abdominal exam assesses primarily for evidence of abdominal wall defects such as omphalocele and for the presence of organomegaly, which is more suggestive of an inborn error of metabolism. When examining the umbilical cord, a 2-vessel cord with only a single umbilical artery may reflect the presence of a renal anomaly. The genitourinary exam assesses external genitalia where anomalies may be associated with internal malformations of the GU tract as well. Patency of the anus and its placement are assessed as this finding may present as part of a recognizable constellation of findings in a syndrome. The extremities are carefully examined for structural integrity of the digits, their formation and placement and palmar creases. Often, limb anomalies particularly those of the hands and feet can be a vital clue to an underlying diagnosis.

A dermatologic evaluation to examine for the presence of phakomatoses or skin manifestations that signal an underlying genetic diagnosis is important. For example, multiple café au lait spots or neurofibromas can be associated with neurofibromatosis type I. The irregular swirly pigmentation encountered with Hypomelanosis of Ito may be the only clue to an underlying chromosomal mosaicism. Here, the skin pigmentation patterns can represent the distinct chromosomal admixture. Hemangiomata are also noteworthy, particularly those of the face and neck as they may signal the presence of other such vascular malformations affecting the airway.

The neurologic exam, while clearly helpful for diagnostic purposes may have added impact on an infant's ultimate prognosis. Evaluation of tone, basic reflexes, involuntary movements, and seizure activity are critical to management of the patient [5].

An Overview of Genetic Testing

Chromosome Analysis

The field of genetics has experienced tremendous technological advances since the completion of the Human Genome Project in 2000. A brief review of techniques currently used in molecular diagnostics and their applications is discussed.

Methodology for identification and microscopic examination of the integrity of chromosomes became routinely available with the development of G-banding techniques in the 1960s. This staining methodology is still used today to identify aneuploidy involving whole chromosomes, or large

(>5–7 Mb) rearrangements such as duplications and deletions within chromosomes. Standard G-banded *karyotypes* are typically performed on peripheral blood from the patient after stimulating the lymphocytes to grow and divide in culture. Usually, after 72 h in culture, a sufficient number of cells can be harvested to perform karyotyping. The process allows the cells to be in the metaphase stage of cell division when the chromosomes lengthen into distinct structures. Special Giemsa-based staining then allows the dark and light colored banding patterns to be discerned by further analysis by a cytogeneticist. This has been the standard technique used for detection and confirmation of common trisomies such as Trisomy 13, 18, or 21 or disorders of the sex chromosomes. Currently, it is still the only clinical diagnostic technique that can detect balanced translocations where chromosomal material from one chromosome is rearranged onto another. A balanced translocation does not result in a change in the dosage or copy number of a chromosomal region or of the genes residing in that region.

It is important to recognize that a normal karyotype (either from a prenatal CVS or amniocentesis specimen or from a postnatal blood sample) does not exclude the possibility of a chromosomal disorder. Due to the advent and rapid adoption of newer microarray technology described below, a large number of *microdeletion/microduplication syndromes* have been recognized, many of which are associated with congenital airway malformations. For example, the 22q11.2 microdeletion syndrome has been associated with cleft palate and laryngeal webs, which may lead to significant airway compromise during the neonatal period. Such submicroscopic gains and losses of chromosomal regions are considered *copy number variations* (CNVs). They may be detected within a chromosome (*interstitial*) or at the ends of the chromosome (*subtelomere*) and can result in change in dosage of a gene or genes located in a given region.

Fluorescence in situ hybridization or FISH is a molecular cytogenetic technique where a specific fluorescent-tagged DNA probe representing a single locus or part of a particular chromosomal region hybridizes to that region of the genome. It is useful in cases where the patient's features are suggestive of a chromosomal disorder that is not typically visible under the microscope. Indeed, these submicroscopic genomic disorders have been, until recently, primarily identified by FISH and are associated with known clinical syndromes. The most frequently occurring microdeletion syndrome is the chromosome 22q11.2 deletion syndrome, associated with the clinical DiGeorge and Velocardiofacial (VCFS) syndromes. In addition, other chromosome-specific deletion syndromes such as those of chromosome 15q11.2 (Prader-Willi Syndrome and Angelman syndrome), chromosome 7q11.2 (Williams syndrome) have historically all been identified using a FISH probe for their respective regions. The disadvantage of this technique is that the clinician must know and specifically order the proper FISH test for a given chromosomal locus and many of the syndromes, even the well-recognized ones, can have atypical presentations or overlap with other diagnoses. In addition, in some cases, a patient may have a rearrangement that does not have the typical breakpoints associated with a given region and may not be detectable using the standard FISH probe. For these reasons, FISH has largely been replaced by chromosomal microarray analysis except for specific applications such as for testing family members of a proband.

FISH continues to be utilized for prenatal genetic testing. This modality can also be used to rapidly assess for trisomy or absence of whole chromosomes even without culturing and stimulating the cells toward metaphase. Such interphase FISH is routinely used as a rapid screen for aneuploidy of chromosomes 13, 18, 21, X and Y on chorionic villus sampling (CVS), amniocentesis, and in postnatal cases where rapid diagnosis may be desired for medical decision making, such as for an infant with features of Trisomy 13 or 18.

Over the last decade, single-locus testing by FISH has given way to chromosomal microarrays. This technique was originally based in comparative genome hybridization where patient DNA is labeled with one fluorescent probe while reference DNA is labeled in another and hybridized together. This allowed detection of regions across the genome, which had changes in copy number relative to the reference DNA and reflecting either gains (duplications) or losses (deletions) in the patient DNA. More recently, this approach has given way to the use of synthesized oligonucleotide probes or single nucleotide polymorphism (SNP)-based probes densely arranged on a microarray chip. Today, over two million such probes are routinely used on clinical diagnostic platforms for genome-wide postnatal testing. This allows the potential to report copy number changes in the 50–100 kb range. The processing is automated and copy number variation is compared against a large panel of standards. As might be expected with such high resolution analysis, changes that are of unknown significance are encountered and require further investigation and often examination of parental samples to help interpret the proband's results.

Chromosome microarrays have provided a rapid, highly reproducible way to assess for submicroscopic chromosome rearrangements that might underlie an airway malformation, in an objective manner across the genome. It tests the regions associated with known syndromes and those not yet described, by identifying regions and groups of genes whose dosage has been changed due to the rearrangement. The widespread use of this technique for postnatal cases has led to the identification of several new genomic disorders. For these reasons, chromosome microarray has been recommended as the first-line study for cases of multiple congenital malformations and unexplained intellectual disability [6]. This recommendation has also been extended to prenatal cases of multiple congenital malformations [7].

The array techniques rely on the detection of copy number change relative to standards from arrays run on control individuals. Structural changes that do not result in copy number variation, such as a balanced translocation or inversion of part of a chromosome, will not be detected by this technique. For example, the presence of an extra copy of material from chromosome 21 will be detected on a microarray for a patient presenting with Down syndrome. However, whether this has occurred due to a trisomy (a free-standing extra chromosome 21) or from a translocation that might also occur in a balanced form and be carried by a healthy parent will not be differentiated by the microarray. Knowledge of the mechanism is necessary to provide an accurate recurrence risk for the parents and further testing and genetic counseling is indicated.

Single Gene Disorders. Many syndromes are due to the disruption of the normal function of a single gene or *single gene disorder*. An alteration of a single base pair in the sequence of the gene leads to a disruption in the gene's functional product. In other cases, insertions or deletions of even a small number of nucleotides can disrupt the gene and subsequently, its protein product. These insertions or deletions may be as small as 2–3 base pairs, or may involve hundreds of base pairs. Neither a standard karyotype nor chromosomal microarray will detect these small sequence changes. These techniques may fail to detect deletions that encompass an entire gene, especially for small genes. Direct sequencing of the target gene will reveal single base pair mutations or small insertions and deletions. Larger deletions or duplications that involve either part or all of the gene are often even more difficult to detect, being too small to detect on a chromosomal microarray, but too large to detect with standard sequencing. These genetic lesions often require PCR-based deletion/duplication testing targeted to a specific gene locus. It is important to consider these potential mutational mechanisms and ensure they have been appropriately tested prior to eliminating a diagnosis from consideration.

Airway malformations can be part of a constellation of findings that result from mutation in a single gene. CHARGE syndrome is a good example, with mutations in the CHD7 gene associated with the clinical findings of CHARGE. Assessment of *single gene disorders* requires different techniques than those described above. Until recently, PCR-amplification and Sanger sequencing were the most commonly used techniques, requiring a gene-by-gene approach. These techniques are designed to examine the DNA at an individual nucleotide level assessing for alterations of one nucleotide for another (e.g., cytosine to adenine, C to A), deletion of one or more individual nucleotides or the insertion of a single or group of nucleotides into the normal sequence. The deletions or insertions have the potential to change the reading frame, resulting in a *frameshift*, which can affect production of the resulting mRNA and protein. A mutation that substitutes one nucleotide for another can result in formation of a premature termination codon and truncation of the putative protein. The mutation then is known as a *nonsense* mutation. An alteration in the DNA sequence that results in substitution of one amino acid for another in the translated protein, is known as a *missense* mutation, and can lead to production of a defective protein product. Gene sequencing can detect a variety of disease-causing mutations but requires that the clinician has selected the correct gene to test, which can be difficult in disorders with variable features.

Sequencing is not the testing method of choice for alterations where large segments of a gene are altered. For example, sequencing may miss cases where an entire exon of a gene is missing and not amplify properly to be sequenced. The exon deletion may be too small for accurate detection on a chromosome microarray. In these situations, specialized techniques involving quantitative PCR or MLPA may be used.

Standard PCR or polymerase chain reaction is commonly used to amplify desired segments of DNA; however, it is not typically quantitative or related to the amount of input DNA. Real-time PCR instead is a kinetic measurement, which assesses amplification in the early linear stages of the reaction and utilizes fluorescent labeling to quantitate products. The higher the copy number of a segment of DNA at the start, the more rapidly a significant increase in fluorescent product can be detected. MLPA or multiplex ligation-dependent probe amplification allows the relative quantitation of dozens of different PCR products of various lengths simultaneously. These two quantitative techniques allow for rapid assessment of copy number of a gene, part of a gene or a group of genes in a specific chromosome region. These diagnostic approaches require the selection of the appropriate target regions and unlike arrays, are not genome-wide. They are however, useful to test for intragenic deletions and duplications that might be below the threshold of reliable detection for microarray-based diagnostic testing and are routinely used in this capacity.

Sequencing

As mentioned, sequencing is the primary diagnostic modality to assess for mutations causing single gene disorders. Sequencing until recently has referred to Sanger-based sequencing of a single gene where typically, PCR is used to amplify the coding regions of a given gene, sequenced and then compared to the reference DNA. In addition, targeted sequencing, to assess a small region of a gene that is known to harbor a specific familial mutation for example, is also in routine use. Both of these techniques require the identification of a specific gene to test and in targeted sequencing, the familial mutation must be known. This has served as the classical method to identify single gene disorders such CHD7 mutations causing CHARGE syndrome for example, or one of the FGFR-based craniosynostosis syndromes. It requires examining the genes one at a time.

Over the last several years, methods for massively parallel sequencing or next-generation sequencing have allowed the availability of next-generation sequencing panels, where multiple genes in a disease pathway can be tested simultaneously. This approach works well for disorders where more than one gene in a developmental or biochemical pathway, when mutated, can cause disease and where clinical overlap in the phenotypes exists. In other words, it may be difficult to determine which of the group of genes to test based on clinical examination. Examples of well-known panels include those used for hypertrophic cardiomyopathy, non-syndromic hearing loss, Noonan syndrome (RAS/MAPK spectrum disorders), and craniosynostosis syndromes.

Over the last 3–4 years, next-generation sequencing has been applied to clinical exome sequencing. Whole exome sequencing (WES) targets the protein-coding regions or exons of the human genome. This includes approximately 20,000 genes and accounts for about 2 % of the total genome [8]. Despite the relatively small percentage of the genome sampled, this strategy is skewed toward the regions that directly result in producing functional protein and has rapidly moved from primarily research-based studies of related cohorts for a specific disease, e.g., Miller syndrome, to clinical diagnostic use and availability for unknown conditions [9]. It is available through commercial diagnostic laboratories.

For exome sequencing, the exons are targeted and captured from the patient's DNA sample. Then the captured material is subjected to massively parallel sequencing. The patient's sequence is then compared to reference DNA sequences, published control individuals and whenever possible, the patient's family members. The typical scenario in a pediatric patient is to analyze a trio, or the patient and both parents to use as comparison. The analysis requires a series of sophisticated bioinformatics analyses often referred to as a pipeline. This reduces the thousands of variants that can be seen with exome analysis and filters the gene list down to the most likely ones. Clinical information and family history that may support a specific mode of inheritance are critical pieces of information for the interpretation of whole exome data. While whole exome sequencing provides an important new diagnostic test, it is not designed to detect larger chromosomal duplications and deletions that microarray is designed for and is limited to the protein-coding regions and splice junctions of the genes.

Whole genome sequencing instead,is designed using next-generation techniques to sequence both introns and exons providing more complete coverage than exome alone. This is, at this time, not routinely available for patient care though applications for cancer diagnosis seem imminent. As might be imagined, interpretation of these massive data sets will require significant bioinformatics and analysis capacity.

As noted above, it is possible to examine cell-free DNA in the maternal circulation that comes from a fetus. Currently analysis is primarily used to assess for aneuploidy of chromosomes 13, 18, 21, and the X and Y chromosome using a sequencing-based approach on the isolated cell-free DNA. This can take place as a peripheral blood draw as early as 10–11 weeks of gestation and is referred to as noninvasive prenatal testing (NIPT) or noninvasive fetal testing (NIFT). These screening tests are reported to have high sensitivity and are now being adapted to screen for common microdeletion syndromes. At this writing, while NIPT screening shows signs of rapid adoption, only invasive testing involving samples taken from CVS or amniocentesis is considered diagnostic and positive NIPT screens prompt one of these diagnostic studies.

Epidemiology, Etiology, and Genetics of Specific Airway Malformations

In the following section, the epidemiology, known etiologies, and genetics of specific airway malformations will be reviewed. In most cases, these anomalies are complex and multifactorial disorders, which may be present as an isolated finding or in association with one or more additional malformations. For each airway anomaly discussed, there is often a substantial list of syndromes that have been associated with that particular anomaly. As a result, it is important to approach each infant with a detailed head-to-toe physical exam, as outlined above, to identify associated anomalies and guide additional diagnostic testing. It is particularly helpful to focus on unique or distinguishing features; such distinctions are highlighted in the discussion below.

Because the airway begins with the nasal and oral passages, any disorder associated with craniofacial abnormalities can present with significant airway compromise shortly after birth. This may range from "classic" craniofacial disorders such as the Crouzon craniosynostosis syndrome, in which the craniofacial structures alone are significantly affected, to multisystemic disorders such as CHARGE syndrome, in which the upper airway anomaly (e.g., choanal atresia or stenosis) is just one of many structural manifestations. Here, the major classes of craniofacial malformations that may lead to significant airway compromise by altering airflow through nasal and oral passages will be delineated, along with important associated syndromes. Next, malformations of the lower airways, including the larynx, trachea, and bronchi, will be discussed.

Zygomatic Hypoplasia/Aplasia

The zygomatic bones, or "cheekbones," form the orbital floor and a portion of the midface. Because of their close proximity to the mandible, maxilla, and ear ossicles, and the common embryologic origin of these structures from the first

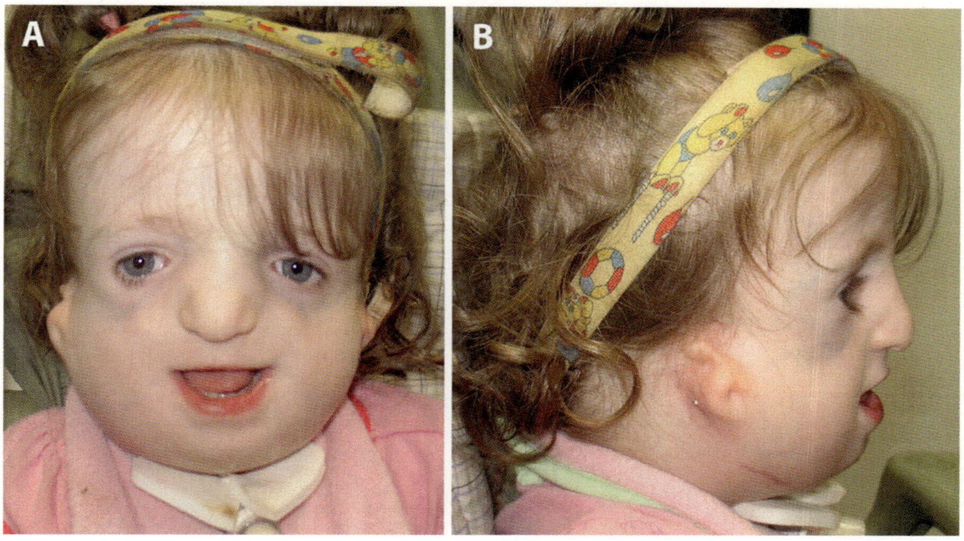

Fig. 3 (**a**, **b**)—Treacher-Collins Syndrome. (**a**)—Front, (**b**)—Side. Striking malar hypoplasia characteristic of Treacher-Collins syndrome is evident. Mandibular hypoplasia is also present. The auricles are malformed and bilateral lower eyelid colobomas are present. Also note the partial absence of the lower eyelids medially. Courtesy of CHOP Craniofacial Program, Permission Obtained

Table 4 Syndromes associated with Zygomatic hypoplasia

Disorder	Key features	Etiology/Gene
22q11.2 microdeletion syndrome	See Table 2	See Table 2
Hallerman-Streiff	Brachycephaly, frontal bossing, micrognathia sparse hair, microphthalmia, cataracts, beaked nose, skin atrophy, dental anomalies, and proportionate short stature	Unknown
Miller	Severe micrognathia, cleft lip/palate, limb anomalies (*including lower limbs*), eyelid colobomas,	DHODH gene (AR)
Nager	Downslanting palpebral fissures, midface retrusion, micrognathia, and radial ray limb defects; *lower limbs typically NOT affected*	SF3B4 gene (AD)
Oculo-auricular-vertebral (OAV) spectrum/Goldenhar	See Table 2	See Table 2
Townes-Brocks syndrome	Ear anomalies (microtia, pits, tags), CHD, GI, GU, and renal anomalies, imperforate anus, bifid or triphalangeal thumb, pre-axial polydactyly	SALL1 (AD)
Treacher-Collins syndrome	Zygomatic and mandibular hypoplasia, microtia, downslanting palpebral fissures, lower eyelid colobomas, choanal stenosis/atresia	TCOF gene (AD)

AD autosomal dominant, *AR* autosomal recessive

branchial arch, hypoplasia of the zygoma is almost never an isolated anomaly. The accompanying midface hypoplasia may be dramatic, and other defects such as cleft palate and micrognathia may be present. In many patients, these combinations of craniofacial findings can lead to significant airway compromise during the neonatal period.

Treacher-Collins syndrome, due to mutations in *TCOF1* (which encodes for the protein treacle), is characterized by striking zygomatic hypoplasia (Fig. 3a, b). Other notable findings include downslanting palpebral fissures, colobomas of the lower eyelids, partial or complete absence of eyelashes on the lower lids, external ear malformations, ear tags, conductive hearing loss, and cleft palate. Airway obstruction may be severe after birth, necessitating early tracheostomy and mandibular distraction [10]. Even those children not requiring aggressive airway management during the neonatal period may have persistent difficulties with obstructive sleep apnea later in childhood [11].

Despite the often highly recognizable features of Treacher-Collins syndrome, a number of other disorders may present with zygomatic hypoplasia and warrant careful consideration before a final diagnosis is made. These disorders are summarized in Table 4. In order to precisely define the craniofacial defects present, for both diagnostic and future therapeutic purposes, a dedicated computed tomography (CT) scan of the maxillofacial structures is indicated. Careful attention to features unrelated to the craniofacial structures will provide important diagnostic clues. Both Miller and Nager syndrome share many features with Treacher-Collins, but are distinguished by the presence of limb anomalies (Fig. 4a, b). In Miller syndrome, postaxial (ulnar side) limb deficiencies and syndactyly may be present, whereas Nager syndrome is

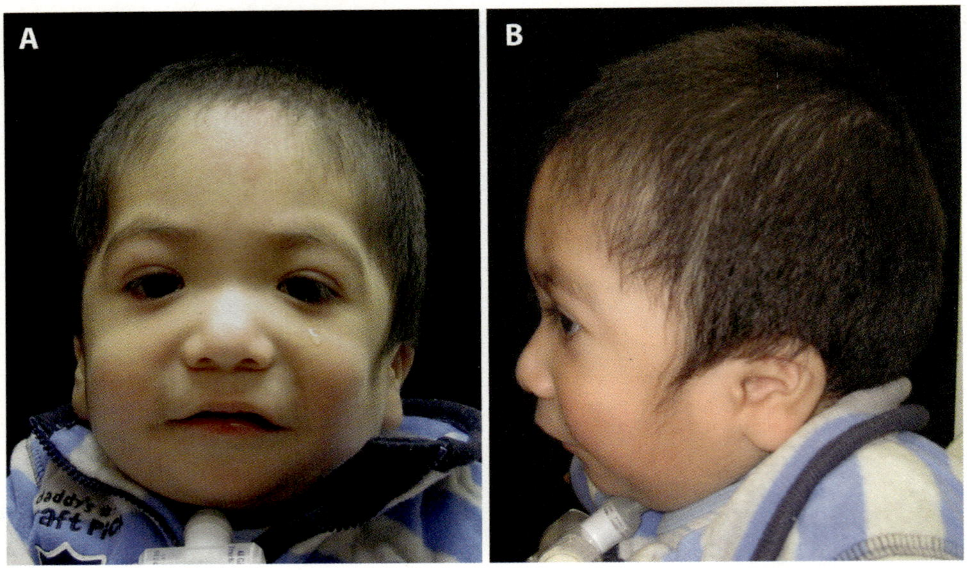

Fig. 4 (**a**, **b**)—Nager Syndrome. (**a**)—Front, (**b**)—Side. Features include microretrognathia, low-set and somewhat posteriorly rotated ears, and downslanting palpebral fissures. There is also sparse-to-absent lower eyelid lashes. Courtesy of CHOP Craniofacial Program, Permission Obtained

characterized by hypoplasia/aplasia of the thumb (radial ray deficiency), radioulnar synostosis, and short forearms. Both disorders may manifest with airway complications similar to those seen in Treacher-Collins syndrome.

Hallermann-Streiff syndrome has very characteristic facies that are quite distinct from Treacher-Collins, Nager, and Miller syndromes, but also includes significant malar hypoplasia. Typical craniofacial features include brachycephaly with frontal bossing, a beaked nose with hypoplastic cartilage, high arched palate, and micrognathia. Microphthalmia, cataracts, dental anomalies, skin atrophy, hypotrichosis, and proportionate stature are commonly seen. Tracheomalacia is often encountered, which in combination with these craniofacial findings can lead to significant respiratory insufficiency and even right heart failure [12]. A minority of patients may have intellectual disability or seizures. The underlying etiology of Hallermann-Streiff syndrome remains unknown.

Midface Hypoplasia

Anterior and medial to the zygomatic processes are the maxilla, nasal bones, and inferior portions of the orbit, which compose the midface. The developmental mechanisms leading to proper formation of the midface involve the interaction of multiple components (e.g., branchial arches, cranial base, neural tissue) in a complex and incompletely understood fashion. As a result, midface hypoplasia may be seen in a relatively large number of developmental and genetic disorders (Table 5). Because hypoplasia or retrusion of the midface commonly leads to obstruction of the nasal passages and feeding difficulty due to malalignment of the maxilla and mandible, respiratory compromise is commonly observed. In infants with severe midface hypoplasia, endotracheal intubation is often required and long-term airway management with a tracheostomy may be necessary until a more definitive craniofacial reconstruction can take place.

Although hypoplasia of the maxillary bone may occasionally be seen as an isolated, autosomal dominant finding (usually associated with prognathism), the vast majority of cases of midface hypoplasia are associated with other anomalies, and are due to a genetic disorder or environmental insult [13]. As emphasized above, the key to a successful diagnosis often relies on identifying unique features and associated anomalies. The craniofacial syndromes Apert, Crouzon, and Pfeiffer syndromes are all characterized by striking midface hypoplasia and craniosynostosis (Figs. 1a–d and 2a, b). While Crouzon and Apert syndromes are both due to heterozygous mutations in the fibroblast growth-factor receptor 2 (*FGFR2*) genes, the mutations seen in each condition and their clinical features are distinct. In Crouzon syndrome, the findings are limited to the craniofacial region and intelligence is normal. Apert syndrome, however, is associated with severe syndactyly of the hands and/or feet, often producing a "mitten hand" appearance, broad distal phalanges of the thumb, and intellectual disability. Pfeiffer syndrome is also associated with limb anomalies, including broad distal phalanges of the thumb with medial deviation and broad first toes. While partial syndactyly may be seen, the complete syndactyly characteristic of Apert syndrome is typically not present. In addition to severe midface hypoplasia, patients also have brachycephaly, coronal synostosis, hypertelorism, and ocular proptosis (see Fig. 4). Pfeiffer syndrome can be

Table 5 Syndromes associated with midface hypoplasia

Disorder	Key features	Etiology/Gene
Acondroplasia	Short limb skeletal dysplasia, frontal bossing, megalencephaly, low nasal bridge, upper airway obstruction	FGFR3 (AD)
Angelman syndrome	Hypotonia, ataxia, seizures, paroxysmal laughter	Maternal deletion of 15q11.2-q13, mutation of UBE3A
Antley-Bixler syndrome	Micro-brachycephaly, frontal bossing, proptosis, hypertelorism, choanal stenosis or atresia, limb anomalies, ± genital anomalies[a]	POR (AR) or FGFR2 (AD) gene
Apert	Craniofacial anomalies (see text) + limb anomalies	FGFR2 gene
Crouzon	Craniofacial anomalies only (see text)	FGFR2 gene
Hallerman-Streiff	See Table 4	See Table 4
OAV spectrum	See Table 2	See Table 2
Pfeiffer syndrome	Craniofacial anomalies (see text), broad thumbs/toes, partial syndactyly, occasional intellectual disability	FGFR1 or FGFR2 genes
Rubenstein-Taybi syndrome	Poor growth, microcephaly, broad thumbs/toes, characteristic facial features, and intellectual disability	EP300 (AD)
Stickler syndrome	Ocular abnormalities (high myopia, vitreoretinal degeneration, retinal detachment, cataracts), midline clefting, Pierre-Robin sequence, flat midface, sensorineural or conductive hearing loss.	COL2A1 gene (AD)
Trisomy 21	See Table 2	See Table 2
Turner syndrome	Short stature, webbed neck, congenital heart disease, premature ovarian failure	45, X0 karyotype

AD autosomal dominant, *AR* autosomal recessive

[a]Cases of Antley-Bixler syndrome with genital anomalies are typically due to mutations in the POR gene, which is involved in steroid biosynthesis

caused by mutations in either FGFR-1 or FGFR-2. Syndromes associated with mutations in the FGFR genes may present with other airway anomalies, such as cartilaginous tracheal sleeves, as discussed below.

Saethre-Chotzen syndrome, due to mutations in the TWIST gene, is associated with a number of clinical findings similar to the FGFR disorders discussed above. Facial features, in addition to midface hypoplasia, include craniosynostosis (coronal, lambdoid, and/or metopic), facial asymmetry, hypertelorism, and shallow orbits (Fig. 5a, b) Mild syndactyly (often of fingers 2–3, or toes 3–4), bifid terminal phalanges of digits 2–3, brachydactyly, and/or radioulnar synostosis may be present. Congenital heart defects are seen in some patients, and although most individuals with Saethre-Chotzen syndrome have normal intelligence, mild to moderate intellectual disability is occasionally seen.

A number of other unrelated syndromes may present with severe midface hypoplasia leading to airway complications in the neonatal period. Stickler syndrome is due to mutations in the type II collagen gene (COL2A1). Disruption of this gene leads to defective production of type II collagen, an extracellular matrix protein specific for cartilage, which leads to abnormal development of the skeleton and facial bones, eyes, and ears. In addition to midface hypoplasia, affected infants may have anteverted nares, a depressed nasal bridge, cleft palate, or Pierre-Robin sequence (see Fig. 6). Sensorineural, and occasional conductive, hearing loss may be present and affected individuals almost always have high myopia. They are at high risk for retinal detachment and resulting blindness. Glaucoma and cataracts may occasionally be seen. Other skeletal findings may include mild spondyloepiphyseal dysplasia, platyspondyly (flattened vertebrae) with anterior wedging, kyphoscoliosis, and arachnodactyly.

Marshall syndrome, due to mutations in the type 11 collagen gene (COL11A1), which also produces a protein found in cartilage, has overlapping features to Stickler syndrome. It was originally identified as a distinct clinical entity from Stickler syndrome, due to subtle differences in the facial appearance between the two disorders. Individuals with Marshall syndrome have thick calvaria, abnormal frontal sinuses and shallow orbits with proptotic eyes. The nose is short and depressed, with a flat nasal bridge and anteverted nares. Falx, tentorial, and meningeal calcifications may be present. Like Stickler, Marshall syndrome is commonly associated with high myopia that may progress to retinal detachment and vitreoretinal degeneration. Sensorineural hearing loss may also be present. Cleft palate and Pierre-Robin sequence may be seen, and the airway complications for the two disorders are similar.

Antley-Bixler syndrome shares many of the same craniofacial features as the FGFR2-related disorders discussed above, and a "purely skeletal" form of Antley-Bixler syndrome has been described due to mutations in this gene. However, the majority of patients with Antley-Bixler syndrome also have defects in steroid hormone production due to homozygous or compound heterozygous mutations in the cytochrome P450 oxidoreductase (POR) gene. Facial features include frontal bossing, midface hypoplasia, a large anterior fontanelle, craniosynostosis, dysplastic ears, and an often severely depressed nasal bridge that may be associated with choanal stenosis or

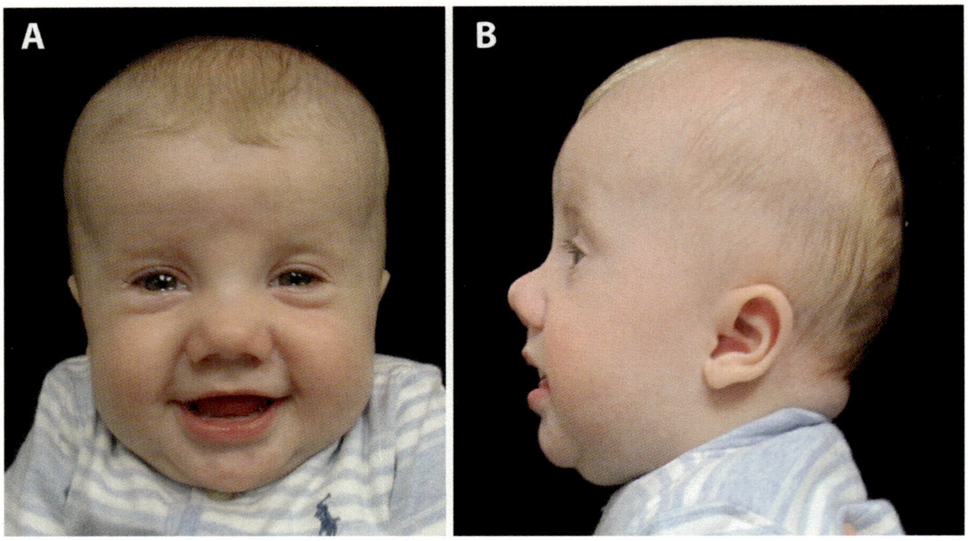

Fig. 5 (**a**, **b**)—Saethre-Chotzen Syndrome. (**a**)—Front, (**b**)—Side. Again note the turribrachycephaly, relatively flat face with high, flat forehead, maxillary hypoplasia, prominent ear crus, low-set ears, and hypertelorism. Courtesy of CHOP Craniofacial Program, Permission Obtained

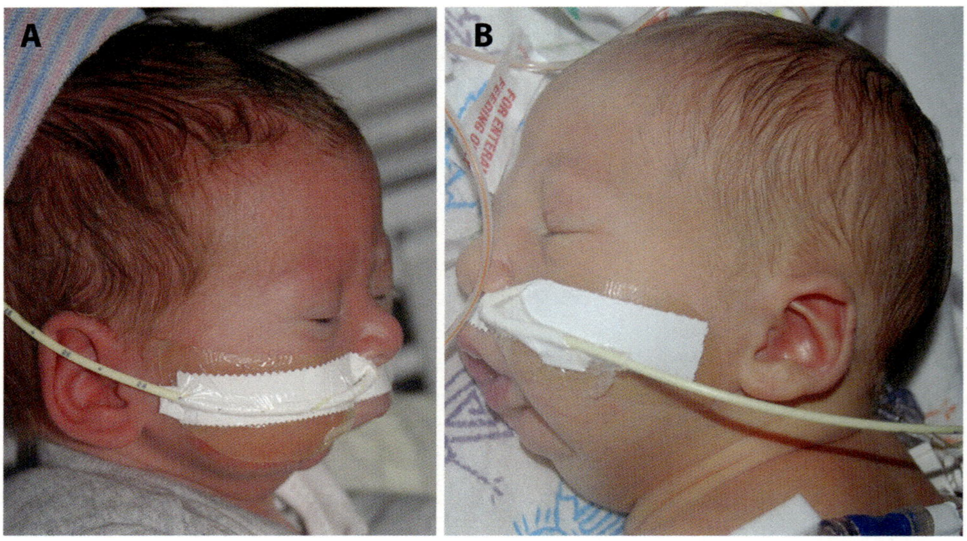

Fig. 6 (**a**, **b**)—Stickler Syndrome. (**a**)—Right side, (**b**)—Left side. Striking microretrognathia is present, along with a flat midface and depressed nasal bridge. Anteverted nares can be appreciated in (**a**). Courtesy of CHOP Craniofacial Program, Permission Obtained

atresia (see Fig. 7). As a result, the mortality rate has been reported to be as high as 80 % in the neonatal period, usually due to airway complications [14]. Other features include tracheobronchomalacia, genitourinary abnormalities, limb and skeletal defects, neurologic findings, and defective steroid hormone production leading to adrenal crisis.

Micrognathia and Agnathia

While micrognathia is a common malformation that may be seen as part of a broader syndrome, complete absence of the mandible (agnathia) is extremely rare. Agnathia may be seen in conjunction with or without holoprosencephaly. Microstomia (small mouth) and aglossia (absent tongue) are seen in both forms of agnathia. Agnathia with holoprosencephaly may be accompanied by synotia, in which the ears are displaced inferiorly and medially, even fusing at the midline. This collection of anomalies is usually lethal in the neonatal period. Agnathia without holoprosencephaly is often associated with middle ear anomalies, cleft lip/palate, and downward slanting palpebral fissures. The precise etiologies of both forms of agnathia, thought to be mechanistically distinct, remain unknown.

In contrast to agnathia, micrognathia is frequently encountered in newborns. While mild micrognathia may often be asymptomatic and even difficult to detect, severe micrognathia

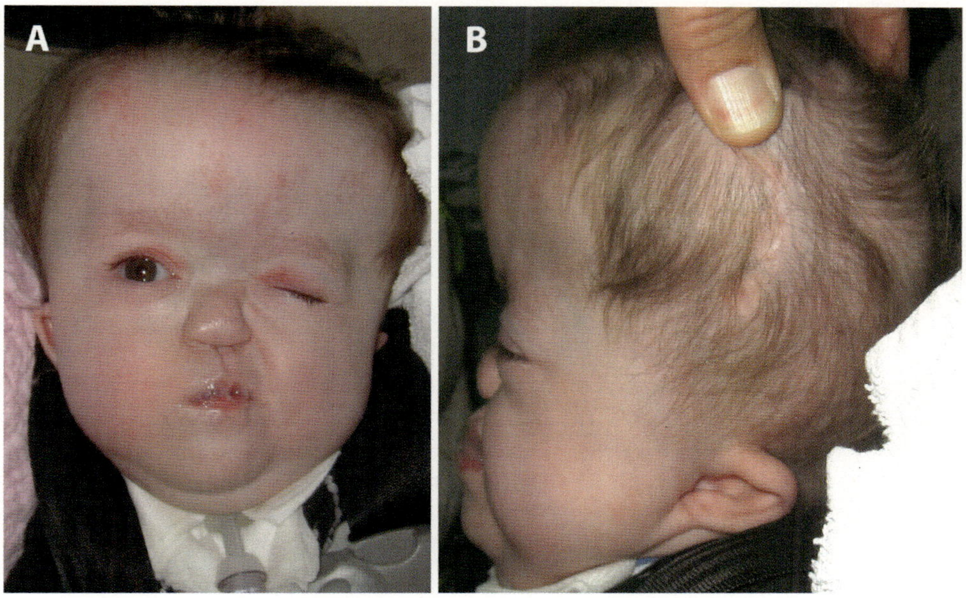

Fig. 7 (**a**, **b**)—Antley-Bixler Syndrome. (**a**)—Front, (**b**)—Side. Note brachycephaly, frontal and temporal bossing, midface hypoplasia, depressed nasal bridge, hypertelorism, and simple, overfolded ears that are low-set and posteriorly rotated. Courtesy of CHOP Craniofacial Program, Permission Obtained

Table 6 Syndromes associated with micrognathia

Disorder	Key features	Etiology/Gene
22q11.2 microdeletion syndrome	See Table 2	See Table 2
Cornelia de Lange	Characteristic facial features (low anterior hairline, arched eyebrows, synophrys, anteverted nares, maxillary prognathism, thin lips), growth retardation, intellectual disability, upper limb anomalies.	Multiple genes involved in the cohesion complex (most common, NIPBL)
Miller	See Table 4	See Table 4
Nager	See Table 4	See Table 4
OAV spectrum	See Table 2	See Table 2
Pallister-Hall syndrome	Hypothalamic hamartoma, pituitary dysfunction, central polydactyly, and multiple visceral malformations	GLI3 gene (AD)
Stickler	See Table 5	See Table 5
Treacher-Collins syndrome	See Table 4	See Table 4

AD autosomal dominant, *AR* autosomal recessive

may lead secondary malformations during development (Pierre-Robin sequence), and life-threatening airway complications in the neonatal period. A large number of syndromes are associated with micrognathia, including aneuploidies (Trisomy 18), microdeletion/microduplication syndromes (del 22q11.2 syndrome), disorders associated with other craniofacial abnormalities as discussed above, and single-gene disorders such as Cornelia de Lange syndrome. See Table 6 for a list of syndromes associated with micrognathia.

Choanal Stenosis/Atresia

Choanal atresia is due to obstruction of the posterior choanae, which is thought to result from failure of the nasobuccal membrane to break down during development. While choanal atresia or stenosis may be an isolated finding, in at least 50 % of cases it is associated with a multiple malformation syndrome. Particular attention should be paid for other features of CHARGE syndrome, an acronym for *C*oloboma, *H*eart defects, *A*tresia choanae, *R*etarded growth/development, *G*enitourinary abnormalities, and *E*ar anomalies/deafness. In additional to choanal atresia, individuals with CHARGE syndrome may have additional airway anomalies, including "anteroposterior flattening of the larynx; short vocal cords; anteriorly positioned, tall and hypertrophic arytenoids obscuring the glottis; uncoordinated movement of the vocal cords, epiglottis and arytenoids; salivary pooling," and abnormal cranial nerve function [15]. As a result, it is not uncommon for patients to require endotracheal intubation in the neonatal period, and some may require a tracheostomy for long-term airway management. This disorder is due to mutations in the

Table 7 Syndromes associated with choanal stenosis or atresia

• 22q11.2 microdeletion syndrome
• Hallerman-Streiff syndrome
• Miller syndrome
• Nager syndrome
• Oculo-auricular-vertebral (OAV) spectrum/Goldenhar syndrome
• Townes-Brocks syndrome
• Treacher-Collins syndrome

chromatin remodeling gene, *CHD7*. In addition to CHARGE syndrome, a number of other disorders, including many of the craniofacial syndromes previously discussed (e.g., Treacher-Collins, Crouzon, Pfeiffer, Antley-Bixler) may also be associated with choanal stenosis or atresia (Table 7).

Piriform Aperture Stenosis

The most anterior aspect of the bony nasal opening, referred to the piriform aperture, is also anatomically the narrowest aspect of the bony nasal passage. In rare instances, this bony opening is stenotic, and may lead to life-threatening respiratory complications in the neonatal period similar to bilateral choanal atresia. Piriform aperture stenosis may be seen as an isolated condition, but it also may be the presenting feature of holoprosencephaly, so a careful examination of the infant and his or her parents is warranted [16]. Additional features suggestive of holoprosencephaly (HPE) may include hypotelorism, absent frenulum, midline defects, or signs suggestive of panhypopituitarism (e.g., hypoglycemia, abnormal newborn screen due to thyroid dysfunction). Variable expression among family members all carrying the same genetic mutation can occur. Thus, subtle findings in an affected parent may include mild hypotelorism or a single central incisor. Brain imaging, either a head ultrasound, or ideally, magnetic resonance imaging (MRI) of the brain, is warranted in the infant with congenital piriform aperture stenosis. Genetic testing should be considered for infants with other signs suggestive of holoprosencephaly, as it can be part of a known syndrome, such as Trisomy 13, or associated with microdeletions and duplications in the genome. HPE has been associated with a growing number of single genes, including those involved in Sonic hedgehog signaling (e.g., *SHH*, *GLI2*, *PTCH1*) [17]. Next-generation sequencing-based multi-gene panels are now available to simplify testing.

Macroglossia

While a variety of tongue abnormalities may be observed, it is usually only when the tongue is significantly enlarged that airway compromise is observed. Tumors and vascular malformations, including dermoid cysts, rhabdomyomas, and lymphatic, venous and capillary malformations, may all develop prenatally and lead to life-threatening airway compromise at birth. Muscular enlargement of the tongue may be seen in overgrowth syndromes, including Beckwith-Wiedemann syndrome. Other characteristic features of this disorder include ear creases/pits, hemihypertrophy, visceromegaly, embryonal tumors, omphalocele, and hypoglycemia due to hyperinsulinemia. This disorder is related to epigenetic abnormalities on chromosome 11p15: (1) 50 % of individuals have loss of methylation of the maternal copy of this chromosomal region (IC2); (2) 20 % have paternal UPD for this chromosomal region (e.g., two copies of this region from father, none from mother); (3) 5 % with gain of methylation on the maternal copy of imprinting region 1 (IC1); and, genetic changes such as (4) mutations within the gene *CDKN1C*. A small number of patients have larger deletions involving this entire chromosomal region.

Macroglossia may be seen in mucopolysaccharidoses. While this is typically a feature later in childhood, it can occasionally present during infancy and should be considered if other suggestive features, such as coarse facies, hepatosplenomegaly, or cytopenias are present.

A number of conditions can also make the tongue appear large, when it is in fact, normal in size. These may include hypoplasia of the surrounding structures (e.g., mandible), or neurologic dysfunction that leads to frequent tongue protrusion. Relative macroglossia is most commonly observed in Trisomy 21, but may also be seen in conditions such as congenital hypothyroidism.

Facial Asymmetry

Development of normal facial structures is dependent upon a complex interplay of multiple tissue types, each signaling to one another during development. The branchial arches, which form many of the facial structures as discussed above, must not only form properly themselves, but also need to interact appropriately with surrounding structures, such as the brain. Any insult or genetic lesion that disrupts these structures or interactions, from the branchial arches themselves to disorders of the developing CNS, may lead to asymmetry of the facial bones. Although it may seem counterintuitive that a genetic syndrome, in which every cell in the body carries the pathologic genetic change, would lead to asymmetry, many genetic disorders have been associated with facial asymmetry, including several of the craniofacial disorders discussed above (Table 8). In other cases, no underlying genetic etiology can be identified. It has been hypothesized that these sporadic cases may result from a vascular insult to the developing brachial arches, such as interruption of blood flow through the stapedial artery [18–20].

Oculo-auriculo-vertebral (OAVS), commonly known as Goldenhar syndrome in its more severe manifestation, is

Table 8 Syndromes associated with facial asymmetry

Disorder	Key features	Etiology/Gene
Apert	See Table 5 (and text)	See Table 5
Craniofrontonasal syndrome	Frontonasal dysplasia, craniofacial asymmetry, craniosynostosis, bifid nasal tip, grooved nails, wiry hair, skeletal anomalies (in females)	EFNB1 gene (X-linked, predilection for females)
McCune-Albright	Craniofacial hyperostosis, polyostotic fibrous dysplasia, and endocrine abnormalities (hyperthyroidism, hyperparathyroidism, Cushing syndrome, acromegaly, hyperprolactinemia)	Mosaic mutation in GNAS1 (AD)
Muenke	Brachycephaly, macrocephaly, hypertelorism, downslanting palpebral fissures, ptosis, coronal craniosynostosis, and hand/foot anomalies (clinodactyly, brachydactyly, broad, middle phalanges, broad 1st toes)	FGFR3 gene (AD)
OAV spectrum	See Table 2	See Table 2
Saethre-Chotzen	Brachycephaly, flat face, maxillary hypoplasia, ear anomalies, shallow orbits, hypertelorism, buphthalmos, ptosis, congenital heart disease, 2–3 syndactyly, bifid terminal phalanges of digits 2–3, absent first metatarsal, 3–4 toe syndactyly	TWIST1 gene (AD)
Townes-Brocks	See Table 4	See Table 4

AD autosomal dominant, *AR* autosomal recessive

Table 9 Syndromes associated with bifid epiglottis

Disorder	Key features	Etiology/Gene
Bardet-Biedl	Obesity, rod-cone dystrophy, retinitis pigmentosa, congenital heart disease, hepatic fibrosis, renal anomalies, learning disabilities, hypogonadism	Multiple genes
Joubert	Retinal disease, disordered breathing (including central apnea), renal disease (including neprhonophthisis), hypotonia, intellectual disability, cerebellar anomalies (*"molar tooth" sign* on MRI)	Multiple genes
McKusick-Kaufman	Pulmonary hypoplasia, Hirschprung disease, imperforate anus, vaginal anomalies, including vaginal atresia, hydrometrocolpos, and rectovaginal fistula, postaxial polydactyly	MKKS gene (AR)
Pallister-Hall	See Table 6	See Table 6
Weyer acrofacial dysostosis	Short stature, single central incisor, conical teeth, brachydactyly, postaxial polydactyly, hypoplastic, or dysplastic nails	EVC gene (AR)

AD autosomal dominant, *AR* autosomal recessive

one of the most frequently encountered disorders presenting with significant facial asymmetry in the newborn period. It is usually sporadic, with no known genetic etiology. However, families with multiple affected members have been reported; both autosomal dominant and autosomal recessive modes of inheritance have been proposed based on these rare families. While both sides of the face may be affected in OAVS, typically one side is more severely affected, leading to asymmetry that can be quite pronounced. There is hypoplasia of the malar, maxillary, and mandibular regions, with hypoplasia of the overlying musculature. The ear on the affected side is often small (microtia) and malformed, and preauricular tags and sinuses may be present. There is typically secondary hearing loss due to these features and atresia of the external auditory canal has been observed. Some patients may also have senorineural hearing loss. Cleft lip/palate may be present with this spectrum. In some patients, microphthalmia or upper eyelid coloboma may be present. When epibulbar dermoids are present, the eponym Goldenhar syndrome is often applied. Vertebral anomalies, including hemivertebrae or vertebral hypoplasia are often seen. Occasionally, malformations of other organ systems may be seen, including congenital heart defects (VSD, Tetralogy of Fallot, aortic coarctation) or lung hypoplasia. Cognitive function is typically unaffected, although individuals with OAVS may occasionally have intellectual disability or structural CNS anomalies, including agenesis of the corpus callosum, Arnold-Chiari malformation, or hydrocephalus. Airway complications in infants with OAVS are similar to those seen in other children with craniofacial disorders, and are often directly related to the degree of mandibular hypoplasia.

Bifid Epiglottis

Bifid epiglottis, consisting of a cleft down the midline of the epiglottis with two distinct halves, is an extremely rare disorder that presents in the neonatal period with stridor, aspiration, or failure-to-thrive [21]. It is most commonly associated with Pallister-Hall syndrome, but has been associated with several other genetic syndromes (Table 9).

Table 10 Syndromes associated with laryngeal hypoplasia or atresia

Disorder	Key features	Etiology/Gene
Fraser	Hairline extends to lateral temples, ear malformations, cryptophthalmos, hypertelorism, cleft lip/palate, GU/renal anomalies, neural tube defects	FRAS1 or FREM2 genes (AR)
Marshall-Smith	Accelerated skeletal maturation, respiratory difficulties, intellectual disability, characteristic facies	NFIX gene (AD)
Nager	See Table 4	See Table 4
Optiz-G BBB	See Table 2	See Table 2
Rhizomelic chondrodysplasia punctata	Short stature (rhizomelic), characteristic facial features, congenital contractures, ocular abnormalities, and intellectual disability	Peroxisomal disorder, multiple genes

AD autosomal dominant, *AR* autosomal recessive

Pallister-Hall syndrome is a complex and often lethal multiple malformation syndrome due to heterozygous mutations in the *GLI3* gene, whose protein product plays a role in Sonic hedgehog (Shh) signaling. Hypothalamic hamartoma with postaxial polydactyly is particularly characteristic of this disorder. The facial features include a short nose, flat nasal bridge, anteverted nares, and small, posteriorly rotated ears. Cleft lip and palate may be present, and the tongue may be small. In addition to bifid epiglottis, laryngeal clefts and abnormal lobation of the lungs may be seen. Other commonly encountered malformations include congenital heart disease (VSD, aortic coarctation, PDA), genitourinary abnormalities (micropenis, renal dysplasia, renal ectopia), imperforate anus, skeletal defects (postaxial polydactyly, synactyly, hemivertebrae), and CNS malformations (holoprosencephaly, hypothalamic hamartoma, pituitary aplasia/dysplasia).

Laryngeal Stenosis/Atresia

While underdevelopment of the larynx has been reported in association with a variety of genetic syndromes (Table 10), true laryngeal atresia is extremely rare and typically lethal unless special measures, such as an EXIT procedure to immediate surgical airway management are undertaken. EXIT, or *ex utero intrapartum treatment*, is a specialized surgical procedure used to deliver babies who have severe airway compromise or other conditions that are unlikely to lead to successful transition to the postnatal environment without significant medical intervention. Laryngeal stenosis is often included under the larger umbrella term, congenital high airway obstruction syndrome (CHAOS), which may include other malformations such as complete tracheal atresia, severe subglottic stenosis, laryngeal webs, or laryngeal masses/cysts that obstruct the upper airway. Laryngeal atresia has been observed in *Fraser syndrome* and *rhizomelic chondrodysplasia punctata*. It has also been observed more commonly in association with encephalocele and limb deformities, but the genetic basis for this observed association remains largely unknown [22].

Fraser syndrome is a severe autosomal recessive disorder due to mutations in the FRAS1, FREM2, or GRIP1 genes, and is associated with cryptophthalmos and syndactyly. There is often a characteristic extension of the hairline onto the temples extending toward the lateral aspect of the eyebrows. The most striking aspect of the facial features in this disorder is the cryptophthalmos. There may also be a broad, low nasal bridge, with hypoplastic, notched nares. Cleft lip and palate can be seen. Genitourinary abnormalities are common (hypospadias, cryptorchidism, vaginal atresia, bicornate uterus, or renal agenesis/hypoplasia) and neural tube defects, including encephalocele and meningomyelocele may be present.

Laryngotracheal Clefts

During the fourth week of development, the respiratory tract begins to bud from a single tube known as the foregut. The trachea and esophagus are progressively separated from one another, starting caudally and progressing toward the larynx. Disruption of this developmental process may lead to clefting or fistula formation between the two structures. Laryngeal clefts are almost always on the posterior aspect of the larynx and trachea with communication to the esophagus and are commonly divided into five types (Table 8):

Type I: Supraglottic interarytenoid cleft
Type II: Partial cricoid cleft extending below the vocal cords
Type III: Complete cricoid cleft extending into the cervical trachea
Type IV: Complete cleft extending into the thoracic trachea
Type V: Cleft to or beyond the carina

While type I clefts may be seen in isolation, more severe laryngotracheal clefts are typically associated with other anomalies. Other abnormalities of the tracheobronchial tree are commonly present, including TEF/EA, focal stenosis of the airway (subglottic stenosis, tracheal stenosis), cysts, or hamartomas. Cleft lip/palate, congenital heart disease, and malformations of the GI or GU tract may be seen.

Laryngotracheal clefts may be seen in association with Down syndrome, Opitz GBBB syndrome, Pallister-Hall syndrome, and mosaic deletions involving the long arm of chromosome 13. Opitz GBBB syndrome may result from mutations in the MID1 gene on the X chromosome, and its features overlap those seen with deletions involving chromosome 22q11.2. Striking hypertelorism is often present in Opitz GBBB and is accompanied by epicanthal folds, a broad, flat nasal bridge, posteriorly rotated ears, and micrognathia. Cleft lip and palate, congenital heart disease (VSD, PDA), and pulmonary hypoplasia may be seen among the midline defects associated with this clinical entity. Genitourinary abnormalities are common, including hypospadias, cryptorchidism, or bifid scrotum in males. Developmental delay and intellectual disability are present, and structural CNS anomalies, including agenesis of the corpus callosum, cerebellar vermal hypoplasia, and ventriculomegaly may be seen Fig. 8.

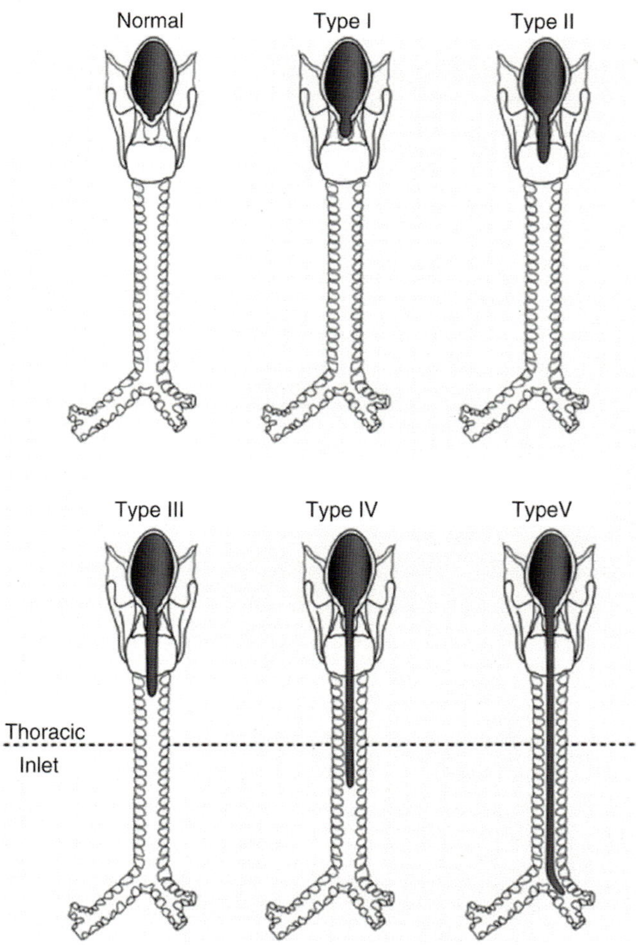

Fig. 8 Laryngotracheal Clefts volume 2: Respiratory cardiovascular and central nervous systems: Shanley, Wheeler and Wong Chapter 3; congenital airway anomalies: Figure 3.1. Classification of posterior laryngotracheal clefts. Type I: Supraglottic interarytenoid cleft. Type II: Partial cricoid cleft extending below the vocal cords. Type III: Complete cricoid cleft extending into the cervical trachea. Type IV: Complete cleft extending into the thoracic trachea. Type V: Cleft to or beyond the carina

Tracheoesophageal Fistula

While tracheoesophageal fistula/esophageal atresia (TEF/EA) is often seen as an isolated and sporadic birth defect, it has long been recognized that TEF/EA may occur in association with multiple malformations, including the VACTERL association. VACTERL is defined as an "association" rather than a "syndrome" because, although these collections of findings occur more frequently together than would statistically be expected to occur by chance, the underlying etiology remains elusive. The VACTERL association includes: *V*ertebral defects, *A*nal atresia/stenosis, *C*ardiac defects, *T*EF or *E*A, *R*enal anomalies, and *L*imb defects. Every infant with TEF/EA warrants a thorough evaluation to exclude the presence of these commonly associated malformations. It is also important to recognize that VACTERL remains a diagnosis of exclusion, and that it can be very easy to mistake many of the well defined genetic syndromes that are also associated with TEF/EA due to their clinical overlap with the VACTERL association (Table 2). For example, the presence of colobomas of the eyes or characteristically shaped ears may indicate a diagnosis of CHARGE syndrome, due to mutations in the CHD7 gene. The presence of a triphalangeal thumb and hypopigmented skin lesions in an infant with TEF/EA may suggest a diagnosis of Fanconi's anemia. This has important implication for future management, as patients with Fanconi's anemia often do not exhibit hematologic manifestations until several years of age. However, these manifestations may be severe and necessitate bone marrow transplant. Patients must also be followed closely later in life due to increased risk of malignancy. Short 2nd and 5th fingers in an infant with "VACTERL-like" features (TEF/EA, vertebral, and/or renal anomalies) may indicate a diagnosis of Feingold syndrome. This disorder is due to heterozygous mutations in the MYCN gene, which can be run through families in an autosomal dominant fashion. This diagnosis will have important implications for genetic counseling, as the risk for recurrence in future children if the parents are also affected will be 50 %, in contrast to an infant with isolated TEF/EA or VACTERL syndrome.

Tracheal Stenosis

Tracheal stenosis, a fixed narrowing of the trachea, often due to complete cartilaginous rings, is quite rare. It is typically accompanied by multiple congenital malformations. Not surprisingly, additional malformations of the tracheobronchial tree and lungs are often seen, including bronchial stenosis, TEF, and pulmonary hypoplasia or aplasia. Congenital heart disease may be present (common AV canal, aortic coarctation, VSD, dextrocardia) and often complicates the management of these patients [23]. Skeletal anomalies may be present, including vertebral and radial ray defects, and a subset of patients

Table 11 Syndromes associated with tracheal stenosis

Disorder	Key features	Etiology/Gene
Trisomy 21	See Table 2	See Table 2
Conradi-Hunermann	Linear or whorled atrophic and pigmentary lesions, striated hyperkeratosis, coarse hair/alopecia, cataracts, skeletal, and craniofacial anomalies.	EPB gene (X-linked dominant)
Frontometaphyseal dysplasia	Generalized skeletal dysplasia, deafness, urogenital defects	FLNA gene (X-linked)
Geleophysic dysplasia	Short stature, short hands/feet, joint limitations, skin thickening, characteristic facial features, progressive cardiac valvular thickening	ADAMTSL2 gene (AR)
Hydrolethalus	Polydactyly, CNS malformations, congenital heart disease, GI & GU malformations, skeletal anomalies	HYLS1 or KIF7 genes (AR)
Keutel	Midface hypoplasia, small nasal alae, depressed nasal bridge, hearing loss, pulmonary artery hypoplasia, peripheral pulmonary stenosis, abnormal ossification	MGP gene (AR)
Larsen	Large-joint dislocations, characteristic craniofacial features, spatula-shaped fingers, cleft palate, short stature, spinal anomalies, hearing loss	FLNB (AD), B3GAT3 (AR)
OAVS spectrum/Goldenhar	See Table 2	See Table 2
Optiz-G BBB	See Table 2	See Table 2
VACTERL association	See Table 2	See Table 2

AD autosomal dominant, *AR* autosomal recessive

will fulfill multiple features of the VACTERL association. A number of the syndromes associated with other malformations of the airways and tracheobronchial tree discussed above may also present with tracheal stenosis, including Goldenhar, Opitz GBBB, and Down syndrome, and mosaic deletion of chromosome 13q. In summary, tracheal stenosis can be an occult finding and is associated with a number of syndromes that are not as familiar to the clinician (Table 11).

Congenital Tracheal Cartilaginous Sleeve

Congenital tracheal cartilaginous sleeve is an unusual condition in which the normally discrete C-shaped cartilaginous rings of the trachea are fused vertically to form a rigid tube with smooth tracheal surface evident at the time of bronchoscopy.

Although rare, it is an important complication of the FGFR2 related disorders (e.g., Crouzon, Pfeiffer, Apert syndromes), as discussed above. Although the complete tracheal rings typically do not affect the length or diameter of the trachea, the increased rigidity alters normal airflow through the upper airways and the mechanics of coughing. As a result, infants may present with biphasic stridor. Mucus clearance is defective, which predisposes to mucus plugging, bronchospasm and respiratory infection. Infants may have sporadic episodes of cyanosis and respiratory distress, and if unrecognized, these events can be fatal.

Other Genetic Syndromes Requiring Neonatal Airway Management

Healthcare providers caring for infants requiring advanced airway management will undoubtedly encounter an overwhelming array of genetic syndromes that do not directly involve abnormal development of the craniofacial structures or tracheobronchial tree. They nonetheless impact the infant's ability to maintain a patent airway. While a complete discussion of all such syndromes is well beyond the scope of this chapter, it is worthwhile to highlight important categories of disorders most likely to require airway management.

Neuromuscular disorders, including malformations of the central nervous system, frequently impair the infant's ability to clear secretions, maintain a patent airway, and deliver effective ventilation. A long and growing list of genes have been linked to structural malformations of the brain, and numerous genes involved in formation of the muscle tissue, which when disrupted, have been implicated in the pathogenesis of congenital myopathies and muscular dystrophies.

Congenital masses of the neck and upper thorax may impinge on the airway, leading to life-threatening airway compromise immediately after birth. Most commonly, these giant neck masses are lymphangiomas or teratomas. These typically occur as isolated findings. In contrast, other lympatic malformations of the neck, such as cystic hygroma, may be associated with a wide range of genetic conditions including Turner and Noonan syndrome. Hemangiomas may involve the airway itself, or may extend from the neck or upper thoracic region to compress the airway. Again, these lesions are often sporadic, but may be associated with other anomalies, including the PHACE association. This association is characterized by *P*osterior fossa abnormalities, segmental *H*emangioma(s), *A*rterial abnormalities of the head/neck region, Congenital heart defects, and Eye abnormalities (cataracts, retinal/vascular abnormalities, visual impairment). The underlying genetic/developmental etiology of PHACE syndrome is currently unknown.

References

1. Graham JM. Smith's recognizable patterns of human deformation. 3rd ed. Philadelphia: Saunders; 2007. p. 384.
2. Stevenson R. Overview: human malformations and related anomalies. In: Stevenson R, Hall JG, editors. Human malformations and related anomalies. New York: Oxford University Press; 2006. p. 3–84.
3. Shashi V, McConkie-Rosell A, Rosell B, Schoch K, Vellore K, McDonald M, et al. The utility of the traditional medical genetics diagnostic evaluation in the context of next-generation sequencing for undiagnosed genetic disorders. Genet Med. 2014;16(2):176–82. PubMed PMID: 23928913.
4. Gripp KW, Slavotinek AM, Hall JG, Allanson JE. Handbook of physical measurements. 3rd ed. New York: Oxford University Press; 2013. p. 592.
5. Haldeman-Englert CR, Saitta SC, Zackai EH. Evaluation of the dysmorphic infant. In: Gleason CA, Devaskar S, editors. Avery's diseases of the newborn. Philadelphia: Saunders; 2012. p. 186–95.
6. Miller DT, Adam MP, Aradhya S, Biesecker LG, Brothman AR, Carter NP, et al. Consensus statement: chromosomal microarray is a first-tier clinical diagnostic test for individuals with developmental disabilities or congenital anomalies. Am J Hum Genet. 2010;86(5):749–64. PubMed PMID: 20466091. Pubmed Central PMCID: 2869000.
7. Wapner RJ, Martin CL, Levy B, Ballif BC, Eng CM, Zachary JM, et al. Chromosomal microarray versus karyotyping for prenatal diagnosis. N Engl J Med. 2012;367(23):2175–84. PubMed PMID: 23215555. Pubmed Central PMCID: 3549418.
8. Bamshad MJ, Ng SB, Bigham AW, Tabor HK, Emond MJ, Nickerson DA, et al. Exome sequencing as a tool for mendelian disease gene discovery. Nat Rev Genet. 2011;12(11):745–55. PubMed PMID: 21946919.
9. Ng SB, Buckingham KJ, Lee C, Bigham AW, Tabor HK, Dent KM, et al. Exome sequencing identifies the cause of a mendelian disorder. Nat Genet. 2010;42(1):30–5. PubMed PMID: 19915526. Pubmed Central PMCID: 2847889.
10. Thompson JT, Anderson PJ, David DJ. Treacher Collins syndrome: protocol management from birth to maturity. J Craniofac Surg. 2009;20(6):2028–35. PubMed PMID: 19881372.
11. Akre H, Overland B, Asten P, Skogedal N, Heimdal K. Obstructive sleep apnea in Treacher Collins syndrome. Eur Arch Otorhinolaryngol. 2012;269(1):331–7. PubMed PMID: 21626120. Pubmed Central PMCID: 3249173.
12. Friede H, Lopata M, Fisher E, Rosenthal IM. Cardiorespiratory disease associated with Hallermann-Streiff syndrome: analysis of craniofacial morphology by cephalometric roentgenograms. J Craniofac Genet Dev Biol Suppl. 1985;1:189–98. PubMed PMID: 3877095.
13. Baxter DJ, Shroff M. Congenital midface abnormalities. Neuroimaging Clin N Am. 2011;21(3):563–84, vii-viii. PubMed PMID: 21807312.
14. McGlaughlin KL, Witherow H, Dunaway DJ, David DJ, Anderson PJ. Spectrum of Antley-Bixler syndrome. J Craniofac Surg. 2010;21(5):1560–4. PubMed PMID: 20818252.
15. Naito Y, Higuchi M, Koinuma G, Aramaki M, Takahashi T, Kosaki K. Upper airway obstruction in neonates and infants with CHARGE syndrome. Am J Med Genet A. 2007;143A(16):1815–20. PubMed PMID: 17630667.
16. Nanni L, Ming JE, Du Y, Hall RK, Aldred M, Bankier A, et al. SHH mutation is associated with solitary median maxillary central incisor: a study of 13 patients and review of the literature. Am J Med Genet. 2001;102(1):1–10. PubMed PMID: 11471164.
17. Solomon BD, Mercier S, Velez JI, Pineda-Alvarez DE, Wyllie A, Zhou N, et al. Analysis of genotype-phenotype correlations in human holoprosencephaly. Am J Med Genet C Semin Med Genet. 2010;154C(1):133–41. PubMed PMID: 20104608. Pubmed Central PMCID: 2815217.
18. Gorlin RJ, Jue KL, Jacobsen U, Goldschmidt E. Oculoauriculovertebral Dysplasia. J Pediatr. 1963;63:991–9. PubMed PMID: 14071056.
19. Poswillo D. The pathogenesis of the first and second branchial arch syndrome. Oral Surg Oral Med Oral Pathol. 1973;35(3):302–28. PubMed PMID: 4631568.
20. Ryan CA, Finer NN, Ives E. Discordance of signs in monozygotic twins concordant for the Goldenhar anomaly. Am J Med Genet. 1988;29(4):755–61. PubMed PMID: 3400721.
21. Stevens CA, Ledbetter JC. Significance of bifid epiglottis. Am J Med Genet A. 2005;134(4):447–9. PubMed PMID: 15782417.
22. Kalache KD, Masturzo B, Scott RJ, Rodeck CH, Chitty LS. Laryngeal atresia, encephalocele, and limb deformities (LEL): a possible new syndrome. J Med Genet. 2001;38(6):420–2. PubMed PMID: 11424928. Pubmed Central PMCID: 1734896.
23. Huang SC, Wu ET, Wang CC. Management of long-segment tracheal stenosis: a continuing surgical challenge. Eur J Cardiothorac Surg. 2014. PubMed PMID: 24699206.

Prenatal Assessment and Perinatal Management of Suspected Airway Compromise in the Fetus and Neonate

Stig Somme and Timothy M. Crombleholme

Introduction

Airway obstruction in the fetus is one of the most important findings that can be prenatally diagnosed, because of the direct impact on management. In some instances complete airway obstruction in the fetus can dramatically alter pulmonary development resulting in hydrops and fetal demise. In other instances the compromise of the fetal airway at the time of delivery may be the cause of mortality due to inability to secure an airway by conventional means. Fetal surgical intervention is often needed to treat the obstruction and secure the airway; it must be meticulously planned and executed. The timing of this intervention may be prenatal, perinatal, or postnatal, depending on the underlying diagnosis, secondary consequences of the airway compromise, and the severity of airway obstruction anticipated at delivery.

The many etiologies of airway obstruction can be categorized into two groups: as intrinsic or extrinsic to the airway. Extrinsic airway obstruction is most commonly caused by a mass external to the airway compromising the lumen or access to the glottis (e.g., epignathus, micrognathia with glossoptosis, cervical teratoma, lymphatic malformations, bronchogenic cysts).

Intrinsic causes of fetal airway obstruction will result in congenital high airway obstruction syndrome (CHAOS) if the obstruction is complete. CHAOS is a prenatal syndrome characterized by non-immune hydrops, which occurs as a result of complete intrinsic obstruction of the airway. Unfortunately, CHAOS carries a high rate of fetal loss. In both intrinsic and extrinsic cases of airway compromise an EXIT-to-airway procedure can prevent death due to inability to establish an airway at delivery.

S. Somme, M.D.
Department of Surgery, The Children's Hospital of Colorado, University of Colorado School of Medicine, Aurora, CO, USA

T.M. Crombleholme, M.D. (✉)
Division of Pediatric General, Thoracic and Fetal Surgery, Colorado Fetal Care Center and the Colorado Institute for Maternal and Fetal Health, Children's Hospital Colorado, 12123 East 16th Avenue, Aurora, CO, USA
e-mail: Timothy.crombleholme@childrenscolorado.org

Extrinsic Airway Compression

There is an extensive list of possible causes of extrinsic airway obstruction at every level of the fetal airway; each carries potential implications for fetal development, as well as compromise of the fetal airway at the time of delivery (see Table 1). Epignathus, micrognathia with glossoptosis, cervical teratoma, and cervical lymphangioma account for the majority of extrinsic airway obstruction. Below we highlight the diagnostic features and management strategies for the most common causes of extrinsic airway obstruction.

Epignathus

Epignathus is an oropharyngeal teratoma arising from the sphenoid bone, palate, or pharynx. The cells of origin are likely pluripotent stem cells derived from cells in Rathke's pouch. The tumor may vary considerably in size but tumors that fill the oral cavity and protrude through the mouth are common, often leading to obstruction of the upper airway. Without prompt intervention at time of delivery, most newborn infants will succumb to airway obstruction and die soon after birth [1]. Epignathus is fortunately a rare tumor with an estimated incidence range from 1:35,000 to 1:200,000 [2]. Large epignathus can present early in the second trimester with polyhydramnios and complete airway obstruction at the level of the oro-pharynx [3]. Polyhydramnios can be severe in this setting and may require serial reduction to avoid premature labor [4]. In addition to ultrasound, an ultra-fast MRI scan can provide important anatomic information about the mass, confirm the origin of the tumor, vascular supply, and secondary effects of the mass on the mandible and other adjacent structures (Fig. 1).

J. Lioy and S.E. Sobol (eds.), *Disorders of the Neonatal Airway: Fundamentals for Practice*, DOI 10.1007/978-1-4939-1610-8_17, © Springer Science+Business Media New York 2015

Table 1 Differential diagnosis of fetal airway obstruction

Causes of extrinsic airway obstruction
Oral
Epignathus
Epulus
Micrognathia
Parotid tumor
Cervical
Cervical teratoma
Lymphangioma
Congenital goiter
Solid thyroid tumor
Cystic anomaly of thyroid
Branchial cleft cyst
Hamartoma
Choristoma
Hemangioma
Lipoma
Anterior neural tube defects
Twins sac of a blighted ovum
Thoarcic
Bronchogenic cyst
Mediastinal teratoma
Pericardial teratoma
Congenital pulmonary airway malformation
Causes of intrinsic airway obstruction
Laryngeal atresia
Laryngeal cyst
Laryngeal web
Laryngeal stenosi
Tracheal atresia
Tracheal stenosis
Bronchial atresia
Bronchial web

Management of the fetus with epignathus depends upon the size of the mass and the degree of airway compromise, gestational age at diagnosis, and the potential physiologic derangements caused by the tumor [4]. In many cases, the epignathus is small and does not obstruct the fetal airway and can be readily managed at the time of delivery by conventional means. In contrast, at the other end of the spectrum, epignathus can grow very rapidly and to large proportions exophytically. This leads to increased blood flow through the tumor, high output congestive heart failure, and fetal hydrops. In addition, these large fetal epignathus can create such large metabolic demands on the fetus that it induces fetal growth arrest. Both of these fetal presentations warrant considering fetal surgery in order to afford the fetus any chance of survival. Despite its large size, the mass invariably arises from a very narrow pedicle at the fetal palate. It may be approached by open fetal surgery (Fig. 2), or if there is a single systemic arterial feeding vessel (usually derived from the palatal arteries), by interstitial laser coagulation of the feeding vessel. If the fetus is at a gestational age ≥ 28 weeks gestation consideration should be given to ex utero intrapartum treatment (EXIT) to resect the mass and secure the airway prior to delivery. See section on EXIT procedure below.

Congenital Epulis

Congenital epulis is also known as Neumann's tumor or gingival granular cell tumor (GGCT) of the newborn [5, 6]. The tumor arises from the mucosa of the gingiva, most commonly from the anterior part of the maxillary or mandibular ridge. Similar to epignathus, epulis of the newborn is an oral mass (or masses), which protrudes through the mouth and can obstruct the airway (Fig. 3). Congenital epulis has a female preponderance of 8:1 and can vary in size from a few millimeters to as large as 7.5 cm. The GGCT seen in newborns has different histologic features than those originating elsewhere [7].

Epulis in the newborn has been reported to spontaneously regress after birth, suggesting that its growth is dependent on maternal hormonal milieu associated with pregnancy [8]. If sufficiently large, these tumors can compromise the upper airway, but these cases are rare. Intervention at birth may be necessary, depending on the size and likelihood of airway obstruction [4]. Epulis usually originate from a pedicled stalk and can often be easily resected before establishing an airway in the controlled environment of an EXIT-to-airway procedure [4]. If the diagnosis has not been made prenatally, and the epulis is large, establishing an airway may be difficult and may require emergency resection or tracheostomy.

Micrognathia

Severe underdevelopment of the fetal mandible can result in Pierre-Robin sequence (PRS) and is associated with microretrognathia and glossoptosis, causing airway obstruction. A small mandible characterizes PRS, and it is typically accompanied by a U-shaped cleft palate [9]. PRS occurs in 1:8,500–1:14,000 births. It can be seen alone or as part of a syndromic presentation [10]. About 40 % of PRS cases occur in isolation and 60 % present with an associated syndrome, most commonly Stickler, Nagger, and velocardiofacial syndromes (see Table 3) [10]. Arthrogryposis multiplex is a rare congenital disease characterized by nonprogressive multiple joint contractures at birth. It is also associated with micrognathia, a small mandible, and cleft palate [11].

Identifying micrognathia with or without associated polyhydramnios or cleft palate leads to the prenatal diagnosis of PRS (Fig. 4). In a fetus with PRS, the severity of micrognathia will determine the likelihood of airway obstruction.

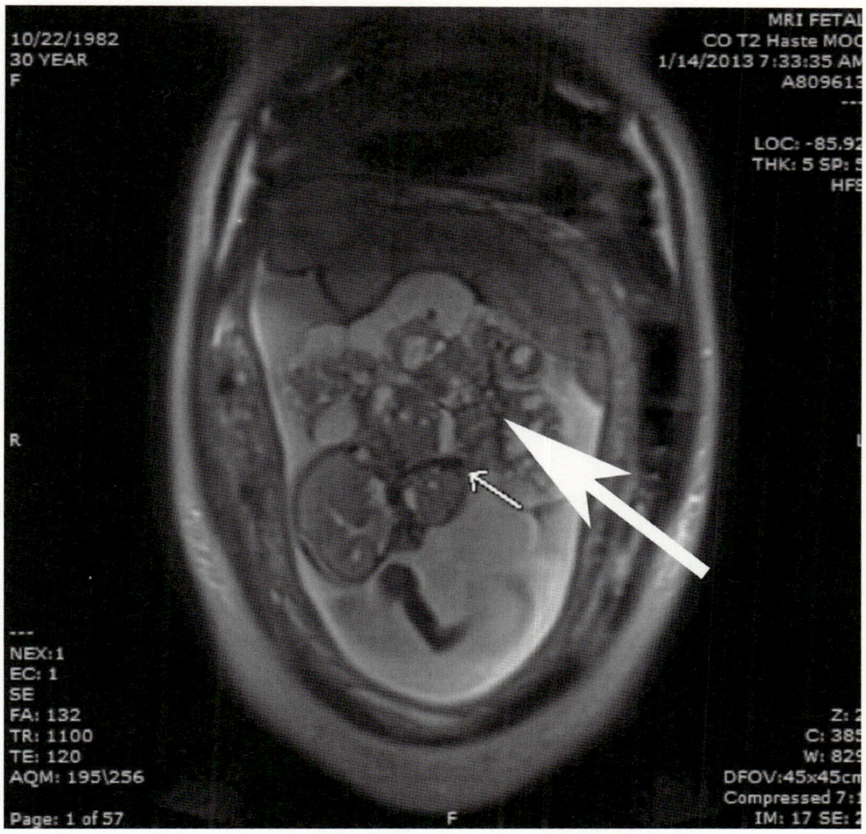

Fig. 1 Fetal MRI in sagittal section of a 25-week gestation fetus with very large exophytic epignathus with mass larger than the fetus but arising from the hard palate in the fetal mouth. The *arrow* points to a large vessel creating a "flow void" consistent with the major systemic blood supply to the epignathus

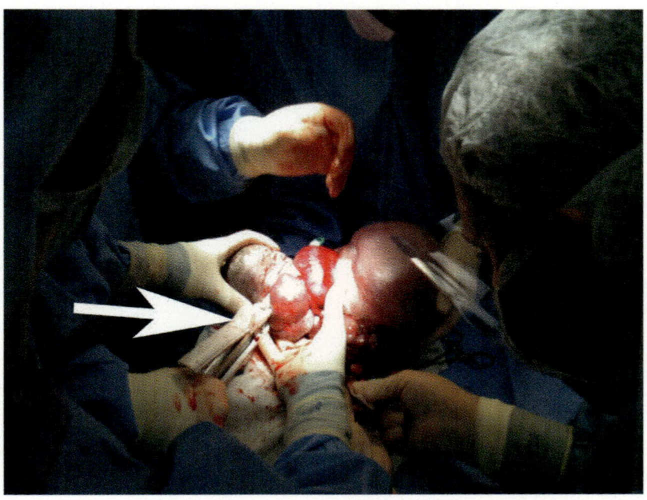

Fig. 2 Intraoperative photograph taken during EXIT-to-airway for giant epignathus. The *arrow* is pointing at a thick tissue stapling device which is being applied to take the mass off at the mouth. The size of the mass makes it near impossible to resect the mass without first debulking. This also allows the airway to be secured either by nasotracheal intubation or tracheostomy tube placement

Airway obstruction is more likely to be present if it is associated with evidence of aerodigestive obstruction, as indicated by polyhydramnios, glossoptosis, or the absence of fluid in the stomach [12]. Ultrasound is most commonly used to assess the presence and severity of micrognathia, which subjectively may be evident on sagittal images of the fetal head. The jaw index (Fig. 5), described by [47] offers a more objective measure of micrognathia and is defined by the ratio of the anterior–posterior length of the mandible divided by the biparietal diameter multiplied by 100. When the jaw index is less than the fifth percentile and is associated with evidence of aerodigestive obstruction, such as glossoptosis, polyhydramnios, or absent stomach bubble, [48] have suggested that an EXIT-to-airway is indicated. In these severe cases of micro-retrognathia a tracheostomy is necessary to establish an airway, and is most safely and effectively achieved as part of EXIT-to-airway procedure.

Cervical Lymphangioma (Vascular Malformation)

Lymphangioma is the former term still commonly used for lymphatic vascular malformations. These benign tumors can grow to large proportions and significantly compromise the fetal airway (Fig. 6). They are often present at birth and usually clinically evident as a soft tissue mass of the neck. Vascular malformations can also present in the axilla, thorax, and lower extremities, although this occurs less frequently [13]. When a vascular malformation of the neck is large and

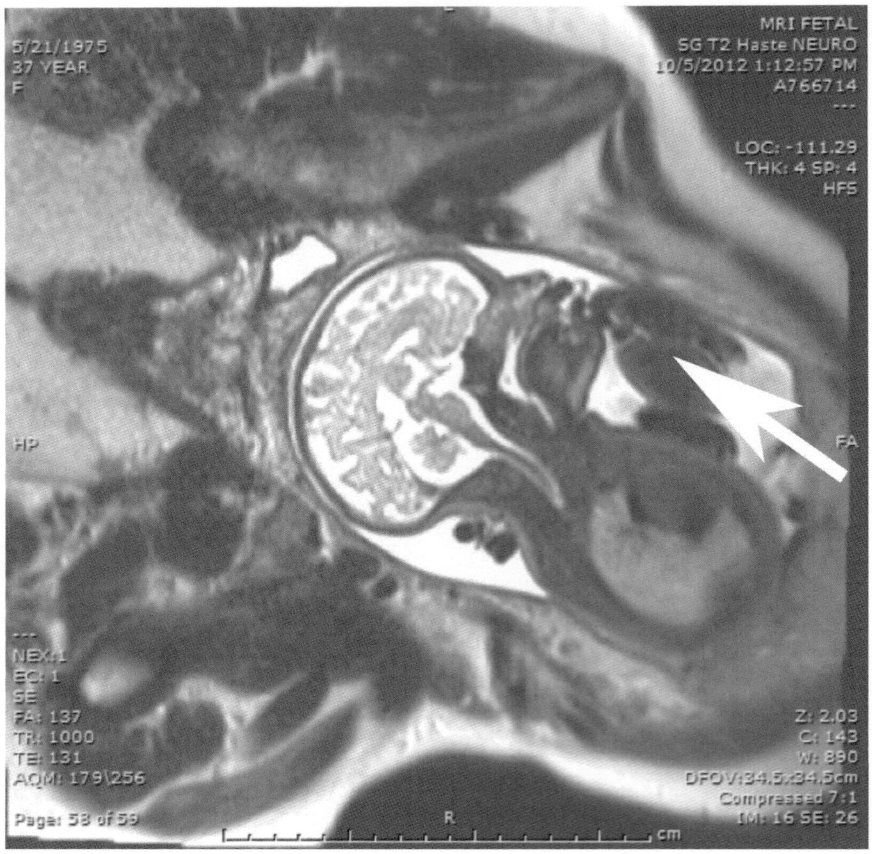

Fig. 3 Not every oral mass requires fetal MRI to demonstrate an oral mass. The image shows a fetus with an epulis, the *arrow* is pointing at the mass, which was not sufficiently large to compromise the airway and did not require the EXIT strategy

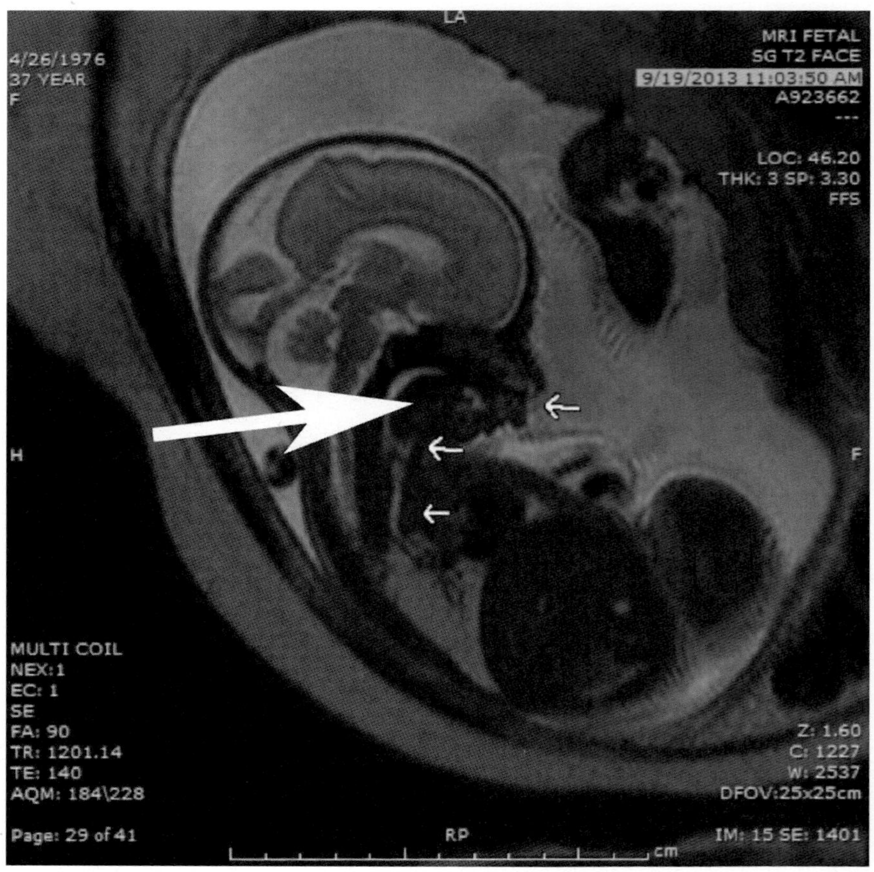

Fig. 4 Fetal MRI image in profile demonstrating severe micrognathia (*small arrows*). This fetus had micrognathia as part of Nager syndrome and had a jaw index of less than the fifth percentile with associated glossoptosis, the *arrow* is pointing at the tongue, as can be seen by the tongue displaced posteriorly. There was also absence of fluid in the stomach by ultrasound indicating inability to swallow amniotic fluid due to the glossoptosis. This is consistent with the presence of a critical airway meeting criteria for EXIT-to-airway strategy

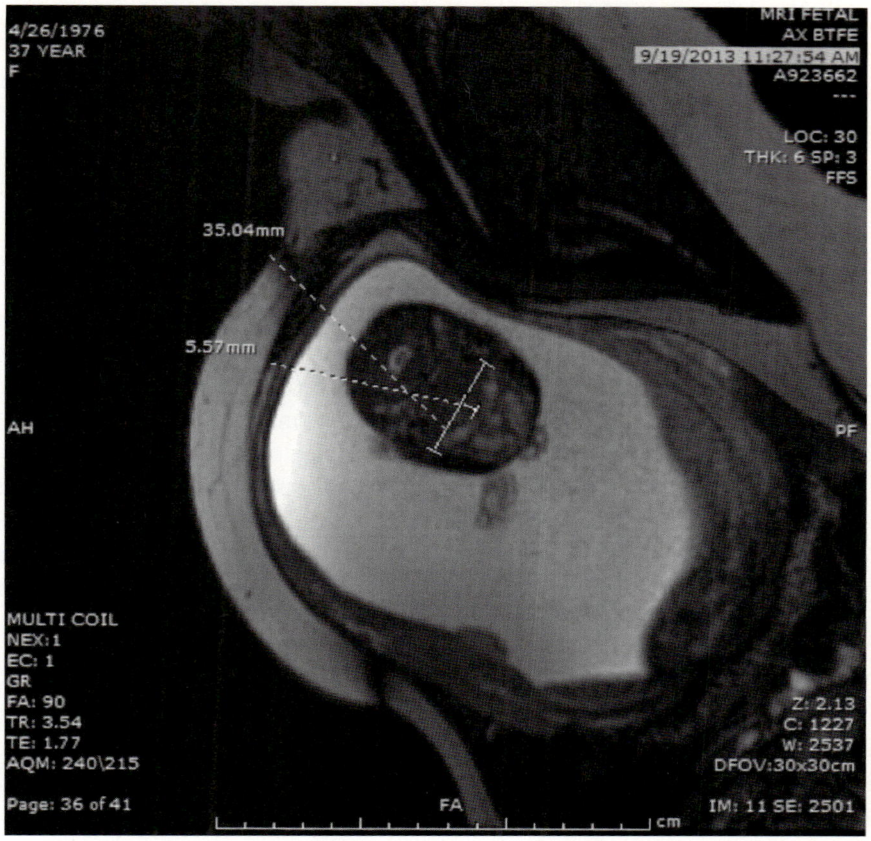

Fig. 5 MRI image demonstrating the technique to obtain the jaw index. A line is drawn from the angles of the mandible and an orthogonal line is drawn to the mentum of the mandible. This later measurement is then divided by the biparietal diameter to yield a ratio that is multiplied by 100. A value less than the fifth percentile (jaw index < 24) would indicate fetuses at highest risk for airway compromise and when associated with glossoptosis and absence of fluid in the stomach would be an indication for EXIT-to-airway

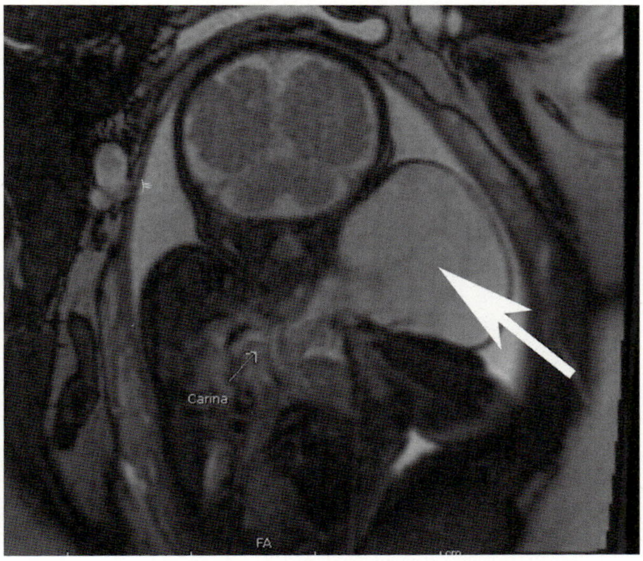

Fig. 6 The coronal section of a fetal MRI demonstrate the appearance of a large cervical lymphatic vascular malformation, an *arrow* is pointing at the malformation, it is extending from the fetal left neck and causes minimal compression of the midline airway. The mass extends into the upper left chest but does not cause significant airway compromise. This vascular malformation was not particularly vascular and would not be expected to critically compromise the airway at delivery. However, rapid enlargement post-delivery is not uncommon. Conventional delivery followed by intubation would be the safest way to prevent development of airway compromise until the vascular malformation can be fully evaluated postnatally

comprised of macrocystic components, it has commonly been referred to as a cystic hygroma.

The lymphatic system develops at the end of the fifth week of gestation as a result of six primary lymph sacs sprouting in the neck, iliac region, and retroperitoneum. One theory on the formation of lymphatic vascular malformations is that they are developmental defects secondary to sequestration of lymphatic tissue in early embryonic life [14]. Cervical lymphatic vascular malformations are believed to result from a failure of cervical lymph sacs to join the lymphatic channels. As a result, endothelial-lined spaces secrete lymph-like fluid, which leads to local distention and gradual enlargement of cysts. Over time the walls of these cysts thicken, and connective tissue septae separate large cysts [15].

The prevalence of prenatally diagnosed lymphatic vascular malformations has been estimated to be 1 in 1,775 live births [16]. The incidence may be as high as 1 in 300 among spontaneously aborted fetuses [17]. The mortality of lymphatic vascular malformations diagnosed prior to 20 weeks is high, due to associated chromosomal anomalies, syndromes, and nonimmune hydrops [18, 19]. The incidence of chromosomal abnormalities may be as high as 60 %, and additional structural abnormalities are common. Lymphatic vascular malformations diagnosed prior to 20 weeks may be associated with Turner syndrome, oligohydramnios, single vessel umbilical cord, Noonan syndrome, fetal alcohol syndrome, Fryn syndrome, trisomies 18 and 21, and hydrops fetalis [18–22]. Lymphatic vascular malformations diagnosed early in gestation are typically located in the posterior triangle of the neck and are associated with lymphangiomatosis. In contrast, isolated cervical lymphatic vascular malformations usually present in the third trimester or after birth, often following a normal ultrasound earlier in pregnancy [18]. Thus, the etiology for early and late appearing lymphatic vascular malformations is suspected to be different.

The natural history of cervical lymphatic vascular malformations is largely determined by the gestational age at the time of diagnosis. Diagnosis early in pregnancy, before 20 weeks gestation, is associated with multiple anomalies, karyotype anomalies, and a high rate of spontaneous abortion with mortality exceeding 90 %. If a lymphatic vascular malformation is diagnosed later in pregnancy, after 20 weeks gestation, no other anomalies are found on prenatal imaging, and the karyotype analysis is normal, the outcome is almost uniformly favorable, with the exception of the impact on the fetal airway. In this subset, careful evaluation of the airway is necessary to assure a safe transition to postnatal life, as this transition often results in rapid enlargement of the vascular malformation. Because most of these later gestation age lymphatic malformations arise from the lateral neck there may be impingement or displacement of the fetal airway (Fig. 6). In many cases conventional management of the airway is possible. However, even in cases in which intubation is not initially deemed necessary, it is important to consider intubation to secure the airway, because of the rapid enlargement of the vascular malformation following delivery. In cases where the size of the lymphatic vascular malformation is large, crossing the midline, and severely compromising the fetal airway, it may be difficult to distinguish from cervical teratoma, and warrants serious consideration of an EXIT-to-airway.

Cervical Teratoma

Teratomas are germ cell tumors composed of tissue foreign to their anatomical location. Teratomas contain tissue from all three germ layers and are most commonly located in the sacrococcygeal region, but can occur in the abdomen, chest, neck, or intracranially. The incidence of teratoma in newborn infants is approximately 1:40,000 [23]. Teratomas of the neck are less common, comprising somewhere between <5 and 13 % of the total number of teratomas in newborns [24, 25]. Cervical teratomas are more often diagnosed prenatally and less often contain yolk sac components [24], which are considered to be a histologic feature suggesting malignancy. There is no gender or race predilection [24]. The most common tissue present in cervical teratomas is neural tissue. However, cervical teratomas contain thyroid tissue in 30–40 % of cases—it is unknown if this represents involvement of the thyroid gland or ectopic tissue [25].

Cervical teratomas are usually bulky, often 5–12 cm in size [26]. They often extend from the mastoid process and body of the mandible to the clavicle and sternal notch, displacing the ear superiorly. Mandibular hypoplasia can occur as a result of a mass effect on the mandible, often with compression of the marginal mandibular branch of the facial nerve and associated droop of the corner of the mouth. The posterior border of cervical teratomas often reaches the anterior border of the trapezius muscle. Cervical teratomas result in polyhydramnios in about 40 % of cases, which is the result of esophageal compression by the mass [27]. An empty stomach indicates that the polyhydramnios present is secondary to a mass effect on the esophagus and can be the initial finding leading clinicians to the diagnosis of a cervical teratoma [28]. Cervical teratomas may also have calcifications within the mass and compared to lymphatic vascular malformations tend to be more solid.

Lymphatic vascular malformations and cervical teratomas can be difficult to differentiate on prenatal ultrasound [26]. Cervical teratomas usually have a well-defined border when compared to the multi-loculated, cystic appearance of a cervical lymphatic vascular malformation. Cervical teratomas are often bulkier tumors and located in the anterior neck (Fig. 7). Alpha feto protein (AFP) is not useful in differentiating lymphatic vascular malformations from cervical teratoma, as less than 30 % of cases of cervical teratomas have an elevated AFP [29].

The majority of cervical teratomas are benign, but the natural history is not well characterized. One case series suggests metastasis occurs in 14 % of cervical teratomas in the form of immature neuroglial elements in regional lymph nodes, but found that only 1.4 % of cervical teratomas had yolk sac components [24]. Many infants have remained free of disease long term after resection, even in the setting of metastatic lesions to regional lymph nodes. This could indicate that the tumor biology behaves more like a benign tumor even in the setting of regional spread of disease [30].

Cervical teratomas are predisposed to develop into large neck masses in utero, which commonly compromise the fetal airway, and often require management by EXIT-to airway at a mean gestational age of 34 weeks [31].

Intra-thoracic Extrinsic Airway Obstruction

Bronchogenic Cyst

Bronchogenic cysts can cause airway obstruction in the fetus and in the neonate immediately after birth. The degree and location of obstruction can be quite variable and this information will inform decisions in regards to delivery and intervention.

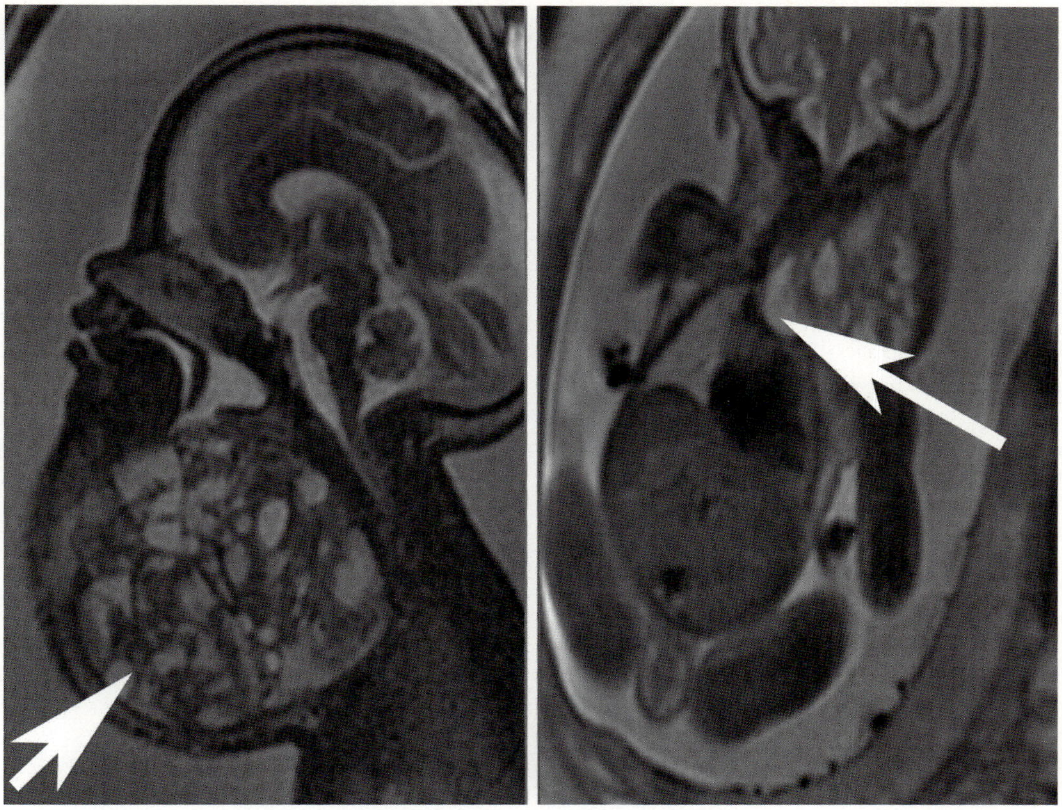

Fig. 7 The *panel* on the *left* shows a sagittal section of a fetal MRI showing a very large cervical teratoma, the *arrow* is pointing at the mass, with both cystic and solid components. Calcifications are difficult to see on MRI but were present on ultrasound. The coronal section seen in the *panel* on the *right* shows a MRI image of the same patient demonstrating extension of the teratoma into the mediastinum through the thoracic inlet, the *arrow* is pointing at the mass. This mass resulted in a SVC syndrome with swelling of scalp and facial edema. The compromise of the cervical airway and the SVC syndrome with associated venous hypertension made EXIT-to-airway through the neck unsafe. In this case a transthoracic retrograde intubation EXIT (TRI-EXIT) allowed an airway to be secured by median sternotomy during the EXIT with retrograde passage of ETT changer over which an ETT was placed and the trachea repaired

If the bronchogenic cyst arises from the trachea or one of the main-stem bronchi, it can cause complete obstruction of the airway. In utero this can cause "hyperinflation" of the lung distal to the obstruction and malacia of the airway at the area of obstruction (Fig. 8). This can result in a ball-valve effect with fluid trapping in the lung before birth and air trapping at delivery. If one of the main-stem bronchi is affected this can result in mediastinal shift and compression of the opposite lung with resultant respiratory collapse. If the trachea is affected, both lungs could be compromised due to surfactant deficiency and inability to clear secretions. Airway obstruction in utero results in less type II pneumocytes and surfactant deficiency.

An EXIT procedure may be the safest approach in the more severe cases. The EXIT procedure is described in detail below. On placental bypass, the airway can be assessed bronchoscopically, and surfactant can be directly administered into the affected area. Consideration should be given to resection of the bronchogenic cyst during an EXIT procedure if the cyst is causing significant airway compromise (Fig. 9). Alternatively, if the cyst affects the trachea only, an endotracheal tube can be inserted and positioned distal to the bronchogenic cyst. The most common location of a bronchogenic cysts is close to the carina, which may preclude simple intubation from being successful in establishing an airway.

Whenever the trachea or bronchi have been exposed to an external mass compressing the airway, the cartilaginous part of the airway may be soft and will be at risk for trachea-bronchial malacia. This may result in symptomatic trachea-bronchial malacia with hypoxic spells secondary to airway collapse. Long term, children with this condition may be prone to recurrent pneumonia and reactive airway disease.

Intra-thoracic Teratoma

Congenital intra-thoracic cystic teratoma is a rare tumor that can cause multiple fetal problems including hydrops and fetal loss because of high flow vascular connections, fast growth of the mass, and compression on intra-thoracic structures. Management of these lesions depends on the location, size, and the perceived effects that mass has on the airway. If the fetus is developing hydrops before viability, fetal surgery with resection of the mass may be the only option.

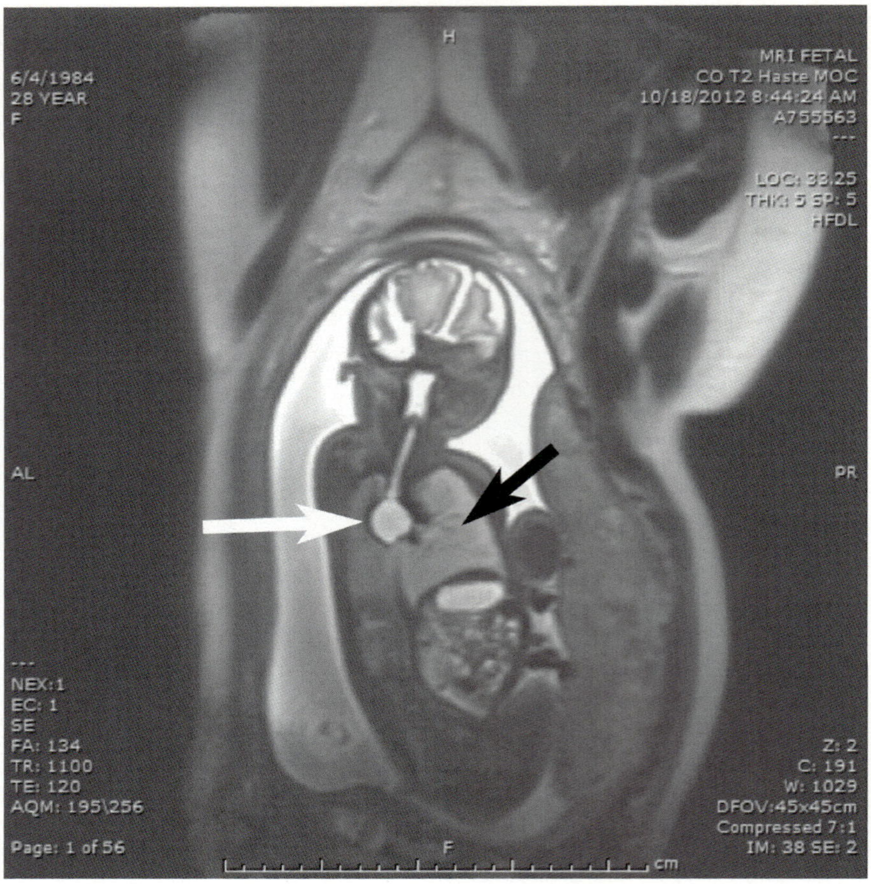

Fig. 8 Fetal MRI demonstrating a large bronchogenic cyst, a *white arrow* is pointing at the cyst, compressing the left main-stem bronchus, the *black arrow* is pointing at the "hyperinflated" left lung. By the time of delivery, the left lung was very enlarged and herniated across the midline into the right hemithorax. EXIT-to-resection was performed allowing time to perform a right thoracotomy and resect the bronchogenic cyst. In addition, bronchoscopy was performed to evaluate the compressed trachea for malacia and to administer surfactant protein selectively to the left lung, which due to obstruction was surfactant deficient from type II pneumocyte down regulation

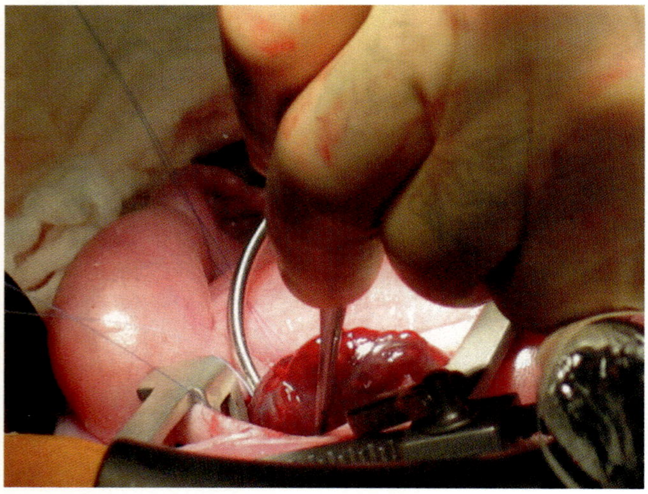

Fig. 9 Intraoperative photo demonstrating the resection of a pericardial teratoma during an EXIT procedure that due to size was compressing the distal trachea

Cystic Pulmonary Airway Malformations

Large cystic pulmonary airway malformations (CPAMs) can cause significant airway compression. CPAMs consist of a range of histologies in the spectrum of congenital adenomatoid malformations (CAMs). These lesions may be diagnosed at the time of the anomaly scan, around 20 weeks post conception, and will often grow exponentially until 28 weeks. During this time period the fetus will need close monitoring. A CAM volume ratio (volume of an ellipse divided by head circumference) (CVR) greater than 1.6 [32] has been shown to accurately predict the risk of hydrops. Recently it has been shown that maternal betamethasone treatment effectively induces growth arrest of cystic CAMs prenatally [33]. Although, it may present as a significant mass with compression of the intra-thoracic airway. In a fetus diagnosed late in pregnancy, perinatal intervention may be necessary to assure safe transition to postnatal life, if the CPAM significantly shifts the mediastinum and compresses the airway.

Evaluation and Intervention

In a fetus with intra-thoracic extrinsic airway compression, we recommend obtaining a fetal MRI to evaluate the location of the lesion, its association with the airway, and the degree of airway obstruction at the time of diagnosis. Also, fetal MRI will aid in differentiating mediastinal teratoma and pericardial teratoma. A mediastinal teratoma tend to compress mediastinal structures in an anterior–posterior direction. In contrast, a pericardial teratoma arises from the pericardium on the anterior surface of the ascending aorta, which is covered by pericardium. Mass effect of the pericardial teratoma tends to displace the heart anteriorly and inferiorly within the pericardium and may have an associated massive pericardial effusion. Because of the size of these masses the fetal airway may be compromised.

Regular ultrasound studies should be performed to evaluate for progression of the disease. Close to term around 34–36 weeks post conception a repeat fetal MRI should be obtained, sooner if the ultrasound studies are indicating progressive increase in the size of the mass or polyhydramnios predisposing to early delivery. A multidisciplinary meeting will facilitate a discussion surrounding the pros and cons of perinatal versus postnatal intervention. The intervention can range from simple aspiration of a cystic component prenatally, to EXIT-to-airway, EXIT-to-resection, or EXIT-to-ECMO. The type of intervention depends on the nature of the airway compromise.

Intrinsic Airway Obstruction in the Fetus

CHAOS is a prenatal diagnosis characterized by large echogenic lungs with flattened or inverted diaphragms, a dilated tracheobronchial tree, ascites, and other findings of non-immune hydrops, due to complete obstruction of the fetal airway and massive enlargement off the lungs [14]. It is a severe condition—no fetus diagnosed prenatally with CHAOS has survived without an intervention [34]. The airway obstruction seen in CHAOS most commonly arises from laryngeal atresia, laryngeal webs, or laryngeal cysts, or more distal obstruction from tracheal or bronchial atresia (Figs. 10 and 11). The pathophysiology of CHAOS is underscored by a combination of a complete high airway obstruction and the lung's ongoing production of fluid, at an estimated rate of 4 mL per kilogram bodyweight per day. The fluid accumulates in the tracheobronchial tree; the lungs become distended, echogenic, and diffusely enlarged [34–36].

There are three types of laryngeal atresia: type I is characterized by supra and infra-glottic atresia; type II denotes the presence of infra-glottic atresia only; and in type III the atresia is located at the glottis. Laryngeal atresia is believed to be secondary to failure of recanalization, but the exact mechanism remains unknown. Tracheal atresia is most likely a result of a failure in the development of the foregut. The foregut normally separates into the esophagus and the trachea. Most cases of tracheal atresia resulting in CHAOS are sporadic without any known risk of recurrence. However, multiple associated anomalies have been seen with laryngeal atresia (Table 2).

Fraser syndrome (cryptophtalmos–syndactyly syndrome) can present with CHAOS. This inherited syndrome is characterized by variable expression of cryptophthalmos, renal agenesis, syndactyly, abnormalities of ears and external genitalia, and laryngeal stenosis or atresia [37]. It is difficult to diagnose Fraser syndrome by ultrasound, but a previously affected pregnancy may trigger close sonographic surveillance knowing that Fraser syndrome is inherited as an autosomal recessive disorder, with 25 % of future pregnancies expected to be affected [38]. The true incidence of CHAOS is unknown; in part due to the severity of this condition, many fetuses will die undiagnosed in utero [39, 40]. With proper diagnosis and delivery planning survival is possible. The first long-term survivor with CHAOS was described by Crombleholme and coworkers in 2000, the fetus was delivered via EXIT and an airway was established via tracheostomy prior to clamping the umbilical cord [41].

CHAOS does not develop in a fetus with tracheal atresia and a fistula to the esophagus, in these cases, the diagnosis of tracheal atresia may go unnoticed until delivery. As a result, the newborn infant may need to undergo emergency tracheostomy to establish an airway [42].

Bilateral cystic adenomatoid malformation is the most common diagnosis that can be mistaken for the findings of CHAOS on prenatal imaging. Bilateral CCAM is even less common than intrinsic high airway obstruction [39] and it is important to thoroughly evaluate a fetus with hydrops and a diagnosis of bilateral CCAM to specifically exclude the diagnosis of CHAOS.

In a fetus with bilateral CCAMs a compressed rim of normal lung can usually be appreciated on fetal imaging. The typical ultrasound findings in CHAOS: uniformly echogenic lungs, flattened or inverted diaphragms, a compressed mediastinum, with a dilated trachea and main-stem bronchus can help differentiate CHAOS from bilateral CCAM.

Diagnosis of Fetal Airway Obstruction

Determining the cause of fetal airway obstruction is important when considering the need for intervention, planning delivery, and counseling family members. Fetal imaging can differentiate between intrinsic and extrinsic airway obstruction and is helpful in determining the severity of airway obstruction. A thorough anatomy scan is essential as many fetuses with congenital airway obstruction will have one or more associated anomalies. An ultra-fast fetal MRI can provide significant information to augment the ultrasound examination. An amniocentesis for karyotype analysis is recommended for all pregnancies with signs of airway obstruction and associated anomalies, especially if fetal intervention is considered. Similarly, fetal echocardiogram is essential to rule out structural heart disease and exclude high output congestive heart failure.

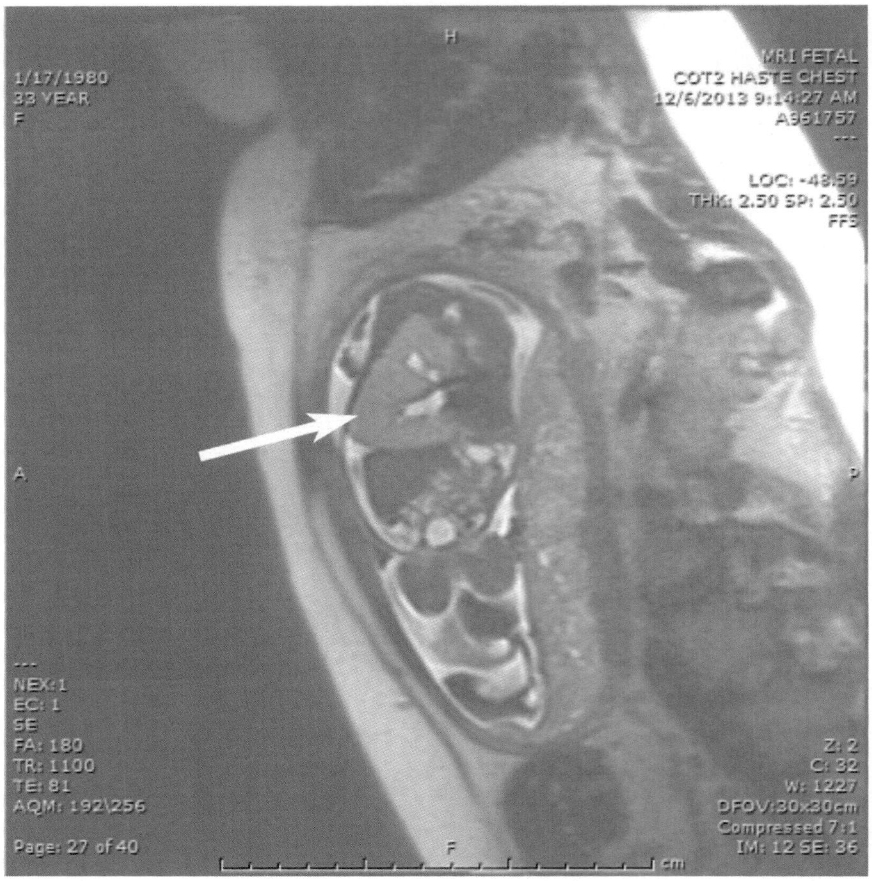

Fig. 10 A coronal fetal MRI image of a fetus with right main-stem bronchial atresia and resulting unilateral CHAOS. The entire right lung is signal intense, an *arrow* is pointing at it, this is due to "hyperinflation" with a dilated right bronchus extending from the bronchus intermedius to the right middle, lower, and upper lobar bronchi. The massive enlargement of the right lung has shifted the medistinum, depressed the ipsilateral diaphragm, and causes ascites

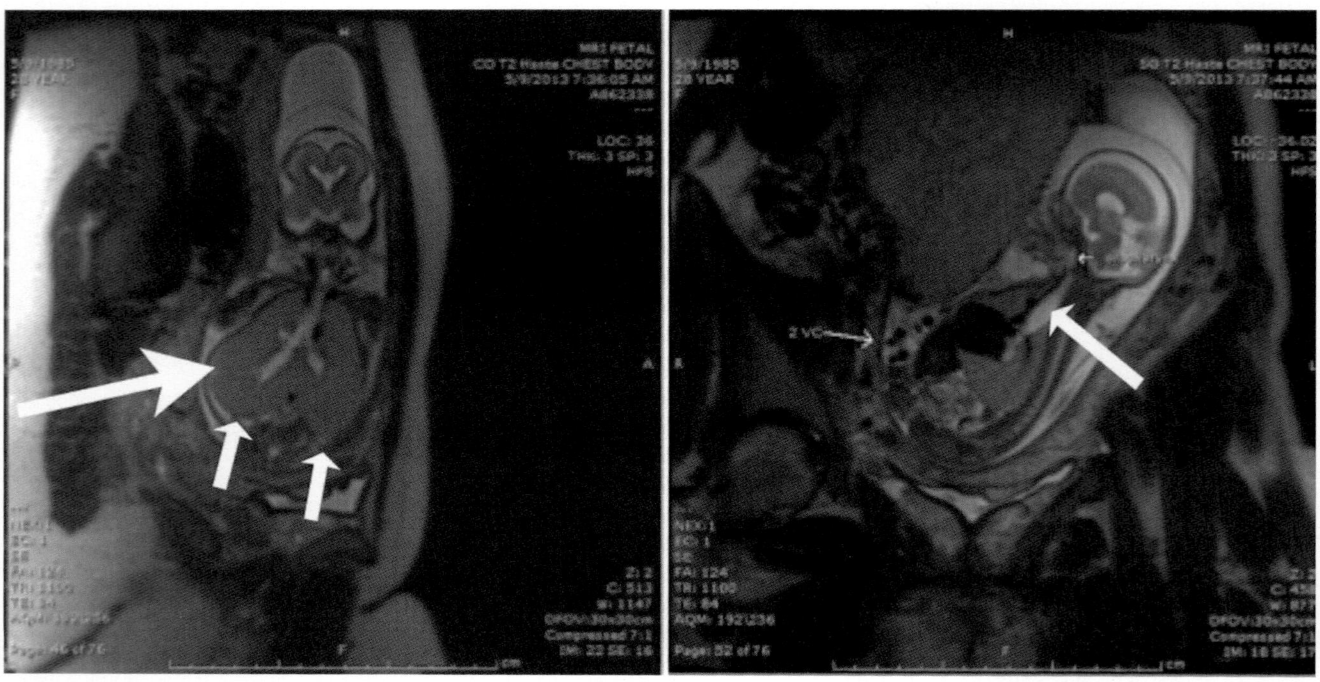

Fig. 11 Fetal MRI images in coronal and sagittal planes demonstrating the characteristic features of CHAOS due to complete obstruction of the larynx due to a laryngeal web; the *large arrow* is pointing at the very enlarged single intense lungs, the *small arrows* are pointing at the inverted diaphragms, narrow compressed heart, and on the *right panel* the *black arrow* is pointing at the dilated trachea and bronchi with severe ascites

Table 2 Anomalies associated with CHAOS

Hydrocephalus
Vertebral anomalies
Absent radius
Bronchotracheal fistula
Esophageal atresia
Genitourinary anomalies
Uterine anomalies
Imperforate anus
Cardiac anomalies
Anophthalmia
Fraser syndrome (syndactyly, cryptophthalmos)

Ultrasound and Differential Diagnosis

The list of conditions that can cause extrinsic fetal airway obstruction is extensive (Table 1). That the management of each condition may be quite different underscores the importance of an accurate prenatal diagnosis. As an example, the presence of a skull or vertebral column defect may suggest the presence of an encephalocele, especially in the setting of hydrocephalus. In contrast, congenital goiter is most commonly seen in mothers taking propylthiouracil for hyperthyroidism. A fetal goiter is homogenous in its echogenicity and is usually symmetrical. Branchial cleft cysts are unilateral and appear as unilocular anterolateral cysts. A lymphangioma of the neck can be identified by fluid filled spaces with fine septations. If it is located in the posterior triangle of the neck, a dense midline posterior septum can often be identified. This is the equivalent of the nuchal ligament. Cysts separated by septae are an important sonographic finding to differentiate a posterior lymphatic malformation from nuchal edema. If there are solid components and there is Doppler evidence of blood flow, a diagnosis of cervical teratoma should be explored. If the diagnosis of a lymphatic malformation of the neck is made, signs of non-immune hydrops should be sought.

Cervical teratomas are typically asymmetrical, unilateral, and well demarcated. Most are multi-loculated, irregular masses with solid and cystic components. About 50 % have calcifications, a pathognomonic finding for a teratoma of the neck [43].

The sonographic findings in a fetus with CHAOS are characterized by extreme distention of the lungs. The lungs appear echogenic and diffusely enlarged, the diaphragm is flat or inverted into the abdomen. The mediastinal structures are compressed, the axis of the heart is altered, and the heart chambers are small because of insufficient filling. The tracheobronchial tree is dilated up to the level of the obstruction, at the level of the trachea or the larynx. In CHAOS there are also findings of non-immune hydrops, the most prominent finding is fetal ascites.

Fetal MRI

The detection of a high-grade airway obstruction in the fetus warrants further investigation with ultra-fast fetal MRI. As reported by Crombleholme et al., fetal MRI provides superior image resolution and adds important information about the level of airway compression when compared to ultrasound [44]. This information can be used to predict which patients are at risk of significant airway compromise and will benefit from undergoing an EXIT-to-airway procedure. Fetal MRI images are improving and the current image resolution is superior to what it was just a few years ago. It is therefore beneficial to also obtain fetal MRI imaging in fetuses with intrinsic obstruction and CHAOS. MRI can also aid in the diagnosis and planning of fetuses with micrognathia. The jaw index can be accurately calculated from MRI images in cases where ultrasound isn't able to do so.

Ex Utero Intrapartum Treatment

It is important to understand how an EXIT procedure is different from a Cesarean section. The principles of performing a safe EXIT and the pitfalls that can occur during this complex procedure have been described in detail elsewhere [45]. Ideally mothers carrying a fetus diagnosed with fetal airway obstruction should be referred to a center with significant experience with EXIT procedures. A multidisciplinary team of experienced anesthesiologists, fetal/pediatric surgeons, neonatologists, maternal fetal medicine specialists, and experienced operating room nurses is required. The operating room environment should ideally have the ability to conduct two operations simultaneously either in the same operating or in two adjacent operating rooms, as well as having equipment for neonatal resuscitation. For EXIT-to-airway procedures, a complete set of airway equipment is necessary, a rigid infant laryngoscope handle, numbers 1 and 2 Miller blades, flexible bronchoscope, rigid ventilating bronchoscopes sizes 2.5 and 3.0, armored endotracheal tubes, tracheostomy tubes, laryngeal mask airways, endotracheal tube extenders for retrograde intubation, and all the instruments needed to perform a tracheostomy or resect a teratoma on a newborn infant must be present. A sterile Mapleson circuit needs to be available on the field for ventilation of the fetus as soon as the airway has been established and allows transition from placental support as uterine tone can then be restored.

Maternal monitoring includes pulse oximetry, electrocardiogram, invasive arterial blood pressure line, urine output, core body temperature, and peripheral nerve stimulation. The EXIT procedure is performed under deep maternal general anesthesia, a necessity to achieve adequate uterine relaxation in order to preserve uteroplacental gas exchange. Intravenous anesthesia is provided during the first part of the operation, until the uterus is exposed, then anesthesia is converted to inhaled anesthesia to induce uterine relaxation [46]. This is done to minimize the duration of exposure to potentially harmful effects of high concentrations of inhaled anesthesia gases on the fetal myocardial function. Maternal hypotension is managed with an alpha-1 agonist as a continuous infusion.

As soon as the uterus is exposed intraoperative sterile sonography is used to map the placental edge. When the uterus is fully relaxed, the hysterotomy is created in an area well away from the placenta, preferably in the lower uterine segment. A hemostatic uterine stapling device (US Surgical, Norwalk, CT), incorporating membranes and full thickness uterine wall, is used to create the hysterotomy. During the procedure, body temperature lactated, Ringer solution is infused via level I device into the uterus to prevent cord compression. The fetal head, upper torso, and arms are gently exteriorized; fetal anesthesia is supplemented by a single intramuscular injection of a muscle relaxant, atropine, and fentanyl. A pulse oximeter and an intravenous catheter are placed on the upper extremity. The fetus is continuously monitored by intraoperative transthoracic echocardiography. Once the fetal head is exposed the airway is evaluated.

The algorithm for airway management depends on the underlying diagnosis. For example, in severe micrognathia, there is little to be gained from evaluation of the airway during the EXIT procedure and we recommend proceeding directly to formal tracheostomy. Conversely, in cases of external compression such as cervical teratoma or lymphatic vascular malformation, we would first evaluate the prospect of obtaining an airway by orotracheal intubation, either directly or over a bronchoscope (Fig. 12). If orotracheal intubation cannot be achieved we would next expose the trachea in the neck for retrograde intubation over an ET tube changer. Lastly, if necessary to secure the airway, the cervical mass can be resected while on placental support. In cases in which the cervical teratoma extends into the mediastinum with associated SVC syndrome, a median sternotomy for transthoracic retrograde intubation (TRI-EXIT procedure) can be performed to allow control of the trachea in the chest and avoid massive hemorrhage from venous hypertension.

In cases with intrinsic obstruction of the airway and CHAOS we start with direct laryngoscopy to evaluate laryngeal involvement and exclude either laryngeal cyst or web, which may respond to incision or excision and simple intubation. If the cause of CHAOS is found to be more extensive, as in laryngeal atresia or tracheal atresia, then the attention can turn to formal tracheostomy.

In all cases the operative team performing the EXIT should be prepared for any and all eventualities, ranging from simple orotracheal intubation, flexible or rigid bronchoscopy, to surgical control of the cervical or mediastinal trachea for retrograde intubation, or formal tracheostomy. As soon as the umbilical cord is clamped, oxytocin (50u) is administered intravenously to induce uterine contractions; the anesthesia is also at that point switched back to primarily intravenous agents.

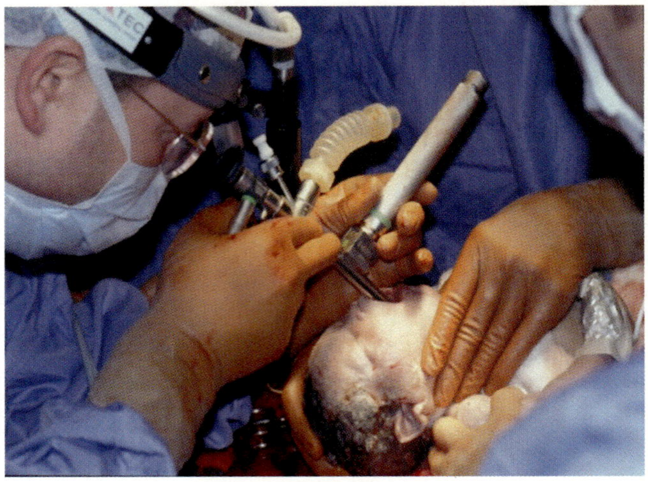

Fig. 12 An intraoperative photograph demonstrating an EXIT-to-airway procedure, the fetus is undergoing continuous monitoring by fetal echocardiogram, and pulse oximetry. IV access will be obtained for crystalloid, blood products, and inotropic agents if needed. The first priority of any EXIT is securing the airway

Postnatal Management

After an airway has been established, the neonate is hand ventilated until the uterine tone is restored, the umbilical cord is then clamped and the baby passed to the neonatologists for evaluation and resuscitation. It is important to secure endotracheal tubes or tracheostomy tubes well, as it may be difficult or impossible to reestablish an airway in a timely fashion if the airway is lost. This is usually accomplished during the EXIT procedure by direct suturing of the ETT to the maxillary plate. We do not transport the infant for additional imaging until the airway is no longer considered critical either because the cervical mass has been resected or the tracheostomy is more than 7 days old.

In cervical masses such as lymphatic vascular malformations and particularly cervical teratomas, hyperextension of the neck pulls the trachea up into the neck, which in turn pulls the lungs into the apices of the chest cavity. This can cause pulmonary hypertension and impair ventilation and oxygenation by either conventional ventilation or even high frequency oscillatory ventilation. It can only be relieved by resection of the mass. In addition, cervical teratoma and some vascular malformations can also be associated with significant consumptive coagulopathies, which may complicate any surgical procedures or airway management.

Small lymphatic vascular malformations can often be managed expectantly if the airway does not appear to be compromised. Since many of these lesions are macrocystic, sclerotherapy should be considered. Cervical teratomas should be resected as soon as the neonate is stable enough to go to the operating room.

Conclusion

The causes for airway obstruction in the fetus are numerous, but can be usefully categorized into two groups, intrinsic and extrinsic to the airway. Accurate diagnosis is imperative to appropriately plan the timing and type of intervention needed. Fetal imaging, primarily fetal ultrasound and MRI have improved diagnosis, monitoring of disease progression throughout pregnancy, and interventional planning. EXIT requires a highly trained multidisciplinary team and can greatly alter the course of previously fatal diagnosis.

References

1. Demajumdar R, Bhat N. Epignathus: a germ-cell tumour presenting as neonatal respiratory distress. Int J Pediatr Otorhinolaryngol. 1999;47:87–90.
2. Vandenhaute B, Leteurtre E, Lecomte-Houcke M, et al. Epignathus teratoma: report of three cases with a review of literature. Cleft Palate Craniofac J. 2000;37:83–91.
3. Nagy GR, Neducsin BP, Lazar L, et al. Early prenatal detection of a fast-growing fetal epignathus. J Obstet Gynaecol Res. 2012;38: 1328–30.
4. Laje P, Howell LJ, Johnson MP, et al. Perinatal management of congenital oropharyngeal tumors: the ex utero intrapartum treatment (EXIT) approach. J Pediatr Surg. 2013;48:2005–10.
5. Neumann E. Ein fall von congaliter epulis. Arch Helik. 1871;12:189.
6. Zuker RM, Buenecha R. Congenital epulis: review of literature and a case report. J Oral Maxillofac Surg. 1993;51:1040–3.
7. Lack EE, Perez-Atayde AR, McGill TJ, Vawter GF. Gingival granular cell tumor of the newborn (congenital "epulis"): ultrastructural observations relating to histogenesis. Hum Pathol. 1982;13:686–9.
8. Jenkins HR, Hill CM. Spontaneous regression of epulis of the newborn. Arch Dis Child. 1989;64:145–7.
9. Gangopadhyay N, Mendonca DA, Woo AS. Pierre Robin sequence. Semin Plast Surg. 2012;26:76–82.
10. Izumi K, Konczal L, Mitchell AL, et al. Underlying genetic diagnosis of Pierre Robin sequence: retrospective chart review at two children's hospitals and a systemic literature review. J Pediatr. 2011; 160:645–50.
11. Epstein JB, Wittenberg GJ. Maxillofacial manifestations and management of arthrogryposis: literature review and case report. J Oral Maxillofac Surg. 1987;45:274–9.
12. Hsieh YY, Chang CC, Tsai HD, et al. The prenatal diagnosis of Pierre-Robin sequence. Prenat Diagn. 1999;19:567–9.
13. Isaacs H. Neoplasms in infants: a report of 265 cases. Pathol Annu. 1983;18:165–71.
14. Goetsch E. Hygroma colli cysticum and hygroma axillae. Arch Surg. 1936;36:394–401.
15. Chervenak FA, Isaacson G, Blakemore KJ, et al. Fetal cystic hygroma: causes and natural history. N Engl J Med. 1983;309:822–6.
16. Howarth ES, Draper ES, Budd JL, et al. Population-based study of the outcome following the prenatal diagnosis of cystic hygroma. Prenat Diagn. 2005;25:286–91.
17. Byrne J, Blanc WA, Warburton D, et al. The significance of cystic hygroma in fetuses. Hum Pathol. 1984;15:61–7.
18. Langer JC, Fitzgerald PG, Desa D, et al. Cervical cystic hygroma in the fetus: clinical spectrum and outcome. J Pediatr Surg. 1990;25:58–61.
19. Welborn JL, Timm NS. Trisomy 21 and cystic hygroma in early gestational age fetuses. Am J Perinatol. 1994;11:19–25.
20. Golden WL, Schneider BF, Gustashaw KM, et al. Prenatal diagnosis of Turner syndrome using cells cultured from cystic hygroma in two pregnancies with normal maternal serum alpha fetoprotein. Prenat Diagn. 1989;9:683–9.
21. Zarabi M, Mieckowski GC, Maser J. Cystic hygroma associated with Noonan's syndrome. J Clin Ultrasound. 1983;11:398–404.
22. Graham JM, Stephens TD, Shepard TH. Nuchal cystic hygroma in a fetus with presumed Robert's syndrome. Am J Med Genet. 1983;15:163–7.
23. Forrester MB, Merz RD. Descriptive epidemiology of teratoma in infants, Hawaii, 1986-2001. Paediatr Perinat Epidemiol. 2006;20:54–8.
24. Isaacs H. Perinatal (fetal and neonatal) germ cell tumors. J Pediatr Surg. 2004;39:1003–13.
25. Jordan RB, Gauderer MWL. Cervical teratomas. An analysis, literature review and proposed classification. J Pediatr Surg. 1988; 23:583–91.
26. Batsakis JG, Littler ER, Oberman HA. Teratomas of the neck. Arch Otolaryngol. 1964;79:619–24.
27. Lloyd JR, Clatworthy HW. Hydramnios as an aid to the early diagnosis of congenital obstruction of the alimentary tract: a study of the maternal and fetal factors. Pediatrics. 1958;21:903–9.
28. Rosenfeld CR, Coln CD, Duenhoelter JH. Fetal cervical teratomas as a cause of polyhydramnios. Pediatrics. 1979;64:174–9.
29. Schoenfeld A, Ovadia J, Edelstein T, Liban E. Malignant cervical teratoma of the fetus. Acta Obstet Gynecol Scand. 1982;61:7–12.
30. Gundry SR, Wesley JR, Klein MD, et al. Cervical teratomas in the newborn. J Pediatr Surg. 1983;181:382–6.
31. Liechty KW, et al. Intrapartum airway management for giant fetal neck masses: the EXIT (ex utero intrapartum treatment) procedure. Am J Obstet Gynecol. 1997;177:870–4.
32. Crombleholme TM, et al. Cystic adenomatoid malformation volume ratio predicts outcome in prenatally diagnosed cystic adenomatoid malformation of the lung. J Pediatr Surg. 2002;37:331–8.
33. Peranteau WH, et al. Effect of maternal betamethasone administration on prenatal congenital cystic adematoid malformation growth and fetal surgery. Fetal Diagn Ther. 2007;22:365–71.
34. Hedrick MH, Martinez-Ferro M, Filly RA, et al. Congenital high airway obstruction syndrome (CHAOS): a potential for perinatal intervention. J Pediatr Surg. 1994;29:271–4.
35. Richards DS, Yancey MK, Duff P, Stieg FH. The perinatal management of severe laryngeal stenosis. Obstet Gynecol. 1992;80:537–40.
36. Weston MJ, Porter HJ, Berry PJ, Andrews HS. Ultrasonographic prenatal diagnosis of upper respiratory tract atresia. J Ultrasound Med. 1992;11:673–5.
37. Schauer GM, Dunn LK, Godmilow L, et al. Prenatal diagnosis of Fraser syndrome at 18.5 weeks' gestation, with autopsy findings at 19 weeks. Am J Med Genet. 1990;37:583–91.
38. Fraser GR. Our genetic load: a review of some aspects of genetic variation. Ann Hum Genet. 1962;25:387–415.
39. Fang SH, Ocejo R, Sin M, et al. Congenital laryngeal atresia. Arch Dis Child. 1989;143:625–7.
40. IL S, Bain AD. Congenital atresia of the larynx: a report of nine cases. Ann Otol Rhinol Laryngol. 1965;74:338–49.

41. Crombleholme TM, Sylvester K, Flake AW, Adzick NS. Salvage of a fetus with congenital high airway obstruction syndrome by ex utero intrapartum treatment (EXIT) procedure. Fetal Diagn Ther. 2000;15:280–2.
42. Okuyama H, Kubota A, Kawahara H, et al. Congenital laryngeal atresia associated with esophageal atresia and tracheoesophageal fistula: a case of long-term survival. J Pediatr Surg. 2006;41:e29–31.
43. Gundry SR, Wesley JR, Klein MD, et al. Cervical teratomas in the newborn. J Pediatr Surg. 1983;18:382–6.
44. Crombleholme TM, Albanese C. The fetus with airway obstruction. In: Harrison MR, Evans MI, Adzick NS, Holzgreve W, editors. The unborn patient: the art and science of fetal therapy. 3rd ed. Philadelphia: WB Saunders; 2000. p. 357–71.
45. Laje P, Johnson MP, Howell LJ, et al. Ex utero intrapartum treatment in the management of giant cervical teratoma. J Pediatr Surg. 2012;47:1208–16.
46. Boat A, Mahmoud M, Michelfelder EC, et al. Supplementing desflurane with intravenous anesthesia reduces fetal cardiac dysfunction during open fetal surgery. Paediatr Anaesth. 2010;20:748–56.
47. Paladini D, Morra T, Teodoro A, Lamberti A, Tremolaterra F, Martinelli P. Objective diagnosis of micrognathia in the fetus: the jaw index. Obstet Gynecol. 1999;93(3):382–6.
48. Morris LM, Lim FY, Elluru RG, Hopkin RJ, Jaekle RK, Polzin WJ, Crombleholme TM. Severe micrognathia: indications for EXIT-to-airway. Fetal Diagn Ther. 2009;26(3):162–6. doi:10.1159/000240162. Epub 2009 Sep 18.

Operative Surgical Management of Fetuses with CHAOS: Management at Delivery

Pablo Laje and Holly L. Hedrick

Introduction

Airway obstruction at delivery is associated with high mortality and anoxic brain injury. The perinatal management of fetuses with airway obstruction changed when prenatal diagnosis became available. Holinger et al. reported in 1985 the first case in which special airway resources were preemptively mobilized to the delivery room for the cesarean delivery of a fetus with a prenatally diagnosed cervical teratoma. The airway was established immediately after delivery via direct laryngoscopy and bronchoscopy [1]. The concept of keeping the fetus under placental support while accessing an obstructed airway was first reported by Kelly et al. in 1990 (the fetus was intubated via direct laryngoscopy before clamping the umbilical cord), and a few months later, Levine et al. reported the first case of a tracheostomy performed while the fetus was under placental support. No intervention was done on the maternal side in either of those cases to prevent uterine contractions, and the fetuses were completely delivered out of the uterus before the airway manipulation [2, 3]. The idea continued to evolve until 1996 when a team at the University of California, San Francisco, reported a standardized procedure for the reversal of the tracheal occlusion in patients with prenatally treated congenital diaphragmatic hernia and named it "Ex Utero Intrapartum Treatment" or "EXIT," for short [4]. The EXIT procedure is now the optimal delivery strategy for fetuses with congenital airway obstruction because it allows access to the fetal airway in an elective, controlled, and secure manner while the fetus is still under placental support (which is only interrupted after adequate ventilation has been established). It was originally developed for the reversal of the tracheal occlusion in fetuses with congenital diaphragmatic hernia treated prenatally, but the indications for an EXIT have expanded over time to include entities as diverse as large lung malformations, conjoined twins, thoracic teratomas, and congenital high airway obstruction syndrome (Fig. 1) [5–7]. Although conceptually simple, the success of an EXIT procedure relies on extensive preoperative planning and the availability of a highly skilled multidisciplinary team.

Prenatal Evaluation

The prenatal identification of a fetus with potential airway obstruction warrants a comprehensive anatomical evaluation to determine the need for a special delivery strategy. Early diagnosis is essential so that the mother can be referred to a center with EXIT and fetal surgery capabilities. The prenatal evaluation not only includes a number of imaging studies (fetal ultrasound, 3D ultrasound, fetal echocardiography, fetal MRI) but also an amniocentesis for fetal karyotype (Fig. 2). Additional genetic studies may be warranted depending on the presence of associated findings. Care must be taken to assess the placenta, as abnormal placentation such as placenta previa or evidence of subchorionic hemorrhage might increase the risk of intraoperative complications (see chapter on "Prenatal Assessment and Perinatal Management of Suspected Airway Compromise in the Fetus and Neonate" for full description).

Multidisciplinary Team and Equipment

In centers prepared to handle post-neonatal airway obstruction, a multidisciplinary team that is familiar with the equipment and surroundings must be present. This team includes anesthesiologists, pediatric surgeons, neonatologists, maternal fetal medicine specialists, and a dedicated

P. Laje, M.D. (✉) • H.L. Hedrick, M.D.
Division of General, Fetal and Thoracic Surgery, The Children's Hospital of Philadelphia, Philadelphia, PA, USA

University of Pennsylvania, Perelman School of Medicine, Philadelphia, PA, USA
e-mail: LAJE@email.chop.edu

J. Lioy and S.E. Sobol (eds.), *Disorders of the Neonatal Airway: Fundamentals for Practice*, DOI 10.1007/978-1-4939-1610-8_18, © Springer Science+Business Media New York 2015

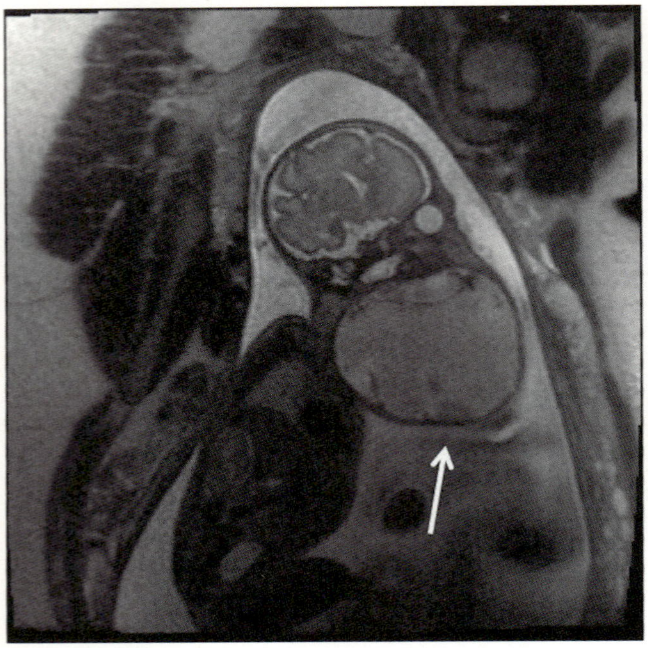

Fig. 1 27-week gestation fetus with a *white arrow* pointing toward a large solid-cystic cervical mass

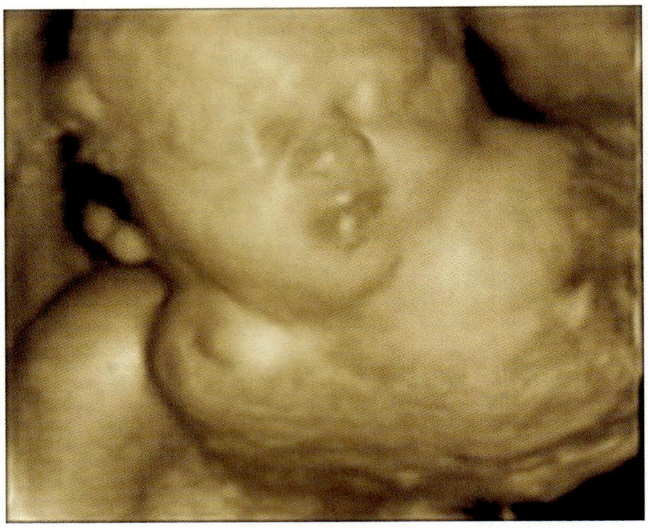

Fig. 2 Three-dimensional ultrasound view of a fetus with large cervical teratomas

Fig. 3 Multidisciplinary team at the operating table

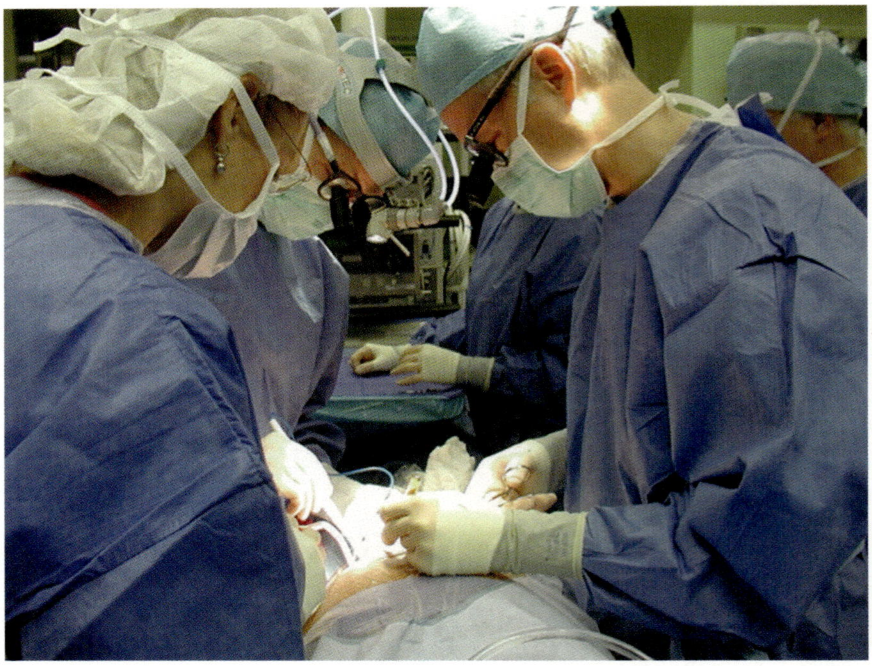

group of diverse nursing staff. Simulation and comprehensive preoperative planning are essential to successfully perform an EXIT procedure and likely surgical resection thereafter (Fig. 3 and Table 1). Our approach includes a mandatory team meeting 1–2 days before the surgery in which the particular case is extensively analyzed; the planned procedure is reviewed step by step; parents are counseled one additional time with all team members present; and informed consent is obtained. A variety of airway equipment needs to be available including a rigid infant-type laryngoscope handle, a set of number 0, 1, and 2 straight Miller blades, a set of rigid ventilating bronchoscopes sizes 2.5 and 3.0, a set of wire-reinforced cuffless endotracheal tubes (ETTs) and tracheostomy tubes, and all surgical instruments required for a neonatal tracheostomy (Fig. 4). In addition, a sterile Mapleson circuit with a manometer and a 1-L bag must be ready on the operating table to manually ventilate the fetus once the airway has been established. In our institution

Table 1 Multidisciplinary teams required for each stage of the EXIT procedure

Preoperative team	Intraoperative team	Postoperative team
High risk obstetrician	High risk obstetrician	Neonatologist
Pediatric surgeon	Pediatric surgeon	Pediatric surgeon
Radiologist	Anesthesiologist	Nurse practitioners
Anesthesiologist	Fetal cardiologist	Nurses
Fetal cardiologist	Scrub nurses	Radiologist
Social worker	Circulating nurses	Standby OR team
Coordinator	Standby ECMO team	Standby ECMO team

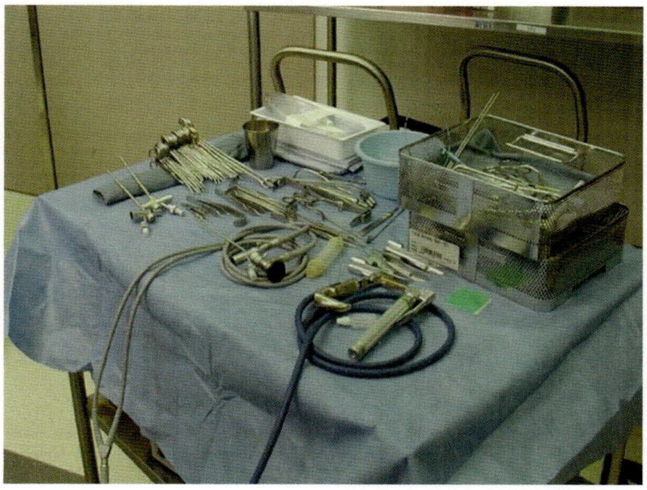

Fig. 4 A separate table with all the airway equipment must be available at the time of the surgery

our operating area includes two large operating rooms (one for the EXIT and one for any potential immediate post-EXIT procedures on the newborn) connected by a neonatal resuscitation room.

Timing of Delivery

Ideally, fetuses with airway obstruction should reach term and be delivered electively. Depending on the cause of the airway obstruction and the effects on the fetal health, this may not be possible. For instance, fetuses with large cervical tumors that compress the airway can also suffer compression of the pharynx/esophagus, which can lead to polyhydramnios and preterm labor. When a fetus with airway obstruction develops signs of impending labor (i.e., severe recurrent polyhydramnios, shortened cervix), it is better to perform an elective preterm EXIT at a time that all the required personnel is available, than waiting for the fetus to reach term at the risk of developing labor at a time that not all the resources necessary for an EXIT are readily available. In a previously large series of fetuses with cervical teratomas, only 23 % of the fetuses reached term [8].

Surgical Technique: The EXIT Procedure

The EXIT procedure must be performed under deep general anesthesia because the general anesthetic drugs are the strongest uterine relaxants known to date. An epidural catheter is placed to facilitate maternal postoperative pain management. Intraoperative maternal monitoring includes pulse oximetry, continuous electrocardiogram, invasive arterial blood pressure monitoring (radial artery angiocatheter), urinary output via a bladder catheter, core body temperature, and peripheral nerve stimulation. The combination of drugs used for induction and maintenance of anesthesia during an EXIT procedure can vary, but the principle of deep inhalational anesthesia must not change. Generally, induction is done with intravenous propofol (2 mg/kg) immediately followed by a muscle relaxant (succinylcholine, 1 mg/kg) for a rapid endotracheal intubation. Maintenance is done with desflurane, titrated between 5 and 10 % according to the uterine tone evaluated by palpation during the operation. Muscle relaxation is maintained with vecuronium (0.1 mg/kg/dose, repeated as needed). The deep maternal anesthesia required to facilitate uterine relaxation can induce maternal hypotension, which is treated with an alpha-1-adrenergic agonist (phenylephrine) as a continuous infusion (10–200 μg/min) throughout the operation to maintain the maternal mean arterial pressure above 60 mmHg. Dopamine can be added as needed, as a continuous infusion. As soon as the procedure is completed and the umbilical cord is clamped, oxytocin (50 U) is given intravenously to the mother to induce uterine contraction. Other drugs can be used if necessary, like methylergonovine and carboprost or misoprostol.

Uterine Exposure

A wide transverse laparotomy halfway between the symphysis pubis and umbilicus is the standard incision for all EXIT procedures because it provides excellent access to the anterior uterine wall, has a low dehiscence rate, and is cosmetically better than a midline laparotomy. Flaps of skin and subcutaneous tissue are raised superiorly and inferiorly. The fascia is divided in the midline from the symphysis pubis to the umbilicus. A Turner-Warwick retractor is placed, and a peritoneal bladder flap is raised. Once the uterus is exposed, intraoperative sterile ultrasonography is used to map the position and edges of the placenta as well as to evaluate the amniotic fluid index. A low-anterior-uterine-segment hysterotomy is the preferred approach for all EXIT procedures. The exceptions are those cases in which the placenta is located in the anterior lower uterine segment. In those cases, a midline laparotomy is performed and the

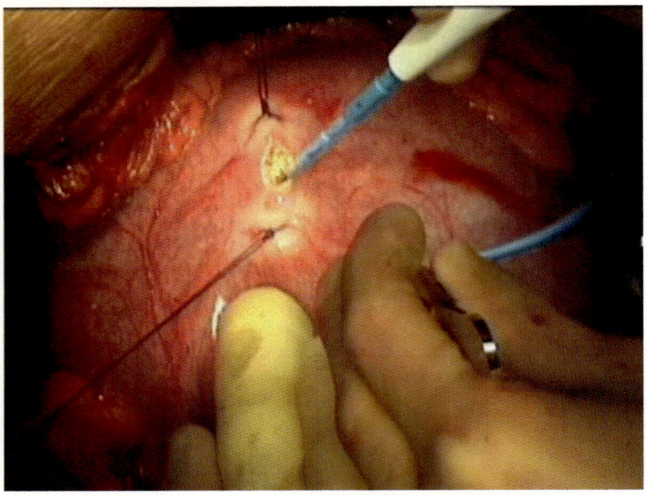

Fig. 5 Hemostatic hysterotomy: two stay stitches are placed under ultrasound guidance far from the placental edge. The uterine wall is incised with electrocautery

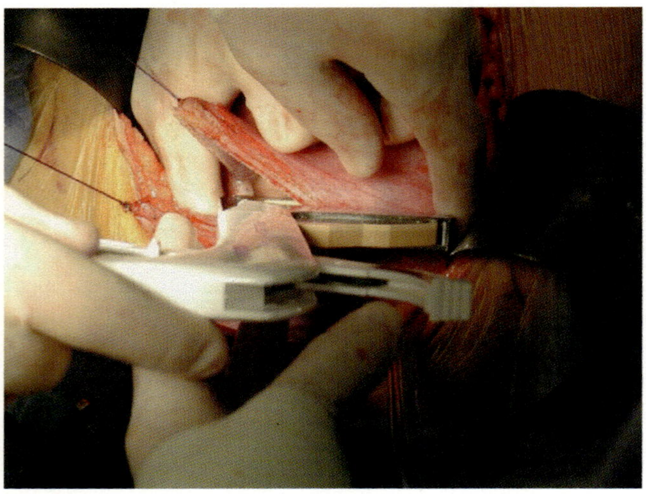

Fig. 6 The hysterotomy is completed in a bloodless manner with a uterine stapler

uterine fundus is exteriorized from the abdomen to perform a fundal or posterior hysterotomy. After the placenta is carefully mapped by ultrasound and marked on the uterine surface, a site is chosen ideally at least 6 cm away from the marked edge. This can be complicated in the setting of polyhydramnios when the placental edge can be difficult to identify. Two monofilament stay sutures (0-PDS; Ethicon, Somerville, NJ) are placed through the uterine wall under ultrasound guidance, and the myometrium and membranes are incised with monopolar cautery (Fig. 5). The hysterotomy is completed in a bloodless manner with a uterine stapling device (Premium Poly CS 57; Covidien Auto suture, Mansfield, MA) (Fig. 6). It is important to carefully inspect the uterine edges and make sure that hemostasis is achieved before manipulating the fetus. After hysterotomy, the uterine cavity is filled continuously with warm (37 °C) lactated Ringer solution using a high-flow fluid warmer/pump (Level I-H1200; Smiths Medical, St. Paul, MN) to maintain adequate uterine volume and prevent compression of the umbilical cord. The tone of the uterine wall must be monitored continuously by palpation, and the inhalational anesthesia adjusted accordingly. After the closure of the hysterotomy and the laparotomy, epidural anesthesia (bupivacaine 0.2 %, 5–10 mL) and opioids (morphine, 4–8 mg) are started, and muscle relaxation is reversed (2.5–5 mg of neostigmine plus 0.4–0.6 mg of glycopyrrolate).

Fetal Exposure

The same concept applies to all EXIT procedures regardless of the indication: only the fetal part that is going to be operated on is exteriorized, whereas the rest of the body must remain within the uterine cavity (until the cord is clamped) to maintain uterine volume and fetal temperature. In cases of airway obstruction, the head, neck, upper extremities, and upper torso are carefully exteriorized. The upper extremities are used to place a pulse oximeter (covered by aluminum foil and a Tegaderm, 3M, St. Paul, MN, USA) and a 24-gauge intravenous catheter (Fig. 7). Fetal vital parameters are monitored by the pulse oximeter and by continuous sterile intraoperative echocardiography. Fetal anesthesia is supplemented by a single intramuscular dose of an opioid (fentanyl, 0.2 μg/kg), and a muscle relaxant (vecuronium, 0.1 mg/kg) immediately after exteriorization. These drugs (and other drugs potentially needed at the time of a code [i.e., atropine, epinephrine, and calcium]) are prepared preoperatively in sterile syringes and are ready for use on the operative table. All drugs as well as crystalloid solutions and blood can be administered to the fetus intravenously as needed. Fetal bradycardia or myocardial dysfunction can occur at any time during the EXIT procedure. They can be directly related to the procedure being performed, such as with the mechanical compression associated with excision of a large lung lesion, or unrelated. The maternal anesthetic drugs cross the placenta and can cause fetal myocardial depression, requiring alterations in dosing of anesthetic, maternal intravenous fluid boluses, or direct administration of drugs, red cells, or crystalloids to the fetus. Acute changes in fetal heart rate prompt immediate investigation, as cord compression can be quickly relieved by fetal repositioning or increased amnioinfusion. Fetal cardiac dysfunction secondary to hypovolemia should be treated with a fetal transfusion.

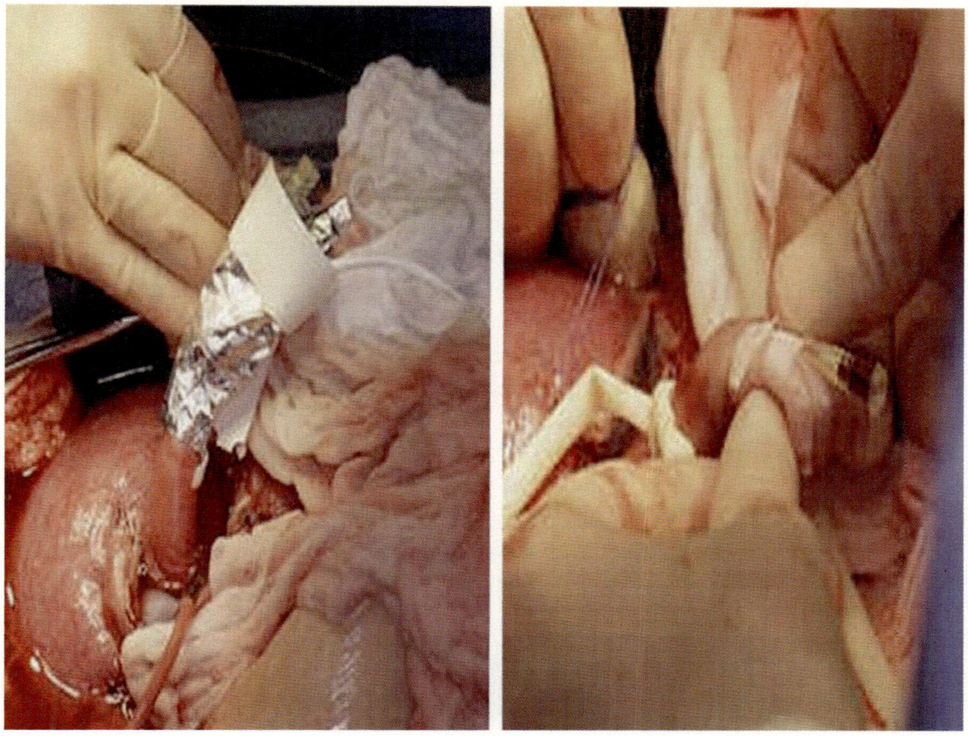

Fig. 7 The fetal upper extremities are used to place an oximeter and a peripheral intravenous catheter

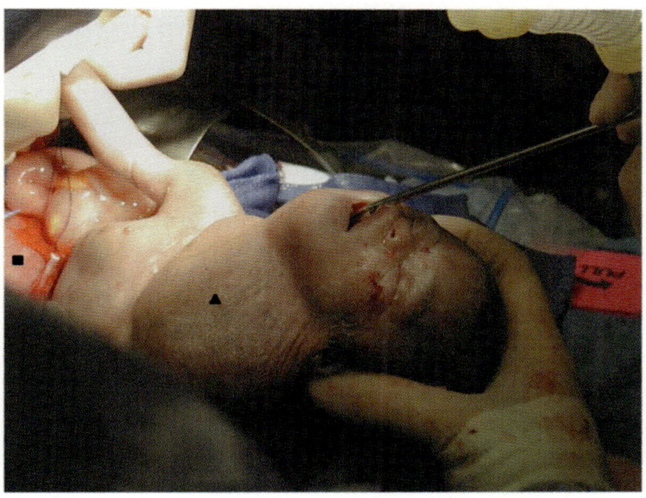

Fig. 8 Fetal bronchoscopy during an EXIT procedure in a fetus with a large cervical mass (*black triangle*)

Airway Management

After the fetal head is exteriorized, it is positioned with a roll under the shoulders to allow access to the airway. The first maneuver is to perform a direct laryngoscopy to try to identify the vocal cords. If there is no invasion of the larynx by a tumor (e.g., lymphangiomas, teratomas) an attempt is made to intubate the trachea exclusively with the help of the laryngoscope. When the airway is not clearly seen by direct laryngoscopy due to deviation, compression, or invasion by a tumor, rigid bronchoscopy must be performed. The rigid bronchoscope allows certain degree of airway manipulation (it can decompress and straighten the airway as it is passed distally) and may serve as a guide to pass a wire into the distal airway to be used as a guide for the endotracheal tube (Fig. 8). Careful external manipulation of the tumor can help accessing the airway with the bronchoscope. Rigid bronchoscopy is also useful to determine the location of the larynx and trachea relative to the tumor should a surgical airway be needed. When the cervical tumor contains large cysts, ultrasound-guided percutaneous drainage during the EXIT can be of great help to decompress the airway and increase the chances of an orotracheal intubation. When the airway is obstructed by pedunculated tumors, the EXIT procedure provides time to do a surgical resection. This is particularly valid for fetuses with a variety of oropharyngeal tumors (e.g., teratomas, epignathus, epulis) (Figs. 9 and 10a, b) [9].

Controlled Emergent Tracheostomy

When laryngoscopy and bronchoscopy fail, the next step is a tracheostomy, which is always a challenging procedure in the setting of large cervical tumors (particularly cervical teratomas). The thorough and extensive preoperative evaluation of the fetal radiologic images is extremely necessary to know, prior to the EXIT, the relationship between the tumor and the airway in order to save valuable intraoperative time [10]. The thorough review of the fetal images also allows determining the cystic or solid nature of the tumor, which helps predict (to certain degree) the likelihood of a successful orotracheal intubation. Specifically, cystic tumors (e.g., lymphangiomas) are usually not invasive and destructive, whereas solid tumors (e.g., teratomas) have a more aggressive behavior. In our experience 53 % of fetuses with cervical teratomas required a tracheostomy at the time of the EXIT, whereas only 8 % of fetuses with a cervical lymphangiomas did. When a tracheostomy is necessary, transverse incision is usually made 1–2 fingerbreadths above the level of the sternal notch and extended to the side of the neck to which the airway is deviated (determined by the preoperative imaging studies). Once the airway is identified, it must be dissected off the tumor to relieve the compression and perform the tracheotomy at the desired level. The tumor usually pulls the trachea superiorly as it grows, and in some cases the carina can be located at the level of the sternal notch, making the interpretation of the anatomy quite difficult. The tracheotomy for airway access should be done at the level of the second or third tracheal ring, but with severe alteration of the anatomy, we have performed initial tracheotomies for airway control at different levels. Although a tracheostomy allows direct access to the airway, it is often difficult to secure the tracheostomy tube to any cervical structures, either while the tumor is still present or in the setting of large skin flaps after the tumor has been removed. To overcome this situation, two different approaches have been used. First, a regular ETT can be tunneled under the skin (via a skin incision lateral to the midline) and used as a tracheostomy tube. Second, once the trachea is dissected off the tumor, a tracheotomy is performed, a 4–8 F nasogastric (NG) tube is threaded retrograde within the airway and retrieved at the mouth, the ETT is sutured to the tip of the NG tube, and the NG tube is pulled back as a guide to slide the ETT antegrade to the desired position in the trachea (Fig. 11). Once the airway is established and secured, manual ventilation is initiated on the operative field. Surfactant is administered if the fetus is less than 34 weeks of gestation. If the fetus is stable, umbilical arterial and venous lines can be placed using an intracatheter technique before the umbilical cord is clamped and divided.

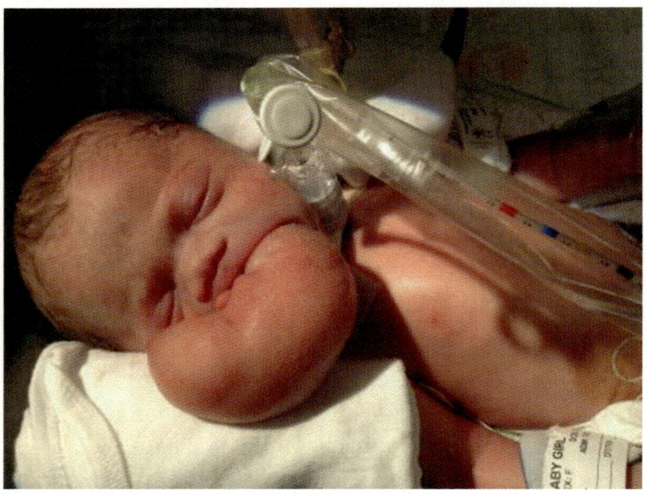

Fig. 9 Neonate with "fetus-in-fetu;" like-teratoma with remnants of twin causing oral obstruction necessitating tracheostomy at delivery. This infant was delivered without time for an EXIT and underwent an emergency lifesaving tracheostomy (Courtesy of Alan Flake-CHOP)

EXIT Procedure

Not all fetuses with oral or neck masses experience airway obstruction. Occasionally, there are situations where a remote, but large birth defect, such as a giant sacrococcygeal teratoma (SCT), may cause difficulty accessing the airway due to positioning of the infant (Fig. 12). When the EXIT is done in a fetus with CHAOS syndrome, the laryngoscopy and bronchoscopy are used to confirm the diagnosis and to evaluate the airway proximal to the obstruction, but a

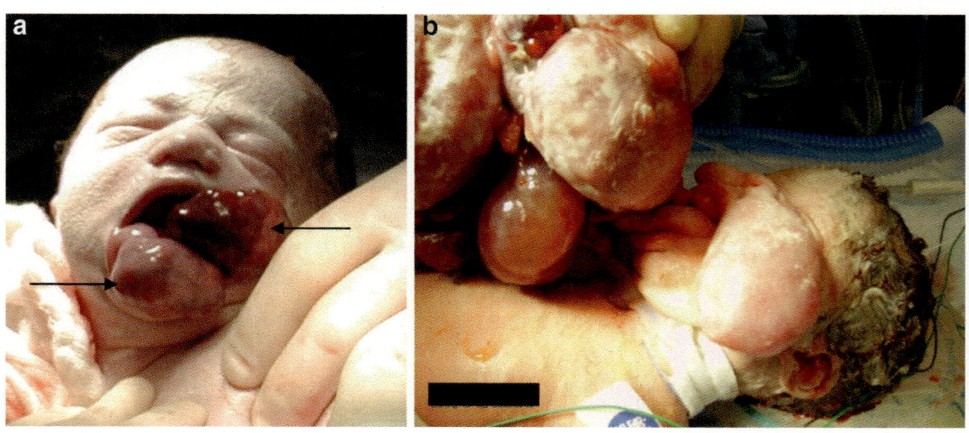

Fig. 10 (**a**) Fetus with multiple epulis arising from the upper and lower gums. (**b**) Fetus with giant epignathus causing airway obstruction (courtesy of Alan Flake, CHOP)

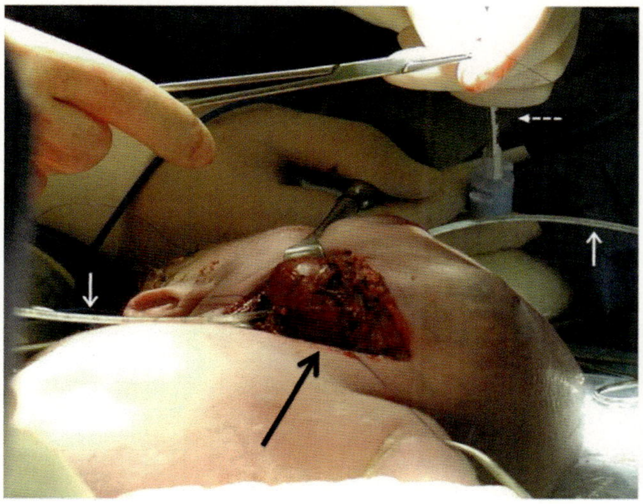

Fig. 11 Retrograde intubation. A nasogastric tube is passed retrograde from the tracheotomy to the mouth and is used to guide the endotracheal tube antegrade into the airway

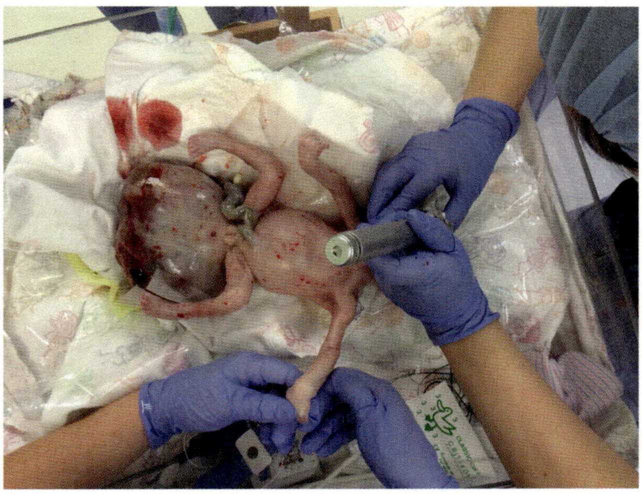

Fig. 12 This premature infant although born with a giant sacrococcygeal teratoma required an EXIT procedure with *black arrow* difficult airway access due to overall size of the teratoma

tracheostomy is mandatory. At this point, the fetal portion of the EXIT procedure ends and the newborn is taken to an adjacent room for further resuscitation and evaluation. The placenta is then delivered, the uterine tone is restored, and the uterus and maternal abdominal wall are closed in a manner similar to that of a cesarean section. In the potential case of a congenital airway obstruction in the context of a twin pregnancy (Fig. 13), the premise of delivering the healthy twin first should prevail, if at all possible [11]. The healthy twin will always require endotracheal intubation and temporary respiratory support due to the exposure to the maternal anesthetic gases.

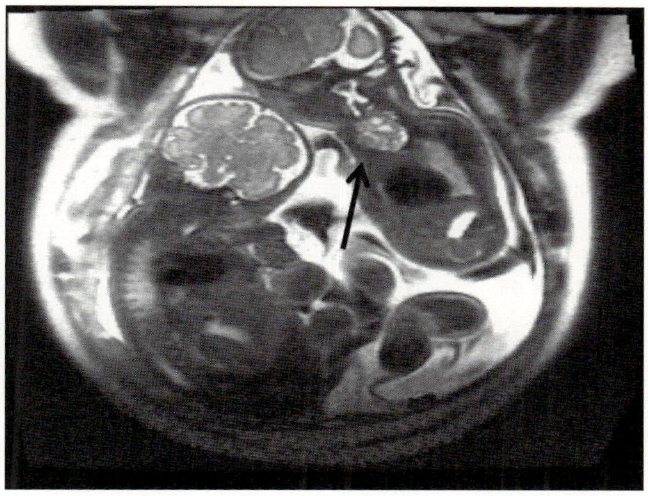

Fig. 13 Congenital airway obstruction in a twin pregnancy (fetus on the right side of the picture has a cervical teratoma) (*black arrow*)

Lung Masses

Fetuses with large lung masses (e.g., congenital cystic adenomatoid malformation, (CCAM), bronchial atresia) and severe mediastinal shift may be delivered by EXIT because of the anticipated postnatal difficulties to oxygenate and ventilate due to deviation of the major airway and compression of the healthy lung. The EXIT procedure will allow securing the airway via endotracheal intubation and resecting the lung mass while the fetus is under placental support [12]. Alternatively, fetuses with lung masses and mediastinal shift may be delivered by cesarean section, intubated immediately after birth and have the lung mass removed right after the initial resuscitation.

From a maternal perspective, the EXIT carries a higher risk of potential complications than a standard cesarean section. Beyond the inherent risks of general anesthesia instead of epidural anesthesia, the purposeful inhibition of uterine contractions is a setup for uterine hemorrhage during the EXIT after the placenta has been detached. The average blood loss for a standard cesarean section is in the 500–600 mL range, whereas in published series of EXITs the average is >1,000 mL. Therefore, the EXIT procedure must be performed by a skilled multidisciplinary team that performs fetal surgery on a regular basis.

Conclusion

Neonatal airway obstruction is a true emergency requiring a team of expert clinicians experienced in high level airway management. Pediatric surgeons, otorhinolaryngologists, neonatologists, respiratory therapists, and nurses are required to create a team approach, which ensures a successful outcome. Equipment that is specific to neonatal infants regarding size and function must be available at each of these deliveries. Ultimately clinician with expertise in tracheostomy must be present at each of these deliveries.

References

1. Holinger LD, Birnholz JC, Bruce DR, et al. Management of an infant with prenatal ultrasound diagnosis of upper airway obstruction. Int J Pediatr Otorhinolaryngol. 1985;10(3):263–70.
2. Kelly MF, Berenholz L, Rizzo KA, et al. Approach for oxygenation of the newborn with airway obstruction due to a cervical mass. Ann Otol Rhinol Laryngol. 1990;99(3 Pt 1):179–82.
3. Levine AB, Alvarez M, Wedgwood J, et al. Contemporary management of a potentially lethal fetal anomaly: a successful perinatal approach to epignathus. Obstet Gynecol. 1990;76(5 Pt 2):962–6.
4. Harrison MR, Adzick NS, Flake AW, et al. Correction of congenital diaphragmatic hernia in utero VIII: response of the hypoplastic lung to tracheal occlusion. J Pediatr Surg. 1996;31(10):1339–48.
5. Hedrick HL. Ex utero intrapartum therapy. Semin Pediatr Surg. 2003;12(3):190–5.
6. Liechty KW. Ex utero intrapartum therapy. Semin Fetal Neonatal Med. 2010;15(1):34–9.
7. Lim FJ, Crombleholme TM, Hedrick HL, et al. Congenital high airway obstruction syndrome: natural history and management. J Pediatr Surg. 2003;38(6):940–5.
8. Laje P, Johnson MP, Howell LJ, et al. Ex utero intrapartum treatment in the management of giant cervical teratomas. J Pediatr Surg. 2012;47:1208–16.
9. Laje P, Howell LJ, Johnson MP, et al. Perinatal management of congenital oropharyngeal tumors: the ex utero intrapartum treatment (EXIT) approach. J Pediatr Surg. 2013;48(10):2005–10.
10. Hubbard AM, Crombleholme TM, Adzick NS. Prenatal MRI evaluation of giant neck masses in preparation for the fetal EXIT procedure. Am J Perinatol. 1998;15(4):253–7.
11. Liechty KW, Crombleholme TM, Weiner S, et al. The ex utero intrapartum treatment procedure for a large fetal neck mass in a twin gestation. Obstet Gynecol. 1999;93(5 Pt 2):824–5.
12. Hedrick HL, Flake AW, Crombleholme TM, et al. The ex utero intrapartum therapy procedure for high-risk fetal lung lesions. J Pediatr Surg. 2005;40(6):1038–43.

Differential Diagnosis of Stridor in the Newborn: Guidelines for a Time-Efficient and Cost-Effective Evaluation

David E. Tunkel and Melissa Ortiz

Introduction and Definitions

Stridor is an audible sound arising during respiration, a noise made by turbulent airflow in the airways. Stridor can be present immediately with the first breaths after birth, and it can also develop in newborns shortly after birth. Stridor is a sign, and not a diagnosis, and persistent stridor in a young infant mandates a diagnostic evaluation. This noise can vary in intensity during the phases of respiration, during inspiration, expiration, or on both phases of respiration (biphasic) depending on the site of the obstruction of the large airways. **Inspiratory stridor** is typically seen with an obstruction at the extrathoracic level, usually at or above the level of the vocal cords. **Expiratory stridor** indicates obstruction at the intrathoracic level, the middle or lower trachea. Obstruction at the subglottic or upper tracheal level often manifests as **biphasic stridor**, both inspiratory and expiratory, although the inspiratory component may be louder and more noticeable than the expiratory sound. Stridor is differentiated from **stertor**, an inspiratory low-pitched sound, guttural or gurgly in nature, produced by obstruction in the nose and/or pharynx. Stridor in a neonate is particularly worrisome because of the limited pulmonary reserve of small infants, the possibility of a progressive airway lesion, and the possible need for prompt diagnosis and intervention. All that said, most infants with stridor have laryngomalacia, which has a generally favorable natural history and limited need for intervention.

D.E. Tunkel, M.D. (✉) • M. Ortiz, M.D.
Department of Surgery, Otolaryngology—Head and Neck Surgery Section, University of Puerto Rico-Medical Sciences Campus, PO Box 365067, San Juan, PR 00936-5067, USA
e-mail: dtunkel@jhmi.edu

History

A detailed history focuses the evaluation of a stridorous neonate, and narrows the number of suspected airway lesions. In fact, many referrals for stridor in a neonate originate from parents and pediatricians in the ambulatory setting. The preliminary history that is obtained by initial phone contact should orchestrate the pace and setting of subsequent evaluation. The growing, noisy but seemingly healthy infant with stridor can have an ambulatory evaluation in an orderly manner. The tachypneic, distressed infant with noisy breathing requires urgent evaluation in the emergency department or on the inpatient unit, where airway support is available as well as rapid diagnostic testing. A detailed history as discussed in the next few paragraphs will allow focus of our examination and precise use of ancillary tests.

The birth history should include determination of birth weight, gestational age at birth, and mode of delivery (vaginal or Caesarean section). Details about duration of labor and need for assisted delivery (forceps, vacuum, etc.) should also be obtained. The improvements in the care of premature and/or low-birth weight infants have allowed survival of infants who have had aggressive and prolonged respiratory support in neonatal intensive care units. This support includes ventilation with endotracheal intubation, noninvasive support with positive airway pressure delivered by nose or face mask, and the use of surfactant to reduce the need for long-term intubation and ventilation. Neonates who have stridor after long periods of endotracheal intubation should be suspected to have subglottic lesions, including subglottic stenosis or less commonly subglottic cysts.

The time of onset of the stridor can give useful clues to etiology as well. Congenital airway lesions can all cause stridor close to the time of birth, but subtle differences in time of onset should be discussed. Laryngomalacia is the most common cause of neonatal stridor, but the high-pitched inspiratory stridor seen with this condition is usually noted a few days to a few weeks after birth. In fact, it usually worsens

J. Lioy and S.E. Sobol (eds.), *Disorders of the Neonatal Airway: Fundamentals for Practice*,
DOI 10.1007/978-1-4939-1610-8_19,

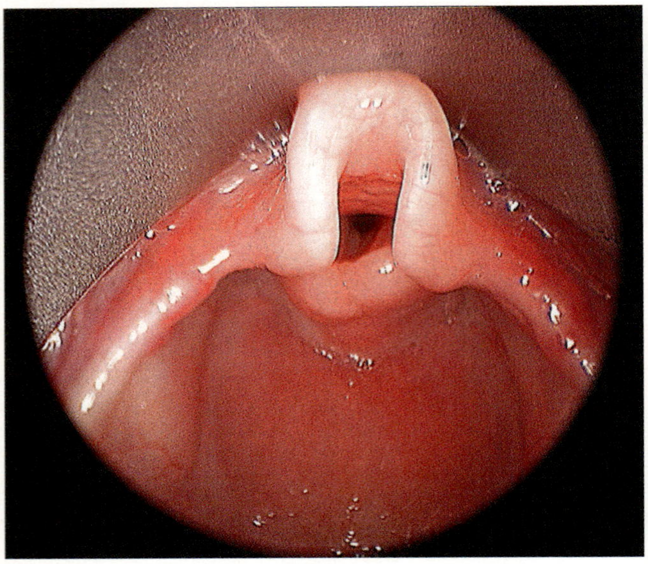

Fig. 1 Endoscopic view of laryngomalacia at time of supraglottoplasty. Note curled epiglottis and anteromedial displacement of supra-arytenoid mucosa

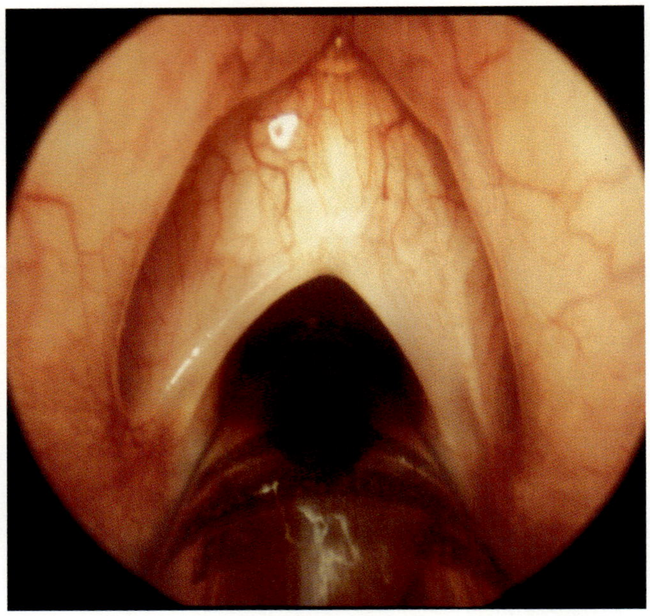

Fig. 2 Anterior commissure web causing dysphonia but almost no stridor, as web extends for about 1/3 of glottis length

over the first few weeks, reflecting dynamic collapse of supraglottic tissues with inspiration that worsens as a more active newborn has increased respiratory effort (Fig. 1). In contrast, congenital bilateral vocal cord paralysis presents as inspiratory stridor close to the time of birth, perhaps immediately after delivery, reflecting a fixed airway lesion from adducted vocal cords during inspiration [1].

If an infant has been intubated or suctioned around the time of birth, details about the mode of instrumentation, size of endotracheal tube, and duration of intubation can also shed light on etiology. A neonate who has been intubated even for a few seconds to suction meconium in the delivery suite can suffer laryngeal trauma. While such trauma is almost always minor, a few infants have developed laryngeal granulomas that cause inspiratory stridor and hoarse cry a few days after birth [2].

The history should also include details about feeding, including changes in stridor quality and intensity during and after feeding. An infant with stridor who has feeding difficulties or poor weight-gain may have more severe airway obstruction. Feeding difficulties may reflect poor coordination of swallow during the increased work of breathing with airway obstruction. Poor feeding in the presence of stridor can occur with laryngotracheal lesions that directly impair swallowing. Infants with large laryngeal clefts can have stridor from inspiratory collapse of the redundant posterior supraglottic tissues surrounding the cleft, as well as the more classic aspiration of feeds through the abnormally patent posterior larynx. Infants with gastroesophageal reflux can develop noisy breathing from an edematous, irritated larynx, or from aspiration of refluxate or swallowed feeds. While neonates with laryngomalacia can have associated esophageal or even pharyngeal reflux of gastric contents, such reflux may result secondarily from increased intrathoracic pressures created by the airway obstruction at the laryngeal level [3].

A history of an abnormal cry, perhaps high-pitched, hoarse, or even aphonia, focuses the evaluation for stridor to glottic (true vocal cord) lesions. Neonates can have inspiratory stridor from unilateral vocal cord paralysis, as the one immobile cord causes relative airway narrowing at the glottic level. These infants have hoarse or weak cry because the immobile vocal cord, usually paralyzed off the midline (the so-called paramedian position), cannot abut the mobile vocal cord during phonation or cry. Neonates with bilateral vocal cord paralysis have more severe stridor and airway obstruction, but the quality of cry may be closer to normal than in those with only one immobile vocal cord. Neonates with abnormal cry can also have abnormalities of vocal cord structure, such as an anterior glottis web that both restricts vocal cord motion and narrows the glottis airway (Fig. 2). Small glottic webs may not cause stridor, but large webs can cause severe airway compromise and stridor, as they have longer lengths of fused vocal cords and are often associated with subglottic stenosis.

A history of barky or croupy cough or history of treatment for recurrent or atypical croup-like illnesses points to a subglottic abnormality. Any history of laryngeal instrumentation suggests the possibility of subglottic stenosis or cysts, although congenital subglottic stenosis can present as recurrent croup-like illness without any history of previous intubation. A subglottic hemangioma can cause barky cough and stridor that may transiently respond to the steroid treatment given for presumed croup. Subglottic hemangiomas usually cause inspiratory or biphasic stridor in the first few months of life, but not at birth, as the airway lesion proliferates early in infancy [4] (Fig. 3).

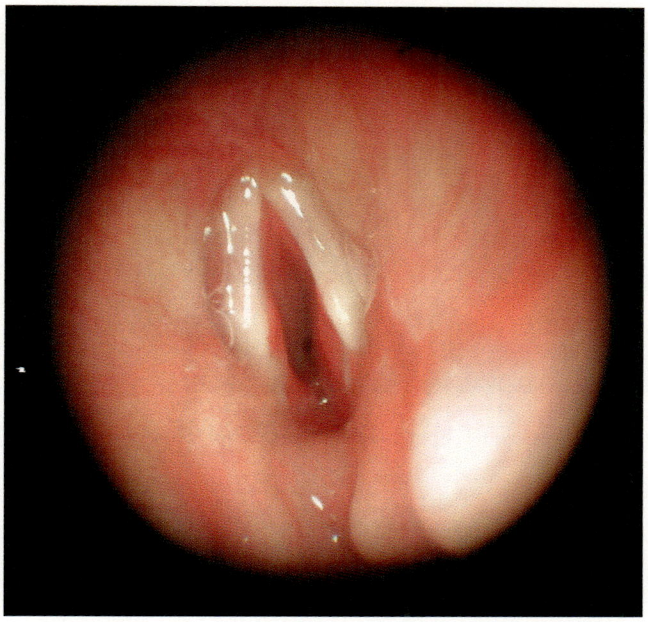

Fig. 3 High-grade airway obstruction from near circumferential involvement of subglottic hemangioma

A detailed history should also elucidate any possible syndromic diagnoses, familial disorders, or multi-system diseases that could explain neonatal stridor. Familial neonatal vocal cord paralysis has been described. Neonates with central nervous system abnormalities such as hydrocephalus or Arnold-Chiari malformation can present with stridor secondary to vocal cord paralysis. Children with congenital heart anomalies can have tracheal compression from cardiac enlargement or from associated anomalous intrathoracic vasculature; unilateral vocal cord paralysis is similarly associated with congenital heart disease. Vocal cord paralysis and subglottic stenosis are both seen in young children after corrective cardiac surgery and postoperative respiratory support [5].

A careful past surgical history is critical to determine the etiology of neonatal stridor, particularly for those who have had intervention to close a patent ductus arteriosus (PDA) or have required extracorporeal membrane oxygenation (ECMO) with cannulation of neck vessels [6, 7]. PDA ligation and ECMO have been associated with unilateral vocal cord paralysis causing neonatal stridor, dysphagia, and dysphonia, by impaired function of the left recurrent laryngeal nerve (PDA) and the cervical vagus nerve (ECMO) motor innervations to the larynx.

The SPECS stridor history mnemonic, described by Hollinger, is a useful construct to focus history-taking, and to determine the speed of subsequent evaluation and need for intervention [8]. The assessment includes: **S—Severity**, **P—Progression**, **E—Eating**, **C—Cyanotic spells**: **Apparent life-threatening events**, **S—Sleep**: **Obstruction so severe that retractions occur even during sleep**.

Severity

The subjective impression regarding the severity of the obstruction and any accompanying respiratory distress, determines the urgency of planned investigations. The seemingly well neonate with mild stridor, no respiratory distress, and good feeding can have an orderly evaluation usually in the office setting, but the infant with signs of severe airway compromise requires immediate intervention for diagnosis and possible intervention. While this assessment is mainly that of the bedside physical examination by experienced observers, the observations of parents and other caregivers are important.

Progression

Stridor that is present at birth suggests a fixed congenital narrowing such as choanal atresia, laryngeal web, vocal cord paralysis, and subglottic or tracheal stenosis. If the stridor progresses during the first few weeks of life, and symptoms change with position and awake/asleep state, a dynamic lesion such as laryngomalacia is possible. If symptoms worsen steadily over time, with louder or more persistent stridor or worsening associated signs and symptoms, an enlarging airway mass such as subglottic hemangioma may be present.

Abrupt onset of stridor, with rapid progression, suggests infectious or inflammatory airway issues, such as viral croup, tracheitis, or epiglottitis. Such laryngeal infection is unusual in neonates. This clinical picture is also seen with airway trauma or foreign body aspiration. While foreign body aspiration is often seen in toddlers and young children, the rare reports of neonatal foreign body aspiration usually involve iatrogenic airway foreign bodies associated with neonatal respiratory support [9].

Eating

Any history of feeding difficulties, symptoms of aspiration, or failure to thrive suggests more severe airway obstruction or an anatomic lesion that affects swallowing as well as airway patency. Lesions of the nasal cavity, nasopharynx, and pharynx are more likely to cause feeding difficulties than those in the lower airways. Slow feeds, frequent pauses for breathing, and cough or spitting-up with feeds may be reported in some stridorous neonates. As discussed above, aspiration and cough can occur in infants with vocal cord paralysis, tracheoesophageal fistula, or laryngeal clefts, each of which can interfere with the necessary exclusion of food from the airways. Additionally, tracheal obstruction and esophageal compression can coexist, particularly with intrathoracic vascular anomalies such as the double aortic arch and other compressive rings (Fig. 4a, b).

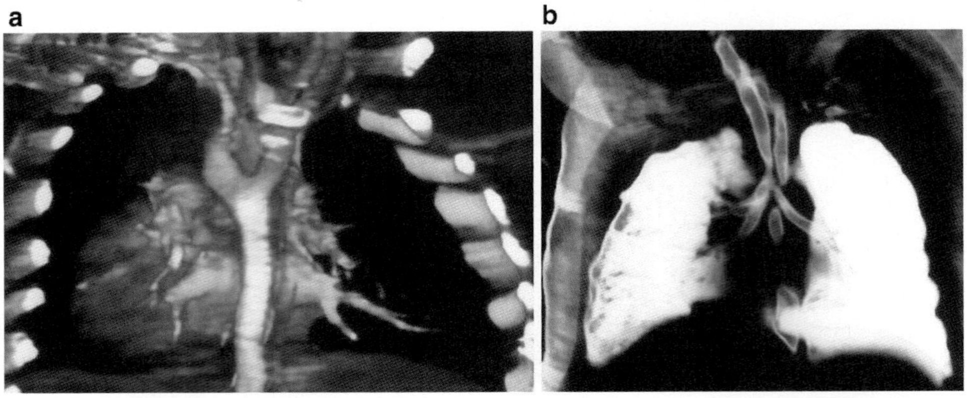

Fig. 4 Enhanced computed tomographic images of (**a**) double aortic arch surrounding the trachea and the esophagus causing (**b**) severe narrowing of the distal trachea

Cyanotic Spells

Any stridorous infant who has cyanotic spells, severe respiratory distress with neck or chest retractions, or with a history of a "near-miss" or apparent life-threatening event (ALTE) requires urgent evaluation and management. These infants are usually admitted for cardiorespiratory monitoring and multidisciplinary work-up. Cardiovascular and central nervous system disorders need to be excluded in the infant with cyanotic spells and ALTE, particularly when stridor is intermittent or absent. However, an infant with a confirmed airway lesion can have concomitant cardiovascular, pulmonary, and/or central nervous system disorders. This is often the case in syndromic infants, as well as in neonates who have had prolonged, complicated intensive care unit stays.

Sleep

Stridor may improve or may worsen during sleep. Some neonates with airway obstruction will suffer from obstructive sleep apnea, with relaxation of upper airway musculature causing multi-level airway obstruction. Airway obstruction at the pharyngeal level often worsens during sleep, most classically demonstrated by infants with glossoptosis and the Pierre-Robin triad. Stridor from laryngeal and tracheobronchial obstruction usually is loudest in the awake and agitated infant, with fewer symptoms during sleep.

Physical Examination

The general examination of the neonate with stridor is a key in determining the severity of airway compromise. In addition to routine vital signs, pulse oximetry may be helpful as a screen for severe respiratory difficulties. One should be cautioned that a normal room air arterial oxygen saturation reading by no means excludes severe airway obstruction, as ventilation may be severely compromised before arterial oxygen desaturation occurs. The nature of the stridor can be determined, with relation to the phase of respiration as well as whether it is high or low-pitched, constant or intermittent, or variable with body position.

The presence of tachypnea, severe retractions, lethargy, cyanosis, or seemingly poor airway movement in an infant with stridor suggests the need for near simultaneous airway evaluation and airway support. In some circumstances this requires urgent transport to the operating room for diagnostic airway endoscopy and support with endotracheal intubation, tracheotomy, or other intervention depending on the nature of the airway lesion. The neonate with stridor who is otherwise stable can usually be evaluated in the clinic setting or at the bedside.

The general examination will include inspection of the head and neck, with attention to presence or absence of craniomaxillofacial deformities. Infants with microtia, absence or deformity of one or both auricles, can have associated mandibular hypoplasia and asymmetry, resulting in relative airway obstruction (Fig. 5). More obvious deformities of the external nose, nasal ala, mouth shape and size, jaw size and position, etc. should be documented. Infants with facial hemangiomas, especially those around the lips, mouth, and chin, may have stridor from laryngeal hemangiomas. Inspection of head and neck, the chest wall anatomy and dynamics, as well as the limbs, may suggest a syndromic diagnosis that includes an airway abnormality. For example, an infant with stridor, misshapen helices, and a submucosal cleft palate may have velocardiofacial syndrome, a condition that is associated with glottic webs and vascular rings.

The nose is examined, looking at size, patency of nostrils, abnormal secretions and masses. The choanal openings can be assessed by passing catheters through the nose, but it is a simple task to assess choanal patency during transnasal fiberoptic laryngoscopy. The oral cavity and oropharynx is inspected for masses, abnormal tongue shape and position,

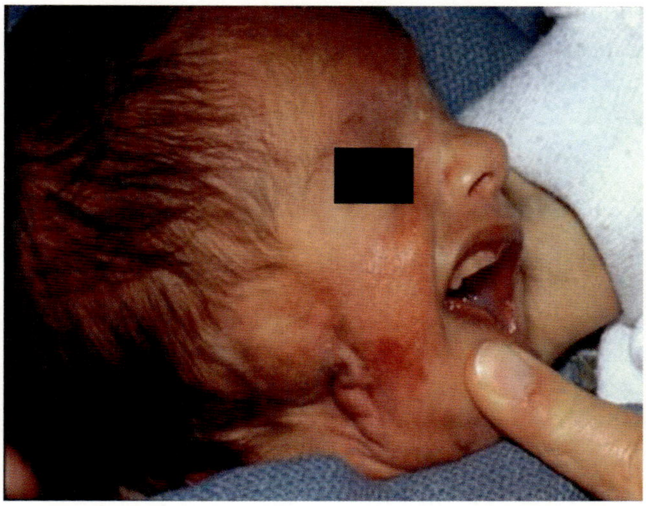

Fig. 5 Infant with severe airway obstruction from mandibular hypoplasia. Note associated ear anomalies

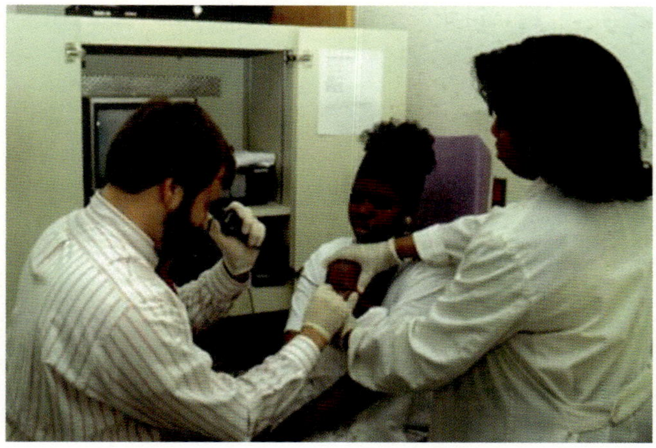

Fig. 6 Awake fiberoptic laryngoscopy to evaluate a young infant with stridor

overt and occult palate clefts, etc. While obstructive airway lesions may not be seen, the clinician may see features to suggest more diffuse issues with neuromotor tone or even syndromic diagnosis.

Auscultation of the lung fields and even over the neck/larynx may amplify features of the stridor, particularly for children with intrathoracic lesions, cardiac disease, or abnormalities of chest wall/lung dynamics. The neck should be examined to look for retractions as well as for masses that may affect airway function.

Symptoms of airway obstruction, including stridor, may vary with position of the infant. The exam can include evaluation while supine, prone, and upright. The infant with laryngomalacia has worsened stridor when supine, improved when upright or prone. Similarly, the micrognathic infant with airway compromise from the Pierre-Robin triad is worse in the supine position, but airway obstruction in this infant worsens when sleeping, unlike infants with laryngomalacia.

When stridor is subtle or not observed in the clinic setting, we ask parents to make audio–video recordings, often using smartphone cameras, to help share concerning observations. Additionally, we will observe for the emergence of stridor in the active/agitated infant, usually during the fiberoptic laryngoscopy described later in this chapter.

Specialized Examinations and Procedures

Fiberoptic Laryngoscopy (FOL)

Fiberoptic laryngoscopy, or flexible laryngoscopy, is the key to our specialized examination to assess both dynamic and fixed lesions of the upper airway, viewing from the nose to the larynx. We routinely perform this in the clinic for the great majority of infants with stridor, once we have ruled out severe airway compromise. While the indication we discuss here is neonatal stridor, fiberoptic laryngoscopy is also used to evaluate stertor, feeding difficulties, cough, or abnormal cry in infants.

Fiberoptic laryngoscopy is most often performed in an awake infant who is held upright on the lap of an assistant (Fig. 6). While topical decongestants such as oxymetazoline can be used to reduce mucosal swelling in the nose, the routine use of topical anesthetics (lidocaine, tetracaine) is avoided in neonates who have respiratory and/or swallowing issues, as impaired pharyngeal sensation may worsen respiratory function. While small caliber scopes (2.7 mm) have been developed for use in neonates, the senior author prefers a 3.5 mm scope for most full-term neonates and young infants, as the larger scope provides better image quality. The small caliber scopes are useful for preterm infants or infants with nasal narrowing such as seen with piriform aperture stenosis. Video recording is routine, and is useful for serial documentation of changing lesions, careful assessment of dynamic issues such as vocal cord motion, and education of parents/caregivers.

The flexible scope is passed through both sides of the nose and advanced to the nasopharynx, assessing for nasal patency and obstructive masses. Nasal masses such as congenital dacryocystoceles can cause airway distress in neonates, who are obligate nasal breathers, as can choanal stenosis or atresia. Soft palate movement can be assessed, nasopharyngeal narrowing can be viewed, and hypopharyngeal anatomy and dynamics can be observed. A detailed view of the anatomy and movement of the base of tongue, the supraglottic larynx, and the vocal cords with respiration should be obtained, The subglottis can often be seen during full abduction of the vocal cords, but most practitioners will not routinely advance the scope below the vocal cords during the evaluation of an awake stridorous neonate in the clinic setting.

This examination can also be performed rapidly at NICU/nursery bedside or in the clinic setting, and requires no sedation or airway control. It is ideal for assessing dynamics of respiration such as pharyngeal tone, tongue position, supraglottic collapse, and vocal cord motion, all of which can be correlated with observed respiratory sounds. The subglottis and trachea are not visualized, so lesions such as subglottic or tracheal stenosis are best diagnosed with operative laryngoscopy and bronchoscopy. Posterior laryngeal clefts can be missed on fiberoptic laryngoscopy because the redundant tissues around the cleft may obscure the lesion.

Fiberoptic endoscopic evaluation of swallowing (FEES) has been introduced as a method to assess swallowing abnormalities in infants with feeding problems, with or without observed airway obstruction and/or stridor. The FOL examination described above is supplemented with real-time observation of the hypopharynx and larynx during swallows of colored boluses of varying consistencies. The ability to exclude the swallowed material from the laryngeal intraoitus and trachea is assessed, and laryngeal and hypopharyngeal sensation can be tested as well. FEES has been used to look for anatomic correlates of swallow dysfunction as a supplement to video-fluoroscopic assessments ("modified" barium swallow). FEES also can be used as a primary assessment of swallow function in neonates to limit exposure to the ionizing radiation of fluoroscopy.

Direct Laryngoscopy/Bronchoscopy

The neonate with stridor may require examination in the operating room under general anesthesia for accurate diagnosis and appropriate treatment of airway obstruction. While a full discussion of operative treatment of neonatal laryngotracheal lesions is outside the scope of this chapter, safe direct laryngoscopy and rigid bronchoscopy in neonates requires coordinated pediatric endoscopic and anesthetic expertise. Except for the most urgent of circumstances, such airway endoscopy is usually done with the most likely diagnoses already considered, with the possible treatments planned before surgery. Consider these examples: (1) an infant who has failed extubation in the NICU, with suspected subglottic stenosis, should undergo confirmation of the diagnosis with direct laryngoscopy and rigid bronchoscopy. The surgeon should be prepared to perform: airway dilation with balloon catheters or other means if a soft, mild subglottic stenosis is found, tracheotomy if multi-level severe airway lesions are found, or excision/drainage of subglottic cysts if these are present; (2) a stridorous infant with failure-to-thrive and severe laryngomalacia observed on awake fiberoptic laryngoscopy should undergo direct laryngoscopy and bronchoscopy to rule out additional airway lesions, and can undergo supraglottoplasty during the same anesthetic.

Operative laryngoscopy and bronchoscopy allows visualization of the airways down to the level of bronchi, palpation of observed lesions, and measurement of the caliber of the airways and the severity of any narrowings. Interventions can be performed, including biopsy or debulking of masses, excision or incision of affected tissues, dilation of narrowed areas, removal of foreign bodies, and stabilization of a compromised airway with endotracheal intubation or with a rigid ventilating bronchoscope. The use of the Hopkins rod telescope and modern video documentation allows high-quality images far superior to conventional fiberoptic scopes. An assortment of laryngoscopes designed for optimal exposure of the neonatal larynx are available, a "favorite" being the Benjamin-Parsons scope (Karl Storz) that allows suspension of the larynx into view for full instrumentation as well as passage of an endotracheal tube (Fig. 7a, b). Rigid ventilating bronchoscopes allow oxygenation and ventilation through the endoscope, examination of the more distal airway into lobar and segmental bronchi, biopsy of lesions through working channels, and removal of foreign bodies with specialized forceps.

This procedure is best suited for evaluation of the subglottis and trachea, when lesions such as subglottic stenosis, tracheal stenosis, subglottic cysts, tracheomalacia, or aspirated foreign bodies are suspected (Figs. 8 and 9a, b). Palpation

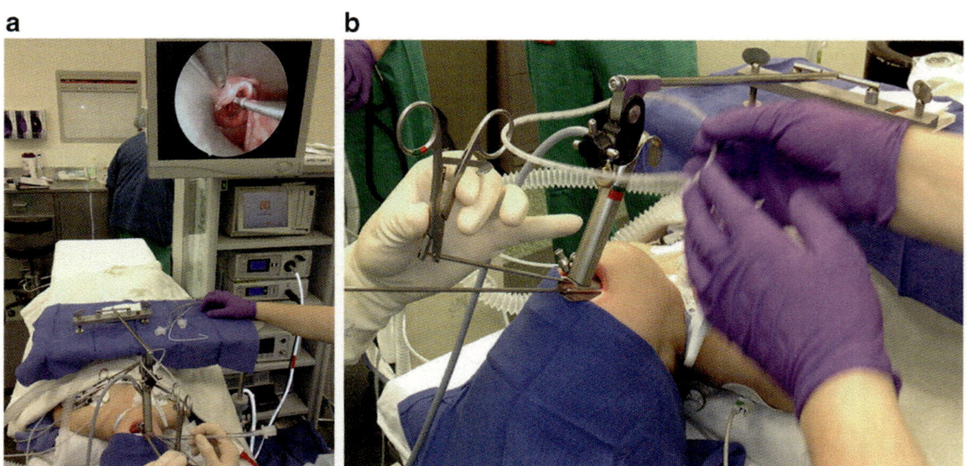

Fig. 7 Suspension laryngoscopy allows (**a**) high-quality real-time images as well as (**b**) two handed instrumentation

and measurement of airway lesions can be performed. Full appreciation of laryngeal/pharyngeal dynamics is not afforded during general anesthesia, so dynamic lesions such as laryngomalacia or vocal cord paralysis are best diagnosed outside the operating room.

Imaging Studies in the Diagnosis of Neonatal Stridor

Radiologic studies are helpful to assess laryngotracheal anatomy as well as neck soft tissues and thoracic structures in relation to the airways. We must make great effort to limit the exposure of young children to ionizing radiation, given the uncertain oncologic risk of even small exposures over a long expected lifetime [10]. With this in mind, selection of the most appropriate imaging modality should be based on clinical suspicion arising from the history and examination outlined above. Imaging studies should be obtained only when the results will impact treatment or prognosis, and the studies should be selected carefully and performed with pediatric protocols to limit exposure.

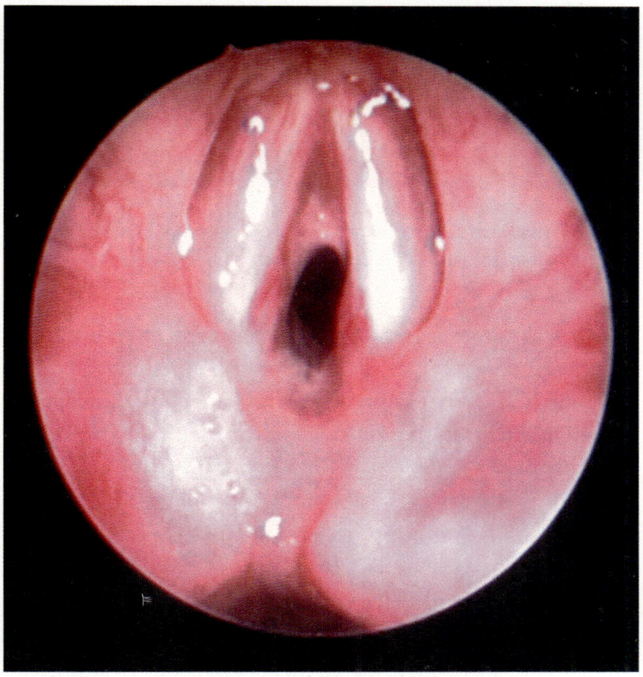

Fig. 8 Acquired subglottic stenosis in an infant with a history of prolonged intubation

Soft tissue neck radiographs, performed with high kV settings, provide information about subglottic and cervical tracheal caliber as well as the relationships of surrounding soft tissue such as the base of tongue and the retropharyngeal tissue. Such films can suggest or diagnose vallecular cysts, subglottic stenoses or masses, and retropharyngeal swellings (Fig. 10). Chest radiographs can detect pulmonary or cardiac pathology and allow a measure of tracheal size. Chest films can be the first clue to the presence of an abnormal aortic arch, a tracheal stenosis, or a cardiac or pulmonary abnormality associated with stridor (Fig. 11).

Technical issues in obtaining such films of diagnostic quality in critically ill neonates often lead to additional or alternative testing, either with endoscopy or other imaging modalities. Airway fluoroscopy can detect dynamic changes in tracheal caliber, such as the collapse of the trachea that is seen in infants with tracheomalacia. Fluoroscopy can also be used to assess diaphragm movement and to look for abnormal mediastinal shifts/pulmonary dynamics seen with bronchial obstruction from an aspirated foreign body or some other bronchial obstruction. The sensitivity and specificity of airway fluoroscopy compared to direct laryngoscopy and bronchoscopy for diagnosis of airway lesions in children have been debated [11–13]. It appears that fluoroscopy is most useful for subglottic and tracheobronchial lesions, and is less helpful for diagnosis of laryngomalacia and other pharyngeal/supraglottic pathology.

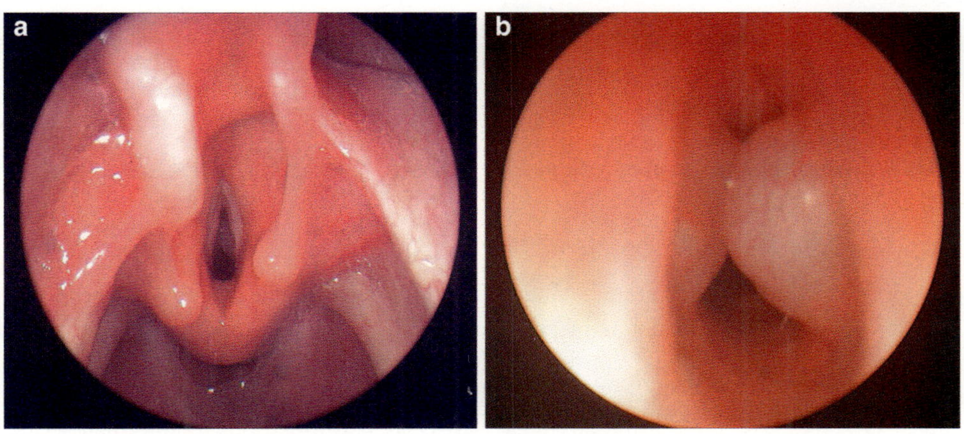

Fig. 9 Subglottic cysts viewed from (**a**) from above the vocal cords and (**b**) below the vocal cords

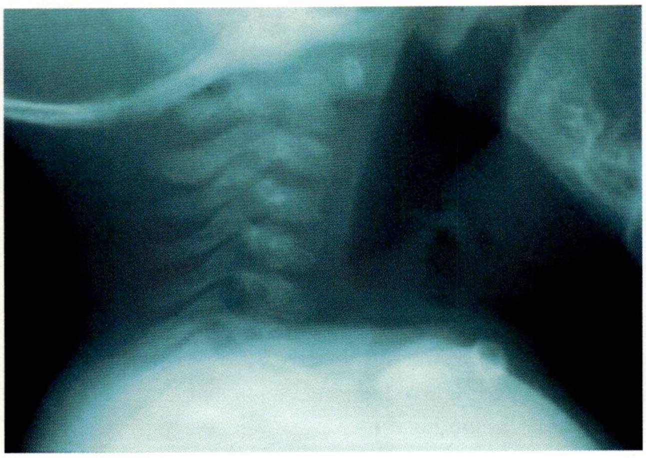

Fig. 10 Lateral neck film of an infant with a vallecular cyst causing inspiratory stridor

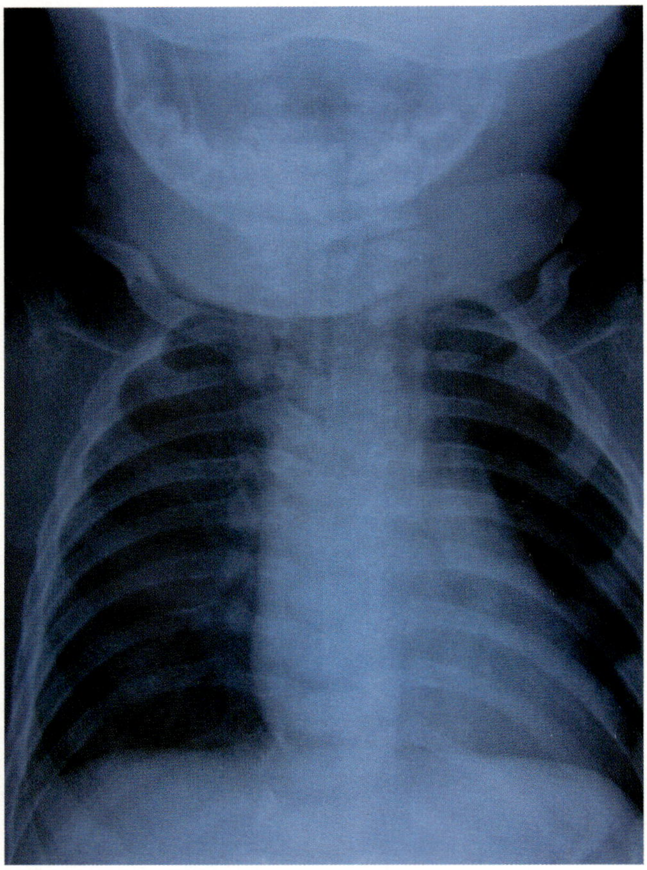

Fig. 11 Chest radiograph showing long-segment tracheal stenosis and calcification in an infant with chondrodysplasia punctata

Contrast esophagrams and modified barium swallow studies are useful studies for infants with stridor and feeding problems. The esophagrams may show focal constriction suggestive of vascular compression in the chest. The modified barium swallows can detect aspiration at the laryngeal level, or lower, that can suggest vocal cord motion impairment, laryngeal cleft, or tracheoesophageal fistula.

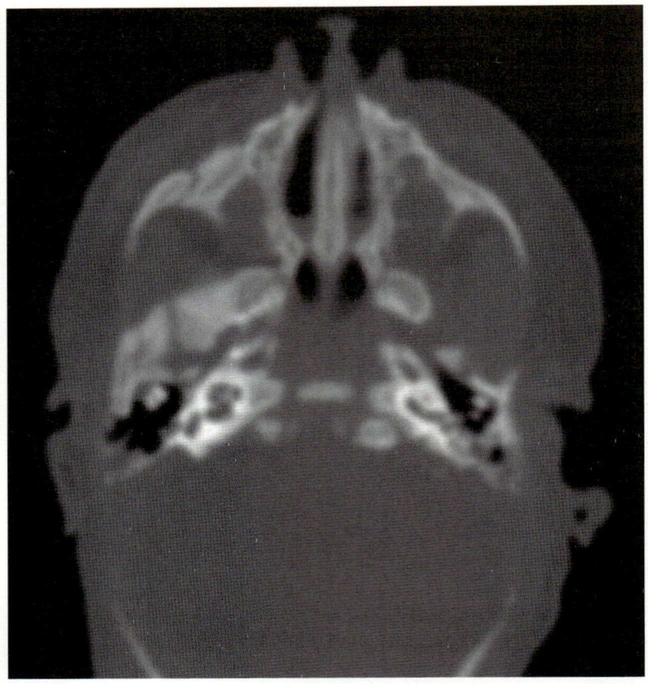

Fig. 12 Axial computed tomography showing bony bilateral choanal atresia in an infant with CHARGE syndrome

Computed tomography (CT) and magnetic resonance imaging (MRI) studies are not first-line studies for diagnosis of stridor in neonates. Computed tomography involves ionizing radiation, and magnetic resonance imaging of infants usually requires general anesthesia with airway control. Such scans should be used to detail anatomy for a diagnosis already suspected based on history, examination, and endoscopy. These scans are often used to plan therapy rather than to diagnose an airway lesion. For example, an MRI or CT angiogram may be used to detail the intrathoracic vascular anatomy when examination or endoscopy is suggestive of a vascular ring. Similarly, a neonate with nasal obstruction in the posterior nasal cavity on nasal endoscopy should undergo axial computed tomography to confirm the diagnosis of choanal atresia, determine whether the atresia plate is bony or membranous, and rule out additional craniofacial anomalies (Fig. 12).

High-resolution "spiral" CT scans can be used to create virtual endoscopic images [14]. These images may help measure tracheobronchial lesions without bronchoscopy. This can avoid multiple bronchoscopies and may be safer than bronchoscopy for infants with high-grade obstruction or long-segment tracheal stenosis. These scans can define the role of intraluminal and extrinsic components of complex airway obstruction in infants.

Imaging of the central nervous system, usually with CT or MRI, is performed when abnormalities of pharyngeal tone are seen or when vocal cord motion is impaired. Congenital bilateral vocal cord paralysis is associated with Arnold-Chiari malformation, usually diagnosed with CT or MRI. Craniofacial CT scans can be performed with reconstructions to analyze the three-dimensional anatomy of complex syndromic anomalies.

Ultrasound has been used to evaluate vocal cord motion in children as well as to study other airway lesions such as recurrent respiratory papillomatosis [15, 16]. While appealing because of the lack of ionizing radiation, this modality has a limited role for diagnosis of stridor in neonates. Ultrasound can play a role in prenatal evaluation of fetal neck masses prior to EXIT procedures and for postnatally diagnosed neck masses. Virtually all infantile neck masses that cause airway obstruction will require anatomic investigation with CT or MRI.

Other Studies for Evaluation of Infants with Stridor

Neonates with stridor may require additional testing to determine the diagnosis of the primary airway lesion, to assess the severity of the airway obstruction, and to rule out concomitant neurologic or aerodigestive disease. Echocardiography may determine the presence of congenital cardiac anomalies, particularly in stridorous neonates with vocal cord paralysis, vascular rings, or syndromic diagnosis. Polysomnography can diagnose and quantify obstructive sleep apnea/hypopnea syndrome in young infants. These sleep studies can help assess the need for intervention for infants with craniofacial anomalies, micrognathia, or laryngomalacia. Infants who have feeding difficulties or signs of gastroesophageal reflux can benefit from specific testing for reflux, most often with esophagogastroduodenoscopy (EGD) with biopsies. EGD often can be done at the time of airway endoscopy under anesthesia.

The evaluation of stridor in young infants is often a multidisciplinary effort, requiring input from neonatologists, otolaryngologists, and pulmonary physicians. Additionally, these diagnostic approaches may require consultations with neurologists, cardiologists, and geneticists. Specific testing for defined genetic syndromes and suspected neurologic/developmental disorders may be needed for complex patients.

The Differential Diagnosis of Neonatal Stridor

This discussion of the specific disease processes and anatomic abnormalities that cause neonatal stridor is organized here anatomically, starting at the nose and mouth and proceeding through the pediatric airway is a manner similar to a well-performed airway endoscopy.

The Nose and Nasopharynx

Neonates are obligate nasal breathers, and nasal obstruction can cause inspiratory stridor, stertor, retractions, and respiratory distress that worsen with feeding. Nasolacrimal duct cysts (dacryocystoceles) arise in the inferior meatus of the nose and can block the nasal airway. While some resolve spontaneously, transnasal excision or marsupialization is curative. Piriform aperture stenosis is narrowing of the bony nasal inlet from overgrowth of the maxillary prominences; this lesion can occur with syndromes and has been associated with feeding disturbance as well as central nervous system disorders such as holoprosencephaly. This rare lesion is diagnosed by nasal endoscopy, and may require surgical drillout through a sublabial approach. Choanal atresia is a bony, membranous, or mixed blockage of the junction of nasal cavity and nasopharynx. Choanal atresia can be an isolated lesion, or in about half of cases is associated with multi-system syndromic disease such as CHARGE syndrome. When catheters cannot pass through the nose into the pharynx, this diagnosis should be confirmed by fiberoptic endoscopy and CT scan. Transnasal endoscopic repair with or without stents is the most popular surgical approach for choanal atresia.

The nasopharynx of an infant can be obstructed by unusual masses such as meningoencephaloceles and teratomas. Surgical excision is the treatment of choice, after thorough investigation of the skull base anatomy, usually with MRI.

The Pharynx and Hypopharynx

Neonatal airway obstruction at the pharyngeal and hypopharyngeal level usually involves combinations of abnormal craniofacial structure, poor neuromotor tone, or malformed/bulky pharyngeal soft tissues. Stertor, inspiratory stridor, obstructive sleep apnea, and feeding difficulties are the key features of obstruction at this level. The standard head and neck examination, fiberoptic laryngoscopy, and polysomnography are the most helpful diagnostic endeavors. A structurally normal pharynx and larynx in the presence of poor pharyngeal tone should lead to a full neurologic evaluation and perhaps central nervous system imaging. Macroglossia associated with syndromic diagnoses (Beckwith-Weidemann, Down), masses in the pharynx (lymphatic malformations, vallecular cysts), and craniofacial anomalies (Pierre-Robin triad, midfacial hypoplasia) all can cause neonatal airway obstruction. Obstruction at this level can be simple or complex, but is often multifactorial. Treatment is based on site of obstruction and severity, ranging from observation and positioning when mild to tracheotomy when severe.

Supraglottic Larynx

Inspiratory stridor is the hallmark of supraglottic obstruction. Laryngomalacia, inspiratory collapse of the supraglottic tissues, is the most common cause of neonatal stridor, causing about 60–70 % of cases. Most infants with laryngomalacia can be managed expectantly, but some severe cases are associated with obstructive sleep apnea, failure to thrive, and even ALTEs. Awake fiberoptic laryngoscopy is diagnostic, but direct laryngoscopy and bronchoscopy, or radiologic imaging, may be necessary to exclude additional airway lesions. The frequency of such secondary airway lesions is debated, with estimates between 7.5 % to more than 65 % [17]. Supraglottoplasty is an effective treatment for the subset of infants that requires intervention. Mass lesions on the epiglottis, saccular cysts, and laryngoceles may mimic laryngomalacia, but these can be distinguished by endoscopy.

The Glottis (True Vocal Cords)

Obstruction at the glottic level causes inspiratory stridor, often accompanied by abnormal cry. Vocal cord paralysis, described previously, can be unilateral or bilateral. This entity is the second most frequent cause of neonatal stridor, but the exact incidence is not known [18]. It is best diagnosed with awake fiberoptic laryngoscopy. Congenital bilateral vocal cord paralysis usually causes inspiratory stridor with severe airway obstruction at birth. Tracheotomy is often but not invariably needed. Laryngeal webs cause dysphonia and airway obstruction with severity of symptoms directly related to the extent of affected vocal folds. Neonatal stridor and hoarse cry is also seen after traumatic or prolonged endotracheal intubation, with vocal cord avulsion, glottic scarring, and secondary granulomas possible.

The Subglottis

The subglottis contains the cricoid ring, the narrowest fixed portion of the pediatric airway. This area is vulnerable to intubation trauma. Subglottic stenosis is third most common cause of neonatal stridor in most series, and presents inspiratory or biphasic stridor, signs of airway obstruction, or history of failed extubation. Acquired subglottic stenosis after intubation can range in extent, and severe cases can include vocal cord motion impairment from posterior glottis fixation. Congenital subglottic stenosis is usually associated with an elliptically shaped cricoid cartilage or an abnormal relation of the cricoid with the first tracheal ring. Other subglottic lesions that cause neonatal airway obstruction are subglottic cysts, usually associated with prior intubation, and subglottic hemangioma. While subglottic lesions can occasionally be seen with awake fiberoptic laryngoscopy, direct laryngoscopy under general anesthesia is the diagnostic procedure of choice for visualization of lesions and assessment of severity.

Trachea

Intrinsic and extrinsic lesions can narrow the trachea of the neonate and cause expiratory stridor that is sometimes low-pitched or goose-like. The presence of such stridor in the face of a normal laryngeal examination should initiate either radiologic studies or direct laryngoscopy and bronchoscopy to fully assess tracheal caliber and function. Tracheomalacia is a dynamic narrowing of the trachea, and it is often associated with extrinsic tracheal compression such as a vascular ring, tracheoesophageal fistula, abnormal chest anatomy, or an enlarged heart. Intrinsic cartilage abnormalities can also cause tracheomalacia. Tracheomalacia is best diagnosed using flexible bronchoscopy during spontaneous respiration.

Tracheal stenosis can vary in both severity of the narrowing and the length of affected trachea; severe lesions may require extensive open surgery with slide tracheoplasty, the most widely performed procedure. Initial work-up should include radiographic imaging, from chest radiographs to spiral CT scans, followed by diagnostic bronchoscopy. Tracheal compression from vascular rings include the double aortic arch (50–60 % of rings) and the right aortic arch with aberrant left subclavian artery and ligamentum arteriosum (12–25 % of rings) [19]. Vascular compression of the trachea can cause neonatal stridor that often does not immediately improve with surgical division of the ring, as the secondary tracheomalacia can take months to resolve. Vascular compression is suspected by echocardiography or bronchoscopy, but precise anatomic features are confirmed by CT angiography or MRI/MR angiography.

Conclusion

Stridor in the neonate can be a sign of a self-limited innocuous problem, like mild laryngomalacia, or it may be the clue to the presence of severe or progressive life-threatening airway obstruction, like long-segment tracheal stenosis. The features of the stridor, the associated symptoms and signs, and examination of a keen observer should focus the subsequent evaluation (Table 1). A focused history and examination should suggest the site of airway obstruction in the noisy infant, and selected endoscopic evaluation and imaging should confirm the precise airway diagnosis.

Table 1 Neonatal stridor: diagnostic tips and tests

Diagnosis/airway lesion	Clinical scenario	Best diagnostic procedure	Additional diagnostic tests	Treatment options
Laryngomalacia	High-pitched inspiratory stridor worse when active, supine	Fiberoptic laryngoscopy	Imaging or direct laryngoscopy/bronchoscopy to rule out second lesions	Observation
				Supraglottoplasty
			Swallowing evaluation	GERD management
			Polysomnography	
Vocal cord paralysis (unilateral)	Inspiratory stridor	Fiberoptic laryngoscopy	Echocardiogram	Observe
	Hoarse cry		MRI	Medialization or reinnervation if persistent
	History of neck/chest surgery			
Vocal cord paralysis (bilateral)	Severe inspiratory stridor at birth	Fiberoptic laryngoscopy	MRI or other CNS imaging	Observe
	Respiratory distress			Tracheotomy
	Normal cry			Cordotomy, arytenoidectomy, or lateralization if persistent
Subglottic stenosis	Inspiratory or biphasic stridor	Direct laryngoscopy/bronchoscopy		Observation
				Dilation
	History of intubation (acquired)			Airway expansion surgery
Subglottic cyst	Inspiratory or biphasic stridor	Direct laryngoscopy/bronchoscopy		Excise or marsupialize cysts endoscopically
	History of intubation			
Subglottic hemangioma	Biphasic stridor at 1–2 months of age	Direct laryngoscopy/bronchoscopy		Propranolol
	Barky cough			Steroids (systemic/intralesional)
	Recurrent croup			Excision (endoscopic > open)
Glottic web	Abnormal cry	Fiberoptic laryngoscopy	Testing for velocardiofacial syndrome	Observation
	Inspiratory stridor variable based on extent of web		Direct laryngoscopy/bronchoscopy	Endoscopic division
				Open repair for severe cases
Craniofacial abnormalities such as Pierre-Robin triad	Stertor or inspiratory stridor	Examination of head and neck	Polysomnography	Positioning
	Obstructive sleep apnea	Fiberoptic exam from nose to glottis	Craniofacial CT scan (3-D reconstruction)	Artificial airways
				Mandibular distraction and other procedures
				Tracheotomy
Tracheomalacia	Expiratory stridor	Flexible bronchoscopy	Airway fluoroscopy	Observation
			Direct laryngoscopy/bronchoscopy	Treat any extrinsic tracheal compression
				Aortopexy or tracheotomy/CPAP for severe cases
Vascular rings	Expiratory Stridor	CT angiogram or MRI/MRA chest	Direct laryngoscopy/bronchoscopy	Surgical division of the ring
	Apneic spells			
	Feeding difficulties		Echocardiogram	

References

1. Berkowitz RG. Neonatal upper airway assessment by awake flexible laryngoscopy. Ann Otol Rhinol Laryngol. 1998;107:75–80.
2. Kelly SM, April MM, Tunkel DE. Obstructing laryngeal granuloma after brief endotracheal intubation in neonates. Otolaryngol Head Neck Surg. 1996;115:138–40.
3. Hartl TT, Chadha NK. A systematic review of laryngomalacia and acide reflux. Otolaryngol Head Neck Surg. 2012;147:619–26.
4. Bajaj Y, Kapoor K, Jephson CG, Albert DM, Harper JI, Hartley BE. Great Ormond Street Hospital treatment guidelines for use of propranolol in infantile isolated subglottic hemangioma. J Laryngol Otol. 2013;127:295–8.
5. Khariwala SS, Lee WT, Koltai PJ. Laryngotracheal consequences of pediatric cardiac surgery. Arch Otolaryngol Head Neck Surg. 2005;131(4):336–9.
6. Schumacher RE, Weinfeld IJ, Bartlett RH. Neonatal vocal cord paralysis following extracorporeal membrane oxygenation. Pediatrics. 1989;84:793–6.
7. Smith ME, King JD, Elsherif A, Muntz HR, Park AH, Kouretas PC. Should all newborns who undergo patent ductus arteriosus ligation be examined for vocal fold mobility. Laryngoscope. 2009;119:1606–9.
8. Zoumalan R, Maddalozzo J, Holinger LD. Etiology of stridor in infants. Ann Otol Rhinol Laryngol. 2007;116:329–34.
9. Chiou HL, Diaz R, Orlino E, Poulain FR. Acute airway obstruction by a sheared endotracheal intubation stylet sheath in a premature infant. J Perinatol. 2007;27:727–9.
10. Goske MJ, Applegate KE, Boylan J, Butler PF, et al. The *Image Gently* Campaign: working together to change practice. Am J Roentgenol. 2008;190:273–4.
11. Rudman DT, Elmaraghy CA, Shiel WE, Wiet GJ. The role of fluoroscopy in the evaluation of stridor in children. Arch Otolaryngol Head Neck Surg. 2003;129:305–9.
12. Berg E, Naseri I, Sobol SE. The role of airway fluoroscopy in the evaluation of children with stridor. Arch Otolaryngol Head Neck Surg. 2008;134:415–8.
13. Huntley C, Carr MM. Evaluation of the effectiveness of airway fluoroscopy in diagnosing patients with laryngomalacia. Laryngoscope. 2010;120:1430–4.
14. Triglia JM, Nazarian B, Sudre-Levillain I, Marciano S, Moulin G, Giovanni A. Virtual laryngotracheal endoscopy based on geometric surface modeling using spiral computed tomography data. Ann Otol Rhinol Laryngol. 2002;111:36–43.
15. Friedman EM. Role of ultrasound in the assessment of vocal cord function in infants and children. Ann Otol Rhinol Laryngol. 1997;106:199–209.
16. Bryson PC, Leight WD, Zdanski CJ, Drake AF, Rose AS. High resolution ultrasound in the evaluation of recurrent respiratory papillomatosis. Arch Otolaryngol Head Neck Surg. 2009;135:250–3.
17. Thompson DM. Laryngomalacia: factors that influence disease severity and outcomes of management. Curr Opin Otolaryngol Head Neck Surg. 2010;18:564–70.
18. King EF, Blumin JH. Vocal cord paralysis in children. Curr Opin Otolaryngol Head Neck Surg. 2009;17:483–7.
19. Kussman BD, Geva T, McGowan FX. Cardiovascular causes of airway compression. Pediatr Anesth. 2004;14:60–74.

Advances in Radiologic Imaging of Neonatal Airway Disorders

Jessica Kurian, David A. Mong, and Monica Epelman

Introduction

Radiology of the airways in newborns and infants is challenging due the small size of their anatomy, their inability to follow breathing instructions, and the concern for long-term effects of radiation exposure. While some patients can be managed with observation or empiric therapy, for other patients the diagnosis may remain uncertain, and imaging is an essential part of management. Radiology serves to detect airway abnormalities, guide therapy, assist with preoperative planning, and help avoid invasive testing. A combination of static and dynamic imaging provides both structural and physiologic information about airway lesions. A variety of imaging modalities is available, but multidetector computed tomography (CT) provides the highest yield of information, and in recent times it became the preferred choice for evaluation of the large airways [1, 2]. This chapter will provide an overview of radiology of the neonatal airway, including available imaging methods, and typical imaging features of specific airway disorders.

Imaging Approach

In neonates with suspected airway disease, a systematic imaging approach begins with conventional radiographs of the neck and chest, which can be performed rapidly and help exclude gross abnormalities. After conventional radiography, further imaging is tailored to the clinical scenario. Airway fluoroscopy is used for real-time observation of the airways in evaluation of tracheobronchomalacia [3]. Contrast esophagogram also uses a fluoroscopic technique, but with oral ingestion of radiopaque material (barium) to assess for esophageal-related disorders such as aspiration, tracheoesophageal fistula (TEF), or vascular ring.

For neonates who require evaluation beyond conventional radiography or fluoroscopy, cross-sectional methods (CT and magnetic resonance imaging (MRI)) offer advanced anatomic imaging. CT is superb for rapid evaluation of the airways, lungs, and mediastinal structures. MRI is also a powerful modality that provides similar information to CT, but it may need use of sedation or general anesthesia, which can be challenging in neonates with airway compromise. Unlike radiography, fluoroscopy, and CT, MRI does not use ionizing radiation.

The following sections of this chapter describe each of these modalities in greater detail.

Imaging Techniques

Chest Radiograph

Conventional radiographs are first-line for imaging airway diseases in neonates. They are relatively cheap and easily accessible, and can be performed as a portable exam in the neonatal intensive care unit. Radiographs of the chest and neck are performed in frontal (anterior–posterior or posterior–anterior) and lateral projections. For assessment of the neck and upper thoracic airway, magnification with a high kilovoltage (kV) selective filter is used [4]. This method decreases overlying bony shadows and improves visualization of the airway. It is important to ensure that the patient is correctly positioned without flexion or rotation, which can affect accuracy of interpretation. Bilateral decubitus views (or in older children, inspiratory and expiratory views) is sometimes helpful

J. Kurian, M.D. (✉)
Department of Radiology, Montefiore Medical Center, Albert Einstein College of Medicine, Bronx, NY, USA
e-mail: jessica_kurian@yahoo.com

D.A. Mong
Department of Radiology, The Children's Hospital of Philadelphia, 34th Street and Civic Center Boulevard, Philadelphia, PA 19104

University of Pennsylvania, Perelman School of Medicine, Philadelphia, PA, USA

M. Epelman, M.D.
Department of Radiology, Nemours Children's Hospital, University of Central Florida and Florida State University, 13535 Nemours Parkway, Suite 0305, Orlando, FL, USA

J. Lioy and S.E. Sobol (eds.), *Disorders of the Neonatal Airway: Fundamentals for Practice*, DOI 10.1007/978-1-4939-1610-8_20, © Springer Science+Business Media New York 2015

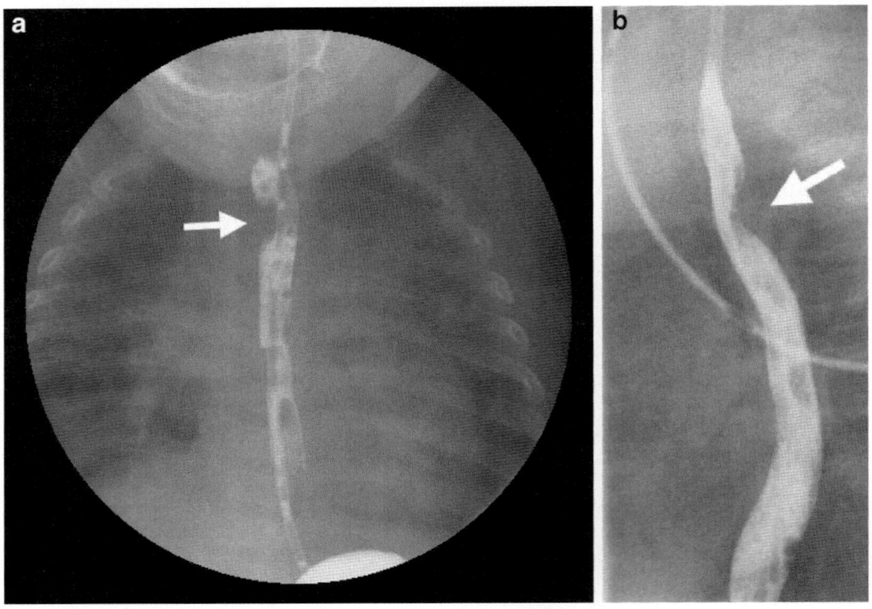

Fig. 1 Frontal view (**a**) from a contrast esophagogram shows a smooth round impression on the right side of the upper esophagus due to a right aortic arch (*arrow*). On the lateral view (**b**) there is a posterior impression on the esophagus due to an aberrant left subclavian artery (*arrow*). These findings constitute a vascular ring

in detecting unilateral air-trapping secondary to bronchial obstruction from foreign body aspiration [3, 5], but has limited utility in the neonatal age group. In general, radiographs are a useful screening tool, and serve to rapidly assess for major abnormalities (e.g., masses, mediastinal shift). However, because radiographs are a planar rather than cross-sectional technique, anatomic detail is limited compared to other types of imaging or compared to direct visualization [5, 6].

Airway Fluoroscopy

Unlike a static chest radiograph, airway fluoroscopy is a dynamic exam, during which the airway is observed typically in frontal and lateral projections throughout the respiratory cycle. Change in caliber or collapse of the airway indicates malacia. During fluoroscopy, the lung fields can also be observed for expiratory air-trapping, and the motion of the diaphragm can be assessed. Abnormal findings on fluoroscopy are specific for diagnosis of laryngomalacia, tracheomalacia, airway stenosis, and even airway masses [7]. However, airway fluoroscopy has extremely variable sensitivities reported for most common neonatal airway diseases, especially glottic or supraglottic lesions [7, 8]. Thus, patients with negative fluoroscopy may require further investigation with other imaging modalities, or with airway endoscopy.

Contrast Esophagography

Fluoroscopic contrast exam of the esophagus (contrast esophagography) is helpful in diagnosis of certain airway-related disorders such as TEF, aspiration, and gastroesophageal reflux.

During a contrast esophagogram, barium is used to opacify the esophagus while the esophagus is observed fluoroscopically in real-time. If needed, this exam can be performed in conjunction with airway fluoroscopy while the patient is in the radiology department. The motility, caliber, and contour of the esophagus are examined in multiple projections, while looking for extrinsic compression that may indicate a vascular ring (Fig. 1a, b). Contrast is administered orally via a baby bottle, or if necessary a catheter-tipped syringe. In small or critically ill neonates, more precise and controlled administration is obtained by injecting contrast through a feeding tube, which is then slowly withdrawn along the length of the esophagus. This method is especially important for demonstrating TEFs [9]. Barium is the preferred contrast agent for fluoroscopic exam of the esophagus, although in select cases such as postoperative patients, a water soluble contrast agent should be used.

Due to the complexity of its mechanism, swallowing is not thoroughly evaluated on a routine esophagogram or upper GI series. Swallowing dysfunction is better assessed with a modified barium swallow (MBS), during which the infant is fed in a semiupright position using barium-impregnated materials of various textures. These exams are recorded in real-time for later playback and detailed review. The MBS is useful for detecting laryngeal penetration and aspiration, and to aid in formulation of feeding plans.

Computed Tomography

Advantages

Recent technologic advances have allowed multidetector CT to become a powerful tool for imaging of the airways in small patients. Unlike bronchoscopy, CT is noninvasive, and can evaluate both the airway wall and the surrounding structures, rather than just the mucosal surface. Also unlike bronchoscopy, CT can demonstrate synchronous airway lesions, as well as demonstrate the distal effects of airway obstruction such as air-trapping and atelectasis [10]. CT offers numerous advantages over other imaging modalities, including a rapid acquisition time, decreased need for sedation, large field of coverage, high spatial resolution, and the ability to generate two-dimensional (2D) and three-dimensional (3D) reformatted images [2]. In addition, paired inspiratory–expiratory imaging and cine imaging can be performed using CT [2].

Technique

Unlike the simple conventional radiographic techniques described earlier, patient preparation is important in CT for maximizing image quality. With the large number of CT detectors available in modern machines, scanning times are relatively fast (in the order of seconds), and the majority of neonates do not require general anesthesia with intubation. Light sedation is recommended for CT exams in older infants [2], which will minimize motion artifact, but still allow the patient to independently maintain an airway.

For patients with suspected tracheobronchomalacia who require both inspiratory and expiratory phase CT, controlled ventilation techniques should be used. In intubated patients, positive pressure is applied during inspiration, and pressure is withheld during expiration [2]. In this way, the patient can be scanned first in "end-inspiration" and then in "end-expiration." In sedated non-intubated patients, hypocarbia can be induced by augmenting inspiration through a face-mask. This results in a short apneic period (via the "Hering-Breuer reflex") during which the patient is scanned at the desired degree of airway distention [10]. In patients for whom a controlled ventilation technique is not feasible, cine CT can be performed by rapidly acquiring axial images at specified levels, with the scan being performed throughout a free breathing respiratory cycle.

Because of the inherent contrast between the airways and soft tissue structures, routine CT evaluation of the airways does not require intravenous (IV) contrast. However in the absence of a specific indication or a previously known airway diagnosis, IV contrast should be used to define the mediastinal structures, and to assess for vascular anomalies such as rings or slings [2]. Note that prior to contrast-enhanced CT, patients must be thoroughly screened for risk factors for adverse reactions to contrast media, including contrast nephropathy and anaphylaxis. The recommended type of contrast material is a nonionic low-osmolar formulation, and the volume administered is calculated based on patient weight (typically 2 cm^3/kg) [2]. The preferred method of contrast administration is through a mechanical power injector. For infants with smaller caliber catheters or central venous lines, contrast can be administered manually ("hand injection") [2].

Technical parameters for performing neonatal chest CT vary by scanner type. In general, the machine with greatest number of CT detectors is best, and the minimum suggested number is 16 detectors. In accordance with the ALARA principle (As Low As Reasonably Achievable), radiation exposure to the patient should be minimized by adjusting CT parameters (milliamperage, kilovoltage) appropriately for the patient's age and weight. Ultra-low radiation dose techniques can still provide high quality, diagnostic CT images of the airways [1, 2, 11]. In patients requiring paired inspiratory–expiratory CT, the second (expiratory) series can be performed using even further dose reduction, without affecting diagnostic confidence [11].

Image Analysis

The first step in interpretation of airway CT is review of the source (axial plane) images. Following this, the radiologist performs several post-processing steps using a specialized workstation, in order to fully understand the nature and extent of the airway lesion, and to define complex anatomy.

2D reconstruction techniques include curved planar reformatting (CPR), in which images can be created as reformations of the curve along the axis of the airway. This allows accurate airway length measurements, which can be used for treatment planning. Another 2D reconstruction technique is minimum intensity projection (MinIP) reformatting, in which images are formed by projecting the voxels with lowest attenuation (e.g., those in air-filled structures such as the airways and lungs). This enhances visibility of the tracheobronchial tree and lung parenchyma [2].

The key 3D reconstruction method used for airway evaluation is volume rendering. In this method, a computer algorithm detects the edges of the airway wall and creates a surface rendering. An external rendering ("virtual bronchography") allows one to view the outer surface of the airway wall, and its relationship to surrounding structures. An internal rendering ("virtual bronchoscopy") allows one to view the inner lumen of the airway, which mimics conventional/direct bronchoscopy. These methods are extremely useful for depicting complex anatomic relationships in three dimensions. Volume rendering provides life-like images, which may preclude the need for conventional bronchoscopy [2, 5] (Fig. 2a).

Magnetic Resonance Imaging

Like CT, MRI is a cross-sectional imaging modality which can provide information about the airway and mediastinal vessels. The major advantages of MRI are its lack of ionizing radiation, high soft tissue contrast, and the ability to image in multiple planes without changing the position of the patient. Cardiovascular MRI has excellent accuracy in diagnosis of vascular anomalies that cause airway compromise [12].

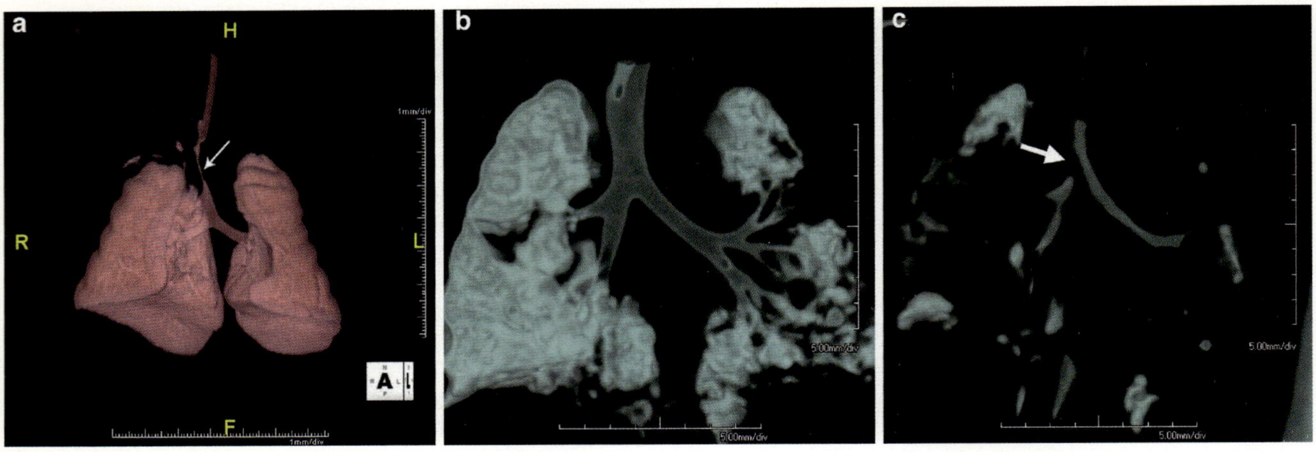

Fig. 2 (**a**) shows CT 3D colorful reconstruction of an infant with long-segment tracheal stenosis previously unrecognized on conventional radiologic modalities. Volume renderings of the airways in a different infant in both inspiratory (**b**) and expiratory (**c**) phases demonstrate diffuse decrease in caliber of the tracheobronchial tree during expiration. There is complete expiratory collapse at the origin of the right mainstem bronchus (*arrow*)

These exams are targeted to evaluation of the heart and major vessels using ECG-gated sequences, as well gadolinium contrast-enhanced angiographic sequences. MRI also has the capability for dynamic ("cine") image acquisition. In current practice, cine MRI is primarily used to evaluate airway motion during sleep studies in older children with suspected obstructive sleep apnea, as well as patients with glossoptosis and hypopharyngeal collapse [5]. Cine imaging is also used in some centers for assessing lung, chest wall, and diaphragm motion in patients with thoracic insufficiency syndrome [1].

There are some disadvantages of MRI which limit its utility in the neonatal age group. Depending on the clinical indication, current MRI protocols may require scan time of up to 30–60 min, and the majority of infants will require sedation or cardiac anesthesia [3]. In young infants (usually less than 6 months old), a "feed and swaddle" method can be attempted, and may obviate the need for anesthesia or deep sedation [12]. Evaluation of the lung parenchyma on MRI is limited due to artifacts from air-tissue interface susceptibility, as well as respiratory and cardiac motion. However, newer techniques such as respiratory triggering, respiratory gating, and motion-insensitive sequences have enhanced the pulmonary imaging capability of MRI. MRI technology is a rapidly evolving field, and future improvement of scan time and image quality will make this a valuable modality for assessment of the neonatal airway.

Fetal Imaging

Although this text is focused on postnatal imaging of the neonatal airway, awareness of fetal imaging is also important for all clinicians involved with management of prenatally diagnosed airway lesions. Airway lesions for which fetal imaging is critical include neck masses (e.g., vascular malformations, teratomas) and congenital high airway obstruction syndrome (CHAOS) [10, 13]. Fetal ultrasound (US) and MRI are used in complement to assess these obstructive airway lesions prior to delivery, and to help determine the need for an ex utero intrapartum therapy (EXIT) procedure.

Fetal US is a real-time examination which allows direct observation of swallowing and respiration, and Doppler US is used for evaluation of vascular structures. Fetal MRI has the added ability to examine the fetus in a large field of view and in multiple planes. MRI is superior to US for soft tissue contrast, characterization of masses and their effect on the airway, and for evaluation of cartilaginous structures such as the oropharynx and nasopharynx [13]. Both modalities are necessary for complete assessment of fetal airway compromise, and for guiding management decisions.

Imaging Features of Specific Neonatal Airway Disorders

Tracheobronchomalacia

TBM of the trachea and mainstem bronchi can be visualized on airway fluoroscopy, but at times the diagnosis is difficult, or the underlying cause cannot be determined. In these patients CT is helpful for more complete evaluation, and is especially useful for evaluating caliber of airways distal to the mainstem bronchi. Since TBM can be missed on static CT images, an additional expiratory series is typically performed to assess for change in size of the tracheobronchial tree (Fig. 2b, c). The criteria for diagnosis of TBM on CT is

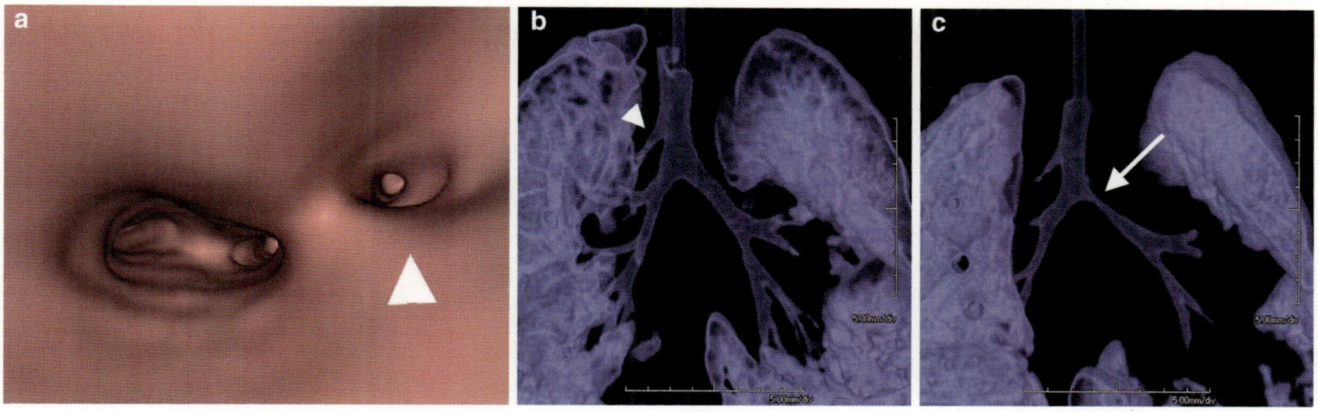

Fig. 3 Internal (**a**) and external (**b**, **c**) volume renderings from an airway CT show an anomalous right upper lobe bronchus arising from the right lateral wall of the trachea (*arrowhead*), consistent with a tracheal bronchus. On the expiratory image (**c**), there is diffuse decrease in caliber of the airways consistent with bronchomalacia, particularly affecting the left mainstem bronchus (*arrow*), and most of the bilateral segmental bronchi

the reduction of airway cross-sectional area by 50 % or more, and this criteria has been shown to be concordant with bronchoscopy results [14]. Cine (4D) CT can depict airway collapsibility in real-time, and is best performed on CT machines with 64 or more detectors [15].

In addition to identifying the presence, location, and severity of airway malacia, CT provides information about predisposing conditions, and offers quantitative measures for preoperative planning. CT also depicts the distribution of expiratory air-trapping and inspiratory alveolar recruitment [16].

Congenital Malformations

Branching Anomalies

There are multiple variant branching patterns of the tracheobronchial tree. Some of the most common are ectopic bronchi, supernumerary bronchi, and tracheal diverticulum [2, 17]. These variants are uncommon and usually found incidentally, but rarely they are responsible for air-trapping, recurrent atelectasis, repeated infections, and aspiration [18]. The most well-known ectopic bronchus is the tracheal bronchus ("bronchial suis" or pig bronchus), which is a small upper lobe bronchus that arises from the lateral wall of the trachea above the carina (Fig. 3a–c). A tracheal diverticulum is a congenital outpouching which arises from the posterolateral wall of the trachea near the thoracic inlet, and has a narrow neck [5]. Acquired tracheal diverticulum may be posttraumatic or due to increased transluminal pressure, and usually have a wide neck [5, 19].

Ectopic bronchi and supernumerary bronchi are small in caliber, and tracheal diverticula usually have a very small communication to the airway. CT is useful for identifying these small structures, which can be missed endoscopically.

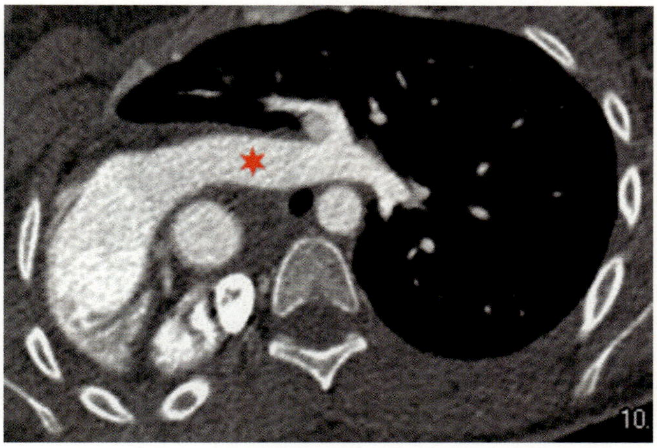

Fig. 4 Axial CT shows dextroposition of the heart. The left pulmonary artery is shown (*), but there is agenesis of the right pulmonary artery. The right lung is congenitally absent

Developmental Anomalies

The spectrum of congenital bronchial underdevelopment includes bronchial agenesis, bronchial aplasia, and bronchial hypoplasia. These anomalies range from complete absence of the bronchus, lung, and pulmonary vasculature (bronchial agenesis), to a small lung with a rudimentary bronchus and variable vascular supply (bronchial aplasia or hypoplasia). A developmental airway anomaly is suggested on a chest radiograph that demonstrates a unilateral opaque lung and ipsilateral mediastinal shift. CT offers more specificity for the diagnosis, by depicting the presence and size of the large airways, the quantity and quality of the lung parenchyma, and size of the pulmonary vessels [2, 14, 20] (Fig. 4).

Congenital Stenoses

Congenital tracheal stenosis is caused by complete or near-complete cartilaginous tracheal rings [10]. Congenital stenosis can be focal/segmental, diffuse, or funnel shaped [5].

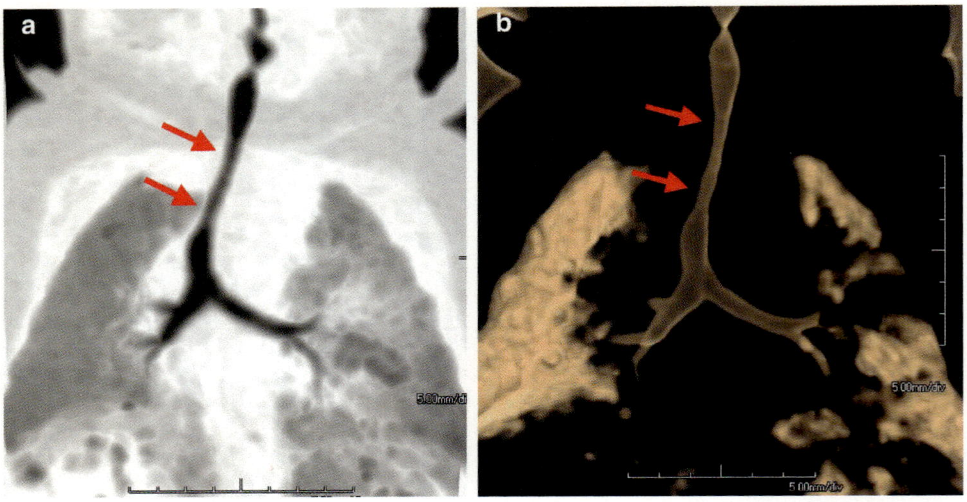

Fig. 5 Coronal minimum intensity projection image (MinIP) (**a**) and 3D volume rendered image (**b**) from an airway CT show an approximately 2 cm-long concentric stenosis (*arrows*) of the trachea. At bronchoscopy, complete tracheal rings were identified

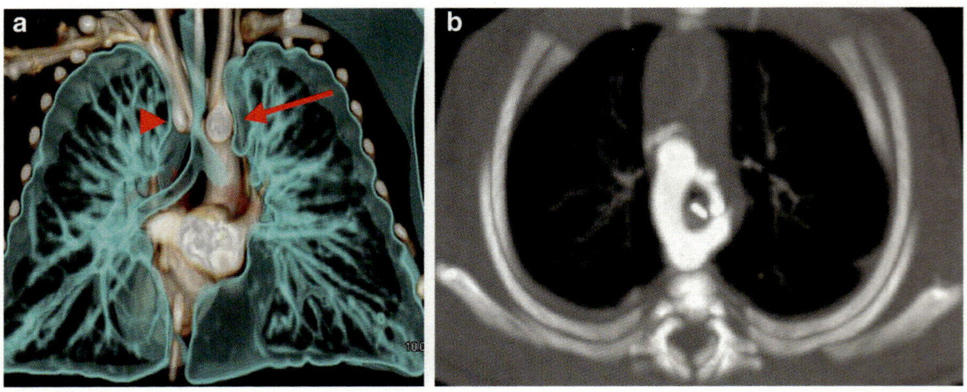

Fig. 6 Posterior view from an external CT rendering of the vessels and airways (**a**) shows a double aortic arch, with a dominant right arch (*arrow*) and smaller left arch (*arrowhead*). There is circumferential narrowing of the trachea at this level. The axial maximum intensity projection (MIP) CT image (**b**) shows how the double arch forms a ring that encircles both the trachea and the esophagus

While tracheal stenosis can be visualized on chest radiographs or airway fluoroscopy, CT is the mainstay for imaging diagnosis (Fig. 5a, b). CT is a powerful tool for surgical planning, in its ability to characterize the location and extent of disease, and provide precise measurement of airway dimensions. The imaging findings of congenital tracheal stenosis include circumferential narrowing of the trachea, often with an "O" shape on axial CT images due to the absence of the posterior membranous wall [10]. CT is also useful for identifying cardiovascular anomalies associated with tracheal stenosis, such as pulmonary sling.

Vascular Compression

Vascular anomalies of the mediastinum can cause extrinsic compression of the airway, and many are also associated with tracheomalacia. Vascular rings result from abnormal fusion or regression of primitive structures during formation of the aortic arch, pulmonary arteries, and ductus arteriosis [10]. The most common vascular rings are a right aortic arch with an aberrant left subclavian artery, and a double aortic arch (Fig. 6a, b). Pulmonary artery sling causes external narrowing of the distal trachea and the esophagus, and is also associated with complete tracheal rings [2] (Fig. 7a, b). Other vascular causes of airway compression include innominate artery compression syndrome and congenital absence of the pulmonary valve.

Signs of a vascular ring on conventional radiographs include leftward deviation of the trachea due to a right aortic arch, or bilateral tracheal indentation due to a double aortic arch. Both of these types of rings may cause anterior tracheal displacement on the lateral chest radiograph. Vascular rings also cause extrinsic compression of the esophagus that can be visualized on a contrast esophagogram (Fig. 1a, b).

While chest radiograph and esophagram findings may be suggestive of a vascular ring, they cannot reliable distinguish between different types of rings, and additional imaging with

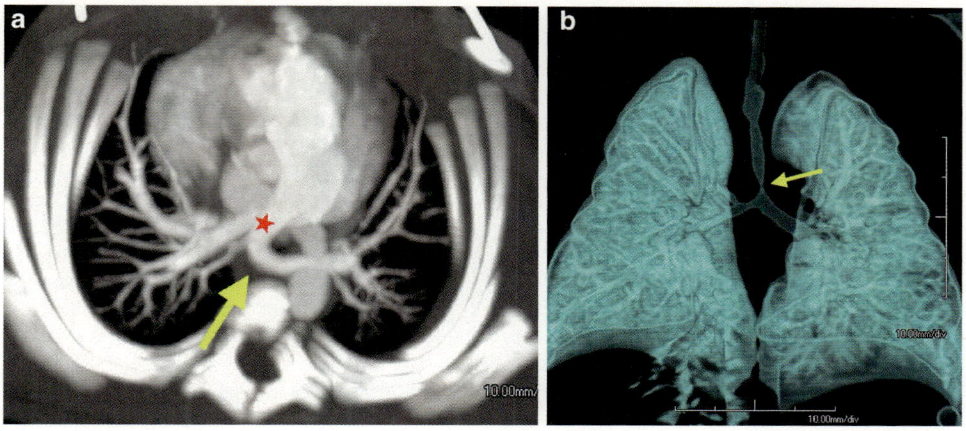

Fig. 7 Axial MIP (**a**) from a CT shows the left main pulmonary artery (*arrow*) arising from the right main pulmonary artery (*). CT 3D volume-rendered image of the airways (**b**) illustrates the associated large airway abnormalities: A flattened carina, and tight narrowing of the lower trachea at the level of the sling (*arrow*)

CT or MRI is necessary for accurate diagnosis [10, 20]. CT or MRI serves to delineate the anatomy of the mediastinum and help plan the surgical approach. For example, in double aortic arch, the position of the smaller arch must be visualized in order to determine the side of thoracotomy (Fig. 6a). The choice between CT and MRI in diagnosis of vascular ring depends on the individual case; the patient's clinical status and need for sedation must be considered. Compared to MRI, CT has the added benefits of improving visualization of the airways and lung fields, and identifying concomitant tracheobronchomalacia [21].

Acquired Abnormalities

Post-instrumentation

Tracheobronchial stenoses can be acquired in neonates after instrumentation or surgery [5]. The majority of these stenoses are located at the site of an endotracheal tube balloon or tracheostomy stoma [5]. The CT findings of acquired stenosis include focal narrowing of the proximal trachea, associated with soft tissue thickening of the tracheal wall due to intimal hyperplasia [2]. When compared to bronchoscopy, CT is 89 % sensitive in diagnosis of post-intubation tracheal stenosis [22]. As with congenital tracheal stenosis, CT depicts the location and extent of disease for planning of surgical resection or stenting.

Conclusion

Radiology is an essential component in diagnosis and management of neonatal airway disorders. Communication between the pediatrician and radiologist is important in order to tailor the diagnostic imaging approach to the specific clinical scenario. A variety of modern imaging techniques are available to provide both structural and physiologic information about the tracheobronchial tree, mediastinum, and lung parenchyma. Of these, multidetector CT approaches the gold standard of bronchoscopy, with the added benefit of being noninvasive. Advances in MRI also make it a useful option in airway imaging while eliminating the risk of radiation exposure. For all types of airway imaging, careful attention should be paid to adequate patient preparation, and the need for sedation or anesthesia should be considered.

References

1. Lee EY, Zucker EJ, Restrepo R, Daltro P, Boiselle PM. Advanced large airway CT imaging in children: evolution from axial to 4-D assessment. Pediatr Radiol. 2013;43(3):285–97. doi:10.1007/s00247-012-2470-7. PubMed PMID: 23417254.
2. Lee EY, Greenberg SB, Boiselle PM. Multidetector computed tomography of pediatric large airway diseases: state-of-the-art. Radiol Clin North Am. 2011;49(5):869–93. doi:10.1016/j.rcl.2011.06.006. PubMed PMID: 21889013.
3. Laya BF, Lee EY. Congenital causes of upper airway obstruction in pediatric patients: updated imaging techniques and review of imaging findings. Semin Roentgenol. 2012;47(2):147–58. doi:10.1053/j.ro.2011.11.006. PubMed PMID: 22370193.
4. Slovis TL. Noninvasive evaluation of the pediatric airway: a recent advance. Pediatrics. 1977;59(6):872–80. PubMed PMID: 865939.
5. Lee EY, Restrepo R, Dillman JR, Ridge CA, Hammer MR, Boiselle PM. Imaging evaluation of pediatric trachea and bronchi: systematic review and updates. Semin Roentgenol. 2012;47(2):182–96. doi:10.1053/j.ro.2011.12.002. PubMed PMID: 22370196.
6. Assefa D, Amin N, Stringel G, Dozor AJ. Use of decubitus radiographs in the diagnosis of foreign body aspiration in young children. Pediatr Emerg Care. 2007;23(3):154–7. doi:10.1097/PEC.0b013e3180328cd8. PubMed PMID: 17413429.
7. Rudman DT, Elmaraghy CA, Shiels WE, Wiet GJ. The role of airway fluoroscopy in the evaluation of stridor in children. Arch Otolaryngol Head Neck Surg. 2003;129(3):305–9. PubMed PMID: 12622539.

8. Berg E, Naseri I, Sobol SE. The role of airway fluoroscopy in the evaluation of children with stridor. Arch Otolaryngol Head Neck Surg. 2008;134(4):415–8. doi:10.1001/archotol.134.4.415. PubMed PMID: 18427008.
9. Beasley SW, Myers NA. The diagnosis of congenital tracheoesophageal fistula. J Pediatr Surg. 1988;23(5):415–7. PubMed PMID: 3379546.
10. Yedururi S, Guillerman RP, Chung T, Braverman RM, Dishop MK, Giannoni CM, et al. Multimodality imaging of tracheobronchial disorders in children. Radiographics. 2008;28(3):e29. doi:10.1148/rg.e29. PubMed PMID: 18299559.
11. Lee EY, Strauss KJ, Tracy DA, Bastos M, Zurakowski D, Boiselle PM. Comparison of standard-dose and reduced-dose expiratory MDCT techniques for assessment of tracheomalacia in children. Acad Radiol. 2010;17(4):504–10. doi:10.1016/j.acra.2009.11.014. PubMed PMID: 20207318.
12. Fogel MA, Pawlowski TW, Harris MA, Whitehead KK, Keller MS, Wilson J, et al. Comparison and usefulness of cardiac magnetic resonance versus computed tomography in infants six months of age or younger with aortic arch anomalies without deep sedation or anesthesia. Am J Cardiol. 2011;108(1):120–5. doi:10.1016/j.amjcard.2011.03.008. PubMed PMID: 21679782.
13. Dighe MK, Peterson SE, Dubinsky TJ, Perkins J, Cheng E. EXIT procedure: technique and indications with prenatal imaging parameters for assessment of airway patency. Radiographics. 2011;31(2):511–26. doi:10.1148/rg.312105108. PubMed PMID: 21415194.
14. Lee EY, Mason KP, Zurakowski D, Waltz DA, Ralph A, Riaz F, et al. MDCT assessment of tracheomalacia in symptomatic infants with mediastinal aortic vascular anomalies: preliminary technical experience. Pediatr Radiol. 2008;38(1):82–8. doi:10.1007/s00247-007-0672-1. PubMed PMID: 18038169.
15. Baroni RH, Ashiku S, Boiselle PM. Dynamic CT evaluation of the central airways in patients undergoing tracheoplasty for tracheobronchomalacia. AJR Am J Roentgenol. 2005;184(5):1444–9. doi:10.2214/ajr.184.5.01841444. PubMed PMID: 15855094.
16. Goo HW. Advanced functional thoracic imaging in children: from basic concepts to clinical applications. Pediatr Radiol. 2013;43(3):262–8. doi:10.1007/s00247-012-2466-3. PubMed PMID: 23417252.
17. Desir A, Ghaye B. Congenital abnormalities of intrathoracic airways. Radiol Clin North Am. 2009;47(2):203–25. doi:10.1016/j.rcl.2008.11.009. PubMed PMID: 19249452.
18. Berrocal T, Madrid C, Novo S, Gutierrez J, Arjonilla A, Gomez-Leon N. Congenital anomalies of the tracheobronchial tree, lung, and mediastinum: embryology, radiology, and pathology. Radiographics. 2004;24(1):e17. doi:10.1148/rg.e17. PubMed PMID: 14610245.
19. Soto-Hurtado EJ, Penuela-Ruiz L, Rivera-Sanchez I, Torres-Jimenez J. Tracheal diverticulum: a review of the literature. Lung. 2006;184(6):303–7. doi:10.1007/s00408-006-0010-7. PubMed PMID: 17086467.
20. Lee EY. MDCT and 3D evaluation of type 2 hypoplastic pulmonary artery sling associated with right lung agenesis, hypoplastic aortic arch, and long segment tracheal stenosis. J Thorac Imaging. 2007;22(4):346–50. doi:10.1097/RTI.0b013e31813fabca. PubMed PMID: 18043391.
21. Lee EY, Zurakowski D, Waltz DA, Mason KP, Riaz F, Ralph A, et al. MDCT evaluation of the prevalence of tracheomalacia in children with mediastinal aortic vascular anomalies. J Thorac Imaging. 2008;23(4):258–65. doi:10.1097/RTI.0b013e31817fbdf7. PubMed PMID: 19204470.
22. Sun M, Ernst A, Boiselle PM. MDCT of the central airways: comparison with bronchoscopy in the evaluation of complications of endotracheal and tracheostomy tubes. J Thorac Imaging. 2007;22(2):136–42. doi:10.1097/01.rti.0000213579.24527.6c. PubMed PMID: 17527116.

Evaluation of the Neonatal Airway: Laryngoscopy and Bronchoscopy

Craig Derkay and Christina Baldasseri

History of Airway Evaluation

As with most great discoveries laryngoscopy and bronchoscopy were designs of necessity, having been developed to treat acute airway obstruction and to reverse its cause. The first recorded direct laryngoscopy and intervention was credited to Horace Green in 1852 who visually examined the larynx of a child with obstructive breathing and removed an obstructing mass [2]. Gustov Killian was an early pioneer of rigid endoscopy and is credited with the first therapeutic rigid bronchoscopy to remove an airway foreign body from the right main stem bronchus in 1897. Shortly thereafter came Chevalier Jackson in 1903 who developed his own version of a laryngoscope and became the first to fashion a direct laryngoscope [3]. Quickly after, driven by necessity, it was adapted to have distal illumination capabilities. Jackson became known as the American father of bronchoesophagology and wrote the first book on the subject in 1907 and dedicated it to Killian whose work greatly influenced his innovation in the one-handed technique and instrumentation of direct laryngoscopy [4, 5].

Once Jackson introduced a laryngoscope with a distal light source the ease and functionality of handling a handheld laryngoscope made it a more practical tool for routine use. The practice of minimally invasive airway endoscopy became a mainstay of otolaryngology practice following that time. Further knowledge and detail of the airway became available with invention of the operating microscope by Kleinsasser. The practice of office-based endoscopy expanded rapidly with the invention of flexible fiberoptic airway visualization beginning in the 1960s. Over the ensuing 50 years, endoscopy has been a key tool for the otolaryngologist in diagnosing and managing airway lesions in infants.

C. Derkay (✉) • C. Baldasseri
Department of Otolaryngology, Children's Hospital of The King's Daughters, Eastern Virginia Medical School, Norfolk, VA, USA
e-mail: craig.derkay@chkd.org

Upper and Lower Airway Embryology and Anatomy

The earliest embryologic development of the respiratory tract involves the appearance of the median pharyngeal grooves at approximately 3 weeks of intrauterine life. The tracheobronchial groove eventually gives rise to the mature infant's larynx, trachea, bronchi, and lungs. By 5 ½ weeks the laryngeal primodium develops from contributions of the III, IV, and VI arches. By the end the embryonic period of development, the larynx, trachea, and esophagus are well formed. Fetal breathing movement has been demonstrated by ultrasound as early as the third month of gestation.

The newborn larynx is arranged to coordinate suckling-type feeding and respiration. The larynx in a neonate is located high in the cervical neck (C2) as compared to a much lower location (C6-7) in teenagers and adults. The epiglottis is short and more curved with thick, bulky arytenoids and aryepiglottic folds. The vocal folds are also oriented more transversely. The narrowest portion of the infantile larynx is the subglottis which has a diameter of 4–5 mm. The infant's trachea is also predisposed to collapse due to increased airway resistance from its increased compliance. This is related to the flexibility of the cartilage and the low tone of the tracheal musculature. All of these features make the newborn larynx adept at protecting the airway while suckling.

The larynx develops rapidly until age 15 when the larynx descends to its final position. The most rapid phase of growth is during the toddler years, up to age three, and then slows until puberty again stimulates further growth. The lengthening of the vocal cords creates a gradual lowering of voice pitch. During puberty the male and female vocal cord undergo separate growth patterns and changes with the male vocal cords lengthening twice as much, creating gender differences of voice pitch. Laryngeal cartilage begins to ossify in teenage years and continues through the third decade of life. The different appearances of the newborn, child, and adult larynx are important to understand and distinguish so

J. Lioy and S.E. Sobol (eds.), *Disorders of the Neonatal Airway: Fundamentals for Practice*,
DOI 10.1007/978-1-4939-1610-8_21, © Springer Science+Business Media New York 2015

that normal can be determined from pathologic appearance during endoscopy.

The larynx functions to provide airway transmission to the lungs, protection of foreign and potential harmful material from entering the lower airway, and as an instrument for phonation. The larynx is able to accomplish this by being a narrow, tightly controlled, muscular organ. The larynx, and specifically the subglottis, is the narrowest portion of the airway. By virtue of this fact, it is a common place of obstruction. The larynx serves to protect the airway by reflexive glottic closure during swallowing, though this function is somewhat immature in newborns. Glottic closure is crucial for swallowing, airway protection, and coughing. Coughing is created by complete or partial closure of the glottis creating high intrathoracic pressure; this is released quickly resulting in a forced expulsion of air. Newborns have an immature cough reflex and limited glottic control and are thus not able to create productive coughs to expel aspirated secretions or milk. The infantile glottis closes in reaction to direct stimulation by chemical, touch, or temperature irritation. As soon as the stimulating signal is removed, the glottis should open to allow the infant to breathe. The neonatal airway is also more disposed to laryngospasms (tight closure of the glottis and obstruction of the airway inappropriately in response to a stimulus). The adult larynx can more easily overcome a laryngospasm once the partial pressure of CO_2 in the blood increases. However, this response is blunted in the infant and can lead to prolonged laryngospasms, airway obstruction, and sometimes death. This is thought to be a cause of sudden infant death syndrome (SIDS) [6].

Office-Based Evaluation

The office is the place where many neonates are seen and evaluated for the first time. They are referred to a variety of airway-related reasons. Infants will present with feeding difficulties, voice changes, noisy breathing, cough, and other symptoms that all have a broad and wide differential diagnosis.

Performing a complete history and physical will allow the otolaryngologist to determine the urgency of the airway complaint, what intervention if any are appropriate for the office, what studies/images would be helpful, and what surgical interventions could be beneficial. It is important to distinguish between a parent's complaints of "noisy breathing" by determining if this represents stridor or stertor. If a true abnormality is suspected, it is then important to differentiate between upper and lower airway obstruction and the degree of airway distress that is present. This differentiation is important for establishing a narrower differential diagnosis and for choosing the appropriate equipment for endoscopic evaluation if necessary.

History

Obtaining a detailed and accurate history can be difficult in the pediatric patient. It is important to know what questions to ask and how to organize information to determine the nature and course of the child's airway history. This will also rapidly allow you to assess the urgency of the condition. The examiner needs to quickly determine if the airway is stable or unstable since the degree and nature of the obstruction will help determine the best intervention and immediate need for supportive care with oxygen, heliox, steroids, or racemic epinephrine. Once a critical airway has been ruled out, a comprehensive history can be obtained.

The neonatal patient's history begins in utero. Elements regarding the mother's pregnancy, prenatal care, and delivery history should be obtained. The history should focus on factors such as prematurity, difficulty of the delivery, use of forceps, meconium aspiration, respiratory distress requiring deep suctioning or endotracheal intubation, and the timing of onset of obstructive symptoms. Gathering this information can lead you to suspect diagnoses such as choanal atresia, laryngomalacia, or vocal cord paralysis. Essential information to gather include: timing of the onset of the child's symptoms (gradual or sudden), age at which the symptoms developed, and whether the symptoms are progressive or static. For instance, if the family describes gradual onset of airway symptoms after several months of life this can point to airway hemangioma, especially if there are other birthmarks that the family have noticed. To gather the most detailed history the otolaryngologist will have to rely on the observations of parents, other family members, and the pediatrician.

It is important to ask questions that allow you to organize your thoughts into a functional manner. Gathering information regarding symptoms or signs along the path of airflow can be beneficial. Questions regarding feeding difficulties, reflux, and changes in breathing or noisy breathing that vary with patient position are particularly helpful. Asking about the child's voice/cry, intubation history, coexisting medical conditions, prior surgeries (i.e., PDA repair), birth/prenatal history, sleeping patterns, and vaccination history are also essential. Questions regarding snoring and noisy breathing during sleep can narrow the differential based on the description of the snoring/breathing pattern. Having the child's family fill out a pre-visit patient form with questions regarding these important questions can give family a chance to think about these things before they see you. As more and more is uncovered regarding genetics and heritability of disease, a detailed family history regarding birthmarks, breathing problems in infancy, recurrent croup, or known airway anomalies add valuable information.

Physical Examination

Inspect and Listen

This element of the exam begins as you enter the room. Take note of the neonate's breathing pattern, their effort and rate of breathing. Tachypnea can point to an underlying infectious cause or hypoxia. Look for symmetry of the neck, airway, and thorax. An infant's neck may be difficult to examine and assess due to its location. The larynx is well protected beneath a low mandible and is located in the high cervical region. It may therefore be difficult to assess the position of the trachea and larynx in relation to midline. It also makes it difficult to find nodes, masses, or neck lesions on first glance and requires further detailed exam with palpation. Make note of any craniofacial abnormalities that may pose a difficulty in examining the child with endoscopy. Babies with micrognathia, cleft lip or palate, nasal vestibular stenosis, or syndromic craniofacial features may complicate access to the airway via endoscopic examination and will require advanced planning.

Palpate

As the newborn larynx develops the external laryngeal skeleton becomes more easily identifiable. With the growth of the internal structures, the larynx moves lower down the cervical spine. In the newborn the laryngeal skeleton is soft and pliable. In contrast to adults, the most prominent structure is the cricoid and not the thyroid cartilage. The examiner should feel for the location of the airway and identify its position as either midline or shifted. If the airway is deviated, one should look for causes such as cysts or masses than can be palpated during the exam.

Auscultate

Make it a point to assess a patient's cry or cough during the initial examination. If the baby has a muffled cry, this can point to a supraglottic or oropharyngeal obstruction or mass that is affecting the voice projection. Hoarseness can be a sign of thickened vocal cords from either swelling or masses such as papillomatosis. An infant with a weak or breathy voice should make one consider vocal cord paralysis or paresis. If stridor is auscultated during the exam, attempt to classify it into inspiratory, expiratory, or biphasic. This can narrow the location of the obstruction to being located in the supraglottis for inspiratory stridor, subglottis for expiratory stridor, and at the level of the glottis for biphasic stridor. There are common lesions associated with each level and knowing this information can help the otolaryngologist build a differential diagnosis. A tip for auscultating directly over the larynx in the high riding larynx of newborns is to remove the diaphragm portion of the stethoscope on a disposable stethoscope and listen directly over the larynx with the tubing. This can help with subtle degrees of stridor as the high location of the newborn larynx may make it difficult to fit even a pediatric stethoscope flat across the larynx.

Flexible Fiberoptic Nasopharyngolaryngoscopy

The first fiberoptic bronchoscope was developed in 1966 by Ikeda in Japan at about the same time that the Hopkins rod telescopic lens system was being developed for use in conjunction with rigid bronchoscopes. Since that time, many advances in optics and digital display have made flexible endoscopy an essential piece of equipment for the otolaryngologist to use in the office, emergency department, ICU, and on hospital consults. Most neonates can safely undergo office-based flexible endoscopy; however, there is some subtly to selecting out the ones that should not be examined with a flexible nasopharyngolaryngoscope in the office. Factors to consider are the child's age, ability to cooperate, as well as the physical exam information you have gathered. If the airway appears to be tenuous, the patient's symptoms are such that a flexible office-based exam cannot be completed safely or the most likely pathology is distal to the larynx, then the child should have the procedure performed in the operating room along with further endoscopy. Flexible nasopharyngolaryngoscopy is often a crucial portion of an operating room exam and should be performed before sedation to assess the dynamic function of the larynx.

Flexible office-based examination is more problematic and technically challenging in infants and neonates than in the older pediatric population due to the posterior position of the mandible relative to the maxilla, inability to swallow on command and handle secretions. The instrument comes in a variety of lengths and diameters and is typically synced to a video system to capture still and video images [7, 8].

Many clinicians recommend decongestion of the nose with oxymetazoline and topical anesthesia with 2–4 % Lidocaine or other topical anesthetic. In our experience, children under the age of 2 years old are better served by use of a topical decongestant alone for the nasal cavity and that foregoing the topical anesthetic avoids the potential complication of laryngospasm or adverse cardiac reaction. We routinely use topical decongestion alone until age two after which time 4 % topical Lidocaine can be added to the decongesting agent to provide topical anesthesia enhancing the older child's ability to cooperate. Once the nose is decongested, the nasal cavity, nasopharynx, and eustachian tube orifices are examined (Drawing 1). In a crying infant with lots of nasal secretions a thorough exam of the nasal cavity can be difficult, and is sometimes best examined at the end of the examination as the flexible scope is being

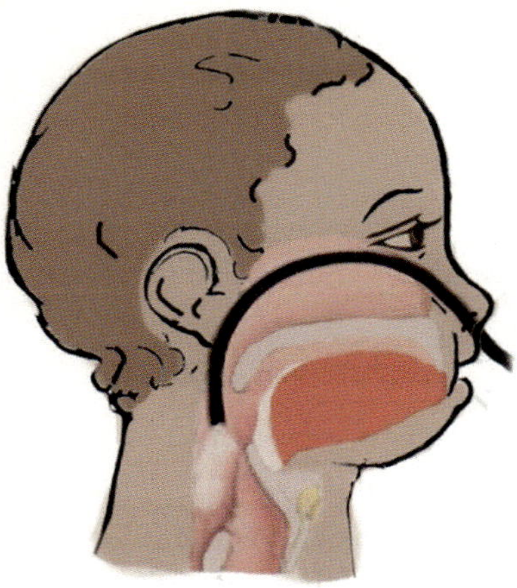

Drawing 1 Flexible nasopharyngolaryngoscopy

removed. After advancing beyond the nasopharynx into the oropharynx, one should begin a systematic examination of the hypopharynx and all its subsites. Of particular interest is an assessment of the epiglottis and aryepiglottic folds as laryngomalacia is the most common cause of stridor in infants. Another crucial aspect of this exam is getting a view of the vocal cords, assessing their mobility and looking for polyps, papillomas, congenital cysts, or other causes for airway obstruction. It is reasonable to attempt to assess the subglottis for stenosis or a shelf, realizing that this can be difficult in a crying or struggling child and that other means of assessment are superior.

The flexible nasopharyngolaryngoscopic exam should not be considered an alternate or equal exam to direct laryngobronchoscopy as the entire airway cannot be examined thoroughly with this modality alone at the bedside. Many noisy breathers, such as those with mild laryngomalacia, can be assessed and followed in the office with flexible nasopharyngolaryngoscopy, although some clinicians advocate that all noisy breathers (even those with mild laryngomalacia), should undergo full endoscopy in the operating room to avoid missing a concomitant secondary airway lesion. This is reported to occur in up to 19–27 % of all patients with laryngomalacia and is even higher in children who need a supraglottoplasty [9]. Due to the fact that the subglottis and lower airway cannot fully be appreciated during a flexible exam a full operating room exam should be planned if the findings on flexible endoscopy do not completely explain the child's airway symptoms. Gonzalez demonstrated that up to 18 % of children who underwent diagnostic laryngobronchoscopy for airway obstruction with or without stridor had two or more synchronous airway lesions [10]. Flexible nasopharyngolaryngoscopy is a useful and invaluable starting point in the evaluation of neonatal obstruction or stridor but may require supplementation with operative endoscopy or further imaging.

Documentation

Photo and video documentation are becoming essential in following and tracking progress over the rapid period of growth that occurs during early infancy. Video can help eliminate repetitive scope examinations and the risk of traumatizing the airway (or the child) from repeat scope exams. In an academic teaching environment, it also provides a tool to provide instruction and information for family, students, trainees, and colleagues. With the advent of smartphones that can capture video, these exams can be easily recorded and shared but HIPAA regulations need to be adhered to. Still pictures are also useful but can fail to provide the dynamic structure and function of the laryngeal apparatus that video provides. Photo and video documentation is also useful for preoperative planning and guidance to determine if imaging is necessary and what modality to obtain.

Operating Room

Preparation is essential to a successful endoscopy. Endoscopy can be used for diagnostic purposes if the etiology and diagnosis are unclear. It can also be therapeutic when combined with operating or rigid microlaryngoscopy. It is important to have a plan for securing and protecting the airway before an emergency can arise. Having open communication and an agreed upon plan with the anesthesia team and operating room support staff is crucial. Each physician should have a clear role in the care so that confusion is avoided. Having the necessary supplies, including laryngoscopes, ventilating bronchoscopes, operating microscope, a selection of Hopkins rod telescopes, and appropriate size and lengths of suction catheters, as well as a tracheostomy tray should be available in the room. If the team is prepared for airway complications and the appropriate equipment is available adverse events can largely be prevented. Approaching the airway in the same systematic manner every time will help operating room staff and anesthesia staff become familiar with the routine and it will help to provide a thorough examination of the oral cavity, oral pharynx, supraglottis, glottis, subglottis, trachea, as well as all subsites. Photo documentation should be performed at multiple levels along the upper airway. Real-time video is helpful for anesthesia and OR staff to follow the progress of the procedure as well as for teaching residents/students/fellows.

Rigid Endoscopy–Direct Laryngoscopy and Rigid Bronchoscopy

Indications

There are numerous reasons to perform airway endoscopy. These include urgent and routine diagnostic or therapeutic interventions or simply to follow a child's chronic airway

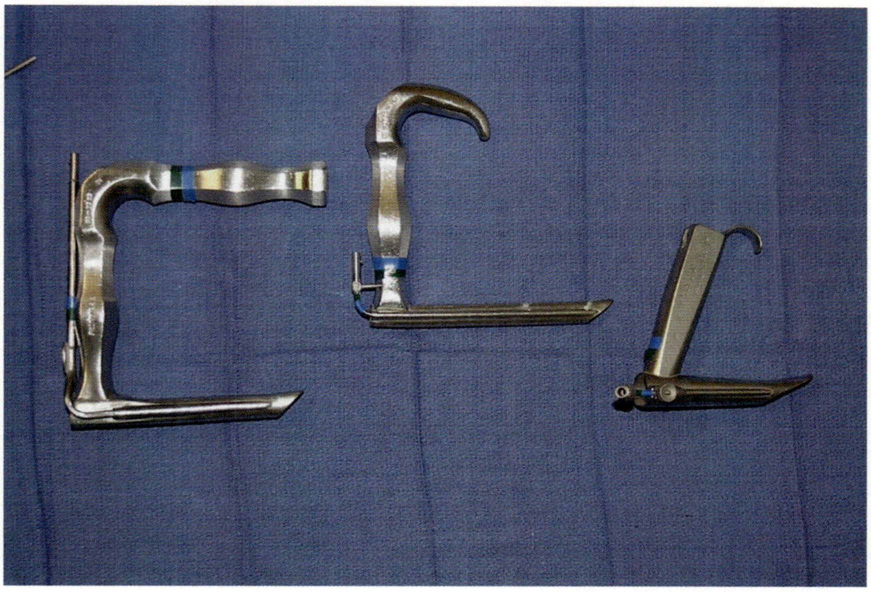

Picture 1 Side view of three common laryngoscopes with light source attachment

conditions through planned, periodic airway examinations. A relatively urgent reason for rigid endoscopy is in the work-up of the neonate with stridor. Stridor is often a sign of a very narrow and tenuous airway. The otolaryngologist should be prepared to discuss the operative plan with the anesthesiologist before any airway manipulation occurs. Once the airway has been examined the otolaryngologist can intubate the patient if there is a need. Rigid bronchoscopy with a ventilating port can be used to examine the lower airway if a culture, biopsy, or bronchoalveolar lavage is to be performed. Rigid bronchoscopy also may provide therapeutic relief if an airway obstruction is identified or if the airway is tenuous and a more secure means of ventilation is necessary. Otherwise, the entire diagnostic exam can be performed with just a telescope.

Another indication for endoscopy is the neonate who is not improving on current therapy, whether that is increasing ventilator pressures or collapse of lung segments due to mucous plugging. Early intervention and airway examination can help to solidify a diagnosis and to establish a treatment plan going forward. If bacterial or infectious etiology is suspected, cultures can be obtained to help direct therapy. If a mucous plug is suspected, a therapeutic suctioning can be performed at the time of endoscopy. Other common reasons for endoscopic airway evaluation are to diagnose abnormalities uncovered on imaging or suspected due to other diagnostic testing.

Maintenance and routine airway endoscopy are indicated in patients with chronic conditions such as chronic indwelling tracheostomy tubes placed to bypass glottic, or subglottic stenosis, for ventilator support or for pulmonary toilet. Tracheostomy-dependent children need regular evaluation as they are at risk for developing suction-induced granulation tissue that can cause distal obstruction and supra-stomal

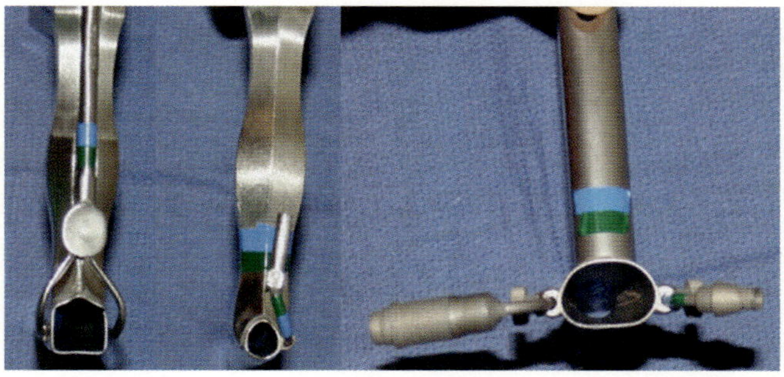

Picture 2 View through a Dedo laryngoscope, anterior commissure laryngoscope, and a Lindholm microlaryngoscope

granulomas. In the growing child, with a tracheostomy, the need for periodic upsizing can best be assessed at the time of endoscopy.

Tools for Rigid Endoscopy

Laryngoscopes

There are several varieties of laryngoscopes, all of which have varying functions and relative indications. In general there are three broad types of laryngoscope: standard laryngoscopes for general examination and intubation; subglottiscopes and anterior commissure scopes for improved view and access to the subglottis and anterior commissure; and suspension microlaryngoscopes which have a wide opening and distal lumen which are ideal for binocular microscopic procedures utilizing microdebriders, lasers, or other microlaryngoscopy instruments (Pictures 1 and 2).

In choosing the best laryngoscope for direct laryngoscopy, the endoscopist will want to consider the size and age of the child and the potential need for performing a therapeutic

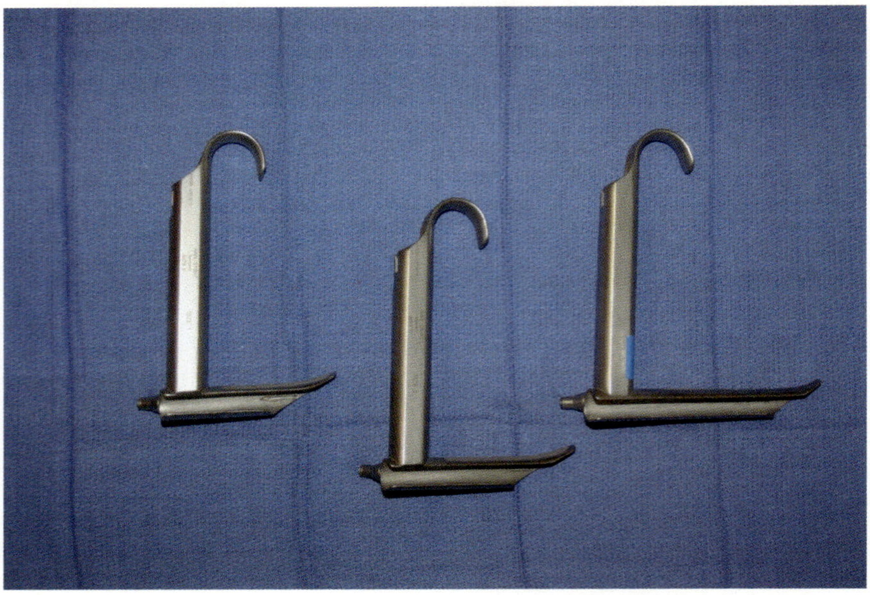

Picture 3 Parsons laryngoscopes three most common sizes from left to right size 8, 9, and 11.5

intervention. The simplest variety of laryngoscope is that routinely used by anesthesia providers for intubation with a Miller or Mac blade. These are all readily available in most operating rooms and crash carts and come in a variety of sizes. They do suffer, unfortunately, from having less than ideal illumination. A common operating laryngoscope for direct evaluation of the newborn larynx in the operating room is the set of Karl Storz laryngoscopes designed for neonatal and pediatric patients, colloquially referred to as the Parsons laryngoscope [11]. Parsons laryngoscopes have a flat superior blade to accommodate a wide and mobile pediatric tongue. They are equipped with a left side adaptor to connect to anesthesia's oxygen supply or inhalational anesthetic. This will help to decrease the incidence of desaturation that can accompany direct laryngoscopy in babies with poor pulmonary reserve. The Parsons laryngoscope is illuminated with a proximal xenon light cable that offers superior visualization over that afforded by a standard anesthesia-intubating laryngoscope with its distal fluorescent bulb. The Parsons set come with a wide proximal opening and an open side channel that easily allows the passage of a Hopkins rod telescope for photo documentation or other instrumentation. This side channel also allows for passage of a rigid ventilating bronchoscope or optical cup forceps. The Parsons has the added benefit of being able to be suspended from a rigid arm off of a side table Mayo tray. This allows the surgeon to have both hands free to operate or to bring in an operating microscope for further intervention. Parsons laryngoscopes come in three common sizes for premature infants, neonates/infants, and toddlers (Picture 3). Older children and adolescents can be exposed with the Benjamin laryngoscope, though it lacks the ventilation port that is present on the Parsons. A better option for suspension laryngoscopy needed in longer or more complex cases in children is the Lindholm microlaryngoscope. This laryngoscope offers a wide operating window to facilitate operative microscopy for interventions such as laser or microdebrider resection of airway lesions.

Using a laryngoscope requires a good understanding of the anatomy of the oral cavity, oropharynx, supraglottis, and glottis. Every time a laryngoscopy is performed the opportunity should be taken to perform a thorough examination as it is often difficult to perform a complete exam on newborns and infants at the bedside. When setting up for the laryngoscopy, it is important to protect the child's eyes, head, and alveolar mucosa. These areas are at risk for iatrogenic injury if care is not taken.

Regardless of what type of laryngoscope you are using the same basic principles apply to the approach. If the patient will tolerate it, the entire procedure can be done through intermittent periods of apnea by rotating between mask ventilation and endoscopy. This generally is preferred if the procedure is relatively short and is referred to as TIVA or total intravenous anesthesia typically with Propofol as the intravenous agent and supplemental oxygen or sevoflurane delivered by way of the ventilation port of the laryngoscope. If a longer procedure is anticipated, then the patient can be intermittently intubated between examinations and therapeutic interventions. The maxilla and mandible can be retracted with a "scissor technique" to maximally open the mouth. The laryngoscope enters the oral cavity with the blade portion oriented toward the lateral portion of the oral cavity (inferior pole of the tonsil) and then gently used to retract the tongue laterally out of the field of view (Drawing 2). Suctioning should be done gently once the glottis is exposed. If the patient is intubated at the time of the initial examination, care should be taken to not dislodge the tube. For right-handed

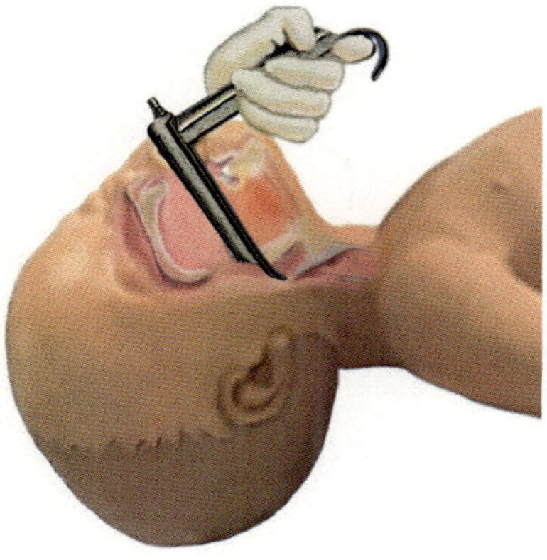

Drawing 2 Proper placement of a Parsons laryngoscope for a right-handed surgeon

surgeons, the tube should be taped to the patient's left oral cavity. The laryngoscope should be advanced along the base of tongue and into the vallecula and then gentle pressure on the lingual-epiglottic ligament is applied to elevate the epiglottis and expose the supraglottis and glottis. An omega-shaped epiglottis or particularly coiled epiglottis, such as those in laryngomalacia and often in premature infants, can be more difficult to elevate. Care should be taken to avoid having the epiglottis fold on itself and cause restricted blood flow to the epiglottis during the exam of the glottis as this can obstruct the glottis as well as being a source for postoperative edema and airway obstruction. Due to the nature of the examination, there is always some degree of edema from the examination that should be expected. Intravenous dexamethasone (0.4–1.0 mg/kg) can be administered to help decrease postoperative airway edema. If another laryngoscope such as a Holinger anterior commissure scope is selected, then you will place the tip of the laryngoscope under the epiglottis to completely remove it from the view of the laryngoscope. Care should be taken to avoid trauma to the anterior commissure of the vocal cords as this can result in scarring and anterior webbing. Once the vocal cords are in view, a weight-based dose of topical Lidocaine can be sprayed onto the vocal cords to allow for topical anesthesia. This helps to reduce the propensity that neonates have for laryngospasm due to stimulation of the glottis and distal airway.

Once the airway is exposed, an age-appropriate sized 0° Hopkins rod telescope can be introduced through the lumen of the laryngoscope and photo documentation can be performed. If the airway is tenuous, a ventilating bronchoscope can be introduced instead of the telescope to secure the airway and allow ventilation during the examination.

A new generation of video-assisted laryngoscopes is becoming more commonly used in the operating room by pediatric anesthesiologists. Video-guided laryngoscopy has become the tool of choice for intubating children with a difficult airway. One study done in adults showed that patients with risk factors for difficult intubation were more likely to be intubated on the first attempt with a video laryngoscope than with conventional direct laryngoscopy [12]. The three most common video laryngoscopes on the market include the C-MAC®, GlideScope, and Bullard video laryngoscopes. The CMAC (Karl Storz, Tuttlingen, Germany) has a laryngoscope blade similar to the Macintosh laryngoscope blade, and can have either a separate video monitor or a video viewer in the handle. The GlideScope® Video Laryngoscope (Verathon, Bothell, Washington, USA) has only one pediatric size and has a separate video monitor screen. The Bullard scope also has only one pediatric size but its handle is specially designed to expose the larynx in children with micrognathia. Video laryngoscopy is frequently being turned to if a difficult intubation is suspected; however, one study showed that although the view of the airway was improved, there was a significantly longer time period between paralytic administration and intubation when using a video laryngoscope [13]. Video laryngoscopy is becoming more commonplace in the operating room and is particularly helpful in teaching institutions where anesthesia providers (residents, fellows, CRNAs, and EMTs) are building their skills in training programs.

Bronchoscopes

With the development of ventilating bronchoscopes able to accommodate Hopkins rod telescopes for improved optics, the use of bronchoscopy for neonates has become a safer and practical procedure (Picture 4).

Bronchoscopy has the ability to simultaneously examine, treat, and ventilate the patient. In combination with an optical telescope, it provides excellent views of the glottis, subglottis, tracheal rings, and bronchi. Through the instrument side port, biopsies, cultures, and assays can be performed. There have been several bronchoscope-specific optical instruments developed that allow one to continue with the telescopic view and ventilate the patient while grasping a foreign body or taking a biopsy. Optical cup forceps are used for biopsy or removal of lesions such as papillomas. Optical alligator or peanut forceps are commonly used for foreign body removal. Other useful tools that can be advanced through the instrument port of a bronchoscope include several types of lasers (CO_2, KTP, ND:Yag) that can feed a laser fiber through the instrument port and under direct visualization shrink or resect lesions. One example is the Omniguide® laser fiber system, a CO_2 laser that can be guided directly to lesions such as papilloma, scar tissue, granulation tissue, and other lesions of the trachea or airway. Another example is the Erbe coagulation catheter which is a plasma laser used for resecting and coagulating vascular lesions.

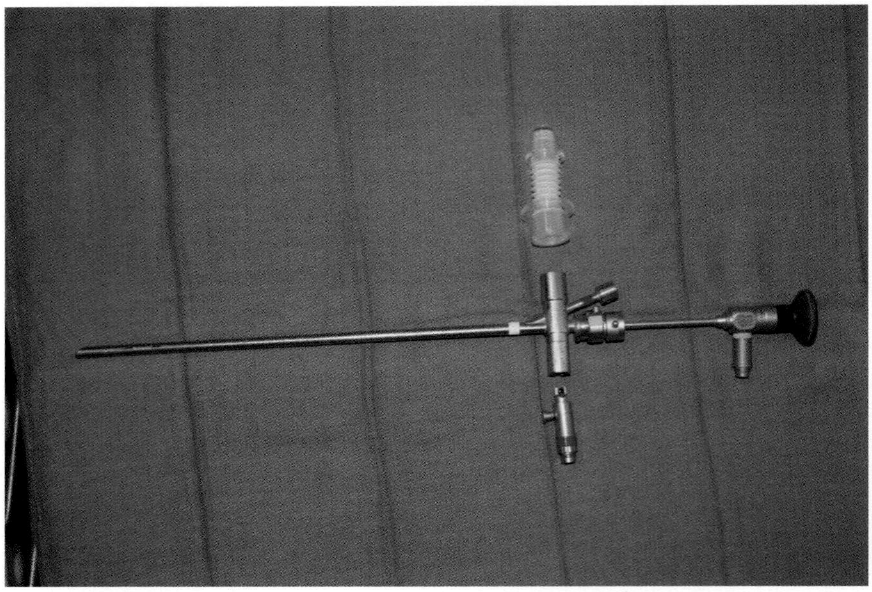

Picture 4 Partially dissembled ventilating bronchoscope

Bronchioalveolar lavage (BAL) is a useful diagnostic adjunct that can easily be performed while performing a rigid or flexible bronchoscopy. A small amount of normal saline can be flushed through the instrument port and then a suction catheter can be passed to collect the secretions and fluid in a sterile trap. The secretions can then be sent for culture and gram stain if infection is suspected. Another useful test is tracheal pepsin (if kept on dry ice) and lipid laden macrophages if extra esophageal reflux and aspiration are suspected.

The zero-degree Hopkins telescopic lens system was developed in 1966. With the addition of angled lens (30°, 70°, and 120°), difficult to examine areas can be viewed that would have previously been unable to be seen because of the rigid nature of the endoscope. Bronchoscopes come in varying lengths and sizes to accommodate even the smallest of premature infants. The size chart below can guide the otolaryngologist in selecting the appropriate bronchoscope and telescope to select based on the child's age and size (Chart 1).

The procedure begins much the same as with laryngoscopy with the additional need to match up the size of the telescope with that of the bronchoscope and the choosing of appropriate length and diameter suctions to fit through the bronchoscope. The head is extended and a shoulder roll can be placed if needed. Care needs to be taken to protect the eyes and upper gingiva. To introduce the bronchoscope into the airway, it is best to gain the needed exposure with a laryngoscope that has an open side port. The bronchoscope should be advanced in through the glottis posteriorly with care to avoid the anterior commissure so as not to cause an abrasion and risk anterior webbing. Turning the bronchoscope slightly to enter with the beveled edge at around the 2 o'clock position usually works the best (Drawing 3). Once in the airway the laryngoscope can be removed. The bronchoscope should be guided through the airway with the thumb and forefinger of the left hand adding tactile support of the hard palate to advance the scope distally. As the bronchoscope is advanced, a detailed examination of the mucosa, tracheal lumen, and integrity of the cartilaginous support structure should be examined while taking note of the quality and color of the secretions. If there is any difficulty in ventilation, the telescope can be temporarily removed offering a more efficient exchange of oxygen and carbon dioxide. In extreme cases, the light source can be directly attached to the bronchoscope prism, though this provides less illumination, no magnification, and no image on the monitor.

The carina will appear in the midline as a sharp inverted "V," dividing the trachea into right and left main stem bronchi. The angle to access the right main stem bronchus is less acute at about 25°, while the left main stem bronchus comes off the trachea at about 75°. Once the carina is identified, some patient adjustments will need to be made to examine the right and left main stem bronchus. It is important to have a good understanding of the anatomy of the bronchial tree system. To more easily access the left main stem bronchus, the patient's head is turned toward the right. This brings the left bronchus into a more linear alignment with the trachea. To fully assess the more distal intermediate bronchus, the telescope can be changed for a 30° or 45° angled telescope. The same technique can be used to examine the right main stem bronchus. However, when examining the right main stem bronchus the patient's head does not need to be turned as sharply to the left because the angle is less acute. The bronchoscope is then advanced into the right main stem bronchus, substituting for an angled telescope (if desired), and the divisions of the anterior, posterior, and apical lobe

Chart 1 Age-directed chart for proper selection of Parsons laryngoscopes, ventilating bronchoscopes, and rigid telescopes along with the attachments for pediatric examination

Age	Parsons laryngoscope	Storz bronchoscope	Hopkins telescope	Bridge	Size	Outer diameter (mm)
Premature–Newborn	8	2.5×20	27017A	Short	2.5	4.2
Newborn–6 month	8	3.0×20 or 3.5×20	27018A/7218A/7219A	Short	3	5
6 month–1 year	9	3.0×26 or 3.5×26	27020A/10020A	Long	3.5	5.7
1–2 years	9 or 11	3.5×26 or 3.7×26	27020A/10020A	Long	3.7	6.4
2–3 years	11	3.7×26 or 3.7×30 or 4.0×30	27020A/10020A 27005A (Hopkins II)	Long Short	4	6.7
3–5 years	11	3.7×40 or 4.0×30	27005A (Hopkins II)	Short	4.5	7.3
5–8 years	11 or 13.5	4.0×30 or 5.0×30	27005A (Hopkins II)	Short	5	7.8
8 years and older	11 or 13.5	6.0×30	27005A (Hopkins II)	Short	6	8.2

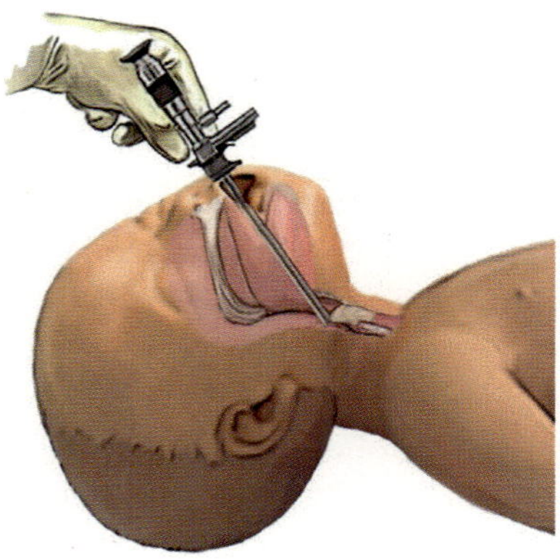

Drawing 3 Rigid bronchoscopy

bronchi can be visualized. Regardless of normal or abnormal findings, it is helpful to document with photographs or videos the findings of the bronchoscopy.

Flexible Endoscopy–Flexible Nasopharyngolaryngoscopy and Flexible Fiberoptic Bronchoscopy

Flexible Nasopharyngolaryngoscopy

Although this topic is covered in more detail in the section regarding office-based procedures, this is an important adjunctive procedure to consider prior to induction of anesthesia in the operating room. Often a quick dynamic assessment of the airway in a controlled environment allows for a more thorough examination that can aid with operating room setup and operative planning prior to induction. We will typically begin with the application of oxymetazoline to both nasal cavities and the establishment of IV access while the baby breathes an inhalational agent such as sevoflurane. Once the IV has been started, we ask the anesthesia provider to turn off the inhalational agent and switch to 100 % oxygen as our preference is to perform this exam in the spontaneously breathing infant to better appreciate dynamic areas of obstruction and to best assess vocal cord mobility. In the premature infant and those with poor pulmonary reserve, an NP trumpet may be placed for the delivery of supplemental oxygen. The flexible examination may require an assistant or nurse to hold the head (and the baby) still and to occasionally perform suctioning of the contralateral nostril to clear secretions in the nasopharynx or hypopharynx.

Flexible Bronchoscopy

Flexible bronchoscopy has the benefit of being able to provide a dynamic assessment of the trachea and bronchial tree. This procedure should be done in the operating room or endoscopy suite with a knowledgeable and prepared anesthesia staff. Although in recent years pediatric and neonatal bronchoscopes have been miniaturized, they still pose a risk of airway occlusion and laryngospasm/bronchospasm during the examination. There are two broad classes of bronchoscopes: those with an operating side port that can be used for suction or biopsy, and those that are without (essentially just a longer nasopharyngolaryngoscope).

The flexible bronchoscope can be introduced into the airway via two methods: transnasally/orally and via an existing endotracheal or tracheostomy tube. When performed transnasally, the baby's nose should be prepared beforehand. The flexible bronchoscope is often of a larger diameter than a nasopharyngolaryngoscope and as such can result in more nasal mucosa trauma. Preparation of the nose with topical decongestants (oxymetazoline) and topical 2 % Lidocaine jelly can help the bronchoscope pass more easily. Orally, the flexible scope can be passed through a special bite guard that allows the instrument to pass without being clamped between the patient's gingiva or damaged by their teeth. Once the bronchoscope is located above the vocal cords, a liquid dose of 4 % Lidocaine can be applied to the laryngeal and subglottic structures through the suction port of the bronchoscope. It is important at this point to clamp the suction so the Lidocaine isn't suctioned away. Communication with your anesthesia colleagues is important regarding a safe weight-based dose of Lidocaine so the proper amount can be titrated throughout the case. Once the topical Lidocaine is placed, the bronchoscope can be advanced slowly through the vocal cords. A thorough 360° exam can take

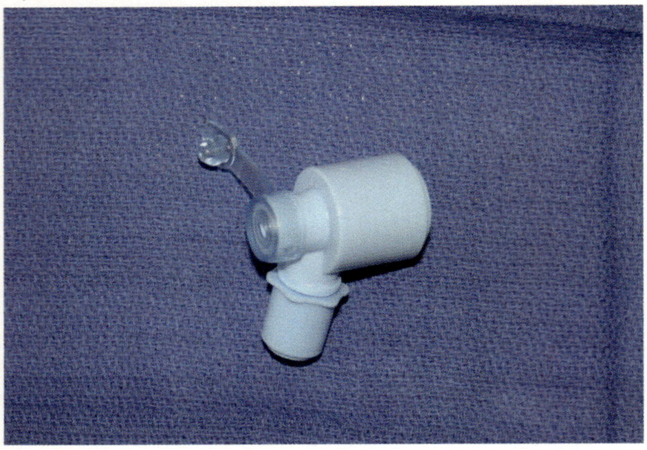

Picture 5 Ventilating adaptor allows for combined flexible bronchoscopy and ventilation

place using the flexibility and maneuverability of the fiberoptic scope. The tip of the scope can be adjusted and guided by the finger control located on the handle. Care should be taken to avoid excess torque as this can put stress on the fiberoptic cables, leading to small black specs (indicating broken fibers) on the video image. The increased utility of the flexible bronchoscope lies in the enhanced ability to assess for distal tracheal or bronchial lesions. Although it is a great tool for performing bronchial alveolar lavage, it has limitations and should rarely be used if a foreign body is suspected. One can perform biopsies but the instrument is unreliable for the removal of larger items as it is limited in its ability to grasp these and it is not possible to ventilate the patient during the procedure. The instrument can also be used to help place an endotracheal tube in a patient with an obstructed upper airway. Using a Seldinger technique, an endotracheal tube is threaded over the bronchoscope which is passed beyond the vocal cords into the trachea. The endotracheal tube is then advanced beyond the tip of the bronchoscope which is then removed.

A common way to perform flexible bronchoscopy is by passing the scope through an existing endotracheal or tracheostomy tube. The smallest diameter flexible bronchoscope that contains a side port for suction has an outer diameter of 2.8 mm and can be passed through a 4.5 endotracheal tube or tracheostomy tube. If a smaller endotracheal or tracheostomy tube is present, you can pass a slimmer flexible endoscope through it (the narrowest outer diameter flexible endoscopy is 1.9 mm and can pass through a 3.0 endotracheal or tracheostomy tube), but you will lose the ability to have a functioning side channel for suction or biopsy. When performing flexible bronchoscopy through an endotracheal or tracheostomy tube, a special ventilating adapter can be used to allow simultaneous ventilation and examination (Picture 5). The scope often fills the large majority of the endotracheal tube and causes partial obstruction of the airway so one needs to keep a careful eye on the oxygen and CO_2 monitors to gauge how much time you have to perform the exam before you need to remove the scope and continue ventilation.

Other Considerations

Ideal neonatal care involves a multidisciplinary approach involving the otolaryngologist, neonatology, anesthesiology, respiratory therapy, feeding therapy, nurses, and family members. Open communication can help to avoid many of the potential pitfalls of neonatal airway management.

Imaging

Imaging can provide a wealth of information for the evaluation of the status of the airway. This can aid in diagnosis and preoperative planning. A lateral and anterior/posterior neck plain film can provide information regarding the mandible, maxilla, cervical spine, nasal cavity, nasopharynx, oropharynx, oral cavity, adenoid/palatine tonsil tissue, tongue base, vallecula, epiglottis, glottis, trachea, and esophagus. The anterior/posterior view offers the best view of subglottic narrowing, which can be caused by prolonged endotracheal intubation, subglottic masses such as hemangioma, or infection (classically referred to as a "steeple sign") These films could be considered as the first line of imaging in the stable child with stridor or signs of airway obstruction.

A barium or gastrograffin swallow study or upper GI series can also provide the otolaryngologist with information regarding the patient's airway. Using radio-opaque contrast a series of images are taken to capture the dynamic process of laryngeal elevation, airway protection, and swallowing. This may aid in the detection of laryngeal clefts with signs of aspiration through the post-cricoid area. A vascular ring may be inferred when compression of the trachea and esophagus is seen on esophagogram. This study may also suggest extra-esophageal reflux as an etiology of the infant's airway abnormality. (Consider adding a sentence or two regarding FEES here though it might not be appropriate for a chapter on neonates).

Computed tomography (CT) can provide a wealth of detailed information regarding the detailed upper and lower airway anatomy. However in children there are several risks that should be weighed before ordering one in a patient with potential airway compromise. A CT scan requires that the patient be still or the scan will have too much motion artifact to be useful. This may require sedation or general anesthesia in younger children, which can potentially worsen the airway obstruction or compromise the airway status. CT also exposes the child to a higher level of radiation than plain films. Many children's radiologic units have protocols in place to limit this exposure through the use of spiral CT technology with subsequent reconstruction of images [14].

CT has become the gold standard in imaging of the lower airway and lungs. It also provides fine detail regarding nasal and sinus anatomy and nasopharyngeal airway narrowing such as with choanal stenosis or atresia.

Magnetic resonance imaging (MRI) is increasingly being used in children to evaluate soft tissue masses and vascular compression of the airway. MRI is the gold standard to assess lymphatic malformations and salivary gland lesions. The benefit of an MRI is that it does not expose the child to radiation. The risk is that the study is much more time consuming and virtually all children will need sedation or a general anesthetic to be compliant enough to obtain a complete exam. This poses a problem when the scan is needed to evaluate possible airway pathology.

Ex Utero Intrapartum Therapy

This procedure came about as a result of continued innovations in diagnostic ultrasound. High-risk obstetricians began to prenatally diagnose conditions such as tracheal occlusion, severe diaphragmatic hernias, laryngeal atresia, large neck masses such as teratomas and lymphatic malformations causing high airway obstruction. Consequently, the ex utero intrapartum treatment (EXIT) procedure was developed to secure the airway before the neonate begins making efforts to breathe in an effort to limit the complications of their congenital airway obstruction. The EXIT procedure allows for the continuation of uteroplacental blood flow and gas exchange during partial delivery of the fetus. It involves providing the mother with tocolytics and high concentrations of inhalation anesthetics to allow continued uterine perfusion and to prevent uterine contraction. Only the head and torso are delivered providing partial exposure for procedures such as laryngoscopy, bronchoscopy, vascular access, and securing the airway with either an endotracheal tube or tracheostomy if needed. It allows a variety of previously near-universally fatal conditions to be managed and controlled in a planned manner giving time for more decision-making and evaluation. The indications for EXIT therapy come from the largest series on the subject from Children's Hospital of Philadelphia, with an experience of 43 fetuses undergoing EXIT procedures [15]. The current indications for EXIT therapy are: neonates with airway obstruction from neck masses, congenital high airway obstruction syndrome (CHAOS), thoracic masses, severe congenital diaphragmatic hernia, and those with an immediate need for extra corporeal membrane oxygenation [16].

Anesthesia

Amongst pediatric anesthesiologists, the general perception is that neonates undergoing a general anesthesia for upper airway procedures are at a higher risk for complications. Two large studies done over an 11-year period that looked at bronchospasm and laryngospasm have demonstrated that the overall incidence of laryngospasm is about 8.7/1,000 patients, with the highest incidence being in babies age 1–3 months undergoing upper airway surgery [17, 18]. Congenital cardiac disease, chronic lung disease, prematurity, and concurrent or recent upper respiratory infection are also associated with increased rates of laryngospasm and bronchospasm.

Working in a children's facility with a familiar group of anesthesia providers adds to the safety of the procedure. Close communication regarding the procedure and operative plan is necessary to avoid intraoperative confusion and complications. Experienced pediatric anesthesiologists will be familiar with otolaryngologic procedures and be ready to assist with multiple modalities of ventilation. It is important for the surgeon to discuss whether apneic procedures will be performed so that adequate levels of anesthesia can be induced.

Jet ventilation can be a useful adjunct in airway cases when an endotracheal tube would obstruct the surgeons view. The patient should be paralyzed to allow for adequate ventilation and the vocal cords need to remain open to prevent air trapping. Care must be taken to titrate the inflation pressures to avoid an iatrogenic pneumothorax.

Laser airway procedures require special considerations in terms of patient and OR staff safety. Oxygen can be delivered via a "laser-safe" endotracheal tube to lessen risk of airway fires. We prefer to use airway lasers in conjunction with apneic anesthesia techniques to avoid the possibility of fire.

The otolaryngologist should assist the anesthesiologist in endotracheal tube size selection, especially if there is prior information available regarding the airway based on clinical evaluation, flexible exam, or previous surgical interventions. There are many different methods for choosing an appropriate ETT size. Age-based systems are used in pediatric patients over 2 years of age, though this has a tendency to overestimate tube size up to 20 % of the time. Neonatal patients require estimation of tube size based on weight and length measurements with length being the most reliable measurement for tube length [19].

Additional airway adjuncts include using nasopharyngeal trumpets and oropharyngeal airways. These useful tools can assist in overcoming obstruction from soft tissue collapse in the nasopharynx and oropharynx.

Heliox is a special helium-oxygen mixture used mostly in the pediatric population in the management of airway obstruction. Helium has the second lowest specific gravity of the gases. Helium's lower density replaces the nitrogen and creates a more effective and less turbulent flow of oxygen capable of bypassing obstructing lesions. This can be used in patients with a tenuous airway in an effort to avoid intubation or to maintain the patient until a more definitive control of the airway can be obtained.

Neonates and infants have lower pulmonary reserve than older children and adult patients and as such a delay in obtaining an airway can result in a more urgent need for intervention. One method that has been used in adults and that can be adapted for the young patient is transtracheal ventilation [20] this method should be reserved as a last case scenario. A 16- or 14 gauge angiocath can be inserted into the cricothyroid membrane; using saline in the attached syringe to confirm location within the airway. Once in the airway a syringe modified with an ETT adapter is connected to the angiocath and connected to oxygen. This can allow enough oxygen to bypass an obstructed airway that is glottic or supraglottic to allow time for the setup of a more definitive intervention to bypass the obstruction or for the establishment of a surgical airway.

Conclusions

Neonatal endoscopy, including rigid and flexible modalities, is an essential and valuable procedure in the diagnosis and treatment of neonatal respiratory disorders. In the hands of an experienced otolaryngologist with the support of an operating room staff familiar with airway procedures and a knowledgeable pediatric anesthesia team, endoscopy can be done safely and effectively. The airway can be controlled throughout the procedure making this a safe and viable option for assessing and treating airway abnormalities in newborns and young infants.

References

1. Becker HD. A short history of bronchoscopy: introduction to bronchoscopy. Cambridge: Cambridge University Press; 2009. p. 1–16.
2. Zeitels SM. Chevalier Jackson's contributions to direct laryngoscopy. J Voice. 1998;12(1):1–6.
3. Koltai PJ, Nixon RE. The story of the laryngoscope. Ear Nose Throat J. 1989;68(7):494–502.
4. Marsh BR. Historic development of bronchoe-sophagology. Otolaryngol Head Neck Surg. 1996;114:689–716.
5. Bailey B. Laryngoscopy and Laryngoscopes—who's first? The forefathers/four fathers of laryngology. Laryngoscope. 1996;106(8):939–43.
6. Sasaki CT. Development of laryngeal function: etiologic significant in sudden infant death syndrome. Laryngoscope. 1979;3:420.
7. Fan LL, Flynn JW. Laryngoscopy in neonates and infants: experience with flexible fiberoptic bronchoscope. Laryngoscope. 1991;91:451.
8. Silberman HD. The use of the flexile fiberoptic nasopharyngolaryngoscope in the pediatric upper airway. Orolarygnol Clin North Am. 1978;11:365.
9. Schroeder JW, Bhandarkar ND, Holinger LD. Synchronous airway lesions and outcomes in infants with severe laryngomalacia requiring supraglottoplasty. Arch Otolaryngol Head and Neck Surg. 2009;133(7):647–51.
10. Gonzalez C, Riley JS, Bluestone CD. Synchronous airway lesion in infancy. Ann Otol Rhinol Laryngol. 1987;96:77.
11. Parsons DS. New set of pediatric laryngoscopes. Ann Otol Rhinol Laryngol. 1990;99(11):892–5.
12. Aziz MF, Dillman D, Fu R, Brambrink AM. Comparative effectiveness of the C-Mac video laryngoscope versus direct laryngoscopy in the setting of predicted airway difficulty. Anesthesiology. 2012;116(3):629–36.
13. McNair D, et al. Pediatric airway management: comparing the Berci–Kaplan Video Laryngoscope with direct laryngoscopy. Pediatr Anesth. 2009;19:577–80.
14. Pearce MS, Salotti JA, Little MP, McHugh K, Lee C, Kim KP, Howe NL, Ronckers CM, Rajaraman P, Sir Craft AW, Parker L, Berrington de González A. Radiation exposure from CT scans in childhood and subsequent risk of leukaemia and brain tumours: a retrospective cohort study. Lancet. 2012;380(9840):499–505.
15. Hedrick HL. Ex utero intrapartum therapy. Semin Pediatr Surg. 2003;10:190–5.
16. Liechty KW. Ex-utero intra partum therapy. Semin Fetal Neonatal Med. 2010;15:34–9.
17. Olsson GL, Hallen B. Laryngospasm during anaesthesia. A computer-aided incidence study in 136,929 patients. Acta Anaesth Scand. 1984;28:567–75.
18. Olsson GL, Hallen B. Bronchospasm during anaesthesia. A computer-aided incidence study in 136,929 patients. Acta Anaesth Scand. 1987;31:244–52.
19. Luten R, Kahn N, Wears R, Kissoon N. Predicting endotracheal tube size by length in newborns. J Emerg Med. 2007;32(4):343–7.
20. Gallagher TQ, Setulr J, Maturo S, Hartnick CJ. Percutaneous transtracheal needle insufflation: a useful emergency airway adjunct constructed from common items found in your anesthesia cart. Laryngoscope. 2012;122:1178–80.

Anesthesia Challenges for the Difficult and Critical Neonatal Airway

John Fiadjoe, Rebecca Isserman, and John McCloskey

Preoperative Preparation

Normal Anatomy and Physiology

The larynx descends as children grow and is most cranially positioned in the neonate [1]. The high cervical position of the larynx is often described as being "anterior" because of the view obtained with direct laryngoscopy. Because of the high location of the glottis, straight blades are thought to offer better exposure of the larynx because of the ability to elevate the base of the tongue. Despite this, some clinicians prefer curved blades and use them successfully. Other consequences of the high location of the neonate's glottis include the tendency for laryngeal masks to become dislodged and inadvertent compression of the airway in the neck during bag-mask ventilation.

The tongue in the neonate is relatively large and may obstruct the airway by adhering to the palate; relief can be obtained by opening the mouth or by applying continuous positive airway pressure (CPAP), to the airway via a bag-mask device. An oral airway is rarely needed to open the airway of a neonate. The neonatal epiglottis is relatively short. This allows one to elevate the tip by simply placing the straight laryngoscope blade in the vallecula much like how a curved blade is used. The glossoepiglottic ligament located in the vallecula should be engaged with the tip of the straight blade in order to gain adequate glottic exposure. The vocal cords in the neonate are slanted rostrally as compared to the vocal cords in the adult. This can cause difficulties in passing an endotracheal tube because the tip is already directed in an upward fashion to the anteriorly located larynx causing it to have a greater chance of being hung up at the anterior commissure or anterior tracheal wall. Classically, it has been taught the neonatal airway is funnel shaped, but a recent study suggests it may be tubular much like the adult airway [2]. Traditionally teaching is that the narrowest part of the neonatal/pediatric airway is at the cricoid ring and not at the vocal cords like the adult airway.

Normal cardiopulmonary physiology can also make the management of the neonatal airway difficult.

In the operating room (OR), the initial approach to a patient with a difficult airway is to perform an inhalational induction with a volatile anesthetic agent to allow for spontaneous ventilation. This can be done successfully in a neonate; however, the response is different due to differences in physiology. Theoretically, uptake of the volatile anesthetic can be delayed due to the relatively higher cardiac output; however, the higher minute ventilation and increased proportion of cardiac output to the brain in the neonate can actually increase the rate of induction. The faster rate of induction and effects on the neonatal brain subsequently leads to a faster decrease in respiratory function as compared to older children and adults (Fig. 1a).

Neonates are also more prone to develop hypoxia during the process of securing the airway due to differences in lung volumes and metabolic rate as compared to children and adults. In neonates, the functional residual capacity is approximately 27 mL/kg versus 43 mL/kg in the adult. Oxygen consumption is approximately 6–8 mL/kg/min in neonates versus 3–4 mL/kg/min. Thus, when a neonate becomes apneic, hypoxia occurs much more rapidly due to the increased metabolism depleting oxygen from the relatively smaller reserve. Attention to the airway management strategy is a central component of the preanesthetic assessment of the neonate. Underlying diagnosis, coexisting diseases, and diagnoses should be reviewed with attention to airway management. If tracheal intubation has previously

J. Fiadjoe, M.D. (✉) • J. McCloskey, M.D. • R. Isserman
Department of Anesthesiology & Critical Care Medicine,
The Children's Hospital of Philadelphia, Philadelphia, PA, USA
e-mail: fiadjoej@email.chop.edu

University of Pennsylvania, Perelman School of Medicine,
Philadelphia, PA, USA

J. Lioy and S.E. Sobol (eds.), *Disorders of the Neonatal Airway: Fundamentals for Practice*,
DOI 10.1007/978-1-4939-1610-8_22, © Springer Science+Business Media New York 2015

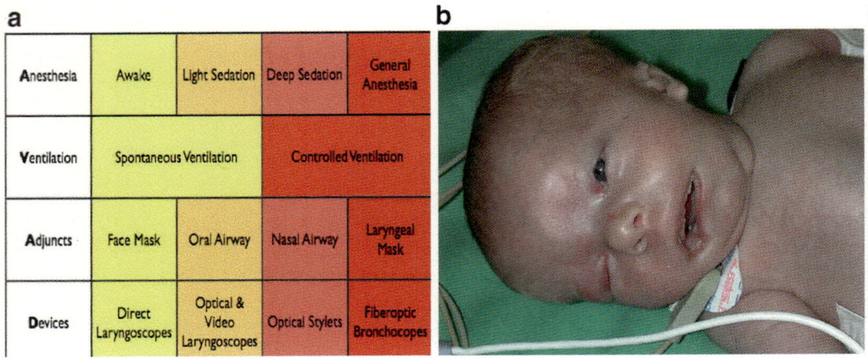

c

Cervical Spine Limitations	Birth injury with cervical spine injury				
Mandibular Disorders	Robin Sequence	Goldenhar Syndrome	Nager's Syndrome	Noonan Syndrome	Treacher Collins
Maxilla & Midface Disorders	Treacher Collins	Pterygium syndrome	Holoprosencephaly		
Limitations in Mouth Opening	Severe Arthrogryposis with TMJ Ankylosis	Trisomy 13 others with small oral opening			
Submandibular space & compliance	Trisomy 13 and others with severe micrognathia	Severe Micrognathia			

Fig. 1 (a) An useful simple framework anticipating level of anesthesia and possible tools for safe airway management. (**b**) Potentially difficult or critical airway with Goldenhars Syndrome. (Courtesy of John McCloskey, The Children's Hospital of Philadelphia, [CHOP]). (c) Conditions associated with difficult airway management in neonates

been performed, the involved providers can be questioned and the medical records reviewed to determine if there were unexpected difficulties. Conditions such as omphalocele and congenital diaphragmatic hernia may indirectly impact airway management causing rapid decompensation during anesthesia. Oxyhemoglobin desaturation follows apnea secondary to pulmonary hypoplasia and reduced functional residual capacity. Special attention to peak inspiratory pressures during anesthetic induction and intubation in particular lung malformations can prevent competing intestinal insufflation prior to intubation while also avoiding pneumothorax following intubation.

Rapid Sequence Intubation in Neonates

The goal of rapid sequence induction is to decrease the risk of pulmonary aspiration of gastric contents. Rapid sequence induction of anesthesia is a technique to minimize the time from anesthetic induction to tracheal intubation and can be challenging in infants. Due to the higher oxygen consumption rates, reduced FRC, and elevated closing volumes compared to older children and adult's desaturations occur much more rapidly following apnea. Consequently, when a classic rapid sequence induction technique is performed and 45–60 s of apnea are allowed to occur before tracheal intubation is attempted, significant Oxyhemoglobin desaturation commonly occurs. Therefore many pediatric anesthesiologists perform a "modified" rapid sequence induction in this population [53–56]. This technique uses facemask ventilation performed under low pressures (<10–15 cm H_2O) while cricoid pressure is applied until enough time has elapsed for complete neuromuscular blockade to occur. In support of this practice, appropriately applied cricoid pressure has been shown to be effective in preventing gastric inflation during gentle bag-mask ventilation in anesthetized infants and children [54–56]. If the initial attempt at intubation fails, gentle facemask ventilation through cricoid pressure should be performed. If ventilation is difficult with cricoid pressure despite the use of noninvasive devices (oral or nasopharyngeal airway, laryngeal mask airway) cricoid pressure should be lessened [54–56].

Abnormal Neonatal Anatomy and Physiology

There are numerous genetic abnormalities that can cause difficulties with airway management, but the most commonly encountered craniofacial syndromes that can cause difficulty right from birth include Treacher–Collins syndrome, the Pierre Robin sequence, and Goldenhar syndrome. Each of these syndromes involves some element of mandibular dysplasia, micrognathia, and retrognathia that can make intubation with a standard laryngoscopy extremely difficult. Goldenhar syndrome is especially challenging since these patients typically have asymmetrical hypoplasia of the mandible which makes it extremely difficult to get a good mask fit for bag-mask ventilation (Fig. 1b, c). In a busy neonatal practice, these syndromes can be seen quite often since the incidence of Treacher–Collins syndrome, Pierre Robin sequence, and Goldenhar syndrome is 1 in 10,000–50,000, 1 in 8,500–10,000, and 1 in 3,000–5,000 live births, respectively. One of the most dreaded situations that can be faced in a neonate with a difficult airway is the neonate who presents with CHAOS—**C**ongenital **H**igh **A**irway **O**bstruction **S**yndrome. This syndrome consists of patients whose upper airways are distorted by either teratomas, hemangiomas, or lymphatic malformations. Due to the high probability of needing a surgical airway, these patients are usually delivered via an EXIT, or ex utero intra partum, procedure. The placental bypass allows for oxygenation of the neonate while securing the airway. In many instances, endotracheal intubation is performed via rigid bronchoscopy or immediate placement of a tracheostomy.

Other examples of abnormal airway anatomy related in neonates potentially include the former premature infant with a past history of prolonged intubation in the neonatal intensive care unit. Although a number of these patients are successfully extubated and no obvious problems with their

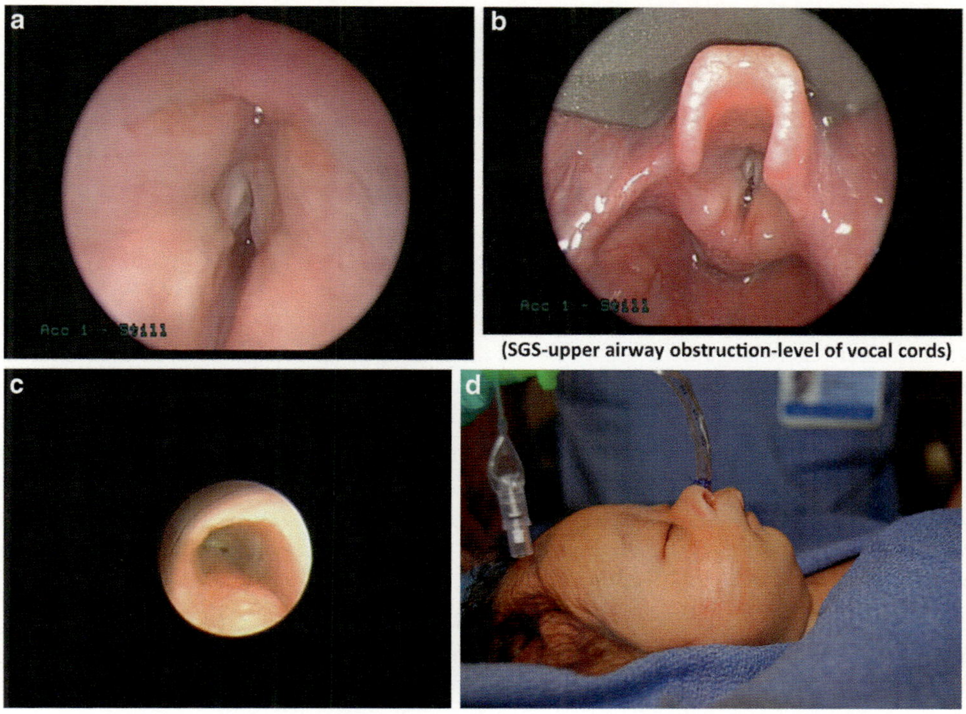

Fig. 2 2 (a), (**b**), (**c**) Bronchoscopy photos showing various forms of glottic and subglottic abnormalities such as subglottic stenosis, vocal cord paralysis and vocal cord atresia posing anesthesia challenges. (Courtesy of Ian Jacobs and Steve Sobol, CHOP). (**d**) Neonate with micrognathia posing anesthesia challenges. (Courtesy of Jesse Taylor, CHOP)

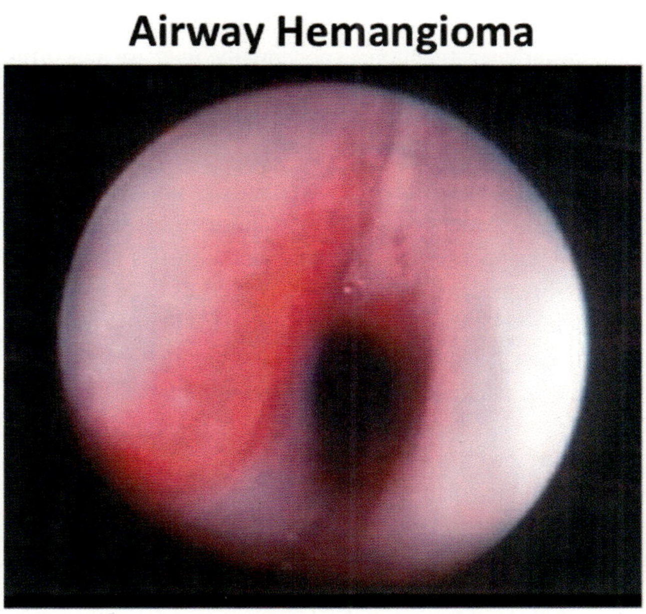

Fig. 3 Airway hemangioma, (Courtesy of Ian Jacobs, CHOP).

airways, careful attention should be made to ascertain any history of stridor/croup; these patients can occasionally present at induction with difficulty to ventilate and intubate due to mild micrognathia or occult subglottic stenosis (Fig. 2a–d). The patient with a history of prolonged intubation while in the NICU can also present months later with stridor secondary to cyst formation. Patients with airway hemangiomas can also present months after birth with stridor since the natural course of these lesions is for them to enlarge before involuting (Fig. 3).

In terms of abnormal physiology, patients with cyanotic cardiac disease not uncommon can have issues with craniofacial syndromes causing airway difficulties due to these lesions being midline defects. These patients are truly challenging when trying to secure their airways since they are hypoxic to begin with and have very little reserve. The patients with an abnormal airway and chronic lung disease secondary to prematurity are also complex to manage due to a limited respiratory reserve. This difficulty can be further compounded by the presence of pulmonary hypertension, which can accompany the chronic lung disease.

Intraoperative Management

Approach to Securing the Airway in Neonate with a Difficult Airway

What is a Difficult Airway?

According to the report by the American Society of Anesthesiologists (ASA) Task Force on Management of the Difficult Airway, a standardized definition of the difficult airway cannot be identified in the literature [3]. The definition suggested by this task force is "The clinical situation in which a conventionally trained anesthesiologist experiences difficulty with face mask ventilation of the upper airway, difficulty with tracheal intubation, or both [3]." As such, the difficult airway is not a single entity or disease state, but a clinical endpoint associated with a wide variety of diseases and conditions. The extant literature on difficult airway management is replete with case series and case reports describing various techniques that have been effective in specific scenarios by specific providers. However, owing to the myriad of clinical conditions associated with the difficult airway in children and the relatively low incidence, systematic studies to determine the optimal management are lacking (Fig. 2b).

Principles of Difficult Airway Management: The ASA Difficult Airway Algorithm

Evaluating some prospective randomized clinical trials that evaluate various management strategies can be problematic, and the approach to the airway must be tailored to the specific airway problem of the available resources. In 1993, the American Society of Anesthesiologists (ASA) Task Force on Management of the Difficult Airway published a set of practice guidelines for difficult airway management in adults which have since been updated again in 2013 [1]. Due in large parts to the paucity of high-level evidence in the literature, these guidelines were developed based on the available information and expert opinion/consensus to provide rational guidance to practitioners. The algorithm included in these guidelines (Fig. 4) has become the gold standard for most adults when managing difficult airway clinical decision-making. As a framework, this algorithm provides an appropriate decision tree for individual patient management. Furthermore, the algorithm represents guidelines that, while widely adopted, do not necessarily represent the standard of care, especially in neonatology. In fact, one of the initial assessments proposed by the ASA guidelines that can affect the decision tree/pathway in the algorithm is whether there is difficulty in patient cooperation or consent. The neonate is similar to the uncooperative adult patient; a two-way dialogue cannot be held with the neonate if one is considering an awake intubation. However, it is common and thought to be a safe practice to intubate a neonate awake. In many pediatric institutions, the ASA Difficult Airway Algorithm has been modified to their specific patients and utilized to create emergency airway algorithms such as we use in our institution (Fig. 5).

In reviewing the ASA algorithm, two basic questions need to be answered when approaching the patient with a potentially difficult airway; can I ventilate? can I intubate? In most situations, where there is a high likelihood that one cannot ventilate then there should be a consideration to either intubate the neonate awake or keep the patient breathing spontaneously with light sedation or through the use of an inhalational anesthetic. Difficult mask fits are typically seen in many craniofacial syndromes. For neonates with these problems, these difficulties can be circumvented with a Laryngeal Mask Airway (LMA) (Fig. 6).

The ASA difficult airway algorithm highlights the use of the laryngeal mask airway (LMA) as a rescue device. First introduced in 1983, the LMA has revolutionized the approach to the patient with a difficult airway not only as a rescue device, but also as a conduit for placement of an endotracheal tube into the trachea [4]. Its use as a rescue device is described in the International Neonatal Resuscitations Guidelines [5, 6]. This device allows for the ability to oxygenate and ventilate a patient while using a fiberoptic bronchoscope. The LMA has also been proven to be useful as a way to perform an inhalation induction in a neonate when it is difficult to get a mask fit such as in patients with Goldenhar syndrome [7]. A topical local anesthetic can be applied to the oropharynx of the patient to reduce airway activation when the LMA is placed awake; however, this is not necessary in most neonates.

In the situation where there is a potential for a difficult intubation, multiple plans for securing the airway with the use of different techniques and standard and advanced devices should be developed prior to attempting to secure the airway.

Preparation for managing the difficult airway should take several factors into consideration such as anatomy, physiology, pharmacology, and equipment choices. As outlined above, congenital anomalies of the face along with masses obstructing the airway are the most common causes of difficulties with the neonatal airway. The unique differences in cardiorespiratory function exponentially increase the difficulty, whether the laryngoscopist is a neonatologist or anesthesiologist sedative, and induction agents have been used successfully during intubations for neonates [8]. For most anesthesiologists, the approach is usually an inhalation induction since the patient can be slowly anesthetized, continue to breath spontaneously, and maintain their airway since muscle tone is still present. The use of large doses of intravenous induction agents and muscle relaxants leads to apnea and can be detrimental if the patient cannot be bag-mask ventilated. In situations where an inhalation induction may still be risky in patients with airway masses or severe anomalies, these patients can be "sedated" with small doses of agents such as ketamine, midazolam, or dexmedetomidine [9] (Table 1). Muscle relaxants, such as succinylcholine, vecuronium, or rocuronium, should only be considered if a patient could be satisfactorily bag-mask ventilated and further use of sedative or induction agents will potentially lead to cardiovascular instability (Table 2). Neuromuscular blockade can be advantageous in some scenarios. The advantages include a motionless patient, jaw relaxation, and removal of the risk of laryngospasm. Some of the potential disadvantages of neuromuscular blockade are essentially the opposites of the advantages for spontaneous ventilation—namely, a greater potential for upper airway soft tissue collapse with loss of the ability to ventilate, and the risk of arterial desaturation rapidly due to apnea during prolonged intubation attempts. Another disadvantage is gastric distension from manual positive pressure ventilation resulting in compromised ventilation (through

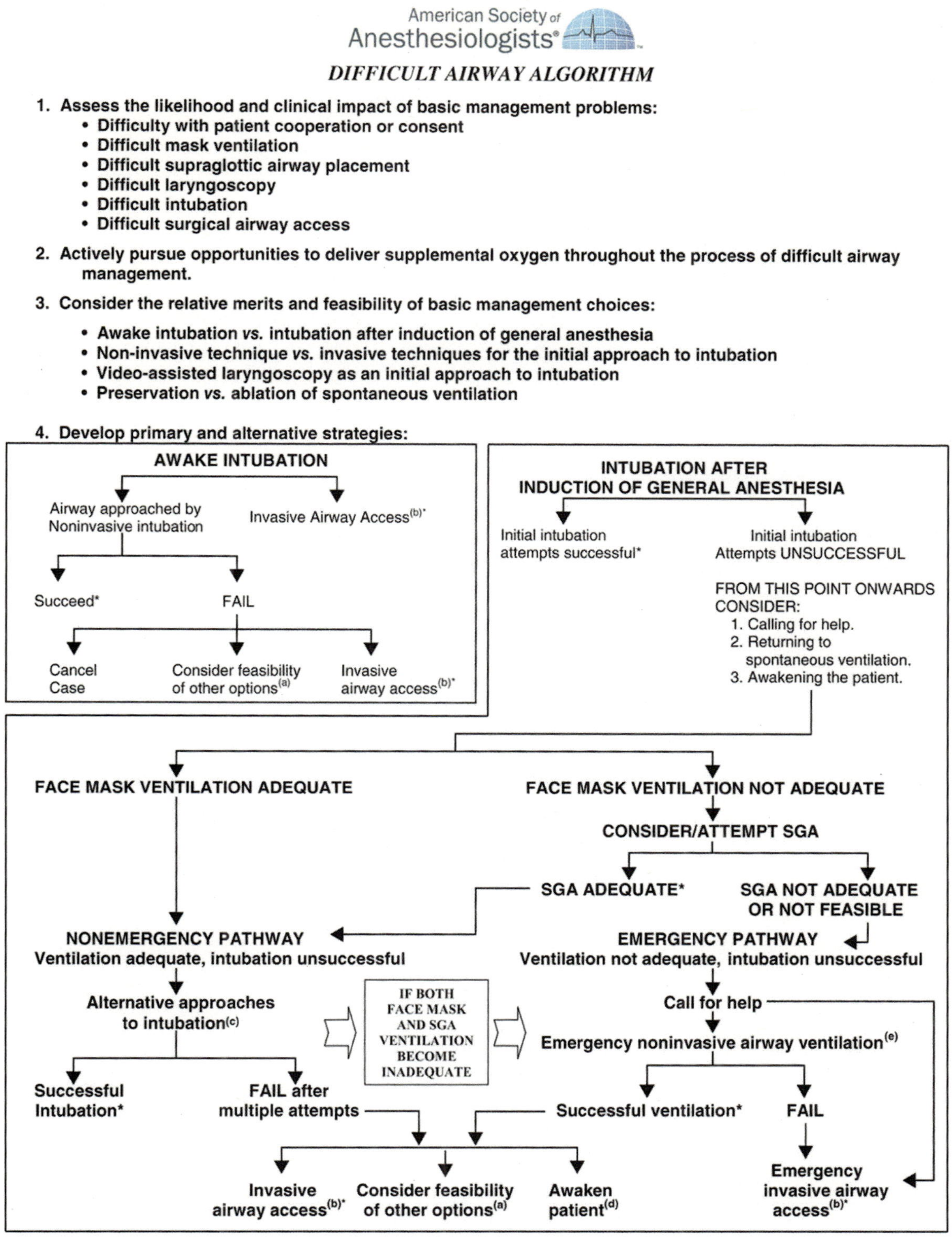

Fig. 4 American Society of Anesthesiologist difficult airway algorithm (Reprinted from [3]. With permission from Wolter Kluwers Health

abdominal competition) and/or regurgitation of gastric contents. This can be particularly problematic in infants and smaller children where an inflated stomach can significantly reduce functional residual capacity

Basic Equipment

With any approach to securing a difficult airway, a primary plan and backup plans need to be formulated. Each approach/plan should define the equipment necessary to secure the

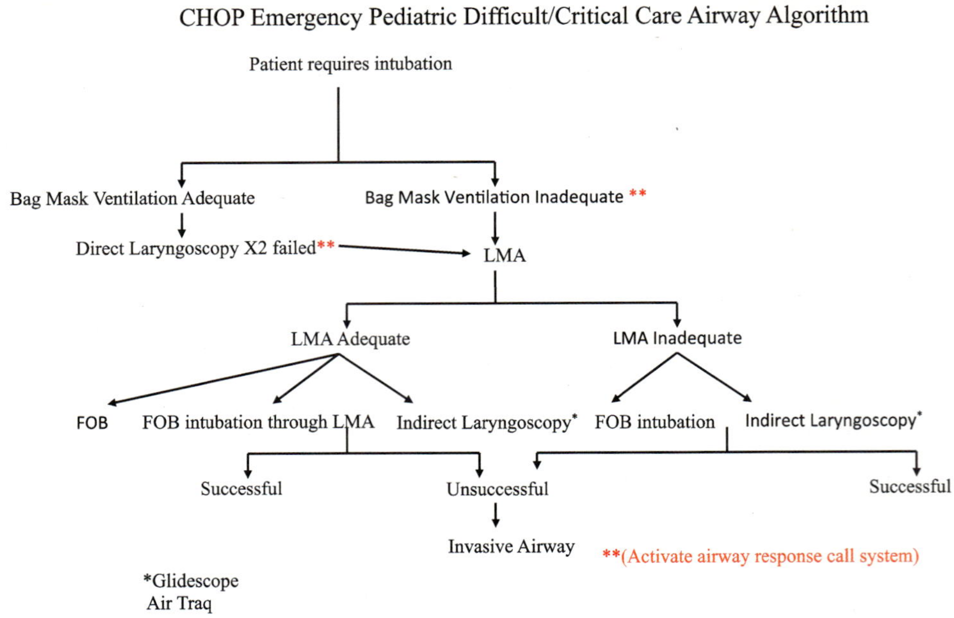

Fig. 5 CHOP difficult/critical airway algorithm

Fig. 6 Variety of laryngeal mask airways, (LMA's), and oral airways

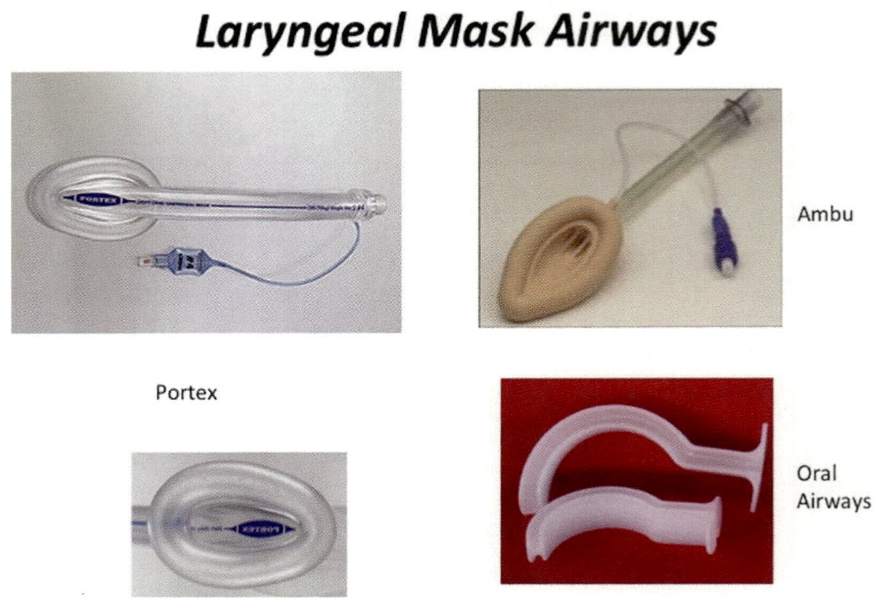

airway, whether it is a supraglottic airway such as an LMA, an endotracheal tube, or a tracheostomy tube. Inherent to any approach is a progression from basic to more complex equipment.

The basic equipment required for any approach to any airway includes airway adjuncts such as oral and nasal airways, laryngoscopes with blades, a bag-mask ventilation system, and an LMA as a rescue device [10] (Fig. 7). For most neonates, there should be two laryngoscopes available with straight blades, Miller #0 and #1. As described above, the anatomical differences allow for the straight blade to be used like a curved blade: the tip of the blade is placed in the vallecula to raise the epiglottis. The Rendell–Baker mask, a hard black rubber mask with little dead space, was the standard mask utilized with a manual bag-mask ventilator system; however, this has been supplanted by the modern clear mask with an inflatable rim. The inflatable rim allows for a tight seal by conforming to almost any contours of the face. It is imperative this rim be checked for function prior to using it; poor inflation or leak of the rim can lead to difficulties in bag-mask ventilation. The next important basic device to have is the LMA. As mentioned before, the LMA serves both

Table 1 Comparison of three sedation regimens for airway management

	Midazolam/ Fentanyl	High-dose dexmedetomidine	Ketamine
Sedation	++	+	++
Analgesia	++	+	+++
Amnesia	++	+/–	+++
Reversible	Yes	No	No
Clinician familiarity	+++	+/–	++
Pt responsive to commands	+	+	No
Respiratory drive	–	++	+
Adjuncts required	No	No	No

Table 2 Drugs used for intubation

Drugs	Doses
Sedatives	
Midazolam	Starting dose: 0.05 mg/kg IV—bolus to a total max of 0.2 mg/kg
Fentanyl	Starting dose: 1 mcg/kg IV—bolus to a total max of 2–3 mcg/kg
Ketamine	Starting dose: 0.5 mg/kg IV—bolus to a total max of 1.5–2.0 mg/kg
Dexmedetomidine	Starting bolus: 1 mcg/kg IV—bolus to a total max of 3 mcg/kg
	Infusion: 0.5 mcg/kg/h IV
Paralytic agents	
Succinylcholine	1–2 mg/kg IV
Vecuronium	0.1 mg/kg IV
Rocuronium	1 mg/kg IV

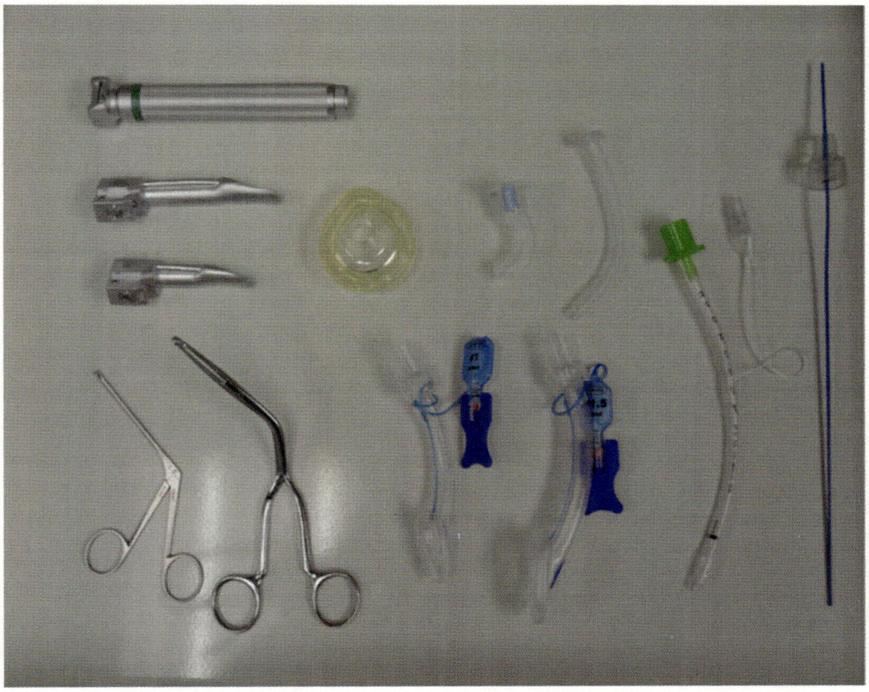

Fig. 7 Neonatal intubating equipment kept handy in an emergency airway cart. (Courtesy of Janet Lioy, neonatal airway program-CHOP)

as a rescue device and a conduit for placing an endotracheal tube [11]. Its basic design as a mask that sits over the larynx allows for easy identification of the vocal cords and displacement of soft tissues of entire airway allowing for easier entry into the trachea with a fiberoptic bronchoscope. An endotracheal tube preloaded on the bronchoscope can then be easily passed into the trachea. Difficulties with earlier versions of the LMA were encountered due to the flexible grill over the aperture of the LMA, which made passing the tube difficult. Furthermore the length of endotracheal tubes was similar to the length of the airway tube of the LMA making it difficult to insert the tube completely through the mask without adjuncts. Also, the pilot balloon on cuff endotracheal tubes would not easily pass through the tube of the LMA. A newer version of a laryngeal mask, the AirQ® (Fig. 8) is designed specifically to allow as a conduit for fiberoptic intubation. It has no grill over the aperture, the airway tube has a relatively greater diameter and shorter length, and the airway connector is easily disconnected. It also comes in a variety of sizes for a variety of sized patients. The #1 size has been used as an adjunct to fiberoptically intubate neonates [12].

Although not usually thought of as a basic device, the fiberoptic bronchoscope is routinely used in the next step to secure a difficult airway, whether either as a stand-alone device or in conjunction with a laryngeal mask. Its ability for the tip to be manipulated makes it an essential piece of

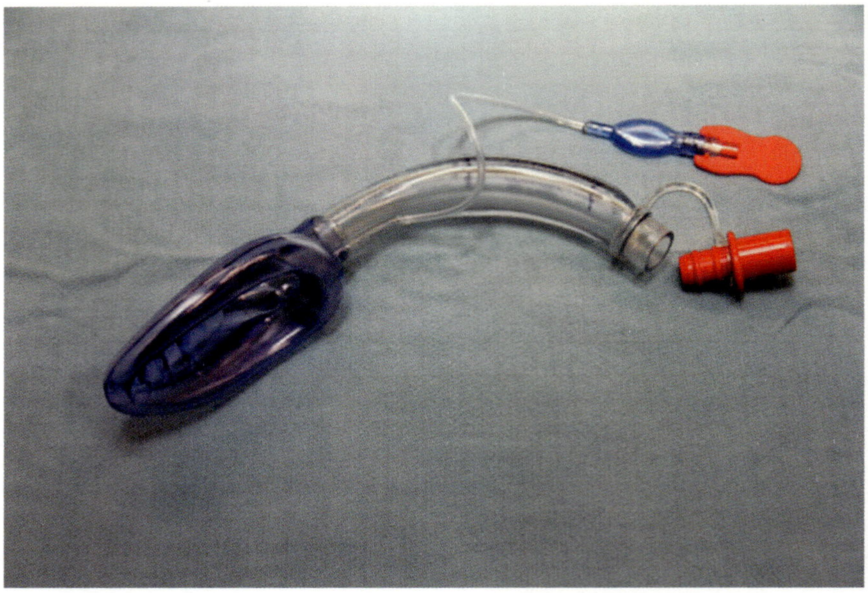

Fig. 8 Air Q LMA for indirect intubation through tube lumen

equipment. For neonates, there are two sizes of scopes that can be used, the 2.2 or 2.8 mm scope. The measurement describes the outside diameter of the scope, thus, the 2.2 scope can accommodate a 2.5 mm inside diameter endotracheal tube and the 2.8 can accommodate an endotracheal tube 3.0 mm or greater. The 2.8 scope has a suction channel to remove secretions which can obscure the view of the airway, but the 2.2 scope does not. Due to the small size of the visual fields it can sometimes be difficult to ascertain anatomic structures by viewing through the eyepiece on the scope. Attaching a camera to the scope will transmit the image to a larger monitor that can enhance the view of the airway. This also allows other individuals at the bedside to help assist in identifying structures. Newer models of scopes are now incorporating a video "chip" at the tip which essentially builds integrates a camera into the scope and allows for a higher resolution.

Typically, in most operating room suites and critical care areas, most of the equipment described above to secure a difficult area are stored together in a difficult airway cart. The cart, as is our institution will include other equipment such as oral airways to facilitate an oral fiberoptic intubation, Magill forceps to allow manipulation of the tip of the endotracheal tube in the posterior pharynx, airway exchangers, tracheostomy dilators, and needle cricothyroidotomy kits. In our own institution, our carts also have an Airtraq camera with screen mounted to the top of the cart and are stored in the same area with fiberoptic bronchoscopes and GlideScopes so they can be easily obtained at the same time (Fig. 9).

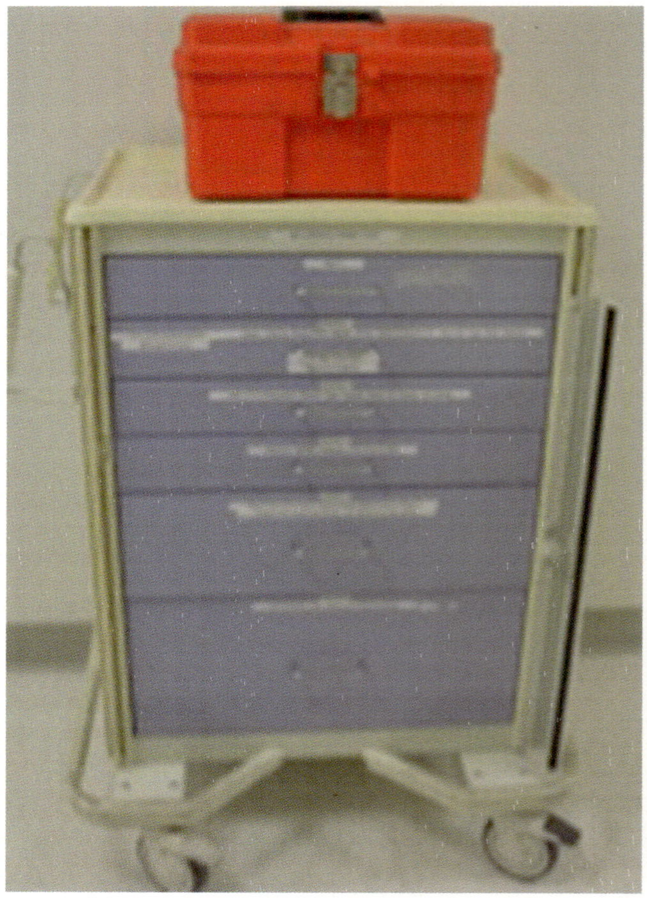

Fig. 9 Emergency airway neonatal cart. (Courtesy of Janet Lioy, neonatal airway program-CHOP)

The rest of this section will now focus on advanced equipment and techniques, specifically indirect laryngoscopic devices that are used to secure difficult airways. Not one device is better than the next device; however, anatomic conditions will dictate the choice of one device versus another. Comfort and skill of the operator will also direct decisions on a device. There are many different devices on the market but the ones presented have been used successfully for securing the airway in a neonate. It is recommended that practice should be obtained with simulation and normal airways prior to incorporating them to secure a difficult airway.

Advanced Equipment and Techniques

Video and Optical Laryngoscopes

Video and optical laryngoscopes have transformed adult airway management. They incorporate a camera into the tip of a curved or straight blade. Their use in neonates has been limited because the earlier designed models were ineffective. Newer designs are now smaller and more appropriate for neonates. Although video and optical laryngoscopy is easier to learn than direct laryngoscopy, a learning curve still remains. Deliberate practice and kinesthetic skill is necessary for successful intubation. Because a camera is placed in the vicinity of the larynx, video-laryngoscopes provide a better view of the glottis and improve intubation success in simulated difficult intubations [13, 14].

GlideScope™

The GlideScope™ is the most popular and most studied video-laryngoscope.

The original GlideScope™ design (GVL 2) was too large for infants and neonates and was associated with repeated failures when used in neonates [15–17]. The analog GlideScope Cobal™t and digital GlideScope AVL™ videolaryngoscopes (GCV; Verathon Medical, Bothell, WA) are newer designs made strictly for pediatric use (Fig. 10a–c). The blades are narrower (10 mm compared to 14.5 mm) and are available in a full complement of pediatric sizes. The Cobalt model consists of a flexible video baton which provides a high-resolution image on a video monitor. This baton is inserted into different-sized disposable plastic blades called Stats. The size 1–2 video baton is most suitable for infants and neonates. Specifically, the manufacturer recommends the following weight-based guidelines for the various blades; size 0 blade (patients <1.5 kg), size 1 blade (patients 1.5–3.6 kg), and size 2 blade (patients 1.8–10 kg). The size 0 blade too is ideal for preterm neonates, size 1 for full-term neonates, and size 2 for infants.

The GlideScope Cobalt™ provides a better view of the airway than standard direct laryngoscopy [18]. Sola et al. found in a cohort of children 3 days to 7 years of age, all patients with poor direct laryngoscopic views (Cormack and Lehane grades 3 and 4), had better views with the GlideScope size 1 blade [19]. Our own study of infants and neonates confirmed this and demonstrated similar intubation success as compared to direct laryngoscopy [20]. Although visualization is improved with the GlideScope™, actual passage of an endotracheal intubation may not be possible. This is usually due to a lack of experience with the indirect approach of inserting the breathing tube.

Technique

Typically, a stylette is placed in the endotracheal tube and shaped to mimic the curve of the selected GlideScope blade. To create more space in the oropharynx, the blade is placed in the left side of the mouth. It is then advanced along the curvature of the tongue into the vallecula. The tracheal tube is inserted directly adjacent to the blade and placed just between the vocal cords. The stylette is withdrawn slightly to reduce the angle of the tip of the tube and allow easier advancement into the trachea.

Common Causes of Failure

Blade size: Selecting the correct blade size is important for successful intubation. An inappropriate blade size will result in a poor view. A blade that is too big may be difficult to insert and may limit the space available to insert the endotracheal tube. A blade that is too small will not allow appropriate tongue control and will not extend far enough into the vallecula.

Blade Tip Position

With standard direct laryngoscopy, the operator usually obtains the best possible view prior to inserting the breathing tube. Counter intuitively; this practice may make tracheal intubation more difficult with the GlideScope™. A Cormack and Lehane grade II view may facilitate tracheal intubation with the GlideScope™. Alignment with the tracheal axis width is enhanced with this grade of view and allows an improved path to advancing the tube. It also reduces the incidence of the tube that is catching on the anterior tracheal wall. A grade 2 view can be artificially created by slightly withdrawing the blade after it is placed in the vallecula. A grade 1 view, despite being the best view with a standard laryngoscopy, often pulls the glottic opening in an anterior direction increasing the angle of incidence between the advancing tube and the tracheal axis.

Bend Angle

The bend angle of the stylleted tube when using the Glidescope™ is critical for successful tracheal intubation. A curve that mimics the selected blade seems to be ideal optimal (Fig. 11). This guarantees the endotracheal tube will be ideally positioned in front of the GlideScope™ camera when inserted.

Tips and Tricks

External laryngeal manipulation (ELM) of the larynx may facilitate intubation with the GlideScope™. ELM is particularly effective when the tip of the endotracheal tube hangs up at the level of the glottis. A second operator is needed to provide effective ELM. It may be beneficial for the second operator to handle the stylleted tube while performing ELM. This allows real time tactile feedback when the tube passes the glottic opening. It is sometimes easier to manipulate a hung-up tube into the trachea by removing the GlideScope while maintaining the tube at the glottis. The nondominant hand manipulates the larynx while the dominant hand advances the tube into the trachea.

Fig. 10 (**a**) GlideScope. (**b**) GlideScope Cobalt blade. (**c**) Bronchoscopes and Special laryngoscopes, (courtesy of Steve Sobol, The Children's Hospital of Philadelphia). (**d**) Specifics of flexible bronchoscopes. (Adapted from Wheeler et al. [ref 58] Springer 2009

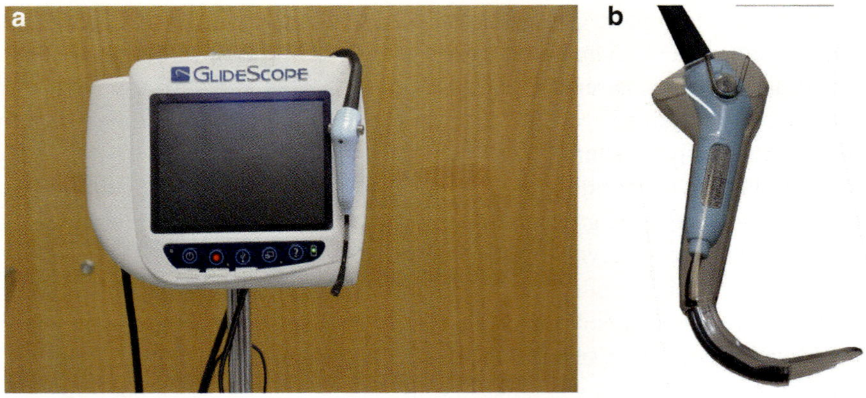

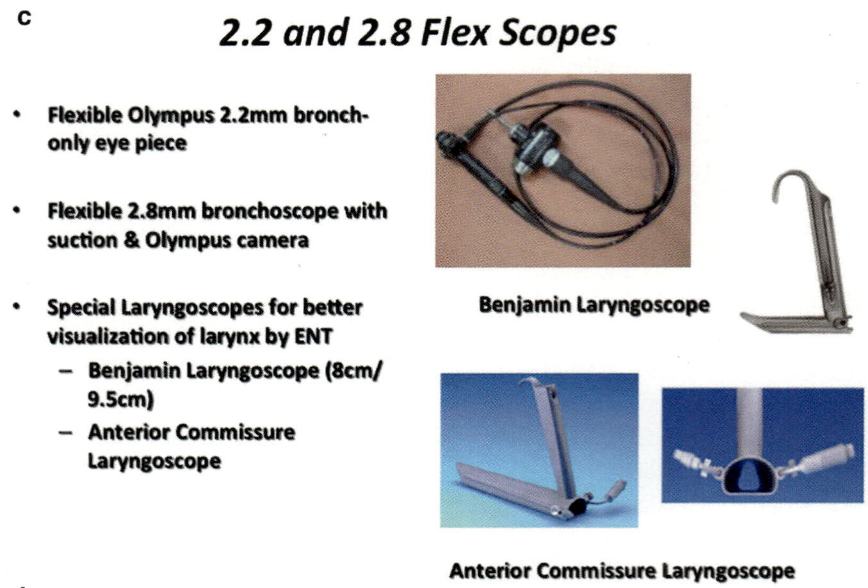

d

TABLE-----Flexible bronchoscopes.*

Diameter (mm)	Suction channel (mm)	Smallest endotracheal tube for intubation (mm)	Smallest endotracheal tube for assisted ventilation (mm)	Smallest endotracheal tube for spontaneous ventilation (mm)	Largest tube that should beused with this instrument for intubation (mm)†
2.2	None	2.5	3.0	3.5	4.0
2.8	1.2	3.0	3.5	4.0	4.5
3.5	1.2	4.5	5.0	5.5	6.0
3.8‡	1.2	5.0	5.0	5.5	7.5
4.4	2.0	5.0	5.5	6.0	7.5
4.9	2.0	5.5	6.0	6.5	NA

*Olympus Corporation. Instruments by other manufacturers may have similar (but not necessarily identical) characteristics.

†Use with larger tubes may result in damage to the instrument.

‡True videoscope; tip diameter is actually closer to 4.4 mm.

Fig. 11 Bend angle for ETT and Glidescope

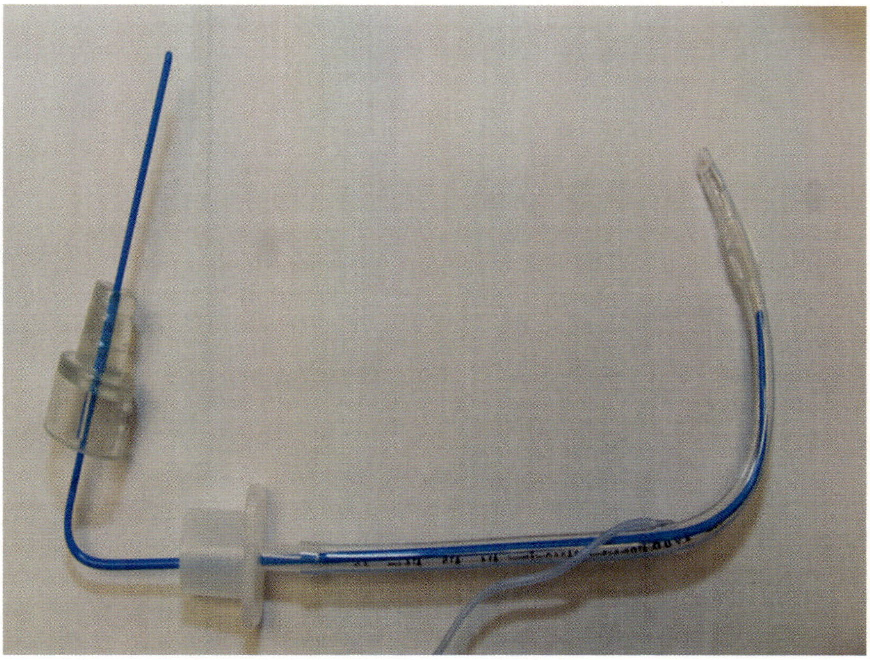

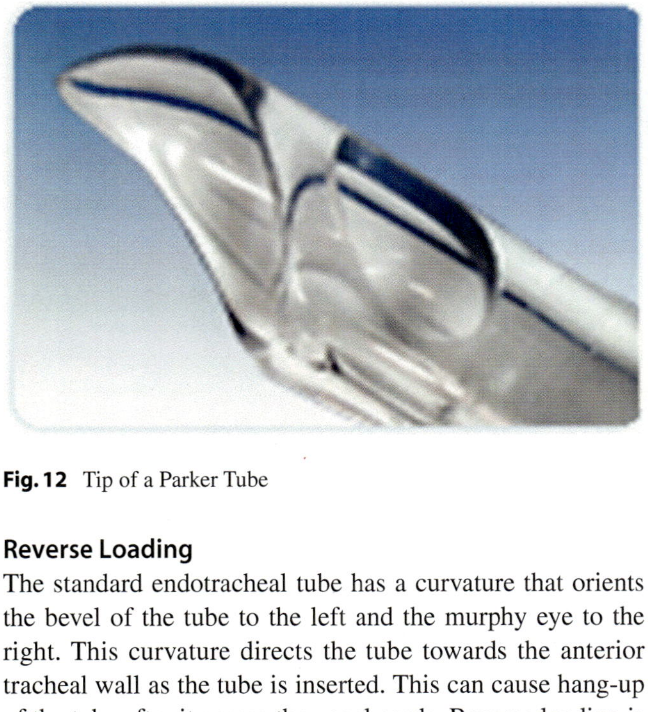

Fig. 12 Tip of a Parker Tube

Reverse Loading

The standard endotracheal tube has a curvature that orients the bevel of the tube to the left and the murphy eye to the right. This curvature directs the tube towards the anterior tracheal wall as the tube is inserted. This can cause hang-up of the tube after it passes the vocal cords. Reverse loading is when the tracheal tube is rotated 90° counter clockwise from the standard orientation.

Endotracheal Tube Type

A Parker ™ type tube may allow the tracheal tube to pass more easily into the trachea. This type of endotracheal tube has a tip that is beveled into the airway, thus making the advancing portion of the endotracheal tube round and smooth. The tip of the tube flexes around obstructions and reduces the incidence of hang-up (Fig. 12).

Cuffed Versus Uncuffed Tracheal Tubes

Historically, the classic teaching in pediatric anesthesia was to use uncuffed tracheal tubes in children under 8–10 years of age. This was recommended because children were often spontaneously breathing and larger tubes meant for lower resistance and decreased work of breathing. Also concerning is the notion that cuffed tubes may be associated with a higher risk of subglottic injury. However, the use of modern tracheal tubes with high volume, low pressure cuffs has not been associated with an increased incidence of subglottic airway injury or an increased incidence of post-extubation croup following their use in anesthetized children [57].

Placement Technique

In patients with limited mouth opening, inserting the GlideScope™ and stylleted endotracheal tube into the airway as a unit may facilitate intubation. Another alternative is to insert the endotracheal tube into the oropharynx before the GlideScope.

Storz Videolaryngoscope

The Storz DCI® ™Video-Laryngoscope (SVL, Karl Storz GmbH Tuttlingen, Germany) integrates a video camera into standard laryngoscope blades. The image is displayed on a portable video screen or on the handle of the blade (Fig. 13). The incorporation of the Miller 0 and Miller 1 blades into video-laryngoscopes has created the option of using of this

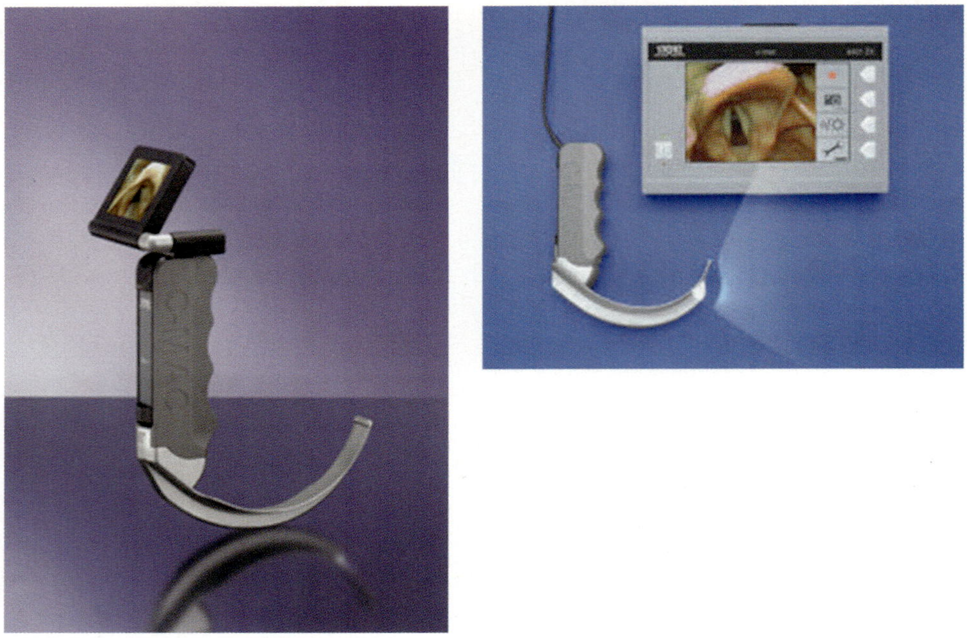

Fig. 13 CMAC Videolaryngoscope

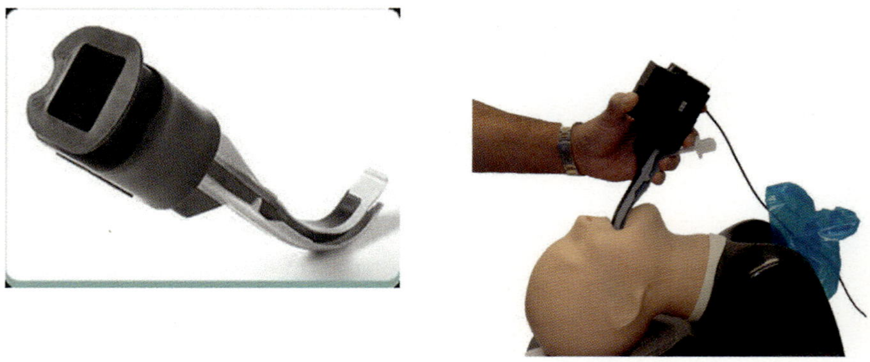

Fig. 14 Adapted from Fiadjoe, et al: In Wheeler DS et al., eds. [46]. Springer 2014

device in neonates. The advantage of this system is that standard blade sizes can be used not only with the usual ability of direct line of site but also an additional video image is provided with the addition of a pocket monitor which sits atop the handle for direct view without turning away from the mouth. There are a number of case studies describing the successful use of SVL in difficult infant intubations after failed direct laryngoscopy [21–23]. In all cases of difficult direct laryngoscopy, a styletted endotracheal tube was required to successfully intubate these patients with the SVL. Some investigators have described tracheal tube placement without a stylette by corkscrewing the tracheal tube through the channel of the SVL. Despite this we routinely prefer to place a stylette for all video intubations with this device [24]. The video-laryngoscope allows the laryngoscopist to perform tracheal intubation exactly in the same manner as a standard direct laryngoscopy. It further allows an instructor to see the same view on a video screen that a trainee is seeing while performing laryngoscopy. This facilitates instruction of the trainee as to how to perform standard direct laryngoscopy [25].

Airtraq

The Airtraq ™ Optical Laryngoscope (Prodol Meditec, Vizcava, Spain) is a disposable, portable indirect laryngoscope that uses lenses, prisms, and mirrors to transmit an image from the tip of a curved blade to an eyepiece [26]. It can be used with a wireless or wired camera that displays the image on 5.7-in. screen (Fig. 14). The device has a channel that holds the tracheal tube in place and directs it towards the center of the image on the screen. It comes in a variety of sizes, but size 0 is ideal for neonates; it accommodates endotracheal tube sizes 2.5–3.5 mm. A minimum mouth opening of 12.5 mm is needed in order to insert the device. Case studies report variable success in normal infants and those who failed direct laryngoscopy [26–29]. Failures were frequently due to posterior displacement of the endotracheal tube and the inability to direct the tube through the vocal cords [30].

Maneuvers to minimize or eliminate this issue included using a stylette, a gum elastic bougie, an Endoflex® Endotracheal tube, or a fiberoptic bronchoscope through the guide channel [30, 31]. Many of these options are not feasible with the smallest tracheal tubes. One manikin study found faster intubations and higher success when using an Airtraq™ as compared to conventional laryngoscopy during infant cardiopulmonary resuscitation [32]. In another comparison study with standard direct laryngoscopy, the Airtraq™ faired well in children less than 6 months with an improved view of the larynx and no statistically significant difference in intubation time [33]. Although the Airtraq's guide channel is designed to reduce difficulty with inserting the breathing tube, this problem still occurs especially in neonates. The relatively large size of the device, as compared to the mouth opening, can also make insertion of the device difficult in the smallest patients.

Truview

The Truview™ EVO2 Infant Laryngoscope (Truphatek International Ltd, Netanya, Israel) integrates lenses and prisms into an angulated blade (Fig. 15). The blade has a built-in port for oxygen insufflation, both to supply oxygen to the patient during intubation, and to prevent fogging of the camera. This infant blade is designed for patients 1–15 kg. The Truview PCD Pediatric™ (Truphatek International Ltd, Netanya, Israel) uses the same design with an attached camera for video capabilities. In addition, four blade sizes are available for use in children of varying sizes. There have been three case reports describing the use of these devices in infants with difficult airways. In all of the cases, intubation was unsuccessful with direct laryngoscopy due to a poor view of the glottis. The Truview devices improved the glottic view and allowed successful intubation in all of the patients [34–36].

In another study, Singh et al performed a randomized, controlled study comparing the Truview EVO2 Infant to direct laryngoscopy with a Miller 0 blade in 60 infants and neonates under 10 kg. They showed a statistically, but not clinically significant difference in intubation time (18.18 s in the Truview group; 16.3 s in the Miller group) and an improved view of the glottis in the Truview group [37].

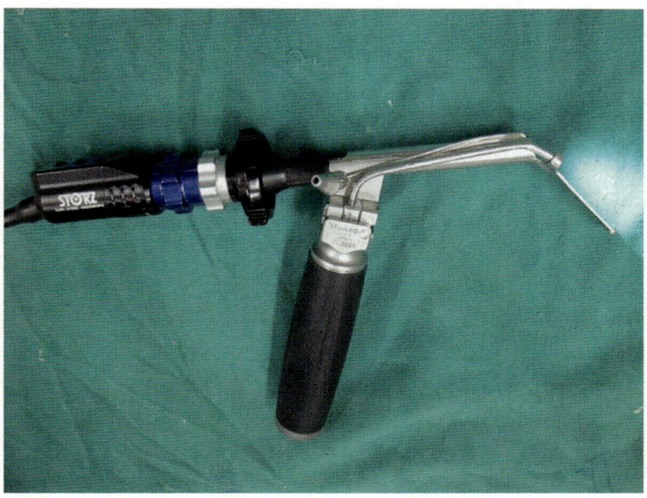

Fig. 15 Truview

Optical Stylletes

The Shikani Optical Stylette™ (Clarus Medical, Minneapolis, MN, USA) is a stainless steel malleable fiberoptic stylette with an eyepiece. The malleable stylette has enough rigidity to maneuver around airway structures [9]. The pediatric version can accommodate endotracheal tube sizes from 2.5 to 5.5. This device has been successfully used to intubate infants with difficult airways due to limited mouth opening, micrognathia, and mandibular hypoplasia [9, 38, 39]. The Storz Bonfils ™ fiberscope (Brambrink Intubation Endoscope; ä Karl Storz Endoscopy, Tuttlingen, Germany) is another optical stylette that is designed for neonatal use. The Bonfils differs from the Shikani in that it is a rigid stylette with a fixed 40° curved tip and a much higher image quality (Fig. 16). It is available in 2, 3.5, and 5 mm external diameters, sizes with the 2 mm being appropriate for most neonatal intubations. Caruselli et al. describe the successful intubation of a small for gestational age full-term neonate with failed direct laryngoscopy using the Bonfils fiberscope using a 2.5 mm endotracheal tube [40]. Bein et al. described their experience with the Bonfils fiberscope

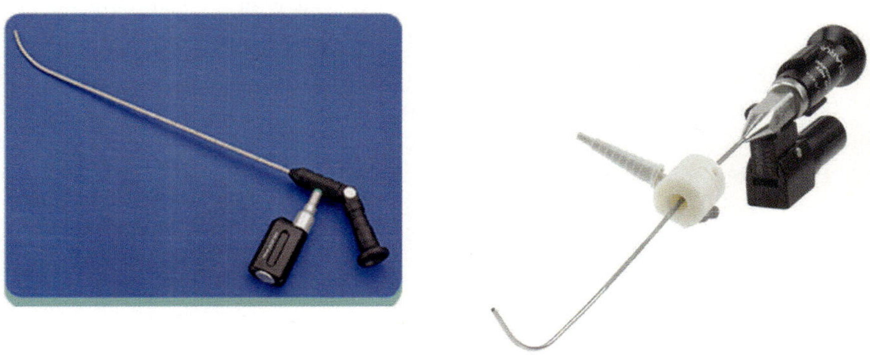

Fig. 16 Bonfils and Shikani

in 55 children (mean age 6 years); they reported an increased failure rate, and increased time to successful intubation in children with normal airways [41]. The authors attributed much of this difficulty to the increased secretions in infants and children, obstructing the view of the lens. One manikin study reported improved view and ease of intubation using the Bonfils fiberscope as an adjunct to direct laryngoscopy in a simulated Cormack-Lahane Grade 3b view of the glottis. Although the view was improved this did not result in an improved intubation time [22].

Video enhanced scopes have transformed the way we perform tracheal intubation in neonates [42–44]. Several options are available but each has unique strengths and limitations.

Video-laryngoscopes enhance trainee education, provide a superior view of the airway and are more successful in patients with difficult airways. Despite their advantages in exposing the airway, challenges still remain such as how to manipulate the endotracheal tube to get into the trachea. Currently, no one device is proven to any other device and the selected device should be based on provider experience and efficiency with the device. Future comparative studies would help to define best practices in this growing area.

Other Methods of Securing the Airway

The ASA practice guidelines also mention alternative methods of securing an airway in adults such as needle cricothyroidotomy, retrograde intubation, percutaneous tracheostomy, and emergency surgical tracheostomy [3]. However, the small size of neonates, especially the premature neonate, preclude the ability to successfully perform these procedures [45].

Postoperative Management

Extubation of the Neonate with a Difficult Airway

Typically, neonates with difficult airways will be left intubated after surgical procedures due to residual effects of the anesthetic. In many institutions, the neonatology staff will ask for an anesthesiologist to be present in the NICU at extubation. In these instances, a difficult airway cart should be readily available.

Neonates with difficult airways will also occasionally be brought to the OR for extubation. This is done to allow for the ENT surgeon to better assess the patient's airway while they are spontaneously awake. This is also done if there is total collapse of the airway, due to laryngo-tracheomalacia or severe subglottic stenosis and the situation warrants an immediate tracheostomy.

Postoperative Apnea and Bradycardia

Neonates and former preterm infants are at increased risk for developing postoperative apnea with or without bradycardia following general anesthesia and sedation [47–49]. Extreme prematurity despite older post-conceptual age and anemia are independent risk factors for this complication [47–52]. Luckily, the improvements in regional and spinal anesthesia have been recommended as a safe means to avoid this increased risk for this complication [49, 50]. Usually those infants with failed spinal anesthetics or spinal anesthetics will then require sedative supplementation are at high risk of apnea [47–49]. Often in neonates and infants at risk of postoperative apnea who receive a general anesthetic, prophylactic caffeine administration can be an effective measure to decrease the incidence of postoperative apnea [51].

Management of Postoperative Airway Obstruction

Airway obstruction in the postoperative period is managed using many of the same techniques used to treat obstruction following the induction of anesthesia. Proper positioning during recovery may help maintain airway patency. Using a soft roll under the shoulders will help maintain and extend the head and neck and insure an open upper airway. If airway obstruction fails to improve with positioning, a soft nasopharyngeal airway can be inserted; if the child is still anesthetized, an oral airway may be preferred. If airway obstruction is incompletely relieved with a nasopharyngeal airway, a 15 mm tracheal tube adaptor can be placed into the external flared end nasopharyngeal airway in the manner described by Beattie [52]. This adaptor can be connected to a portable mapleson circuit for the delivery of CPAP. When the respiratory and central nervous system depressant effects of opioids are suspected to be the primary causes of postoperative airway obstruction, naloxone can be cautiously administered to test and treat this possibility. Incremental doses of 0.5–1 mcg/kg can be carefully titrated to reverse the excessive depressant effects without reversal of analgesic effects. Infants who fail these measures to restore patency of their airway may require tracheal intubation.

Role of the Anesthesiologist in Managing the Difficult Neonatal Airway Outside of the OR

As experts in airway management, anesthesiologists are typically called to other areas of a hospital, such as the NICU, to secure an airway. In our own institution, we have a rapid response airway team comprised of both anesthesiologists and ENT surgeons to address issues with difficult and critical airways. Through the work of the Difficult/Critical Airway Committee, standards were developed to make this response timely and efficient. These standards included:

- Standardization of difficult airway carts in every critical care area with bronchoscopes and Glidescopes coupled to these carts
- Development of definitions of difficult and critical airways
- Development of notification system to activate the team
- Standards for documentation of issues with the airway and tools/techniques used to secure the airway
- An emergency algorithm which highlights a decision point for notifying the Airway team
- A quality assurance program to evaluate the efficacy of the team

This initiative allows for the appropriate personnel with advanced airway skills to be notified promptly and proceed directly to the bedside of the patient without requiring to bring equipment to the bedside. This had decreased the rate of adverse events associated with airway emergencies and indirectly decreased the incidence of airway emergencies due to better recognition of airway problems and earlier calls to anesthesiologists and ENT surgeons prior to an emergency.

Occasionally, the neonate with severe airway issue and comorbidities cannot be safely transported to the OR for a tracheostomy. In these situations, the procedure needs to be performed at the bedside. OR personnel and equipment can easily be brought to the bedside. The only disadvantage in this process is that the lighting is typically not as the OR lighting. Despite the plan to place a tracheostomy, the difficult airway cart with appropriate scopes needs to be readily available in the event of losing the airway during the procedure.

Summary

The neonate with a difficult airway can present unique challenges to an anesthesiologist in and out of the OR. Unlike the adult or older child, the anatomy and physiology of a neonate with a difficult airway requires much different thinking and planning when attempting to secure the airway. However, with the advancement and miniaturization of airway devices, such as the AirQ, bronchoscopes, Glidescope, videolaryngoscopes, AirTraqs, many more options are available to help facilitate intubation. Securing the airway outside of the OR in emergency situations also requires much anticipatory planning and availability of airway equipment at a moment's notice. Simulation and practice with this equipment will allow for the laryngoscopist to be skilled and comfortable with securing the airway in these most unique patients.

References

1. Holzman RS. Chapter 12—Airway management. 8th ed. Elsevier; 2011. p. 344–64.
2. Litman RS, Weissend EE, Shibata D, Westesson PL. Developmental changes of laryngeal dimensions in unparalyzed, sedated children. Anesthesiology. 2003;98(1):41–5.
3. Apfelbaum JL, Hagberg CA, Caplan RA, Blitt CD, Connis RT, Nickinovich DG, et al. Practice guidelines for management of the difficult airway: an updated report by the American Society of Anesthesiologists Task Force on Management of the Difficult Airway. Anesthesiology. 2003;98(5):1269–77. Revised 2013;118(2):251–70.
4. Brain A. The laryngeal mask—a new concept in airway management. Brit J Anesth. 1983;55(8):801–5.
5. Perlman JM, Wyllie J, Kattwinkel J, Atkins DL, Chameides L, Goldsmith JP, et al. Part 11: Neonatal resuscitation: 2010 international consensus on cardiopulmonary resuscitation and emergency cardiovascular care science with treatment recommendations. Circulation. 2010;122(16 Suppl 2):S516–38.
6. Paterson SJ, Byrne PJ, Molesky MG, Seal RF, Finucane BT. Neonatal resuscitation using the laryngeal mask airway. Anesthesiology. 1994;80(6):1248–53; discussion 27A.
7. Stricker PA, Budac S, Fiadjoe JE, Rehman MA. Awake laryngeal mask insertion followed by induction of anesthesia in infants with the Pierre Robin sequence. Acta Anaesthesiol Scand. 2008;52(9): 1307–8.
8. Simons SH, van der Lee R, Reiss IK, van Weissenbruch MM. Clinical evaluation of propofol as sedative for endotracheal intubation in neonates. Acta Paediatr. 2013;102(11):e487–92.
9. Stricker P, Fiadjoe JE, McGinnis S. Intubation of an infant with Pierre Robin sequence under dexmedetomidine sedation using the Shikani Optical Stylet. Acta Anaesthesiol Scand. 2008;52(6):866–7.
10. Schmölzer GM, Agarwal M, Kamlin CO, Davis PG. Supraglottic airway devices during neonatal resuscitation: an historical perspective, systematic review and meta-analysis of available clinical trials. Resuscitation. 2013;84(6):722–30.
11. Somri M, Barna Teszler C, Tome R, Kugelman A, Vaida S, Gaitini L. Flexible fiberoptic bronchoscopy through the laryngeal mask airway in a small, premature neonate. Am J Otolaryngol. 2005;26(4): 268–71.
12. Fiadjoe JE, Stricker PA. The air-Q intubating laryngeal airway in neonates with difficult airways. Pediatr Anesth. 2011;21(6):702–3.
13. Narang AT, Oldeg PF, Medzon R, Mahmood AR, Spector JA, Robinett DA. Comparison of intubation success of video laryngoscopy versus direct laryngoscopy in the difficult airway using high-fidelity simulation. Simul Healthc. 2009;4(3):160–5.
14. Kaplan MB, Hagberg CA, Ward DS, Brambrink A, Chhibber AK, Heidegger T, et al. Comparison of direct and video-assisted views of the larynx during routine intubation. J Clin Anesth. 2006;18(5): 357–62.
15. Fonte M, Oulego-Erroz I, Nadkarni L, Sanchez-Santos L, Iglesias-Vasquez A, Rodriguez-Nunez A. A randomized comparison of the GlideScope videolaryngoscope to the standard laryngoscopy for intubation by pediatric residents in simulated easy and difficult infant airway scenarios. Pediatr Emerg Care. 2011;27(5):398–402.
16. Iacovidou N, Bassiakou E, Stroumpoulis K, Koudouna E, Aroni F, Papalois A, et al. Conventional direct laryngoscopy versus videolaryngoscopy with the GlideScope(R): a neonatal manikin study with inexperienced intubators. Am J Perinatol. 2011;28(3):201–6.
17. Trevisanuto D, Fornaro E, Verghese C. The GlideScope video laryngoscope: initial experience in five neonates. Can J Anaesth. 2006;53(4):423–4.

18. White M, Weale N, Nolan J, Sale S, Bayley G. Comparison of the Cobalt Glidescope video laryngoscope with conventional laryngoscopy in simulated normal and difficult infant airways. Paediatr Anaesth. 2009;19(11):1108–12.
19. Sola C, Delous E, Raux O, Capdevila X, Dadure C. GlideScope(R) Cobalt with disposable blades: series of 121 intubations in young children. Ann Fr Anesth Reanim. 2011;30(5):447–8.
20. Fiadjoe JE, Gurnaney H, Dalesio N, Sussman E, Zhao H, Zhang X, et al. A prospective randomized equivalence trial of the GlideScope Cobalt(R) video laryngoscope to traditional direct laryngoscopy in neonates and infants. Anesthesiology. 2012;116(3):622–8.
21. Hackell RS, Held LD, Stricker PA, Fiadjoe JE. Management of the difficult infant airway with the Storz Video Laryngoscope: a case series. Anesth Analg. 2009;109(3):763–6.
22. Vlatten A, Aucoin S, Litz S, MacManus B, Soder C. A comparison of bonfils fiberscope-assisted laryngoscopy and standard direct laryngoscopy in simulated difficult pediatric intubation: a manikin study. Paediatr Anaesth. 2010;20(6):559–65.
23. Wald SH, Keyes M, Brown A. Pediatric video laryngoscope rescue for a difficult neonatal intubation. Paediatr Anaesth. 2008;18(8): 790–2.
24. Fiadjoe JE, Stricker PA, Hackell RS, Salam A, Gurnaney H, Rehman MA, et al. The efficacy of the Storz Miller 1 video laryngoscope in a simulated infant difficult intubation. Anesth Analg. 2009;108(6):1783–6.
25. Vanderhal AL, Berci G, Simmons CF, Hagiike M. A videolaryngoscopy technique for the intubation of the newborn: preliminary report. Pediatrics. 2009;124(2):e339–46.
26. Vlatten A, Soder C. Airtraq optical laryngoscope intubation in a 5-month-old infant with a difficult airway because of Robin Sequence. Paediatr Anaesth. 2009;19(7):699–700.
27. Hirabayashi Y, Shimada N. Airtraq optical laryngoscope: initial clinical experience in 20 children. J Anesth. 2010;24(1):148–9.
28. Holm-Knudsen RJ, White J. The Airtraq may not be the solution for infants with difficult airways. Paediatr Anaesth. 2010;20(4):374–5.
29. Sbaraglia F, Lorusso R, Garra R, Sammartino M. Usefulness of Airtraq in a 3-month-old child with Apert Syndrome. Paediatr Anaesth. 2011;21(9):984–5.
30. Xue FS, He N, Liu JH, Liao X, Xu XZ, Zhang YM. More maneuvers to facilitate endotracheal intubation using the Airtraq laryngoscope in children with difficult airways. Paediatr Anaesth. 2009;19(9):916–8.
31. Xue FS, Liu HP, Xiong J, Liao X. A useful suggestion to facilitate tracheal intubation using the Airtraq® laryngoscope in the infants with difficult airways. Pediatr Anesth. 2010;20(7):678–9.
32. Komasawa N, Atagi K, Ueki R, Nishi S, Kaminoh Y, Tashiro C. Comparison of optic laryngoscope Airtraq((R)) and Miller laryngoscope for tracheal intubation during infant cardiopulmonary resuscitation. Resuscitation. 2011;82(6):736–9.
33. White MC, Marsh CJ, Beringer RM, Nolan JA, Choi AY, Medlock KE, et al. A randomised, controlled trial comparing the Airtraq optical laryngoscope with conventional laryngoscopy in infants and children. Anaesthesia. 2012;67(3):226–31.
34. Al-Abri AS, Khan RM, Haris A, Kaul N. Successful airway management in patient with Goldenhar's syndrome using Truview PCD (R) laryngoscope. Paediatr Anaesth. 2012;22(12):1229–31.
35. Gomez-Rios MA, Serradilla LN, Alvarez AE. Use of the TruView EVO2 laryngoscope in Treacher Collins syndrome after unplanned extubation. J Clin Anesth. 2012;24(3):257–8.
36. Khan RM, Kaul N, Gupte S, Al Hinai FS. Truview PCD eases laryngoscopy and tracheal intubation in patient with cleft lip, palate, and protruding premaxilla. Paediatr Anaesth. 2011;21(12):1279–81.
37. Singh R, Singh P, Vajifdar H. A comparison of Truview infant EVO2 laryngoscope with the Miller blade in neonates and infants. Paediatr Anaesth. 2009;19(4):338–42.
38. Jansen AH, Johnston G. The Shikani Optical Stylet: a useful adjunct to airway management in a neonate with popliteal pterygium syndrome. Paediatr Anaesth. 2008;18(2):188–90.
39. Shukry M, Hanson RD, Koveleskie JR, Ramadhyani U. Management of the difficult pediatric airway with Shikani Optical Stylet. Paediatr Anaesth. 2005;15(4):342–5.
40. Caruselli M, Zannini R, Giretti R, Rocchi G, Camilletti G, Bechi P, et al. Difficult intubation in a small for gestational age newborn by bonfils fiberscope. Paediatr Anaesth. 2008;18(10):990–1.
41. Bein B, Wortmann F, Meybohm P, Steinfath M, Scholz J, Dorges V. Evaluation of the pediatric Bonfils fiberscope for elective endotracheal intubation. Paediatr Anaesth. 2008;18(11):1040–4.
42. Kalbhenn J, Boelke AK, Steinmann D. Prospective model-based comparison of different laryngoscopes for difficult intubation in infants. Paediatr Anaesth. 2012;22(8):776–80.
43. Orliaguet GA, Blot RM, Bourdaud N, Egan M, Dogaru E, Salvi N, et al. Endotracheal intubation with the GlideScope(R), the Airtraq(R), the McGrath(R) videolaryngoscope and direct laryngoscopy: a comparative study on an infant manikin. Ann Fr Anesth Reanim. 2013;32(12):844–9.
44. Sorensen MK, Holm-Knudsen R. Endotracheal intubation with airtraq(R) versus storz(R) videolaryngoscope in children younger than two years—a randomized pilot-study. BMC Anesthesiol. 2012;12:7.
45. Navsa N, Tossel G, Boon JM. Dimensions of the neonatal cricothyroid membrane—how feasible is a surgical cricothyroidotomy? Paediatr Anaesth. 2005;15(5):402–6.
46. Fiadjoe J, Sticker P, Kilbaugh T. Pediatric difficult airway management: principles and approach in the critical care environment. In: Wheeler DS et al., editors. Volume 1: Care of the critically ill or injured child. London: Springer; 2014. p. 329–43 [Chapter 28: Pediatric Critical Care Medicine].
47. Cote CJ, Zaslavsky A, Downes JJ, Kurth CD, Welborn LG, Warner LO, Malviya SV. Postoperative apnea in former preterm infants after inguinal herniorrhaphy. A combined analysis. Anesthesiology. 1995;82:809–22.
48. Krane EJ, Haberkern CM, Jacobson LE. Postoperative apnea, bradycardia, and oxygen desaturation in formerly premature infants: prospective comparison of spinal and general anesthesia. Anesth Analg. 1995;80:7–13.
49. Walther-Larsen S, Rasmussen LS. The former preterm infant and risk of post-operative apnoea: recommendations for management. Acta Anaesthesiol Scand. 2006;50:888–93.
50. William JM, Stoddart PA, Williams SA, Wolf AR. Post-operative recovery after inguinal herniotomy in ex-premature infants: comparison between sevoflurane and spinal anaesthesia. Br J Anaesth. 2001;86:366–71.
51. Henderson-Smart DJ, Steer P. Prophylactic caffeine to prevent postoperative apnea following general anesthesia in preterm infants. Cochrane Database Syst Rev. 2001;4:CD000048.
52. Beattie C. The modified nasal trumpet maneuver. Anesth Analg. 2002;94:467–9.
53. Weiss M, Gerber AC. Rapid sequence induction in children—it's not a matter of time! Paediatr Anaesth. 2008;18:97–9.
54. Moynihan RJ, Brock-Utne JG, Archer JH, Feld LH, Kreitzman TR. The effect of cricoid pressure on preventing gastric insufflation in infants and children. Anesthesiology. 1993;78:652–6.
55. Landsman I. Cricoid pressure: indications and complications. Paediatr Anaesth. 2004;14:43–7.
56. MacG PJH, Ball DR. The effect of cricoid pressure on the cricoid cartilage and vocal cords: an endoscopic study in anaesthetised patients. Anaesthesia. 2000;55:263–8.
57. Murat I. Cuffed tubes in children: a 3-year experience in a single institution. Paediatr Anaesth. 2001;11:748–9.

Surgical Challenges for the Critical Airway

Nicholas Smith and Brian J. Wiatrak

Fetal Imaging

Fetal ultrasonography (US) and magnetic resonance imaging (MRI) allow for prenatal evaluation of extrinsic and intrinsic etiologies of airway obstruction, such as cervical teratomas and laryngeal atresia. With this knowledge, parental counseling can ensue and management can proceed with specific surgical resources available for establishing the airway in the delivery room.

Fetal US evaluation is helpful to identify cervical pathology that could hinder fetal adaptability to extra-uterine life. Imaging is initially performed at 20 weeks gestation and can be repeated serially throughout the duration of pregnancy in order to obtain measurements of a lesion's growth, consistency, and vascularization. The amniotic sac can also be examined for the development of polyhydramnios, an indicator of possible airway obstruction [1].

Fetal MRI adds sensitivity to the imaging of the fetal airway due to high soft-tissue contrast. Intrinsic causes of airway obstruction can be better characterized, and the level of obstruction can be localized. When extrinsic tumors are diagnosed, the extent and relationship to the airway can also be determined. This facilitates treatment planning and helps guide the decision to utilize the ex utero intrapartum treatment (EXIT) procedure [2].

N. Smith, M.D.
Department of Otolaryngology—Head and Neck Surgery, University of Alabama at Birmingham, Pediatric ENT Associates, Children's of Alabama, 1600 7th Avenue South, Lowder Building Suite 320, Birmingham, AB 35244, USA

B.J. Wiatrak, M.D. (✉)
Department of Otolaryngology-Head and Neck Surgery, University of Alabama at Birmingham, Pediatric ENT Associates, Children's of Alabama, Birmingham, AB, USA
e-mail: brian.wiatrak@childrensal.org

Ex Utero Intrapartum Treatment

EXIT involves the partial delivery of the newborn, allowing for uteroplacental circulation to remain intact while a stable airway is obtained. Halogenated anesthetic agents promote uterine relaxation allowing uteroplacental gas exchange to be maintained while the airway is being secured. The newborn can remain hemodynamically stable for approximately 45 min, which facilitates airway management by laryngoscopy, bronchoscopy, intubation, and/or tracheostomy.

A multidisciplinary team including anesthesiologists, pediatric surgeons, otolaryngologists, neonatologists, maternal fetal medicine specialists, and dedicated operating room nurses and personnel are part of the EXIT team and are essential for successful outcomes.

Nasal/Nasopharyngeal Obstruction

Considering that newborns are obligate nasal breathers, obstruction of the nasal cavity may present with severe respiratory distress in the neonatal period. A number of abnormalities may result in distress requiring early surgical intervention.

Pyriform Aperture Stenosis (PAS)

The pyriform aperture is the narrowest bony portion of the anterior nasal airway. Stenosis of the pyriform aperture is a rare cause of upper airway obstruction in neonates. It is believed to occur secondary to overgrowth of the medial nasal processes of the maxilla. Although initially thought to be an isolated anomaly, this entity is now felt to be part of a spectrum of midface anomalies and holoprosencephaly.

PAS is associated with a solitary, central median maxillary incisor, a finding also seen up to 60 % of the time in patients with holoprosencephaly (Fig. 1). Clinically, PAS

J. Lioy and S.E. Sobol (eds.), *Disorders of the Neonatal Airway: Fundamentals for Practice*,
DOI 10.1007/978-1-4939-1610-8_23, © Springer Science+Business Media New York 2015

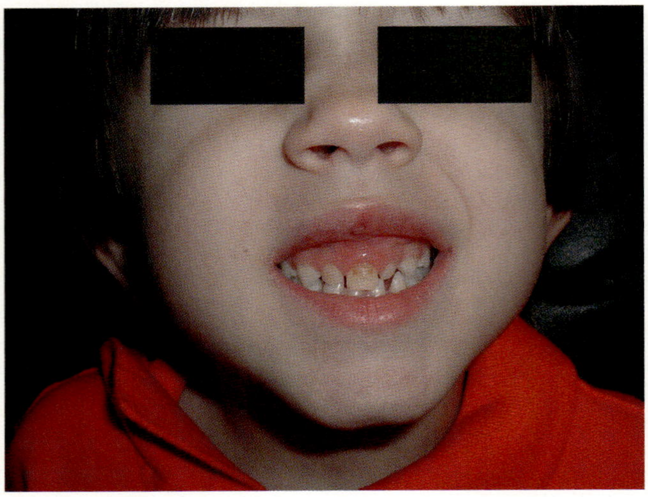

Fig. 1 Eight-year-old male h/o pyriform aperture stenosis with an associated solitary central median maxillary incisor

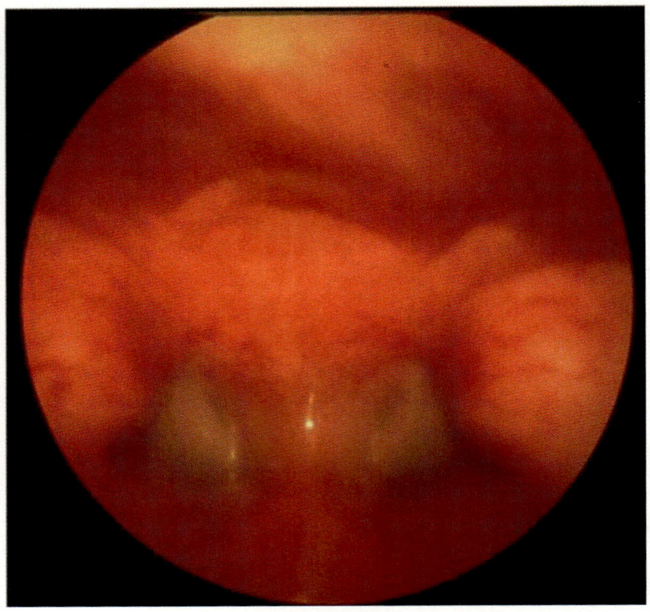

Fig. 2 Bilateral choanal atresia viewed from the oropharynx with a 120° scope

mimics the features choanal atresia, with cyanosis during feeding, respiratory distress, and failure to thrive. Diagnosis is confirmed with axial computed tomography (CT) showing narrowing at the pyriform aperture with normal anatomy at the choanae [3–5].

Mild cases of PAS may be treated conservatively with humidification and topical nasal decongestants. Severe cases require surgical management, which is most frequently approached via a sublabial incision in infants. The aperture is widened using drills, shavers, and/or bony curettes. Occasionally, a portion of the anterior head of the inferior turbinate is removed to improve the airway. Stenting may be recommended for a period of 1–4 weeks.

Nasolacrimal Duct Cyst

Obstruction of the nasolacrimal duct is common, occurring in approximately 30 % of infants. Although most cases are asymptomatic, severe obstruction can occur resulting from the formation of cysts, which can herniate into the nasal cavity causing obstruction. Bilateral cysts form in 14 % of cases causing symptoms of respiratory distress prompting airway evaluation. Diagnosis is made with nasal endoscopy showing cystic masses in the inferior meati. CT can be used to aid in the diagnosis and may reveal dilation of the lacrimal duct and sac. Treatment of intranasal cysts involves an above-and-below approach with ophthalmologic probing of the duct and endonasal marsupialization of the cyst [6, 7].

Septal Deviation/Midnasal Stenosis

Septal deviation or dislocation of the cartilaginous septum can occur during traumatic delivery predisposing infants to severe nasal airway obstruction with nasal rhinitis. Diagnosis is made with anterior rhinoscopy revealing displacement of the septal cartilage into the obstructed side of the nose. Conservative treatment involves humidification, nasal steroids, and suctioning. If conservative treatment fails, manual reduction of the cartilaginous septum back into the septal groove of the maxillary crest can improve the nasal airway [8].

Choanal Atresia

The choanae connect the nasal cavity to the nasopharynx. When this connection fails to develop, choanal atresia (CA) results. CA is unilateral in 65–75 % of cases, typically causing only mild respiratory symptoms and chronic unilateral rhinorrhea. In bilateral CA, the nasal cavity is completely separated from the nasopharynx, resulting in more significant symptoms of cyanosis during feeding, respiratory distress, and failure to thrive. Bilateral CA is also associated with other congenital abnormalities, most notably CHARGE association, in approximately 50 % of patients. Nasal endoscopy shows a blind pouch with lack of connection between the nasal cavity and pharynx (Fig. 2). Axial CT confirms the diagnosis showing thickening of the posterior bony septum and medialization of the lateral nasal walls (Fig. 3) [9].

Surgery is the primary treatment for CA. Timing varies dependent upon unilateral versus bilateral atresia with bilateral atresia needing attention in a more urgent fashion due to symptoms of respiratory distress. Multiple surgical options exist including transnasal puncture and/or dilation, transnasal approach with removal of bony stenosis with/without stenting, and transpalatal approach with/without stenting.

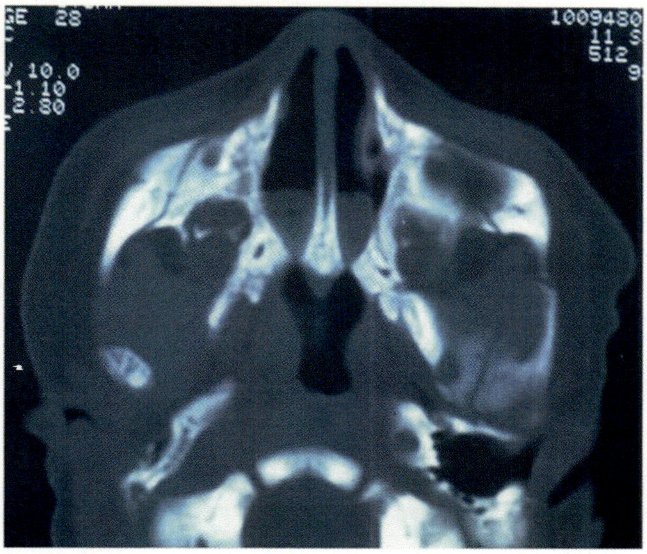

Fig. 3 Axial CT showing bilateral choanal atresia

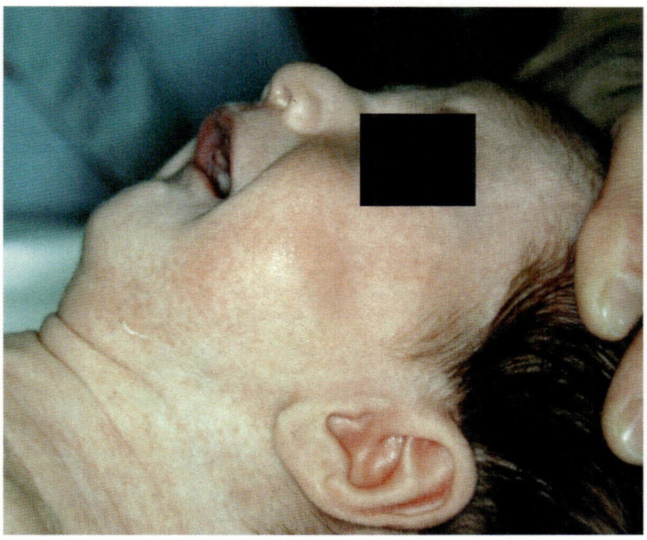

Fig. 4 Micrognathia in a child with Pierre-Robin sequence

Oropharyngeal Obstruction

Newborns may present with obstruction at the level of the oral cavity and oropharynx. Obstruction at this level may cause respiratory distress immediately at birth, necessitating early airway intervention, including laryngoscopy to establish endotracheal intubation or tracheotomy.

Micrognathia/Base of Tongue Obstruction

Hypoplasia of the mandible, or micrognathia, with posterior displacement of the tongue base can cause significant obstruction of the oropharyngeal airway. Micrognathia can occur in isolation or in combination with several congenital craniofacial syndromes, most notably Pierre-Robin sequence (PRS) (Fig. 4). Characteristics of PRS include micrognathia, glossoptosis, or posterior displacement of the base of tongue, and cleft palate. Clinically, infants present with upper airway obstruction and feeding difficulties. Lack of weight gain despite adequate nutritional intake is an indicator of persistent airway obstruction. Severe airway obstruction is manifested by suprasternal and subcostal retractions, cyanosis, and carbon dioxide retention. Physical exam along with sleep endoscopy can confirm the diagnosis.

Management depends on the degree of upper airway obstruction and feeding difficulties. Nonsurgical treatments include prone positioning and nasopharyngeal tube/stenting. Surgical options include tongue–lip adhesion, mandibular distraction osteogenesis, and tracheostomy [10, 11].

Macroglossia

Tongue function is important for deglutition, phonation, and respiration. Macroglossia is defined as a resting tongue that protrudes beyond the teeth or alveolar ridge. Congenital macroglossia is seen in pediatric overgrowth disorders, most commonly Beckwith–Wiedemann syndrome. Low- and high-flow vascular anomalies with tongue involvement can also cause tongue enlargement. Clinically, severe macroglossia in the newborn can obstruct the oropharyngeal airway with symptoms of obstructive sleep apnea with CO_2 retention, retractions, and respiratory distress. Surgical treatment options include tongue reduction surgery and/or tracheostomy [12, 13].

Congenital Pharyngeal Mass

Tumors obstructing the nasal/nasopharyngeal airway are exceedingly rare. Differential includes teratoma, epidermoid cyst, rhabdomyosarcoma, Rathke pouch cyst, lingual thyroid, vallecular cysts, and other rare neoplasms. Presenting signs include stridor with recurrent respiratory distress. CT and/or MRI are recommended to evaluate the extent of the lesion. Treatment involves securing the airway, occasionally with endoscopic assistance, and is subsequently dependent upon the primary etiology.

Laryngeal Obstruction

Obstruction at the level of the larynx can present with severe neonatal obstruction, which can result in death if not recognized early on. With severe obstruction at the level of the larynx, intubation is often not achievable, requiring urgent tracheotomy in order to establish the airway.

Laryngeal Atresia

Atresia of the larynx is a rare anomaly causing respiratory distress in the newborn resulting from failure of recanalization of the larynx in utero at approximately 10 weeks gestational age. It is commonly associated with other abnormalities, including tracheoesophageal fistula, esophageal atresia, and tracheal agenesis.

Diagnosis of laryngeal atresia can be made with prenatal US and MRI. Congenital high airway obstruction syndrome (CHAOS) results when laryngeal atresia is associated with large hyperechogenic lungs, flattened or inverted diaphragms, and ascites. Failure to recognize this anomaly in utero can result in rapid neonatal demise due to complete airway obstruction at delivery. Treatment involves the use of the EXIT procedure with tracheotomy performed immediately upon delivery [14, 15].

Tracheal Obstruction

As with laryngeal anomalies, obstruction at the level of the trachea can present with severe neonatal obstruction, which can result in death if not recognized early on. With severe obstruction at the level of the trachea, intubation may be challenging and tracheotomy may not be an option. Urgent bronchoscopy is often necessary in order to evaluate the airway and plan care.

Tracheal Stenosis

Complete tracheal rings (O-rings) are found in almost all cases of congenital tracheal stenosis with resultant narrowing of a segment or the full length of the trachea. Other anomalies are common and include a right upper lobe bronchus originating from the trachea ("pig" bronchus), hypoplasia/aplasia of the lung, and left pulmonary artery sling. Treatment is dependent upon the degree of obstruction, with most patients presenting with respiratory distress symptoms during the neonatal period and a history of difficult intubation.

In a patient with suspected tracheal stenosis, diagnosis should be made with judicious bronchoscopy as well as imaging in order to assess for vascular and cardiac anomalies. Different techniques of tracheoplasty, including slide and patch, have been used for repair with slide tracheoplasty being the currently preferred method of repair. For short segment stenosis, resection can be considered [16].

Vascular Anomalies

Vascular anomalies with compression of the airway can result in respiratory distress in newborns and occur in 1–2 % of children with congenital heart disease. Innominate artery compression is not a true anomaly, but can result in airway symptoms. Vascular rings and slings are also included in the category of vascular anomalies. The double aortic arch is the most common symptomatic true vascular ring. The left pulmonary artery sling can also cause compression of the right mainstem bronchus. Treatment will be discussed in detail in later chapters [17].

Extrinsic Cervical Lesions

Extrinsic compression of the airway by a mass is rare but potentially lethal if not recognized and treated. Masses include tumors, such as a cervical teratoma and vascular malformations, which are discussed in detail in a separate chapter.

Cervical Teratoma

Teratomas are rare congenital malformations occurring in 1:20,000–40,000 live births. The head and neck is the second most common site of teratoma formation in the neonate. Teratomas consist of tissue from all three germ layers and usually have solid and cystic components. Calcifications on US or MRI are nearly diagnostic but are only present in approximately 50 % of cases.

Cervical teratomas can cause hypopharyngeal compression and disruption of fetal swallowing of amniotic fluid leading to polyhydramnios. Polyhydramnios can lead to preterm labor and placental abruption, and if severe, intraoperative amnioreduction is indicated. Airway obstruction secondary to undiagnosed teratomas is associated with high mortality and anoxic brain injury. Prenatal imaging and EXIT procedures for postnatal management have dramatically improved survival of these patients. Once the airway is obtained, further management is primarily determined by the amount of pulmonary hypoplasia [18].

References

1. Iserte PP, Perez AS, Folch BF, et al. Ultrasound evaluation of congenital cervical teratoma and therapeutic management (ex utero intrapartum treatment). Case Rep Obstet Gynecol. 2012;2012: 597489.
2. Courtier J, Poder L, Wang ZJ, et al. Fetal tracheolaryngeal airway obstruction: prenatal evaluation by sonography and MRI. Pediatr Radiol. 2010;40:1800–5.

3. Brown OE, Myer CM, Manning SC. Congenital nasal pyriform aperture stenosis. Laryngoscope. 1989;99:86–91.
4. Arlis H, Ward RF. Congenial nasal pyriform aperture stenosis: isolated abnormality vs developmental field defect. Arch Otolaryngol Head Neck Surg. 1992;118:989–91.
5. Van Den Abbeele T, Triglia JM, Francois M, et al. Congenital nasal pyriform stenosis: diagnosis and management of 20 cases. Ann Otol Rhinol Laryngol. 2001;110:70–5.
6. Gnagi SH, Schraff SA. Nasal obstruction in newborns. Pediatr Clin North Am. 2013;60(4):903–22.
7. Leonard DS, O'Keefe M, Rowley H, et al. Neonatal respiratory distress secondary to bilateral intranasal dacrocystoceles. Int J Pediatr Otorhinolaryngol. 2008;72:1873–7.
8. Tasca I, Compadretti GC. Immediate correction of nasal septum dislocation in newborns: long term results. Am J Rhinol. 2004;18:47–51.
9. Myer CM, Cotton RT. Nasal obstruction in the pediatric patient. Pediatrics. 1983;72:766–77.
10. Sesenna E, Magri AS, Magnani C, et al. Mandibular distraction in neonate: indications, technique, results. Ital J Pediatr. 2012;38:7.
11. Myer CM, Reed JM, Cotton RT, Willging JP, Shott SR. Airway management in Pierre Robin sequence. Otolaryngol Head Neck Surg. 1998;118:630–5.
12. Kacker A, Honrado C, Martin D, et al. Tongue reduction in Beckwith-Wiedemann syndrome. Int J Pediatr Otorhinolaryngol. 2000;53:1–7.
13. Kadouch DJM, Maas SM, Dubois L, van der Horst CM. Surgical treatment of macroglossia in patients with Beckwith-Wiedemann syndrome: a 20-year experience and review of the literature. Int J Oral Maxillofac Surg. 2012;41(3):300–8.
14. Ambrosio A, Magit A. Respiratory distress of the newborn. Int J Pediatr Otorhinolaryngol. 2012;76(11):1685–7.
15. Elliot R, Vallera C, Heitmiller ES, et al. Ex utero intrapartum treatment procedure for management of congenital high airway obstruction syndrome in a vertex/breech twin gestation. Int J Pediatr Otorhinolaryngol. 2013;77(3):439–42.
16. Wright C. Treatment of congenital tracheal stenosis. Semin Thorac Cardiovasc Surg. 2009;21:274–7.
17. Erwin EA, Gerber ME, Cotton RT. vascular compression of the airway: indications for and results of surgical management. Int J Pediatr Otorhinolaryngol. 1997;40(3):155–62.
18. Laje P, Johnson MP, Howell LJ, et al. Ex utero intrapartum treatment in the management of giant cervical teratomas. J Pediatr Surg. 2012;47(3):1208–16.

Effects of Prematurity, Prolonged Intubation, and Chronic Lung Disease on the Neonatal Airway

Huayan Zhang, Jason Gien, and Kevin Dysart

Introduction

Over the past four decades, advances in neonatal intensive care have led to the survival of smaller and more immature infants. The improved survival of very low birth weight infants (VLBW) is associated with long-term respiratory morbidity, most commonly in the form of bronchopulmonary dysplasia (BPD). The preterm birth rate (less than 37 completed weeks of gestation) rose by more than one-third from 1981 to a peak in 2006 in the USA. While there has been a continuous fall in this rate over the last 6 years, there were still over 300,000 infants delivered prematurely in the USA in 2012 [1]. Currently there are over 75,000 infants born at less than 32 weeks postmenstrual age (PMA) and over 50,000 having birth weights <1,500 g each year [1, 2]. In this chapter, we will describe the developmental characteristics of the immature airway, and discuss the pathogenesis as well as management of commonly seen acquired airway disorders associated with prematurity, prolonged intubation, and ventilation.

H. Zhang, M.D. (✉)
Division of Neonatology, Medical Director, Chronic Lung Disease Program The Children's Hospital of Philadelphia, University of Pennsylvania, Perelman School of Medicine, Philadelphia, PA, USA
e-mail: ZhangH@email.chop.edu

J. Gien, M.D.
The Children's Hospital of Colorado, University of Colorado School of Medicine, Aurora, CO, USA

K. Dysart, M.D.
Division of Neonatology, The Children's Hospital of Philadelphia, University of Pennsylvania, Perelman School of Medicine, Philadelphia, PA, USA

Background

The lungs of preterm infants born at 24–28 weeks gestation are both structurally and biochemically immature. The capillaries of the distal pulmonary circulation are only starting to form and during the saccular stage of lung development primitive air spaces are just beginning to bud off the terminal bronchioles. The endogenous surfactant system is not yet activated and antioxidant defense mechanisms are immature. Supplemental oxygen and ventilatory support are often essential for survival for these extremely premature infants. Unfortunately with these therapies and interventions, lung and airway damage results with the subsequent development of chronic lung disease of infancy or BPD. Along with interrupted alveolar development, BPD is characterized by increased airway muscle thickening as well as abnormalities of elastic fiber architecture, elastin deposition, and elastic recoil. It is these anatomic abnormalities that result in long-term impairment of lung function and the prolonged effects of prematurity on the developing lung and airways.

When first described by Northway et al. in 1967 [65], BPD occurred mainly in larger preterm infants born at 30–34 weeks' gestation. These infants were born at the time that ventilators were first being adapted for use in the newborn, and before the introduction of antenatal steroids or postnatal surfactant replacement therapy. Infants with this type of classic, or "old" BPD usually have a history of severe respiratory distress requiring high levels of ventilator support and oxygen therapy for a prolonged period of time. The pathological features of the "old BPD" are characterized by extensive injury including varying degrees of pulmonary fibrosis involving proximal and distal portions of the airway, necrotizing bronchiolitis, peribronchial smooth muscle hypertrophy, pulmonary artery muscularization, and severe large airway injury. Since this time, there has been dramatic improvements in the area of perinatal care, which included the wide spread use of antenatal steroids for mothers in preterm labor before 34 weeks gestational age (GA), postnatal

J. Lioy and S.E. Sobol (eds.), *Disorders of the Neonatal Airway: Fundamentals for Practice*,
DOI 10.1007/978-1-4939-1610-8_24,

surfactant replacement therapy, more advanced ventilators, better monitoring of oxygen saturations, and the introduction of "gentle" ventilation concept with a variety of noninvasive ventilation strategies. As a result of these evolving clinical practices and the survival of smaller and more immature infants, a new form of BPD has been described [3]. This "new BPD" typically affects smaller (<1,000 g) and more immature infants (<32 weeks). The incidence of BPD in VLBW infants ranges between 15 and 65 % and this incidence increases as the gestational age decreases [4, 5]. These infants often start out with only minimal or mild respiratory distress syndrome (RDS) requiring low levels of respiratory support and then display deterioration in lung function with increased ventilator and/or oxygen requirements within a few days or weeks after birth. Instead of extensive injury as seen in "old BPD," the hallmark pathological feature of the "new BPD" is delayed alveolar and lung vascular development. Some author reports these infants represent more than 80 % of all infants diagnosed with BPD.

Development and Embryology

At 6–8 weeks of gestation, airway smooth muscle cells appear in the trachea and main and lobar bronchi. Muscle then develops sequentially along segmental, terminal, and respiratory bronchioles and alveolar ducts. The human fetal airway smooth muscle contracts spontaneously in the first trimester; it also responds to pharmacologic manipulation [6]. During fetal life and childhood, there is an increase in the amount of bronchial smooth muscle relative to the size of the airways. The amount of bronchial smooth muscle (square millimeter per millimeter) is greater in the hilar region than in the main bronchus in all infants. Muscle could not be identified in airways distal to the small bronchi in the fetus at 22 weeks of gestation, but it could be seen at 24 weeks of gestation. In more distal airways destined to become the terminal and respiratory bronchiole, muscle could not be measured in the lungs of fetuses at less than 26 weeks of gestation. All types of airway showed a significant linear increase in the area of muscle per millimeter airway perimeter with post-conceptual age. About 3 % of the bronchial wall is occupied by bronchial smooth muscle in both the child and adult, whereas in bronchiole it is 20 % of the wall in the adult and only 10 % in the child [7]. Examination of airways in full term and premature babies suggests that there is a more rapid increase in the amount of bronchial smooth muscle immediately after birth, probably as a result of transition to air breathing. This means that premature babies have a larger amount of muscle than normal for both their post-conception age and their airway size. At autopsy in the human fetus, the relative amount of bronchial smooth muscle in all types of airway was greater than expected for their post-conceptual age, especially in the premature infants who had been ventilated, and localized to the bronchi large and small and not in the more peripheral airways [8, 9]. This muscle is reactive and responsible for bronchoconstriction in infants. In a study of 10 normal infants younger than 15 months of age, Tepper [10] demonstrated airway reactivity to methacholine and subsequent bronchodilation with metaproterenol. Other studies [11] have demonstrated the presence of functional beta-adrenergic receptors in the airways of infants 3–12 months of age. Excessive amounts of bronchial smooth muscle in the lungs of ventilated premature infants might help explain the elevated resistance since airway resistance in adults correlates well with bronchial smooth muscle volume [12]. In children who have been ventilated, functional abnormalities may persist. Airway obstruction and bronchial hyper-reactivity have been described in children up to 12 year of age [13, 14].

Between 8 months postnatal age and adult life, the amount of muscle continues to increase in the proximal airways, with a small increase in the amount of muscle in the peripheral airways.

Anatomically, the airway is divided into the upper and lower airways, which combine with the purpose of carrying air to the gas exchanging units or alveoli in the lung. Developmentally the upper and lower airways form from distinct embryologic origins, with the upper airway forming from the branchial arches and lower airways forming from the primitive foregut. The upper airway extends from the nose to the trachea and functionally is involved in deglutition, respiration, and phonation. Upper airway structures consist of the nose, nasal cavity, choanae, oral cavity, hypopharynx, larynx and supraglottis, vocal cords, and subglottic space. Lower airway begins with the trachea and undergoes a series of divisions to the terminal airways. Lower airway structures consist of the trachea, bronchi, bronchioles, terminal bronchi, respiratory bronchi, alveolar ducts, and alveoli.

Development of the Upper Airway

Development of the craniofacial and upper airway structures is a complex choreography of mesenchymal and epithelial tissues responding to soluble growth factors and transcription factors in a tightly regulated sequence. Interruption of the development process or mutation of required transcription or growth factors leads to congenital anomalies of the facial and airway structures. The development of the nasal cavity dates into the sixth post-conceptual week. The primitive nasal cavity is formed by deepening of the original nasal pits and is separated from the primitive oral cavity by the oronasal membrane. Behind the primary palate, the primitive choanae connect the nasal and oral cavities. The final choanae form with the development of the secondary palate at the junction of nasal cavity and pharynx. At the same time, the nasal conchae (upper, middle, and lower) develop, emerging from the lateral wall of the nasal cavity. The nasal septum forms from the fused nasal processes and grows caudally, finally merging with the palatine shelves [15].

The development of the larynx embryologically is an integral part of the development of the lower airways. At 4 weeks post-conception, a bud outgrows from the ventral part of the foregut forming the respiratory diverticulum such that the epithelium of the larynx and the epithelium of the whole system of lower airways originate from the endoderm. Originally, the respiratory diverticulum communicates widely with the foregut, however with the formation of two longitudinal esophagotracheal ridges, the process of separation of trachea and esophagus begins, which is concluded by the fusion of these two ridges and formation of the esophagotracheal septum. The laryngeal orifice remains as the only communication between the oropharynx and the respiratory system. The laryngeal cartilages and muscles form from the mesenchyme of the fourth and sixth pharyngeal arches. Cartilaginous tissues from the fourth and sixth pharyngeal arches fuse and form the arytenoid, thyroid, cricoid, corniculate, and cuneiform cartilages. The laryngeal cartilages, including the epiglottis, originate from the mesenchymal tissue adjacent to both entoderm and endoderm. Around the same time, rapid proliferation of the laryngeal epithelium leads to temporary occlusion of the lumen. After recanalization of the lumen at about the age of 10 weeks, there remains a pair of lateral recesses (laryngeal ventricles). Around them, both true and false vocal cords differentiate. Within a further 6 weeks, the larynx develops almost its definitive appearance with the formation of thyroid, cricoid, and arytenoid cartilages from the mesenchyme, and further differentiation of epiglottis and arytenoids. At birth, the relative position of the larynx is much higher than in older children and adults and facilitates transition to spontaneous breathing. The postnatal descent of the hyoid and larynx is unique to humans and important for establishing the final shape of the vocal tract, which is vital for appropriate development of speech. The lower position of the larynx in humans may, however, lead to lack of sealing of the larynx during deglutition and an increased risk of food aspiration [15].

Development of the Lower Airway

The airways of the lung begin their development 22–26 days after fertilization as a ventral diverticulum budding from the foregut and lined by epithelium of endodermal origin. Normal airway branching requires both epithelium and mesenchyme. If the mesenchyme is stripped away, the airway tube will elongate but not divide [16]. The lobar and segmental bronchi appear at about the fifth week. And division of intrasegmental airways is fastest between the 10th and 14th week, by which time about 70 % of the airway generations present at birth have formed [17]. The pattern of airway branching is complete by about the 16th week of intrauterine life after which airway size changes but no further branching occurs [8]. From 22 weeks to birth, there is a linear increase in diameter in all airways from the bronchus to the terminal bronchiole. This growth continues after birth and the airways double or triple in diameter and length between birth and adulthood. With an increase in the size of the airways, the amount of cartilage, gland, and muscle increases such that the ultimate size and structure of the airway does not appear to be affected by premature delivery [9]. Premature infants who require artificial ventilation show a discrepancy in airway and alveolar development as the respiratory region of the lung is markedly altered by premature birth with arrested lung development resulting in fewer alveoli and increased interstitial collagen and elastin [9]. While airway size and structure is unaffected by prematurity, the functional effects of prematurity on the upper and lower airway as well as large and small airways can be significant. Airway morbidities related to prematurity include vocal cord paresis or dysfunction, subglottic stenosis (SGS), tracheal or bronchomalacia, airway inflammation secondary to reflux or aspiration. Along with these upper and large airway morbidities, other studies have reported excessive amount of bronchial smooth muscle in the lungs of ventilated premature infants, which may account for the airway obstruction [14] and bronchial hyper-reactivity [13] demonstrated into adolescence after premature birth.

Epidemiology of Acquired Airway Disorders in Premature Infants

SGS is a common injury secondary to endotracheal intubation of neonates. The reported prevalence of SGS has decreased in the past 30 years. Based on a single year review of NICU admissions in their institution and a literature review from 1960 to 1999, Walner et al. estimated an incidence of 0–2 % [18]. However the incidence of SGS is likely underestimated due to the retrospective nature of the studies. Using prospective flexible fiber-optic nasolaryngoscopy evaluation, a recent study reported a high incidence of 11.38 % in pediatric patients intubated for more than 24 h [19]. Even higher incidence of 16–24.5 % has been reported in VLBW infants who underwent intubation and mechanical ventilation for more than 7 days [20, 21]. Factors that have been associated with the development of SGS in the neonates include birth weight, gestational age, endotracheal tube size, route of intubation (nasal vs. oral), trauma of intubation, the number of ETT inserted, presence of infection, and duration of mechanical ventilation [21]. In addition, the need for additional doses of sedation appears to be an important factor for the development of SGS during endotracheal intubation [22].

Acquired subglottic cysts (SC) after intubation have been described by several studies [23, 24]. The estimated

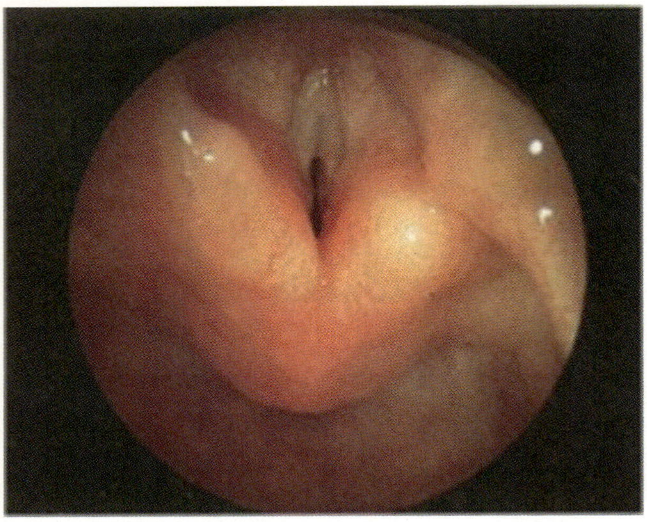

Fig. 1 Vocal cord paralysis. Upper airway obstruction due to vocal cord paralysis noted on bronchoscopy. Courtesy of Steve Sobol, (The Children's Hospital of Philadelphia)

incidence of SC is 1.9 per 100,000 live births. However the true incidence of SC in neonates is difficult to determine due to the selection bias of the studies. Downing et al. reported 11 cases (7.2 %) in 153 premature infants who were intubated for 7 days or longer over a 30-month period [23]. In another study, Halimi et al. identified 17 cases (9.3 %) in 172 premature infants over a 10-year period [24]. The majority of SC cases were reported in premature newborns with gestational age between 24 and 28 weeks.

Traumatic injury of the vocal cords as a result of short- or long-term intubation has been well recognized. Post-intubation laryngeal injuries have been reported in as many as 73 % of patients and vocal cord avulsion in neonates leading to dysphonia has also been reported [25, 26]. Unique to the premature infants, left vocal cord paralysis (LVCP) after patent ductus arteriosus (PDA) ligation has been well documented. Several studies reported incidence in the range of 0.7–17 %. However rate as high as 40–67 % has been reported in ELBW infants [27–29]. This condition may persist well beyond the newborn period. Using flexible laryngoscopy examination, a recent study found 54 % of young adults who was born at ≤28 weeks GA or ≤1,000 g birth weight had LVCP at the time of examination between 23 and 27 years of age [30]. The single most significant risk factor associated with LVCP after PDA ligation is low birth weight (Fig. 1).

Tracheobronchomalacia (TBM) is a dynamic airway narrowing disorder that is difficult to diagnose. The estimated incidence is between 1 in 1,500 and 1 in 2,500 in children, which is thought to be a significant underestimation of the true incidence. This condition has been reported in up to 15 % of infants and 30 % of young children (≤3 years old) who have undergone bronchoscopy for evaluation of respiratory distress [31–33]. In the selected population of premature infants with BPD, incidence between 16 and 50 % has been reported [34]. Identified risk factors associated with the development of secondary TBM include lower gestational age at birth, prolonged intubation, higher mean airway pressures during mechanical ventilation, infection, long-standing extrinsic airway compression (from vascular structures, cardiac and skeletal abnormalities, and tumors/cysts), and chronic inflammation [20, 35].

The incidence of small airway disease varies with BPD with an incidence of 68 % in children with history of BPD, 30 % demonstrating moderate degrees of obstruction and 10 % demonstrating severe obstruction on lung function tests.

Pathogenesis

In comparison with tracheas of infants who have not been ventilated mechanically, tracheas of those who have been ventilated are less compliant, being more difficult to expand but easier to collapse. Both tracheomegaly [36] and tracheomalacia [37] have been described in preterm infants who required mechanical ventilation in the neonatal period. Tracheomalacia may occur as a consequence of epithelial disruption with loss of an epithelial relaxant and an intensive bronchoconstrictor response to inhaled agonists [38, 39]. Disruption of the muscle–cartilage junction may reduce the ability of the trachea to resist compressive forces such as high supra-atmospheric pressures produced in infants with airflow obstruction. Pressure-induced alterations in the orientation of airway smooth muscle fibers may affect the forcefulness of smooth muscle contraction and the effectiveness with which muscle contraction stiffens the airway and helps it resist deformation. It is also possible that pressure-induced alterations in the alignment of cartilage components (i.e., proteoglycan/collagen configuration) results in cartilage providing less structural support for the trachea in newborns who have been mechanically ventilated.

The trachea and large airways are very compliant during development, with compliance of the airway determined largely by the tracheal smooth muscle contained in the posterior wall [40, 41]. During mechanical ventilation, alterations in tracheal smooth muscle mechanics in preterm [41], newborn lamb [42], and adult dog [43], often parallel changes in tracheal compliance seen with lung development. The role of tracheal cartilage in determining tracheal compliance is less well defined. The primary contribution of tracheal cartilage in determining tracheal compliance and dimensions appears to involve its role in limiting evagination of the posterior wall when transmural pressure is positive and invagination when transmural pressure is negative. During spontaneous respiration and lung inflation, a decrease in intrathoracic pressure increases transmural pressure in the intrathoracic trachea, causing the posterior tracheal wall to evaginate and the cartilaginous tips to be pulled further apart.

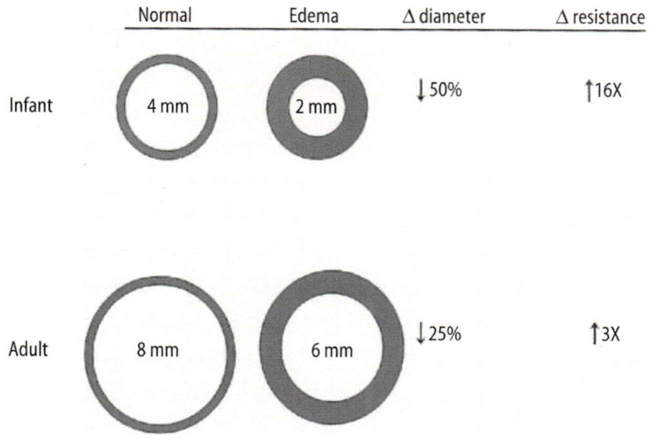

Fig. 2 Differences in luminal size and airway resistance with 1 mm circumferential edema: Changes in airway resistance with intraluminal swelling are more pronounced in infants compared with adults. (Adapted from Wheeler et al. [117]. In Wheeler et al., Resuscitation and Stabilization of the Critically Ill Child)

The increasingly inward forces generated by the cartilaginous tips resist this expanding force, thereby limiting the increase in intraluminal area in the intrathoracic trachea. During exertional expiration, when intrathoracic pressures are relatively positive and transmural pressures in the intrathoracic trachea may be negative, posterior wall invagination and tracheal compression is limited by an outward, and therefore stabilizing, force exerted by the ring [14]. In the immature animal, a reduced ability of the cartilaginous ring to exert these forces may contribute to age-related differences in tracheal compressibility and inflatability. The net effect of increased airway compliance is a change in the pressure-flow relationship, which contributes to the high airway resistance and limitation to airflow [41]. Along with high airway resistance and limitation to airflow, increased airway compliance allows for acute and chronic airway deformation with exposure to positive pressure. With exposure to positive pressure tracheal cross-sectional area, circumference, and mean diameter were found to be significantly greater. The greater circumference was mainly due to the greater length of the trachealis muscle whereas the cartilage length remained essentially unchanged [44]. Other studies have subsequently confirmed these findings with demonstrating with 4 h of ventilation a time-dependent decrease in posterior wall thickness, indicating a thinning of the trachealis muscle and no detectable change in anterior wall thickness, indicating a relative stability of the cartilage component of the tracheal boundary [45]. The radius of the trachea from preterm infants is approximately half that of the adult. The LaPlace relationship, therefore, suggests that the preterm trachealis needs to generate a tension half that of the adult to withstand an equal deforming pressure (Fig. 2).

When immature airways are exposed to distending pressures associated with positive pressure ventilation (PPV), they become deformed, although adult airways do not [46]. This pressure-induced injury to the immature airway may arise in part because of the inability of the preterm trachealis muscle to generate enough tension to withstand that level of barotrauma. The clinical consequences of decreased airway compliance include increased dead space, flow limitation, elevated airway resistance and work of breathing, and higher risk of gas trapping. Thus, the limited ability of immature airway smooth muscle to generate tension may help explain why preterm neonates who require PPV are at risk for developing structural injury to the central airways.

Contrasting the trachea, where compliance progressively decreases from the early fetus to the adult, studies have shown no difference between 1-month-old and adult bronchi with respect to deflation-specific compliance [47]. However as a fetus and in the first month of life, the bronchi are twice as distensible as they are at a month of life. Airway morphology was investigated in an attempt to identify structural changes that might produce the observed maturation of specific compliance. Bronchi from 1-week-old pigs had a significantly lower total wall area and cartilage area than the fetus and 4 week olds. However, the percentage of cartilage in the wall of fetal, 1- and 4-week-old pigs was the same. The mechanism for age-related changes in compliance could involve either a change in composition of the wall (e.g., more cartilage) or a change in the mechanical properties of some wall component (e.g., stiffer cartilage), but is not related to changes in airway smooth muscle tone. Fetal pig bronchi had the same proportion of cartilage as 4 week olds but were significantly less compliant, implying that the maturational change in compliance was not explained by changes in the amount of bronchial cartilage. Cartilage and smooth muscle stiffness are important determinants of the maturational change in tracheal compliance [48, 49], but in bronchi the structures determining specific compliance are unknown. Both immature and adult bronchi showed a change in the internal area (Ai) with inflation, however, no statistically significant change in the outer area (Ao) or total wall area (WAtot) of adult bronchi was detected with inflation. As with the adult, no difference in Ao was detected between inflated and uninflated bronchi from 1-week-old piglets; however, inflation to 20 cmH_2O did produce significant reductions in the wall thickness and total wall area (WAtot) of 1-week-old bronchi; therefore, at this pressure, part of the increase in lumen volume occurs by compression of the airway wall. Some expansion of Ao and movement of the cartilage plates may occur, but at least in bronchi from immature pigs, airway wall compression is a factor in determining lumen volume and specific compliance. Airway mucosa and smooth muscle are incompressible structures [50]; therefore, the region of wall compression may lie in the submucosa between the muscle and cartilage layers. This region can expand during muscle constriction in vitro, suggesting that it may also be compressible [51]. In vitro, fluid appears able to enter the wall of isolated bronchi across their adventitial surface, whether this can occur in the lung in vivo, is questionable.

Ventilatory strategies such as continuous positive airway pressure (CPAP) and mechanical ventilation have been implicated in the pathogenesis of diverse airway disorders [44, 46, 52]. While necessary to sustain life at the extremes of prematurity, positive airway pressure imposes physical forces on the airway that are not normally present during development. Relatively stiff lungs are mechanically ventilated through relatively compliant airways resulting in marked airway deformation. Pressure-induced stretch and high shear forces alter the normal structure and function of the airway. Anatomically positive airway pressure increases the dimensions of the trachea in the anterior–posterior diameter and the tracheal volume resulting in tracheomegaly and increasing dead space [36, 45, 53, 54]. The greatest deformation in trachea dimension is associated with the posterior region where the cartilaginous tips are spread apart. The hinged area is a high stress point where tension (outer region of trachea) and compression (inner region of trachea) simultaneously applied during exposure to positive pressure. Ultrasound technology allows precise measurement of tracheal dimensions in vivo; allowing for a comparison between changes in mechanical properties of the airway and structural changes of the airway [45, 53]. Cartilage plays a major role in the structure of the airway and while the net effect is an increase in the dimensions of the trachea, controversy exists as to whether mechanical stress during ventilation, is damaging to the chondrocytes or if this stress has an impact on airway chondrocytes and extracellular matrix (ECM) expression. Recently published data proposes changes in airway chondrocytes and ECM secondary to the effects of positive pressure on the airway as responsible for acquired tracheomegaly [55] and increased dead space. Histologically, applying positive pressure to the airway results in a thinner and stretched, pseudostratified, ciliated columnar epithelium wall as well as radial expansion of the entire tracheal cartilage and muscle [55]. Fourier transform infrared imaging spectroscopy is a novel imaging methodology that has been utilized to examine various types of natural tissues including bone, cartilage, and tissue-engineered, cartilage-like tissue, and biomaterials. The specific molecular components in cartilage contribute to its infrared spectrum, and these can be detected using FT-IRIS methodology. An FT-IRIS spectrometer, when coupled with a light microscope, enables one to identify intensity and distribution of tissue compositions. FT-IRIS technology allows for assessments of functional alterations in trachea dimensions and mechanical properties. Utilizing this technology, tracheal cartilage can be assessed with respect to collagen, PG, and integrity of newly synthesized collagen [55]. FT-IRIS analysis demonstrated differences in intensity and distribution of ECM in the tracheal cartilage with an increase in the collagen and proteoglycan content and increased signal for collagen integrity (new tissue formation). These findings demonstrate that exposure to positive pressure changes the ECM composition and the level of constitutive ECM components in the neonatal tracheal cartilage, suggesting both airway damage and a concomitant repair.

Another component of pulmonary mechanics is described in terms of compliance of an elastic organ as volume (strain) per unit of pressure (stress), where compliance is lower when the elasticity is greater. Moduli of elasticity are typically used to describe material not intended to be compliant, in this case a large conducting airway. Bulk and elastic moduli represent the amount of force (stress) to achieve a degree of deformation (strain), and thus if something is less elastic, it requires more stress per unit of distortion and has a greater moduli of elasticity. The trachea normally has some degree of elasticity, however over time, with exposure to positive pressure more force is needed to distend the airway. In this regard, the airways are loosing elasticity in response to positive pressure whereby the enlarging internal diameter is associated with the breakdown of elastic components and airway distention is accomplished through stretch of the nonelastic structural components.

Collapsibility of the airway is determined by the contribution of airway cartilage and smooth muscle. Studies of the trachea in preterm lambs demonstrate that the preterm trachea is responsive to ACh by becoming stiffer, less deformable organs. However the magnitude of compliance and resistance changes consequent to smooth muscle contraction is small when compared to the full term and adult trachea suggesting a limited influence of airway smooth muscle on airway function in the preterm trachea. The mechanical properties (both tensile and compressive) of airway cartilage and smooth muscle are determined by the material composition of each tissue. Alterations in tissue composition with development may therefore explain differences in airway compliance. Proteoglycans are important constituents of the cartilaginous matrix and are known to confer rigidity to cartilage. Histochemical analysis by Bucher and Reid [17] has shown that the cartilaginous matrix of proximal human airways stains more basophilic near full term compared with a 16 weeks gestational age, suggesting increasing amounts of chondroitin sulfates with development. Considered collectively, these studies suggest that a relative lack of proteoglycans in immature airway cartilage may contribute to the collapsible nature of preterm lamb tracheae demonstrated in the present study. Additional factors that may contribute to developmental changes in the forcefulness of contraction of airway and non-airway smooth muscle in the preterm infant when compared to the full term and adult trachea includes:

1. Developmental changes in types of contractile proteins (actin and myosin, including isoforms) and concentration per unit area [56, 57].
2. Developmental changes in orientation of smooth muscle cells in the airway vessels from circular to oblique relative to the long axis of the vessel wall [58].

3. Developmental changes in synthetic activity of vascular smooth muscle cells from primarily secretory (producing the extracellular proteins collagen and elastin) during the neonatal period to primarily contractile (producing the intracellular protein actomyosin) after 4 weeks of age in rats [59].
4. Developmental changes in shape and function of airway smooth muscle cells (length and thickness doubled with age, although velocities of shortening were similar, in lambs vs. sheep) [60].

Forced expiration in the intact lung is typically associated with dynamic compression of the central airways, high resistance to airflow, and the establishment of a "flow-limiting segment" (FLS) of airway. Several studies have emphasized the importance of the compliance of the FLS in determining expiratory flow rate and have demonstrated how experimentally increasing or decreasing FLS compliance may respectively decrease [61–63] or increase [62] maximum expiratory flow. Accordingly, preterm infants with highly compliant airways might be expected to exhibit relatively greater airway compression, higher resistance, and severe flow limitation, which may exacerbate problems of gas exchange and breathing common in preterm infants. In the preterm trachea, relatively small compressive pressures are required to create significant airway compression and elevated resistance. The intrathoracic airways possess similar properties and are subject to similar dynamic compression at low efforts and flow limitation demonstrated in the preterm trachea [64] and as a consequence expiratory flow reserve is small. Complications associated with prematurity such as BPD [65–67] or the effects of mechanical ventilation [7, 8] may serve to further limit the preterm infant's physiological range of breathing [66] and exacerbate problems of clinical management. Reflex constriction of airway smooth muscle plays an important physiological role during forced expiration, serving to stiffen the central airways and improve conditions for flow [68]. This mechanism might be particularly useful to the premature infant whose airways are extremely compliant; however, studies have suggested that the effect of ACh on airway mechanics is age dependent and that the ability of airway smooth muscle to decrease airway compliance and increase expiratory flow in the intact lung may be limited in the preterm trachea. As a result, reflex constriction of the airway smooth muscle results in relatively small changes in airway circumference in the preterm infant, and this lack of effectiveness may be a contributing factor to the relatively severe flow limitation observed in preterm infants.

The airway epithelium plays an important role in the modulation of smooth muscle function. Studies of adult airways have shown that airway epithelium generates relaxant and contractile factors that modulate the tone of the underlying smooth muscle [69–72]. Epithelial damage has also been associated with bronchial hyper-reactivity [73] as de-epithelialized smooth muscle cells exhibit greater force of contraction in response to acetylcholine stimulation than did a strip of tracheal smooth muscle with epithelium intact [38]. The magnitude of the effect was as great in the preterm as adult trachea, demonstrating that even during late gestation, epithelial integrity may be an important determinant of smooth muscle function, bronchial hyper-reactivity, and bronchodilator responsiveness.

When one assesses the effect of mechanical ventilation of airway structure and function the effect on the proximal and distal airways may be quite distinct. Histological studies of ventilated neonatal human and animal lungs found that, in addition to tracheomegaly, the peripheral airways were wider in lungs of neonates and animals that had been mechanically ventilated. The mechanisms responsible for this difference are not known, but may include distal/proximal (regional) airway differences, age-related differences in amount of cartilage, orientation of muscle fibers, forcefulness of contraction of muscle fibers, and receptor sensitivity of airway smooth muscle fibers. These differences would lead to mechanical ventilation affecting the more compliant distal and less compliant proximal airways differently.

Clinical Presentation

Improved care of premature infants in the NICUs has led to fewer rate and days of intubation and mechanical ventilation. In infants who required prolonged intubation, failed extubation is often the first clue of developing acquired airway problems. Suspicion of upper airway obstruction should be higher when an infant with minimum ventilator support develops significant respiratory distress soon after extubation. Studies such as direct laryngoscopy and bronchoscopy (DLB) can uncover findings of granuloma formation at infraglottic surfaces and grade 2 membranous SGS in a premature infant who failed multiple extubation attempts (Fig. 3). In a retrospective study, Pereira et al. reviewed 63 infants who underwent DLB for failed extubation between 1998 and 2006. In this study, more than 90 % of these infants had abnormal airway findings at the time of DLB with 39.7 % had either subglottic edema or edema. Infant who were born at 30 weeks GA or less, low birth weight and with history of chronic lung disease were twice likely to have these findings. In addition, the group of infants who required tracheostomy had double the number of days of ventilation, failed extubations, and incidence of subglottic compromise as compared with the group of infants who did not require tracheostomy [74].

Stridor usually indicates an obstruction at the laryngotracheal airway. It may be inspiratory, expiratory or biphasic depending on the location of the obstruction: supraglottic lesions usually present with a coarse, inspiratory stridor, glottis and subglottic lesions often have stridor that described

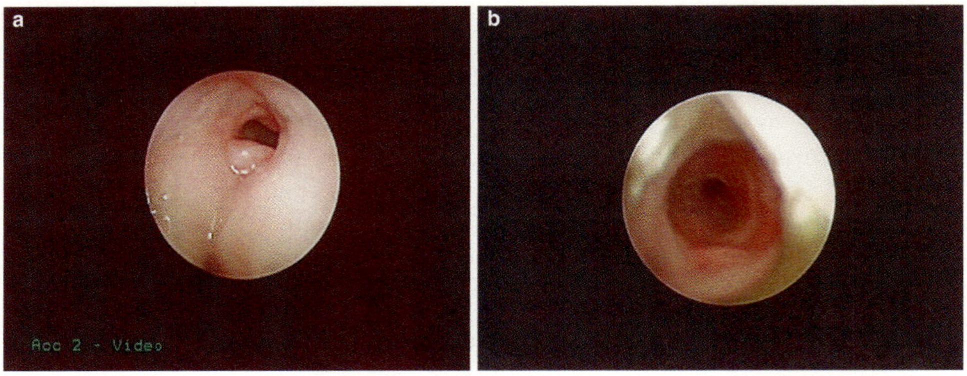

Fig. 3 Multiple failed extubation due to airway obstruction in an infant was born at 26 weeks gestation, receiving mechanical ventilation for 11 weeks. Bronchoscopy was performed at 37 weeks corrected age after multiple failed extubation attempts and showed (**a**) infraglottic granuloma formation; (**b**) membranous subglottic stenosis. Courtesy of Steve Sobol, (CHOP)

as musical and biphasic, whereas a pure tracheal lesion frequently produces expiratory stridor with a prolonged expiratory phase. However stridor is not always present in young infants with airway disorder. Some infants present with a weak, aphonic, or hoarse cry instead. Other infants may present with coughing and desaturation during feeds. In these cases, stridor may be intermittent and only become obvious or worse when the infant is agitated, crying, or during feeds (Fig. 4).

Patients with known BPD often exhibit episodic cyanotic spells known as "BPD" or "blue" spells. The etiology of these spells is often attributed to the exacerbated ventilation/perfusion (V/Q) mismatch during periods of agitation or pulmonary hypertension crisis. However, the "BPD" spells in some patients are actually caused by airway collapse due to severe TBM. During these episodes, the infants often have severe desaturation with bradycardia requiring PPV with high pressures. In non-intubated patients, signs of TBM may include coughing, respiratory distress with or without stridor, or episodes of apnea/bradycardia/desaturation (A/B/D). These A/B/D events in premature infants may be hard to differentiate from the events caused by apnea of prematurity. In addition to the cyanotic spells, TBM in infants with BPD can present with other nonspecific signs that are considered classic signs of BPD. These may include worsening hypoxia, hypercarbia, increasing oxygen requirement, increasing need for sedation, or simply as inability to wean respiratory support (Fig. 5). Often severe TBM in an infant may present as repeated inability to wean from positive pressure sometimes leading to progressively worsening pulmonary hypertension. In contrast to the diffuse, high-pitched and musical wheeze in asthma, wheeze in TBM is typically expiratory, central, low pitched and homophonous in nature [75] and mostly intermittent that worse during feeds and agitation.

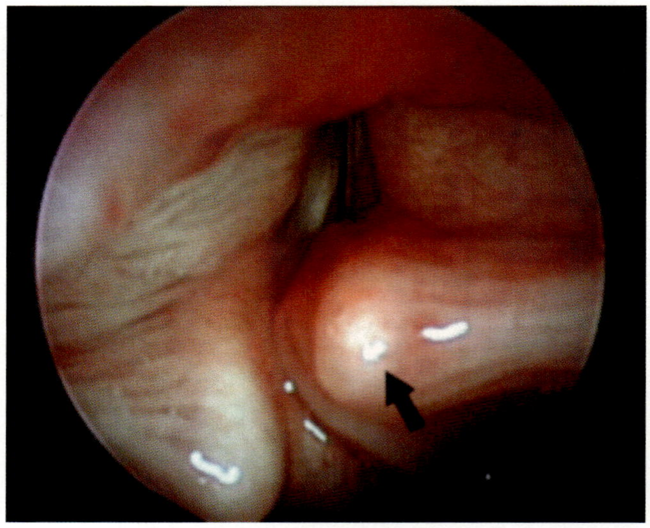

Fig. 4 Saccular cyst with prolapsed arytenoid causing airway obstruction with stridor. Courtesy of Luv Javia, (CHOP)

Evaluation and Diagnosis

The diagnosis of acquired airway disorders in premature infants is difficult due to the small caliber of the airway, the rapid respiratory rate, and intolerance to various diagnostic procedures. When choosing diagnostic methods, issues such as reliability, the need for intubation, radiation dose, and contrast administration need to be considered.

Pulmonary Function Measures

Dynamic pulmonary compliance can be measured using an esophageal balloon and pneumotachometry. In infants who later develop chronic lung disease, compliance is significantly

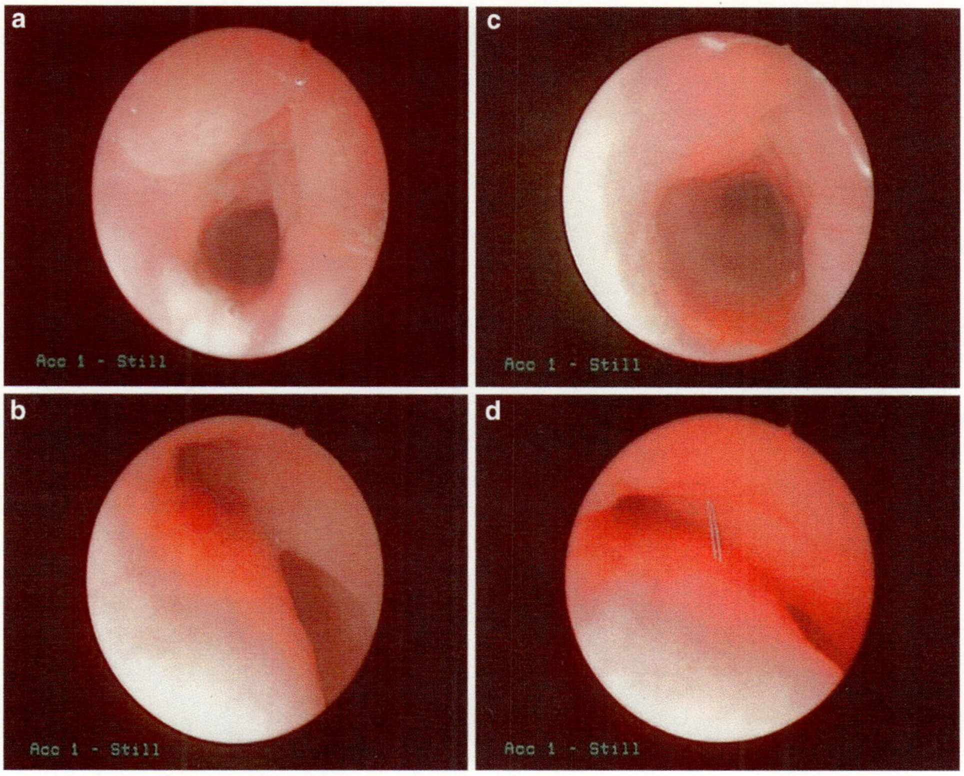

Fig. 5 Born at 23 weeks infant developed chronic respiratory failure and pulmonary hypertension due to severe airway malacia. (**a** & **b**): Bronchoscopy showing open trachea and bilateral bronchi during inspiration. (**c** & **d**): severe tracheal and bronchial collapse during expiration

lower when compared with infants who recover uneventfully from neonatal respiratory distress. In addition to reflecting the elastic properties of the lung to some degree, the dynamic pulmonary compliance time-constant serves to indicate how equally various regions of the tracheobronchial tree are being ventilated. A high value for dynamic compliance in an infant with chronic lung disease probably indicates some degree of airway obstruction. Quasi-static methods of measuring respiratory system compliance in infants with BPD have verified that alterations in the elastic properties of the lung contribute significantly to the lower compliance values measured in these lungs. Static and dynamic compliance measurements have not been compared in this group of infants, so it is not clear whether the improvement in dynamic compliance seen in infants with moderate to severe BPD studied longitudinally represents a change in the characteristics of the lung parenchyma, a decrease in respiratory rate, or improvement in airway obstruction. Interestingly, both static and dynamic measurements of compliance have predictive value regarding the development of BPD in mechanically ventilated preterm infants [76, 77].

Resistance measurements, include airway resistance and is determined by plethysmography, pulmonary resistance measured by the esophageal balloon and pneumotachometry technique, or respiratory system resistance determined by the airway occlusion technique, are significantly elevated in infants with BPD [78–82]. However, when measurements of resistance or its reciprocal, conductance, have been made serially, values have approached normal by age 2 or 3 years [78, 79]. These developmental improvements in resistance values can reflect either resolution of airway obstruction or an increase in airway diameter related to growth. Specific conductance corrects for changes in resistance or conductance without the confounding variable of growth (lung size). Specific conductance is defined as conductance divided by lung volume at forced reserve capacity (FRC). Elevated specific conductance confirms the presence of airway obstruction in infants with BPD [78, 83].

Forced expiratory flow (FEF) measurements can be obtained using either the rapid thoracic compression technique [66, 81, 84] or the rapid deflation technique [85, 86]. Measurements with either technique better reflect flow in small airways and demonstrate significant small airways obstruction in infants with BPD. Longitudinal assessments of (FEF) demonstrate that infants with BPD have significant airway obstruction that does not resolve completely with growth. Maximal expiratory flow-volume (MEFV) demonstrates severe small airway obstruction as determined by a marked reduction in $Vmax_{FRC}$. Among patients with moderate BPD who were weaned from mechanical ventilation before 5 months of age, $Vmax_{FRC}$ increased with increasing age to approximately 40 % of predicted value by 3 years of age [86]. In contrast, patients who required extended periods (10 months) of mechanical ventilation showed increase in Vmax25 over the same time period. Partial expiratory flow-volume (PEFV) curves generated over the tidal range of breathing showed that young infants with BPD had lower maximal flow at FRC ($Vmax_{FRC}$) than young infants without BPD. Furthermore, the separation between tidal and forced-flow curves, which was interpreted as a measure of expiratory flow reserve [66], indicated that infants with BPD had a smaller expiratory flow reserve compared with normal infants. The FEF rates in infants with BPD were only half those of the normal infants and had not increased by 14.5–22 months of age [66]. These findings suggest that early exposure to PPV and high concentrations of oxygen not only caused early airway damage but also interfered with subsequent normal airway growth. Values of $Vmax_{FRC}$ have been used to estimate ventilation of small airways. However, studies have shown that collapse of central airways (i.e., tracheomalacia or bronchomalacia) can cause a marked reduction in values of $Vmax_{FRC}$. When FEF measurements demonstrate marked reductions in $Vmax_{FRC,}$ repeating the measurement in the presence of CPAP is indicated to confirm if the reduction is related to central airway collapse or small airway obstruction. Functionally these airway abnormalities have been shown to persist in children and young adults with a history of BPD [87, 88].

Abnormalities in both tidal mechanics and FEF measurements confirm that airway reactivity is increased in infants with BPD. Taking this into consideration, airway reactivity testing becomes key in the evaluation and management of small airways disease in BPD. Acute decreases in pulmonary respiratory system and airway resistance have been reported in response to a variety of agonist and anticholinergic drugs [80, 81, 89–93]. The magnitude of this response was even more dramatic when forced flows were tested. Several other studies have confirmed airway reactivity in response to bronchodilator therapy.

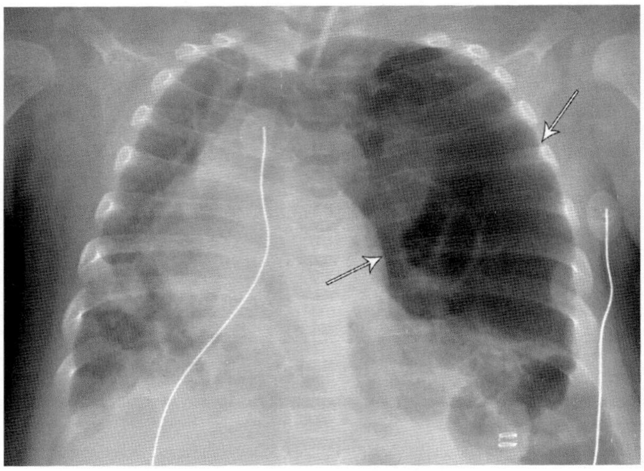

Fig. 6 Acquired lobar emphysema. Severe segmental hyperinflation in a premature infant requiring prolonged mechanical ventilation

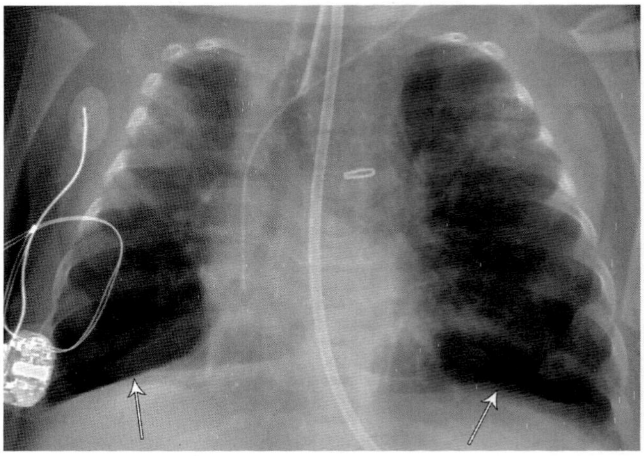

Fig. 7 Severe air trapping from severe tracheobronchial malacia due to persistent respiratory failure with oxygen requirement of 100 %

Chest X-Ray

Chest X-ray (CXR) is the most widely used radiographic tool in the assessment of respiratory issues in premature infants. Many infants on mechanical ventilation require frequent CXR, sometimes daily, assessments to evaluate ETT position and lung expansion. Careful examine of these chest radiographs may provide important clue in the diagnosis of acquired airway anomalies in these young infants. Bhutani et al. reported roentgenographic appearance of acquired tracheomegaly in VLEW infants who required mechanical ventilation. They reported 91 % greater tracheal volume in the ventilated group as compared to weight-matched non-ventilated controls [36].

Some authors have suggested using combined inspiratory and expiratory plain radiographs for the diagnosis of TBM and reported sensitivity as high as 62 % when compared to microlaryngoscopy and bronchoscopy [94]. However, good inspiratory and expiratory films may be difficult to obtain in a premature infant with rapid respiratory rate. Nonetheless, significant segmental hyperinflation (Fig. 6) or air trapping (Fig. 7) on the plain CXR should raise the suspicion for TBM.

Fluoroscopy and Bronchography

Both fluoroscopy and bronchography have been used to diagnose TBM. However both methods have significant limitation such as radiation exposure, difficulty fully visualizing the airway especially in the lateral plane, underestimating the degree of tracheal collapse, and difficult to perform in a small premature infant with borderline respiratory reserve and small airways [95]. Sanchez et al. compared fluoroscopy with flexible bronchoscopy in 22 children

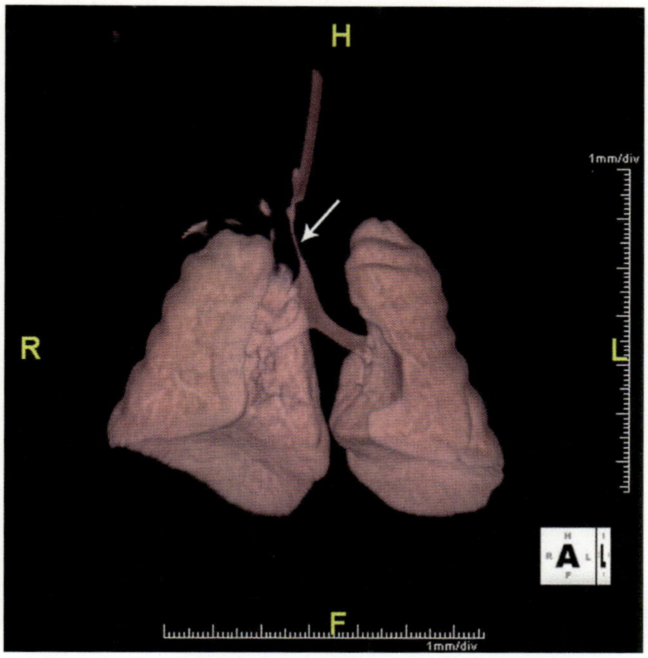

Fig. 8 CT evaluation of tracheal anatomy demonstrating long segmental tracheal stenosis in an infant. Courtesy of Andrew Mong, (CHOP)

at 1 month to 8 years of age. They found that airway fluoroscopy was poorly sensitive (23.8 %) but highly specific (100 %) in the diagnosis of tracheomalacia [96].

CT

CT is a noninvasive method that enables precise and objective delineation of the location, extent, and depth of tracheobronchial pathology (Fig. 8). When compared to bronchoscopy, concordant rate as high as 83–100 % has been reported in the diagnosis of TBM. Figure 9 shows significantly decreased tracheal size during expiration phase in an infant with severe bronchomalacia. In addition, evaluation of the adjacent cardiovascular system and lung parenchyma can be simultaneously obtained, especially when combined with CT angiography (CTA) (Figs. 10, 11, and 12). In recent years, newer CT techniques such as dynamic, volumetric imaging using wide-range multi-detector CT have increased the sensitivity and accuracy in the diagnosis of airway stenosis and malacia. These techniques have been successfully used in young infants [97, 98]. Although CT is becoming increasingly popular as a diagnostic

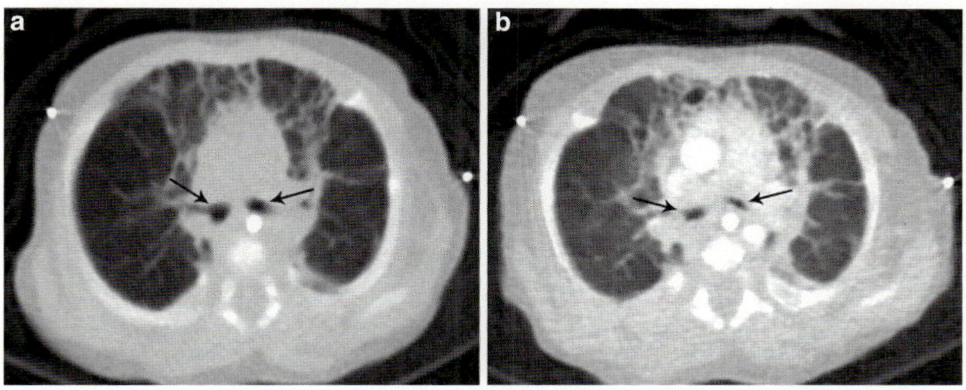

Fig. 9 CT angiography demonstrating severe bronchomalacia. Significantly decreased size of bilateral bronchus during expiration (**b**) as compared to inhalation (**a**) in an infant with BPD

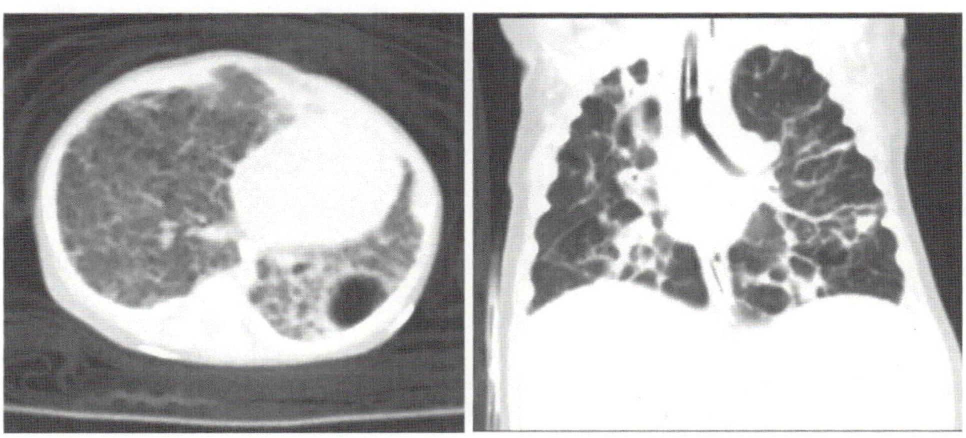

Fig. 10 Evaluating lung parenchyma disease with CTA. *Left*: severe BPD with bulla (*arrow*); *right*: another BPD patient with intercostal bulging and parenchymal bands (*arrow*)

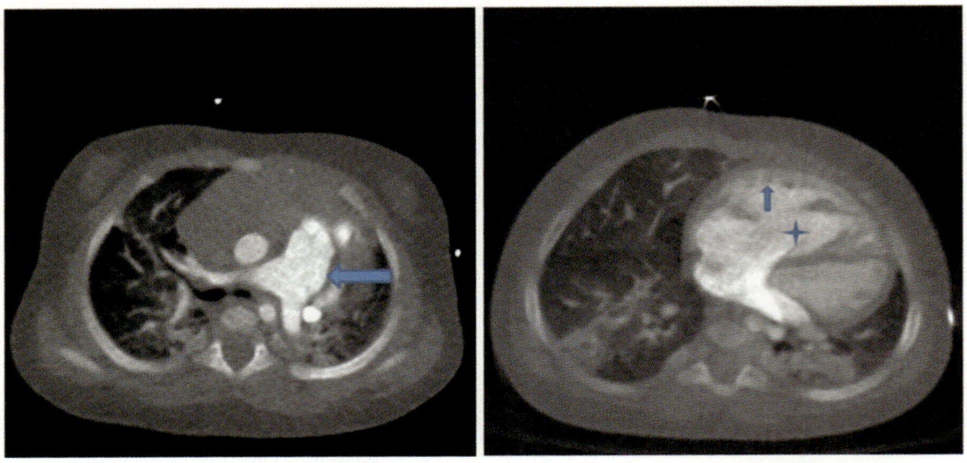

Fig. 11 Evaluation of cardiovascular system in patients with BPD using CTA. Signs of pulmonary hypertension in a patient with mild to moderate BPD: *Left*—enlarged pulmonary artery (*arrow*); *right*—enlarged right ventricle (*star*) with hypertrophy (*arrow*). Courtesy of Andrew Mong, (CHOP)

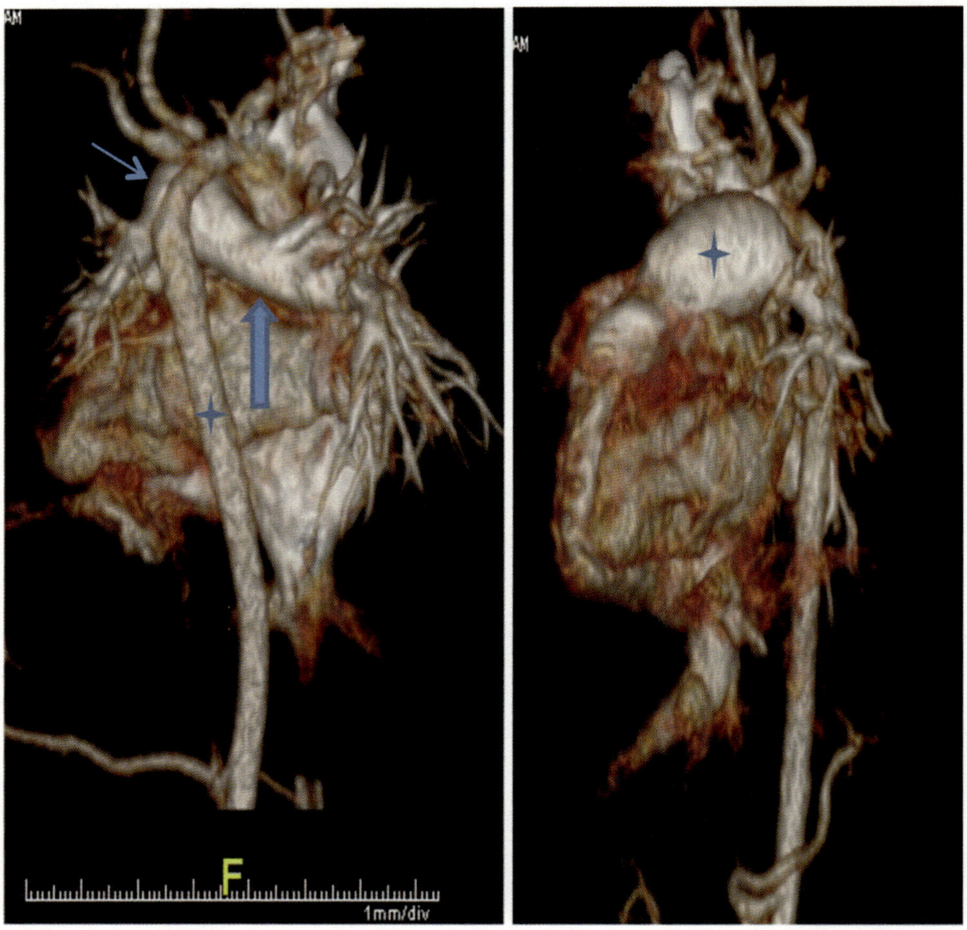

Fig. 12 Use of CTA reconstruction to evaluate pulmonary hypertension in infants with BPD. *Right*: lateral view showing enlarged main pulmonary artery (PA) (*star*); *left*: posterior view showing enlarged right PA (*blue thick arrow*), enlarged left PA (*thin arrow*), and descending aorta (*star*). Courtesy of Andrew Mong, (CHOP)

tool for the noninvasive evaluation of respiratory tract disorders in pediatric patients, attention needs to be paid to reduce the exposure to radiation. This requires each scan to be carefully planned in accordance to body size, respiratory rate, cooperation, and IV access. Using a standardized dose reduction protocol, radiation dose from a CTA has been reduced from 3.2 mSv in 2007 to the current level of 0.2–0.4 mSV at the Children's Hospital of Philadelphia.

Magnetic Resonance Imaging

MRI has the major advantage of lack of ionizing radiation as compared to other imaging modalities and can be used to evaluate central airways in children [99]. However, due to its limitations of longer scan time, need for sedation, and inferior spatial resolution relative to CT, its use as a diagnostic tool for airway disorders has been limited in the premature infants.

Endoscopic Evaluation

Airway endoscopy is useful for the diagnosis of anatomic lesions from the supraglottic, glottic, and subglottic regions down to the tracheal and segmental bronchial level.

Nasopharyngolaryngoscopy (NPL)

Nasopharyngolaryngoscopy (NPL) using a flexible fiberoptic endoscope is commonly used in the neonatal ICUs to achieve more thorough examination of the larynx and the vocal cord. Although the procedure is in general well tolerated and despite the relatively high incidence of LVCP after PDA ligation, most institutions do not routinely examine for vocal cord paralysis after the surgery. In 1 case series of 111 premature infants who underwent PDA ligation, Rukholm et al. found only 27.9 % had NPL to evaluate for vocal cord paralysis [27]. Major argument against routine postoperative examination is that it brings patient discomfort and unnecessary costs to the system as well. However, as high as 14 % of infants with LVCP have been reported initially being asymptomatic [28]. In addition, LVCP may have long lasting health effects into adulthood [30]. Given these reasons, some authors advocate for routine postoperative NPL examination of all PDA ligation patients.

Bronchoscopy

Many have considered bronchoscopy the gold standard for central airway evaluation. Flexible bronchoscopy (FB) is usually performed in sedated but spontaneously breathing patients, whereas rigid bronchoscopy (RB) or a magnified microscopic laryngoscopy bronchoscopy (MLB) requires general anesthesia. Therefore, FB is superior to RB in the evaluation of dynamic airway changes and may provide better visualization of the distal airways. In comparison, RB provides better airway control in infants with borderline respiratory reserve, but may underdiagnose the central airway collapse due to the absence of patient's breathing effort resulting in completely passive exhalation (Fig. 13).

Currently, there is no universally agreed-upon criterion for evaluating the results of bronchoscopy. Some authors proposed using percentage of airway narrowing during exhalation to categorize severity of TBM. For example, Sanchez et al. categorized tracheomalacia severity as: mild, 50–75 % occlusion; moderate, >75 % occlusion; and severe, near or complete occlusion [96].

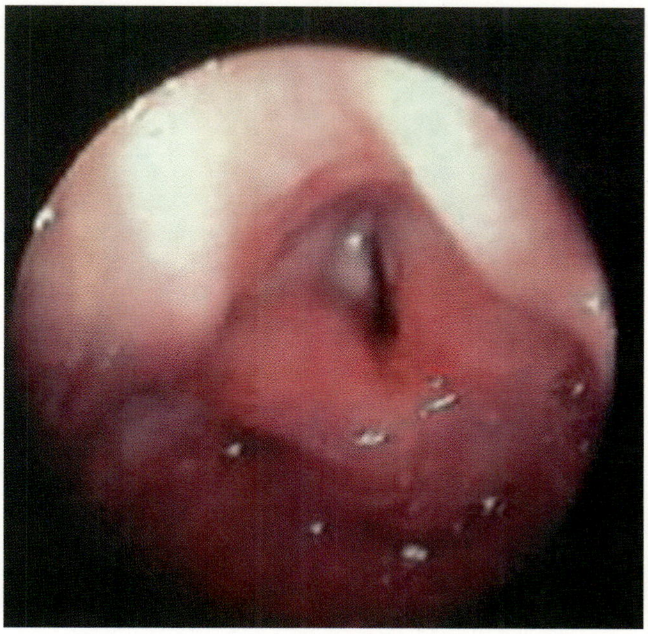

Fig. 13 Nasopharyngeal laryngoscopy showing glottic edema and swelling

Although bronchoscopy is generally well tolerated, it is invasive and have several limitations: (1) the assessment is subjective and dependent on the technique and experience of the operator; (2) inability to pass the instrument to distal airways (especially in small premature infants), or beyond a point of narrowing. Therefore, distal airway involvement tend to be poorly assessed; (3) airway dynamics are affected by the presence of the instrument and its ventilation pressure. Therefore bronchoscopy tends to underestimate the degree of airway collapse as compared to other imaging techniques such as dynamic CTA or bronchography.

Management

Many infants with acquired airway lesions may require surgical intervention. Various surgical techniques such as balloon dilatation, stenting, supraglottoplasty, laryngotracheal reconstruction, cricotracheal resection, and slide tracheoplasty have been well described in the literature [100, 101] as well as other chapters of this book.

The various lesion and conditions that affect the upper as well as the lower airway may be difficult to diagnose in the

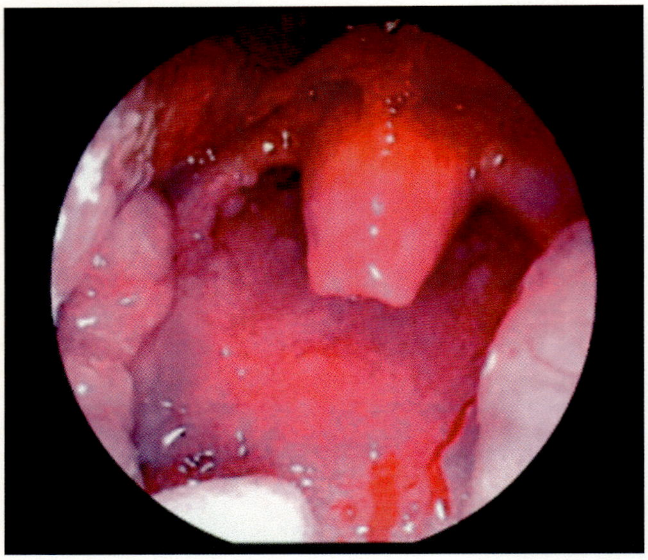

Fig. 14 Inflammation with retroflexed epiglottis causing significant stridor and upper airway obstruction. Courtesy of Ian Jacobs, (CHOP)

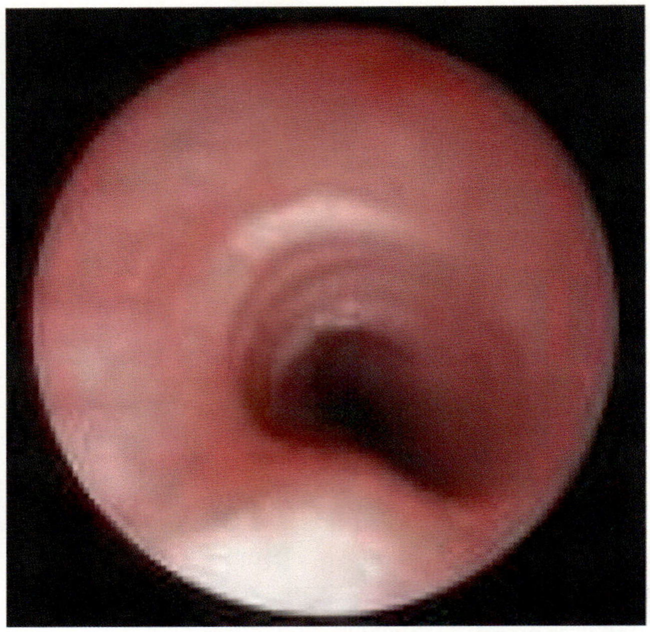

Fig. 15 Picture of bronchoscopy with severe tracheomalacia likely requiring high PEEP. Courtesy of Ian Jacobs, (CHOP)

premature infant with multiple comorbidities, but often a flexible bronchoscopy or rigid bronchoscopy can uncover the major offender (Fig. 14).

The medical management of premature infants requiring respiratory support is complex and often requires a multidisciplinary approach often with pediatric otolaryngology and later pediatric pulmonology. When taking care of small premature infants, every attempt should be made to prevent injury, allow healing after injury has occurred and promote optimum growth. Good nursing care and hygiene are therefore paramount. Instead of tracheal intubation, multiple clinical trials have proven noninvasive respiratory support measures, including NCPAP (Nasal CPAP), NIPPV (Nasal Intermittent Positive Pressure Ventilation), HFNC (High Flow Nasal Cannula), to be feasible and effective in the immediate postnatal days of ELBW infants with RDS [102–104].

In infants who require endotracheal intubation, the procedure should be performed in as controlled an environment as possible. Many studies have demonstrated that premedication for intubation of the newborns can improve intubation conditions and minimize the potential for intubation-related airway trauma. Based on these studies, the American Academy of Pediatrics (AAP) has recommended that premedication should be used in all endotracheal intubations in newborns except for emergent intubation during resuscitation [105]. Currently no consensus guidelines exist regarding the optimal drug or drug combination. Medications with rapid onset and short duration of action are preferable and each unit should develop protocols to improve compliance and minimize medication errors.

Clinicians need to have high index of suspicion for acquired airway problems in premature infant requiring prolonged respiratory support, especially in infants with BPD [106]. Appropriate imaging and bronchoscopy should be considered in infants with stridor, persistent localized atelectasis, segmental or lobar hyperinflation, recurrent respiratory distress, and episodic hypoxemia spells. In addition efforts should be made to eliminate factors that cause ongoing lung and airway injury. These factors include excessive ventilation, recurrent infection, and inflammation from hyperoxia and chronic aspiration.

Although weaning off ventilator support and early extubation are important for the majority of patients, providing adequate respiratory support is also critical to many infants with chronic respiratory insufficiency. Too fast of a wean of the respiratory support may result in significant increase in work of breath and energy expenditure, and therefore hinder growth, healing process and in some cases exacerbate lung disease and pulmonary hypertension. For example, infants with severe airway malacia often require high PEEP (positive end expiratory pressure) for a prolonged period of time to help stent the airway open. In these cases, tracheostomy placement with adequate PEEP may provide a stable airway and improve the hypoxia spells due to airway collapse. Tracheostomy placement has been shown to be safe in premature infants, even in infants with severe BPD [107, 108]. Although tracheostomy in very preterm infants is associated with adverse neurodevelopmental outcome, earlier tracheostomy placement (before 120 days of life) may be associated with better outcomes among infants with tracheostomies [109] (Fig. 15).

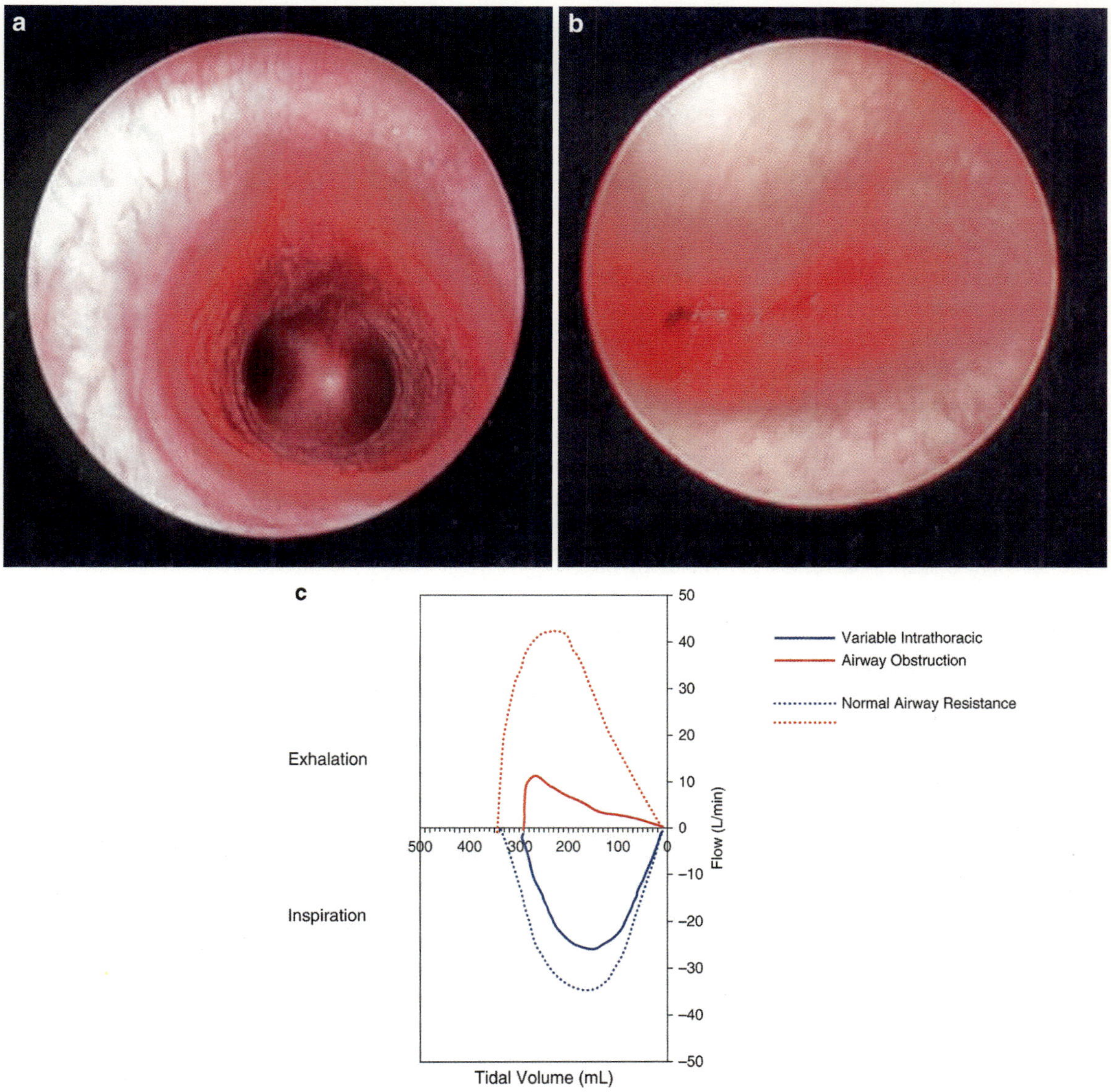

Fig. 16 Severe airway malacia causing expiratory obstruction and potential air trapping. Adapted from Wheeler et al. Life Threatening Disorders of the Respiratory Track: Pediatric Critical Care Medicine: Volume 2: Respiratory, Cardiovascular and Central Nervous Systems. Shanley, et al, eds. 2nd edition. Springer 2014

The approach to management of small airways disease in BPD depends on many factors with the most important factors being whether or not the infant is mechanically ventilated and whether the infant demonstrates a response to bronchodilator therapy. For the patient that is mechanically ventilated, the interplay between large and small airways disease complicates management. Large airway issues contributing to the pathogenesis of BPD include increased large airway compliance, tracheomegaly, and tracheo-bronchomalacia (Fig. 16).

With respect to the small airways, obstruction is the predominant feature, which when present can exacerbate the severity of large airways disease, and potentiate large airway collapse, but also impact ventilation and gas exchange. The interplay between small and large airways disease results in higher airway resistance and decreased compliance with resultant higher peak airway pressures for a given tidal volume. High airways resistance results in a need for longer inspiratory times. Along with increased resistance and decreased compliance, airways obstruction with decreased emptying, necessitates an increased expiratory time. Transitioning from the high rate, low inspiratory time and low tidal volume approach often employed early in the course in preterm infants, to a mode that addresses this complex interaction between small and large airways disease as well as heterogeneity of lung parenchymal disease, is indicated with the development of established BPD, and results in significant improvements in gas exchange and clinical stability. Optimally utilizing a low rate, with a high inspiratory time and larger tidal volume to offset the effects of a lower rate, but also to compensate for increased dead space with acquired tracheomegaly and allow for more even gas distribution throughout the lung. The optimal PEEP is determined by the interplay between the severity of airway collapse or TBM and severity of parenchymal lung disease. Applying enough PEEP to "stent" the airway, without exposing the distal lung parenchyma to excessive PEEP is key. The PEEP can be titrated at the bedside with the use of bronchoscopy and direct visualization of the large proximal airways, applying a stepwise increase in PEEP to the airways and with direct visualization determining the effect of increased PEEP on airways collapse. Once the optimal PEEP is determined by bronchoscopy, serial CXR are needed to determine the effect of the PEEP on the distal lung parenchyma. High airways resistance, decreased compliance, and the need for increased tidal volume results in higher peak pressures for a given tidal volume, and a permissive approach to the increased peak pressures is indicated if optimal gas exchange is to be achieved. This approach allows for optimal management of central large airways disease, addresses the issues of poor lung compliance and increased airways resistance, allows for more even distribution of gas throughout the lung, and provides the infant with sufficient time for the slow emptying component in the lung to empty.

Airway obstruction due to small airway constriction is present in all infants with established BPD and as mentioned there is subset of 30–50 % of infants that will respond to bronchodilator therapy with β-agonists [87, 110, 111]. A trial of bronchodilator therapy is indicated in all patients with established BPD to assess response and optimize management. If available and practical, an assessment of lung function after a bronchodilator trial is the most accurate way to assess response, however when not practical or possible as would likely be the case in most infants with established BPD in the first few weeks of life, one could utilize other parameters to assess response. These include reductions in peak airway pressure due to decreased resistance, improvements in tidal volume for a given peak pressure, due to improved compliance and decreased resistance and improved ventilation and gas exchange with a trial of bronchodilator therapy. Management of bronchodilator responsiveness involves the use of steroids either inhaled or systemic, as well as use of agonists and the muscarinic antagonist ipratropium bromide. Pediatric studies have demonstrated that with alternate day systemic steroids in children with asthma, similar control of asthma symptoms could be achieved with fewer side effects especially effects on growth and adrenal function [112, 113]. Studies of inhaled steroids in preterm infants have demonstrated a decreased need for systemic steroids with no effect on the prevention of BPD [114, 115]. In patients who demonstrate responsiveness to agonists, steroids upregulate adrenergic receptors, improve the response to agonists and reduce airway inflammation [116]. For these reasons, inhaled steroids are indicated in patients with established BPD who demonstrate agonist responsiveness. Where absorption of inhaled steroids is questionable, one should consider 0.5 mg/kg/day alternate day systemic oral prednisone. In addition to the effects on airway obstruction, a recent study demonstrated that patients with established BPD maintained on steroids and bronchodilators demonstrate significantly higher pulmonary function measurements of FRC [111]. While multiple studies have demonstrated no benefit with respect to facilitating extubation and preventing the development of BPD, in the setting of responsiveness to inhaled-agonists, inhaled steroids remain indicated.

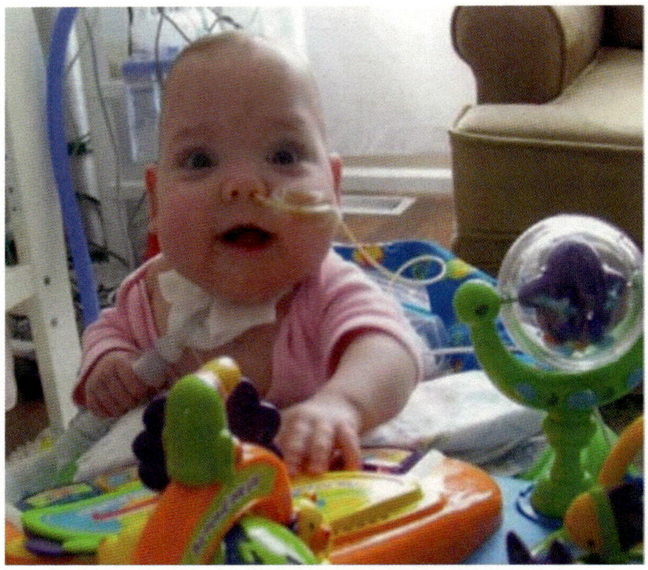

Fig. 17 Former 24-week preterm infant with the diagnosis of acquired grade 3–4-subglottic stenosis now thriving at home with tracheostomy. Courtesy of Janet Lioy, (CHOP Neonatal Airway Program)

Ultimately, many of these infants with severe BPD will require tracheostomy and are then able to transition from one phase of chronic illness to another. Many of these infants without significant comorbidities are able to thrive, grow new lung tissue, and leave the hospital with their families. Fortunately, many will eventually decannulate and live without significant morbidity as they reach childhood years (Fig. 17).

Future Directions

Despite many advances in neonatal care in the past 40 years, significant practice variations and many controversies exist in the care of premature infants. Some key issues include the oxygen saturation target, best strategies of respiratory support, and the role of GER in respiratory diseases. Future biomedical research and clinical studies will undoubtedly provide more valuable insights into the mechanisms of airway dysfunction in premature infants and identify ways to improve the management of neonatal airway disorders. Easier access to multicenter comprehensive databases will provide opportunities to analyze large amount of clinical data and help answer many clinical management questions.

References

1. Hamilton BE, Martin JA, Ventura SJ. Births: preliminary data for 2012. Natl Vital Stat Rep. 2013;62(3):1–20.
2. Martin JA, Hamilton BE, Ventura SJ, Osterman MJ, Mathews TJ. Births: final data for 2011. Natl Vital Stat Rep. 2013;62(1): 1–69, 72.
3. Charafeddine L, D'Angio CT, Phelps DL. Atypical chronic lung disease patterns in neonates. Pediatrics. 1999;103(4 Pt 1): 759–65.
4. Walsh MC, Yao Q, Gettner P, Hale E, Collins M, Hensman A, et al. Impact of a physiologic definition on bronchopulmonary dysplasia rates. Pediatrics. 2004;114(5):1305–11.
5. Stoll BJ, Hansen NI, Bell EF, Shankaran S, Laptook AR, Walsh MC, et al. Neonatal outcomes of extremely preterm infants from the NICHD Neonatal Research Network. Pediatrics. 2010;126(3): 443–56.
6. McCray Jr PB. Spontaneous contractility of human fetal airway smooth muscle. Am J Respir Cell Mol Biol. 1993;8(5):573–80.
7. Matsuba K, Thurlbeck WM. A morphometric study of bronchial and bronchiolar walls in children. Am Rev Respir Dis. 1972;105(6): 908–13.
8. Hislop A, Muir DC, Jacobsen M, Simon G, Reid L. Postnatal growth and function of the pre-acinar airways. Thorax. 1972; 27(3):265–74.
9. Hislop AA, Haworth SG. Airway size and structure in the normal fetal and infant lung and the effect of premature delivery and artificial ventilation. Am Rev Respir Dis. 1989;140(6):1717–26.
10. Tepper RS. Airway reactivity in infants: a positive response to methacholine and metaproterenol. J Appl Physiol. 1987;62(3): 1155–9.
11. Prendiville A, Green S, Silverman M. Airway responsiveness in wheezy infants: evidence for functional beta adrenergic receptors. Thorax. 1987;42(2):100–4.
12. Dalquen P, Oberholzer M, Wyss H, Specht H, Rohr HP, Herzog H. Bronchus morphometry. Correlations between morphometric data and lung function parameters in obstructive airway disease. Respiration. 1977;34(3):121–30.
13. Bertrand JM, Riley SP, Popkin J, Coates AL. The long-term pulmonary sequelae of prematurity: the role of familial airway hyperreactivity and the respiratory distress syndrome. N Engl J Med. 1985;312(12):742–5.
14. Borkenstein J, Borkenstein M, Rosegger H. Pulmonary function studies in long-term survivors with artificial ventilation in the neonatal period. Acta Paediatr Scand. 1980;69(2):159–63.
15. Pohunek P. Development, structure and function of the upper airways. Paediatr Respir Rev. 2004;5(1):2–8.
16. Masters JR. Epithelial-mesenchymal interaction during lung development: the effect of mesenchymal mass. Dev Biol. 1976; 51(1):98–108.
17. Bucher U, Reid L. Development of the intrasegmental bronchial tree: the pattern of branching and development of cartilage at various stages of intra-uterine life. Thorax. 1961;16:207–18.
18. Walner DL, Loewen MS, Kimura RE. Neonatal subglottic stenosis—incidence and trends. Laryngoscope. 2001;111(1):48–51.
19. Schweiger C, Marostica PJ, Smith MM, Manica D, Carvalho PR, Kuhl G. Incidence of post-intubation subglottic stenosis in children: prospective study. J Laryngol Otol. 2013;127(4):399–403.
20. Downing GJ, Kilbride HW. Evaluation of airway complications in high-risk preterm infants: application of flexible fiberoptic airway endoscopy. Pediatrics. 1995;95(4):567–72.
21. Sherman JM, Lowitt S, Stephenson C, Ironson G. Factors influencing acquired subgottic stenosis in infants. J Pediatr. 1986; 109(2):322–7.
22. Manica D, Schweiger C, Marostica PJ, Kuhl G, Carvalho PR. Association between length of intubation and subglottic stenosis in children. Laryngoscope. 2013;123(4):1049–54.
23. Downing GJ, Hayen LK, Kilbride HW. Acquired subglottic cysts in the low-birth-weight infant. Characteristics, treatment, and outcome. Am J Dis Child. 1993;147(9):971–4.
24. Halimi C, Nevoux J, Denoyelle F, Garabedian EN, Leboulanger N. Acquired subglottic cysts: management and long term outcome. Int J Pediatr Otorhinolaryngol. 2012;76(4):589–92.
25. Tadie JM, Behm E, Lecuyer L, Benhmamed R, Hans S, Brasnu D, et al. Post-intubation laryngeal injuries and extubation failure: a fiberoptic endoscopic study. Intensive Care Med. 2010;36(6): 991–8.
26. Bray D, Cavalli L, Eze N, Mills N, Hartley BE. Dysphonia secondary to traumatic avulsion of the vocal fold in infants. J Laryngol Otol. 2010;124(11):1229–33.
27. Rukholm G, Farrokhyar F, Reid D. Vocal cord paralysis post patent ductus arteriosus ligation surgery: risks and co-morbidities. Int J Pediatr Otorhinolaryngol. 2012;76(11):1637–41.
28. Clement WA, El-Hakim H, Phillipos EZ, Cote JJ. Unilateral vocal cord paralysis following patent ductus arteriosus ligation in extremely low-birth-weight infants. Arch Otolaryngol Head Neck Surg. 2008;134(1):28–33.
29. Benjamin JR, Smith PB, Cotten CM, Jaggers J, Goldstein RF, Malcolm WF. Long-term morbidities associated with vocal cord paralysis after surgical closure of a patent ductus arteriosus in extremely low birth weight infants. J Perinatol. 2010;30(6):408–13.
30. Roksund OD, Clemm H, Heimdal JH, Aukland SM, Sandvik L, Markestad T, et al. Left vocal cord paralysis after extreme preterm birth, a new clinical scenario in adults. Pediatrics. 2010;126(6): e1569–77.
31. Boogaard R, Huijsmans SH, Pijnenburg MW, Tiddens HA, de Jongste JC, Merkus PJ. Tracheomalacia and bronchomalacia in children: incidence and patient characteristics. Chest. 2005;128(5): 3391–7.
32. Jacobs IN, Wetmore RF, Tom LW, Handler SD, Potsic WP. Tracheobronchomalacia in children. Arch Otolaryngol Head Neck Surg. 1994;120(2):154–8.
33. Mair EA, Parsons DS. Pediatric tracheobronchomalacia and major airway collapse. Ann Otol Rhinol Laryngol. 1992;101(4):300–9.
34. Doull IJ, Mok Q, Tasker RC. Tracheobronchomalacia in preterm infants with chronic lung disease. Arch Dis Child Fetal Neonatal Ed. 1997;76(3):F203–5.
35. Carden KA, Boiselle PM, Waltz DA, Ernst A. Tracheomalacia and tracheobronchomalacia in children and adults: an in-depth review. Chest. 2005;127(3):984–1005.
36. Bhutani VK, Ritchie WG, Shaffer TH. Acquired tracheomegaly in very preterm neonates. Am J Dis Child. 1986;140(5):449–52.
37. Sotomayor JL, Godinez RI, Borden S, Wilmott RW. Large-airway collapse due to acquired tracheobronchomalacia in infancy. Am J Dis Child. 1986;140(4):367–71.
38. Panitch HB, Wolfson MR, Shaffer TH. Epithelial modulation of preterm airway smooth muscle contraction. J Appl Physiol. 1993;74(3):1437–43.
39. Mirmanesh SJ, Abbasi S, Bhutani VK. Alpha-adrenergic bronchoprovocation in neonates with bronchopulmonary dysplasia. J Pediatr. 1992;121(4):622–5.
40. Penn RB, Wolfson MR, Shaffer TH. Effect of ventilation on mechanical properties and pressure-flow relationships of immature airways. Pediatr Res. 1988;23(5):519–24.
41. Penn RB, Wolfson MR, Shaffer TH. Effect of tracheal smooth muscle tone on collapsibility of immature airways. J Appl Physiol. 1988;65(2):863–9.
42. Koslo RJ, Bhutani VK, Shaffer TH. The role of tracheal smooth muscle contraction on neonatal tracheal mechanics. Pediatr Res. 1986;20(12):1216–20.

43. Palombini B, Coburn RF. Control of the compressibility of the canine trachea. Respir Physiol. 1972;15(3):365–83.
44. Deoras KS, Wolfson MR, Bhutani VK, Shaffer TH. Structural changes in the tracheae of preterm lambs induced by ventilation. Pediatr Res. 1989;26(5):434–7.
45. Miller TL, Zhu Y, Altman AR, Dysart K, Shaffer TH. Sequential alterations of tracheal mechanical properties in the neonatal lamb: effect of mechanical ventilation. Pediatr Pulmonol. 2007;42(2):141–9.
46. Bhutani VK, Rubenstein SD, Shaffer TH. Pressure–volume relationships of tracheae in fetal newborn and adult rabbits. Respir Physiol. 1981;43(3):221–31.
47. McFawn PK, Mitchell HW. Bronchial compliance and wall structure during development of the immature human and pig lung. Eur Respir J. 1997;10(1):27–34.
48. Penn RB, Wolfson MR, Shaffer TH. Developmental differences in tracheal cartilage mechanics. Pediatr Res. 1989;26(5):429–33.
49. Panitch HB, Deoras KS, Wolfson MR, Shaffer TH. Maturational changes in airway smooth muscle structure-function relationships. Pediatr Res. 1992;31(2):151–6.
50. James AL, Hogg JC, Dunn LA, Pare PD. The use of the internal perimeter to compare airway size and to calculate smooth muscle shortening. Am Rev Respir Dis. 1988;138(1):136–9.
51. Mitchell HW, Sparrow MP. Video-imaging of lumen narrowing; muscle shortening and flow responsiveness in isolated bronchial segments of the pig. Eur Respir J. 1994;7(7):1317–25.
52. Bhutani VK, Rubenstein D, Shaffer TH. Pressure-induced deformation in immature airways. Pediatr Res. 1981;15(5):829–32.
53. Miller TL, Altman AR, Tsuda T, Shaffer TH. An ultrasound imaging method for in vivo tracheal bulk and Young's moduli of elasticity. J Biomech. 2007;40(7):1615–21.
54. Keszler M, Nassabeh-Montazami S, Abubakar K. Evolution of tidal volume requirement during the first 3 weeks of life in infants <800 g ventilated with volume guarantee. Arch Dis Child Fetal Neonatal Ed. 2009;94(4):F279–82.
55. Kim M, Pugarelli J, Miller TL, Wolfson MR, Dodge GR, Shaffer TH. Brief mechanical ventilation impacts airway cartilage properties in neonatal lambs. Pediatr Pulmonol. 2012;47(8):763–70.
56. Sparrow MP, Mitchell HW. Contraction of smooth muscle of pig airway tissues from before birth to maturity. J Appl Physiol. 1990;68(2):468–77.
57. Kawamoto S, Adelstein RS. Characterization of myosin heavy chains in cultured aorta smooth muscle cells. A comparative study. J Biol Chem. 1987;262(15):7282–8.
58. Cliff WJ. The aortic tunica media in growing rats studied with the electron microscope. Lab Invest. 1967;17(6):599–615.
59. Wolinsky H. Long-term effects of hypertension on the rat aortic wall and their relation to concurrent aging changes. Morphological and chemical studies. Circ Res. 1972;30(3):301–9.
60. Driska SP, Laudadio RE, Wolfson MR, Shaffer TH. A method for isolating adult and neonatal airway smooth muscle cells and measuring shortening velocity. J Appl Physiol. 1999;86(1):427–35.
61. Herzog H, Keller R, Maurer W, Baumann HR, Nadjafi A. Distribution of bronchial resistance in obstructive pulmonary diseases and in dogs with artificially induced tracheal collapse. Respiration. 1968;25(5):381–94.
62. Jones JG, Fraser RB, Nadel JA. Effect of changing airway mechanics on maximum expiratory flow. J Appl Physiol. 1975;38(6):1012–21.
63. McCormack GS, Moreno RH, Hogg JC, Pare PD. Lung mechanics in papain-treated rabbits. J Appl Physiol. 1986;60(1):242–6.
64. Croteau JR, Cook CD. Volume-pressure and length-tension measurements in human tracheal and bronchial segments. J Appl Physiol. 1961;16:170–2.
65. Northway Jr WH, Rosan RC, Porter DY. Pulmonary disease following respirator therapy of hyaline-membrane disease. Bronchopulmonary dysplasia. N Engl J Med. 1967;276(7):357–68.
66. Tepper RS, Morgan WJ, Cota K, Taussig LM. Expiratory flow limitation in infants with bronchopulmonary dysplasia. J Pediatr. 1986;109(6):1040–6.
67. Wolfson MR, Bhutani VK, Shaffer TH, Bowen Jr FW. Mechanics and energetics of breathing helium in infants with bronchopulmonary dysplasia. J Pediatr. 1984;104(5):752–7.
68. Olsen CR, Stevens AE, McIlroy MB. Rigidity of tracheae and bronchi during muscular constriction. J Appl Physiol. 1967;23(1):27–34.
69. Cuss FM, Barnes PJ. Airway smooth muscle and disease workshop: epithelial mediators. Am Rev Respir Dis. 1987;136(4 Pt 2):S32–5.
70. Aizawa H, Miyazaki N, Shigematsu N, Tomooka M. A possible role of airway epithelium in modulating hyperresponsiveness. Br J Pharmacol. 1988;93(1):139–45.
71. Flavahan NA, Aarhus LL, Rimele TJ, Vanhoutte PM. Respiratory epithelium inhibits bronchial smooth muscle tone. J Appl Physiol. 1985;58(3):834–8.
72. Stuart-Smith K, Vanhoutte PM. Airway epithelium modulates the responsiveness of porcine bronchial smooth muscle. J Appl Physiol. 1988;65(2):721–7.
73. Laitinen LA, Heino M, Laitinen A, Kava T, Haahtela T. Damage of the airway epithelium and bronchial reactivity in patients with asthma. Am Rev Respir Dis. 1985;131(4):599–606.
74. Pereira KD, Smith SL, Henry M. Failed extubation in the neonatal intensive care unit. Int J Pediatr Otorhinolaryngol. 2007;71(11):1763–6.
75. Vicencio AG, Parikh S. Laryngomalacia and tracheomalacia: common dynamic airway lesions. Pediatr Rev. 2006;27(4):e33–5; discussion e5.
76. Dreizzen E, Migdal M, Praud JP, Saby MA, Chambille B, Dehan M, et al. Passive total respiratory system compliance and gas exchange in newborns with hyaline membrane disease. Pediatr Pulmonol. 1989;6(1):2–7.
77. Bhutani VK, Abbasi S. Relative likelihood of bronchopulmonary dysplasia based on pulmonary mechanics measured in preterm neonates during the first week of life. J Pediatr. 1992;120(4 Pt 1):605–13.
78. Gerhardt T, Hehre D, Feller R, Reifenberg L, Bancalari E. Serial determination of pulmonary function in infants with chronic lung disease. J Pediatr. 1987;110(3):448–56.
79. Morray JP, Fox WW, Kettrick RG, Downes JJ. Improvement in lung mechanics as a function of age in the infant with severe bronchopulmonary dysplasia. Pediatr Res. 1982;16(4 Pt 1):290–4.
80. Kao LC, Durand DJ, Phillips BL, Nickerson BG. Oral theophylline and diuretics improve pulmonary mechanics in infants with bronchopulmonary dysplasia. J Pediatr. 1987;111(3):439–44.
81. Kao LC, Durand DJ, Nickerson BG. Effects of inhaled metaproterenol and atropine on the pulmonary mechanics of infants with bronchopulmonary dysplasia. Pediatr Pulmonol. 1989;6(2):74–80.
82. Wilkie RA, Bryan MH. Effect of bronchodilators on airway resistance in ventilator-dependent neonates with chronic lung disease. J Pediatr. 1987;111(2):278–82.
83. Arad I, Bar-Yishay E, Eyal F, Gross S, Godfrey S. Lung function in infancy and childhood following neonatal intensive care. Pediatr Pulmonol. 1987;3(1):29–33.
84. Panitch HB, Allen JL, Alpert BE, Schidlow DV. Effects of CPAP on lung mechanics in infants with acquired tracheobronchomalacia. Am J Respir Crit Care Med. 1994;150(5 Pt 1):1341–6.
85. Motoyama EK, Fort MD, Klesh KW, Mutich RL, Guthrie RD. Early onset of airway reactivity in premature infants with bronchopulmonary dysplasia. Am Rev Respir Dis. 1987;136(1):50–7.

86. Mallory Jr GB, Chaney H, Mutich RL, Motoyama EK. Longitudinal changes in lung function during the first three years of premature infants with moderate to severe bronchopulmonary dysplasia. Pediatr Pulmonol. 1991;11(1):8–14.
87. Baraldi E, Bonetto G, Zacchello F, Filippone M. Low exhaled nitric oxide in school-age children with bronchopulmonary dysplasia and airflow limitation. Am J Respir Crit Care Med. 2005;171(1):68–72.
88. Lum S, Kirkby J, Welsh L, Marlow N, Hennessy E, Stocks J. Nature and severity of lung function abnormalities in extremely pre-term children at 11 years of age. Eur Respir J. 2011;37(5): 1199–207.
89. Denjean A, Guimaraes H, Migdal M, Miramand JL, Dehan M, Gaultier C. Dose-related bronchodilator response to aerosolized salbutamol (albuterol) in ventilator-dependent premature infants. J Pediatr. 1992;120(6):974–9.
90. Cabal LA, Larrazabal C, Ramanathan R, Durand M, Lewis D, Siassi B, et al. Effects of metaproterenol on pulmonary mechanics, oxygenation, and ventilation in infants with chronic lung disease. J Pediatr. 1987;110(1):116–9.
91. Gomez-Del Rio M, Gerhardt T, Hehre D, Feller R, Bancalari E. Effect of a beta-agonist nebulization on lung function in neonates with increased pulmonary resistance. Pediatr Pulmonol. 1986;2(5):287–91.
92. Kao LC, Warburton D, Platzker AC, Keens TG. Effect of isoproterenol inhalation on airway resistance in chronic bronchopulmonary dysplasia. Pediatrics. 1984;73(4):509–14.
93. Sosulski R, Abbasi S, Bhutani VK, Fox WW. Physiologic effects of terbutaline on pulmonary function of infants with bronchopulmonary dysplasia. Pediatr Pulmonol. 1986;2(5):269–73.
94. Walner DL, Ouanounou S, Donnelly LF, Cotton RT. Utility of radiographs in the evaluation of pediatric upper airway obstruction. Ann Otol Rhinol Laryngol. 1999;108(4):378–83.
95. Tan JZ, Ditchfield M, Freezer N. Tracheobronchomalacia in children: review of diagnosis and definition. Pediatr Radiol. 2012;42(8):906–15; quiz 1027–8.
96. Sanchez MO, Greer MC, Masters IB, Chang AB. A comparison of fluoroscopic airway screening with flexible bronchoscopy for diagnosing tracheomalacia. Pediatr Pulmonol. 2012;47(1):63–7.
97. Malhotra A, Armstrong D, Ditchfield M. Evolution of acquired tracheobronchomalacia in an infant studied by multidetector computed tomography. Pediatr Pulmonol. 2013;48(7):728–30.
98. Tan JZ, Crossett M, Ditchfield M. Dynamic volumetric computed tomographic assessment of the young paediatric airway: Initial experience of rapid, non-invasive, four-dimensional technique. J Med Imaging Radiat Oncol. 2013;57(2):141–8.
99. Suto Y, Sugihara S, Yoshida K, et al. Dynamic study of tracheal cavity by fast MRI with coughing in patients with trache- omalacia. Yonaga Acta Med. 1996;39:183–7.
100. Maeda K, Ono S, Baba K. Management of laryngotracheal stenosis in infants and children: the role of re-do surgery in cases of severe subglottic stenosis. Pediatr Surg Int. 2013;29(10):1001–6.
101. Bajaj Y, Cochrane LA, Jephson CG, Wyatt ME, Bailey CM, Albert DM, et al. Laryngotracheal reconstruction and cricotracheal resection in children: recent experience at Great Ormond Street Hospital. Int J Pediatr Otorhinolaryngol. 2012;76(4):507–11.
102. Network SSGotEKSNNR, Finer NN, Carlo WA, Walsh MC, Rich W, Gantz MG, et al. Early CPAP versus surfactant in extremely preterm infants. N Engl J Med. 2010;362(21):1970–9.
103. Morley CJ, Davis PG, Doyle LW, Brion LP, Hascoet JM, Carlin JB, et al. Nasal CPAP or intubation at birth for very preterm infants. N Engl J Med. 2008;358(7):700–8.
104. Kirpalani H, Millar D, Lemyre B, Yoder BA, Chiu A, Roberts RS, et al. A trial comparing noninvasive ventilation strategies in preterm infants. N Engl J Med. 2013;369(7):611–20.
105. Kumar P, Denson SE, Mancuso TJ, Committee on F, Newborn SoA, Pain M. Premedication for nonemergency endotracheal intubation in the neonate. Pediatrics. 2010;125(3):608–15.
106. Greenholz SK, Hall RJ, Lilly JR, Shikes RH. Surgical implications of bronchopulmonary dysplasia. J Pediatr Surg. 1987; 22(12):1132–6.
107. Mandy G, Malkar M, Welty SE, Brown R, Shepherd E, Gardner W, et al. Tracheostomy placement in infants with bronchopulmonary dysplasia: safety and outcomes. Pediatr Pulmonol. 2013;48(3):245–9.
108. Overman AE, Liu M, Kurachek SC, Shreve MR, Maynard RC, Mammel MC, et al. Tracheostomy for infants requiring prolonged mechanical ventilation: 10 years' experience. Pediatrics. 2013; 131(5):e1491–6.
109. DeMauro SB, D'Agostino JA, Bann C, Bernbaum J, Gerdes M, Bell EF, et al. Developmental outcomes of very preterm infants with tracheostomies. J Pediatr. 2014;164(6):1303–10.e2.
110. Fawke J, Lum S, Kirkby J, Hennessy E, Marlow N, Rowell V, et al. Lung function and respiratory symptoms at 11 years in children born extremely preterm: the EPICure study. Am J Respir Crit Care Med. 2010;182(2):237–45.
111. Fakhoury KF, Sellers C, Smith EO, Rama JA, Fan LL. Serial measurements of lung function in a cohort of young children with bronchopulmonary dysplasia. Pediatrics. 2010;125(6):e1441–7.
112. Sheikh S, Goldsmith LJ, Eid N. Oral-steroid sparing effect of inhaled fluticasone propionate in children with steroid-dependent asthma. Paediatr Child Health. 2000;5(3):156–60.
113. Allen DB. Growth suppression by glucocorticoid therapy. Endocrinol Metab Clin North Am. 1996;25(3):699–717.
114. Onland W, Offringa M, van Kaam A. Late (>/=7 days) inhalation corticosteroids to reduce bronchopulmonary dysplasia in preterm infants. Cochrane Database Syst Rev. 2012;(4):CD002311.
115. Shah V, Ohlsson A, Halliday HL, Dunn MS. Early administration of inhaled corticosteroids for preventing chronic lung disease in ventilated very low birth weight preterm neonates. Cochrane Database Syst Rev. 2000;(2):CD001969.
116. Johnson M. Interactions between corticosteroids and beta2-agonists in asthma and chronic obstructive pulmonary disease. Proc Am Thorac Soc. 2004;1(3):200–6.
117. Wheeler D, Spaeth J, Mehta R, Hariprakash S, Cox P. Assesment and management of pediatric airway. In: Wheeler D, Wong H, Shanley T. (eds.). Resuscitation and Stabilization of the Critically Ill Child. 2009. Springer 2009.

Tracheostomy for the Neonate and Infant: Indications, Complications, Timing, and Outcomes

Sara B. DeMauro, Henry Akinbi, and Kathryn Maschhoff

Introduction

Decisions about tracheostomy in neonates and young infants involve careful consideration of a number of factors, including mortality, potential short- and long-term morbidities, prospects for home ventilation therapy, alternatives to tracheostomy, and the impact of tracheostomy and home ventilation on the family. This chapter reviews indications for tracheostomy, complications, mortality, functional and developmental outcomes after infant tracheostomy, and incidence and timing of decannulation, all of which should influence decisions about whether and when neonatal tracheostomy is performed.

Indications for Tracheostomy in the First Year of Life

Among all tracheostomies placed in children, at least a third and perhaps more than half are performed in infants less than 1 year of age (Fig. 1) [1–3]. The indications for tracheostomy vary by age group and are quite different in neonates compared to older children or adults [4–6]. In the immediate neonatal period, congenital anomalies associated with airway obstruction are the most common indications. Airway malfunction or obstruction leading to requirement for tracheostomy can result from anatomic or physiologic occlusion at any level of the airway (Table 1). Obstruction of the nasal passages could result from choanal atresia, piriform aperture stenosis, and rarely from tumors such as glioma, encephalocele, teratoma, or dermoid. These usually manifest as respiratory distress immediately after delivery and can often be relieved with the use of an oral airway. Other life-threatening causes of airway obstruction in the immediate postnatal period include cervical teratomas and lymphatic malformations. Another rare cause of airway obstruction in the neonate is congenital high airway obstruction syndrome (CHAOS.) CHAOS results from laryngeal or tracheal obstruction, which can be due to tracheal or laryngeal atresia, or obstruction due to a laryngeal cyst or intraluminal web (Fig. 2a). Regardless of the cause of the obstruction, common features include distension of the tracheal bronchial tree by fetal lung fluid that is not able to leave the trachea, and enlarged, echogenic lungs [7]. Because of the possibility of complete airway obstruction, fetuses diagnosed in utero with CHAOS require ex-utero intrapartum treatment (EXIT) at delivery to secure the airway [8].

Vocal cord paralysis may occur secondary to central nervous system abnormalities including Arnold-Chiari malformation, cerebral palsy, hydrocephalus, myelomeningocele, spina bifida, or hypoxia (Fig. 2c). In contrast to anatomic airway obstruction, laryngomalacia may not present until the second week of age or beyond (Fig. 3).

Airway and lung diseases that arise as sequelae of postnatal therapies tend to account for most of the tracheostomies in older infants. The specific indications for tracheostomy placement in preterm infants have evolved as modalities for respiratory support for early preterm infants have changed over the years. Such new interventions and new approaches include less invasive respiratory support (continuous positive airway pressure (CPAP), high-flow nasal cannula), increased use of steroids (both systemic and inhaled) in the peri-extubation period and lung-protective ventilation strategies, such as permissive hypercarbia [9]. These newer therapies and changes in neonatal practice have resulted in decreased prevalence of iatrogenic laryngeal tracheal stenosis (LTS), which was long the most common indication for tracheostomy placement in the preterm population [10–13] (Fig. 2b). Today, the most common

S.B. DeMauro, M.D., M.S.C.E. (✉) K. Maschhoff, M.D., Ph.D.
Division of Neonatology, The Children's Hospital of Philadelphia, Philadelphia, PA, USA

The University of Pennsylvania Perelman School of Medicine, Philadelphia, PA, USA
e-mail: demauro@email.chop.edu

H. Akinbi, M.D.
Division of Neonatology, Cincinnati Children's Hospital Medical Center, University of Cincinnati School of Medicine, Cincinnati, OH, USA

J. Lioy and S.E. Sobol (eds.), *Disorders of the Neonatal Airway: Fundamentals for Practice*,
DOI 10.1007/978-1-4939-1610-8_25, © Springer Science+Business Media New York 2015

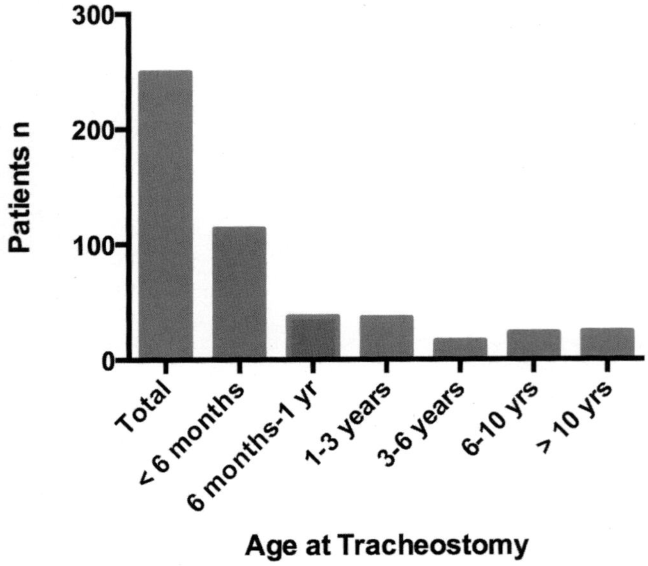

Fig. 1 Age at which tracheostomy was performed. Stratification by age group. Reprinted from Perez-Ruiz et al. [3]. Copyright 2012. with permission from the European Respiratory Society.

indication for tracheostomy in preterm infants is prolonged ventilation secondary to bronchopulmonary dysplasia, rather than pure airway disease [4, 14, 15] (Fig. 4). Murthy et al. report a study of over 5,500 infants born before 32 weeks gestation who were referred to regional NICUs [16]. Eight hundred and ninety eight of these infants were diagnosed with severe bronchopulmonary dysplasia (sBPD), defined as receiving more than 30 % oxygen with a flow rate more than 2 L per minute or positive-pressure ventilation at greater than 36 weeks post menstrual age. Of the infants with sBPD, 107 (12 %) infants received a tracheostomy to facilitate long-term ventilatory support. The median time from referral to tracheostomy was 52 days. Analysis of this large cohort of preterm infants has provided some insight into risk factors for requirement of tracheostomy (or for the competing outcome of death) in these infants. Surprisingly, infants with sBPD who were born at a later gestational age were more likely to die or require a tracheostomy. Thus, while infants born at a later gestational age are less likely to develop sBPD, those that do have a worse

Table 1 Indications for Tracheostomy

Indication	Examples
Structural anomalies	*Anomalies of the Nasal Passages*
	Congenital arhinia
	Severe nasal deformity
	Epignathus
	Encephalocoele
	Pharynx/Larynx
	Pharyngeal cyst
	Subglottic stenosis
	Laryngeal atresia
	Laryngeal cleft
	Laryngotracheal hemangiomas or papillomas
	Bilateral vocal cord paralysis
	Trachea
	Tracheomalacia
	Tracheal stenosis
	Tracheal atresia
	Craniofacial anomalies
	Head or neck mass obstructing the upper airway (e.g., giant cervical teratomas with airway obstruction)
	Pierre-Robin sequence/retrognathia/micrognathia
Medical Problems	Laryngotracheal stenosis from prolonged intubation
	Bronchopulmonary dysplasia
	Need for prolonged continuous positive airway pressure (CPAP)
	Chronic aspiration syndrome
	Seizures with airway complications
	Spastic quadriplegic cerebral palsy
	Osteogenesis imperfecta
	Chiari II malformation
	Diaphragmatic paralysis
	Neuromuscular diseases, e.g., Spinal Muscular Atrophy type 1
Medical support following other treatment	Post cardiac surgery
	Other congenital anomalies associated with difficulty with airway toileting, giant omphalocele with pulmonary hypoplasia, congenital diaphragmatic hernia, other congenital lung malformations

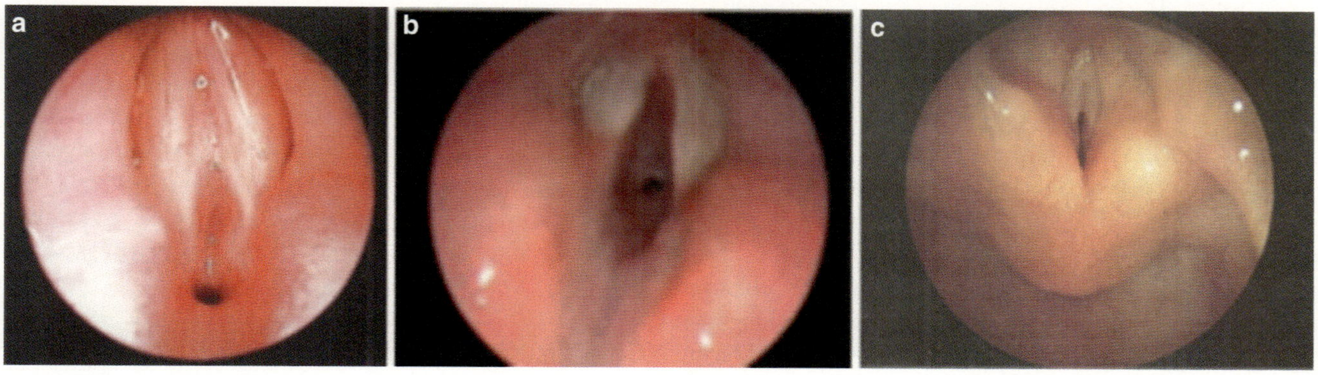

Fig. 2 Examples of airway anomalies necessitating tracheostomy. (**a**) near-complete glottic web. (**b**) laryngotracheal (subglottic) stenosis, (**c**) bilateral vocal cord paralysis. (Courtesy of Steve Sobol, The Children's Hospital of Philadelphia (CHOP), Neonatal Airway Program)

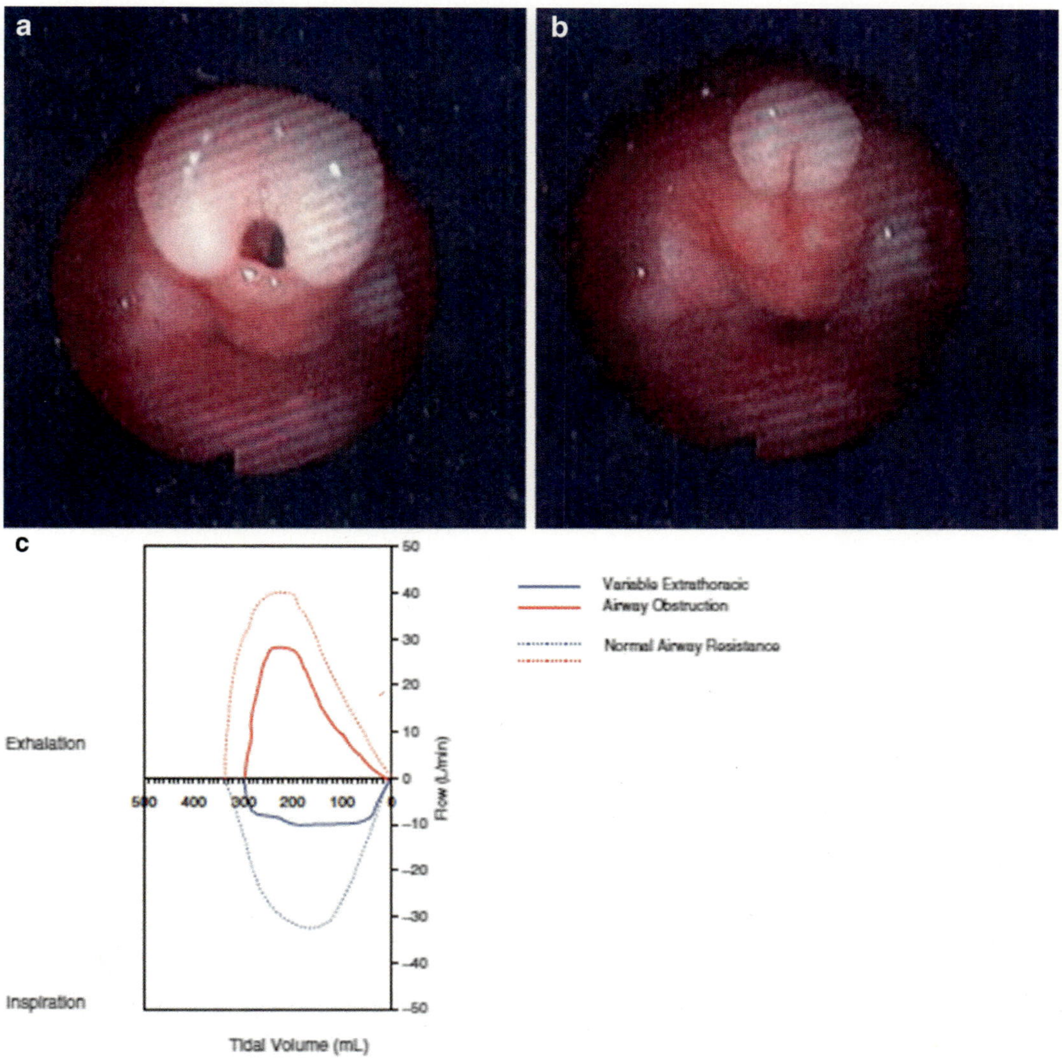

Fig. 3 Endoscopic appearance of the larynx in a patient with dynamic airway compression secondary to laryngomalacia. (**a**) Severe laryngomalacia during expiration. (**b**) Same patient during inspiration with total collapse of the airway. (**c**) Flow-volume loops further demonstrating evidence of worsening extra-thoracic airway obstruction during inspiration (Reprinted from Shanley et al. [66]. Copyright 2014 with permission from Springer)

prognosis. Other risk factors include being born small for gestational age or having sBPD complicated by pulmonary hypertension and cor pulmonale. Pulmonary vascular disease leading to pulmonary hypertension is a life-threatening complication of sBPD that often contributes to the need for prolonged ventilation in preterm infants. Because of improvements in neonatal care leading to improved survival of very preterm infants, and advances in the surgical management of congenital and iatrogenic airway disorders, the need for prolonged ventilatory support for BPD is likely to remain an important indication for tracheostomy in the first year of life (Fig. 5a, b).

Below are a variety of CT angiography (CTA) images showing the extensive different types of lung damage seen in premature infants who remain ventilator dependent. One can see both atelectasis and hyperinflation with cystic formation in the same lung.

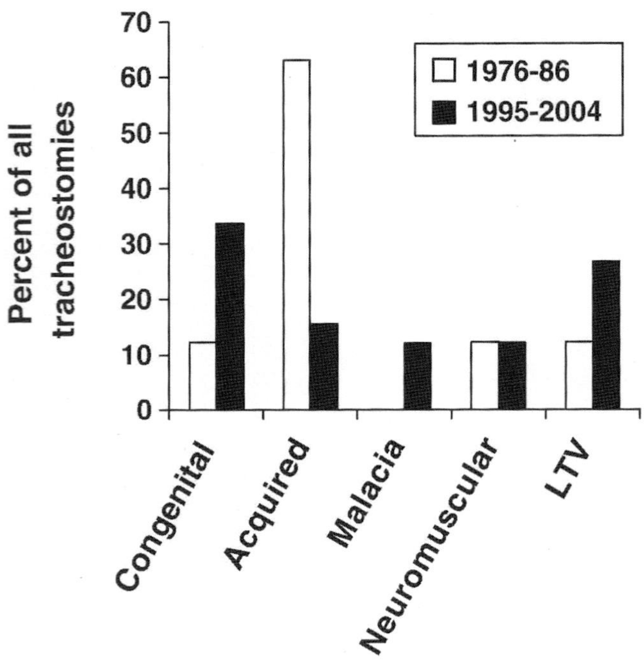

Fig. 4 Changes in indications for tracheostomy over time. From Corbett et al [65] Copyright 2007 with permission from Elsevier

Also, evidence of pulmonary hypertension and airway disease can be seen simultaneously on the same image (Fig. 5c–m).

In addition to BPD, other chronic medical conditions, including congenital heart disease or neuromuscular disorders such as spinal muscular atrophy (SMA), congenital giant omphalocele, congenital diaphragmatic hernia and congenital cystic adenomatous malformation all can result in a need for long-term ventilation via tracheostomy (Table 1).

Complications of Tracheostomy

While tracheostomy-related deaths are uncommon, complications of tracheostomy are not infrequent. (Table 2). In studies where complication rates are reported, the rates of tracheostomy complications in infants less than 1 year of age ranged from 29 to 77 % [14, 17–21]. Most studies show an increased incidence of complications in younger, smaller patients. Complications can be classified by timing: intraoperative; early (usually defined as the first postoperative week); late; and post-decannulation. Intraoperative complications are rare, and range from desaturations to cardiopulmonary arrest. Complications in the first post-tracheostomy week include bleeding, cannula obstruction or mucous plugging, stomal erosion, and infection or cellulitis at the tracheostomy site. Accidental decannulation can occur as well, and has the potential to result in malposition of the cannula outside the trachea or creating of a tracheal false passage. Air leak, including pneumothorax, pneumomediastinum, and subcutaneous emphysema have been reported.

Overall, granulation tissue in the trachea or at the stoma site is the most common complication of tracheostomy. Tracheal wall granulomas occur in 4–80 % of pediatric tracheostomies [22]. Granulomas are frequently found at the superior margin of the tracheostomy tube due to irritation and inflammation of the tracheal mucosa by the cannula (Figs. 6 and 7). Granulomas may also be found at the distal tip of the tracheostomy tube, usually caused by malposition of the tube or by irritation from traumatic suctioning. Small

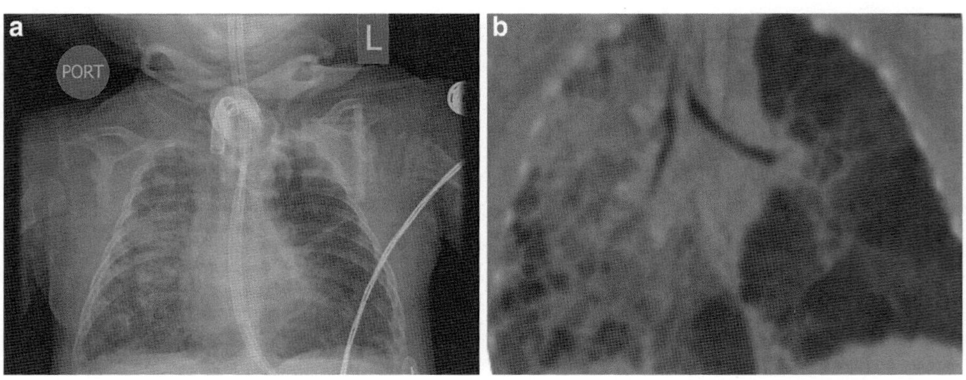

Fig. 5 Infant with severe BPD. (**a**) Plain chest radiograph. (**b**) CT angiogram showing severe cystic changes (Courtesy of, (CHOP), Chronic Lung Disease program

Table 2 Complications of tracheostomy

Timing	Complication
Intraoperative	Cardiopulmonary arrest
	Posterior tracheal wall tear
Early	Hemorrhage
	Mucous plugging
	Infection
	Accidental decannulation
	Pneumothorax
	Subcutaneous emphysema
	Tracheostomy malposition/false passage
Late	Granulation tissue at stoma
	Tracheal granulomas
	Mucous plugging
	Accidental decannulation
	Stoma infection
	Tracheitis
	Hemorrhage
	Suprastomal collapse
	Subglottic stenosis
	Tracheomalacia
	Tracheoinnominate artery fistula
Post-decannulation	Tracheocutaneous fistula
	Hypertrophic scar
	Recurrent stridor
	Granulation tissue

to moderately sized asymptomatic granulomas can be managed expectantly, while large or symptomatic granulomas usually need to be excised. Pressure placed on the tracheal rings by the tracheostomy tube can cause chondritis, inflammation, and deterioration of the cartilage, resulting in suprastomal collapse. (Figs. 7c and 8). The collapse is usually moderate and does not need treatment prior to decannulation. When severe, treatment may be needed before successful decannulation can be achieved.

As discussed above, Laryngotracheal stenosis (LTS) is a common indication for tracheostomy, particularly in preterm infants who have undergone prolonged endotracheal intubation. LTS can also be caused by irritation of the laryngotracheal tissues by the tracheostomy cannula. Whether it is an indication for or the result of the tracheostomy, the presence of LTS often necessitates laryngotracheal reconstruction (LTR) prior to decannulatio.

Similarly, Tracheomalacia, the result of a deficiency of support by cartilage rings, often contributes to the need for tracheostomy in infants (Fig. 9). Long-term tracheostomy can also result in tracheomalacia. There is currently no definitive treatment for tracheomalacia in infants and young children. If severe enough to prevent successful decannulation, the presence of this complication may therefore result in the need for prolonged tracheostomy.

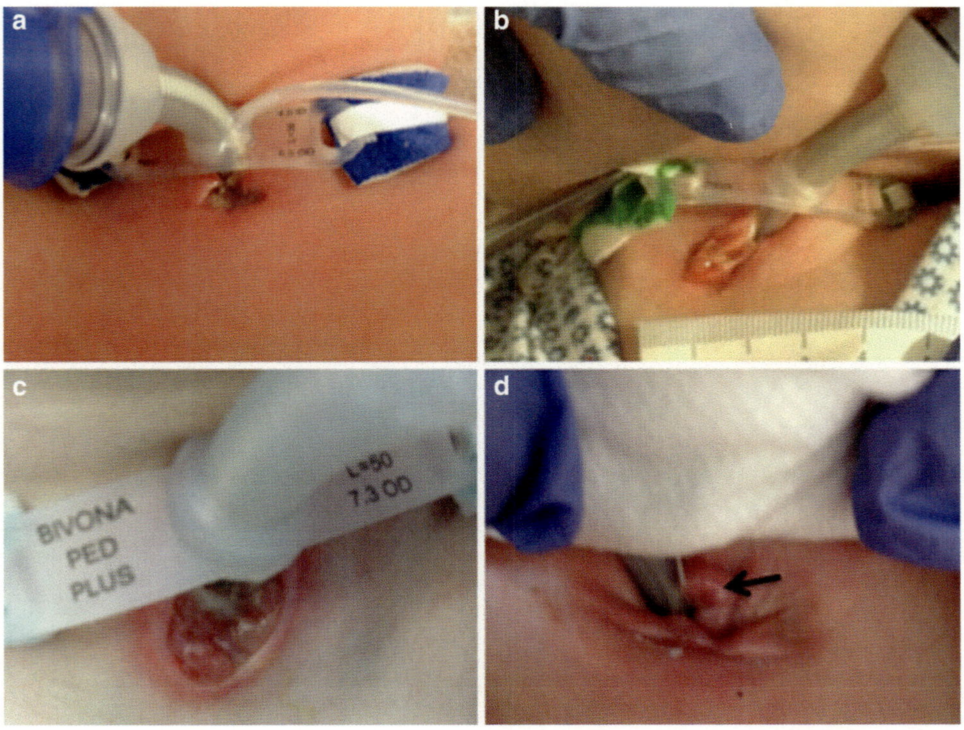

Fig. 6 Tracheostomy stomas. (**a**) Normally healing stoma. (**b**) Stomal breakdown. (**c**) Severe stomal breakdown due to excess secretions. (**d**) Stomal granuloma. (Courtesy of Steve Sobol, (CHOP), Neonatal Airway Program)

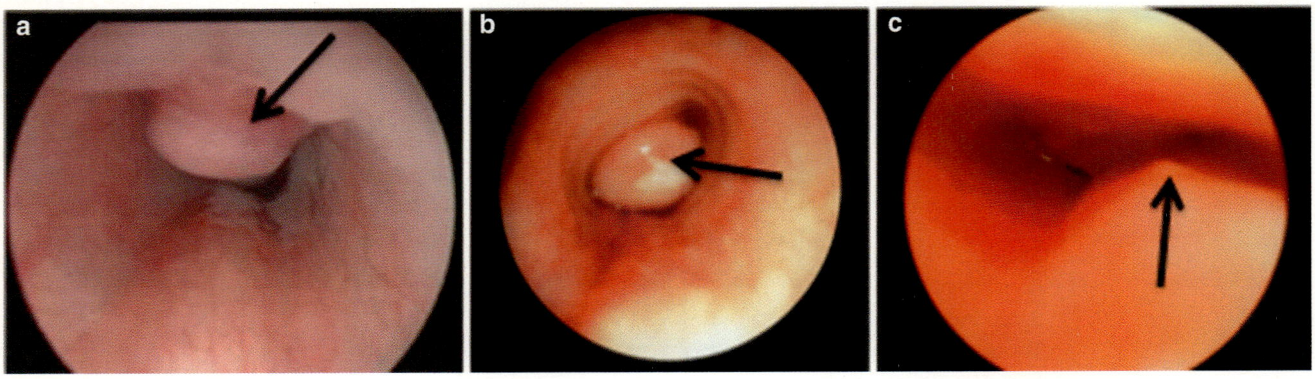

Fig. 7 Suprastomal collapse and granuloma (Courtesy of Michael Rutter, Department of Otolaryngology, Children's Hospital Medical Center, Cincinnati, OH)

Fig. 8 Airway complications. (**a**) suprastomal granuloma (*black arrow*). (**b**) Subglottic granulomas (*black arrow*). (**c**) Suprastomal collapse (*black arrow*). (Reprinted from Zur et al. [63]. Pediatric Otolaryngology: The Requisites in Pediatrics, (Wetmore ed). Copyright 2007 with permission of Elsevier

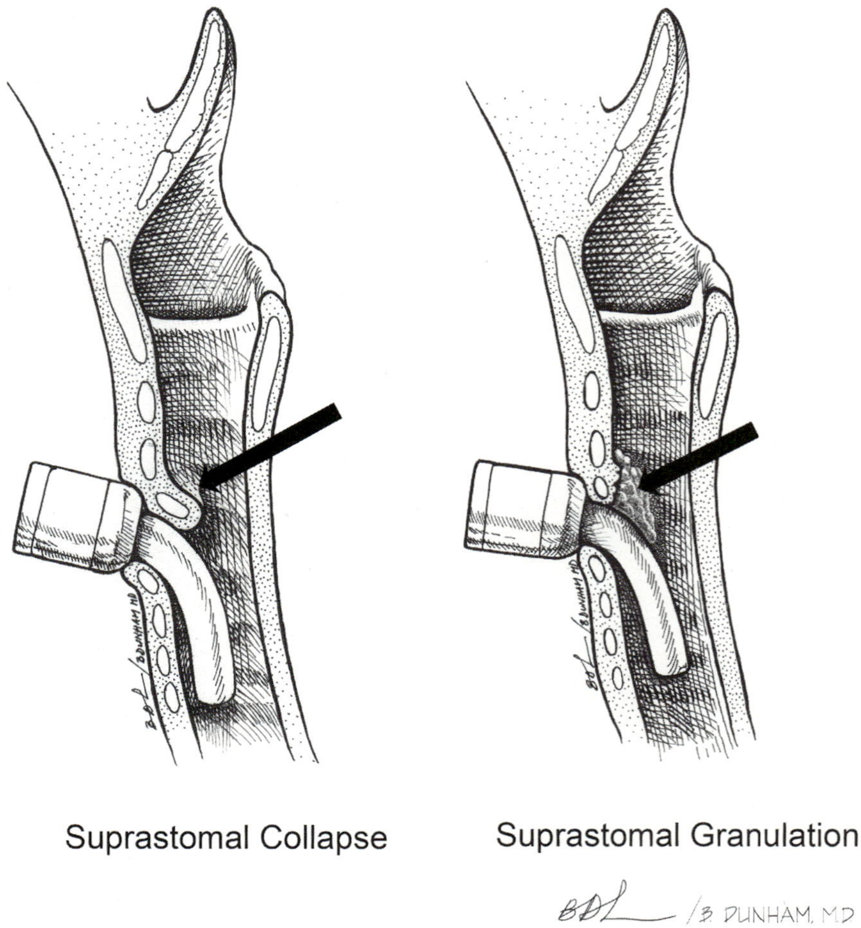

Tracheostomy can be complicated by infection, either at the stomal site or in the trachea (Fig. 10). Stomal site infection represents a localized skin infection and is treated as cellulitis. A tracheostomy tube bypasses the normal host defenses against infection found in the nose, mouth, and upper airway, leaving children with tracheostomies more susceptible to infection of the trachea with a variety of bacterial, fungal, and viral pathogens. Tracheitis can often be difficult to distinguish from microbial colonization that is universally seen in children with long-standing artificial airways. The diagnosis depends on combining signs of clinical illness or respiratory deterioration with evidence of inflammation and identification of a pathogen.

Although tracheostomy-related deaths are less common than once thought, cannula occlusion by mucous plugs, accidental decannulation, malpositioning of cannulas into false

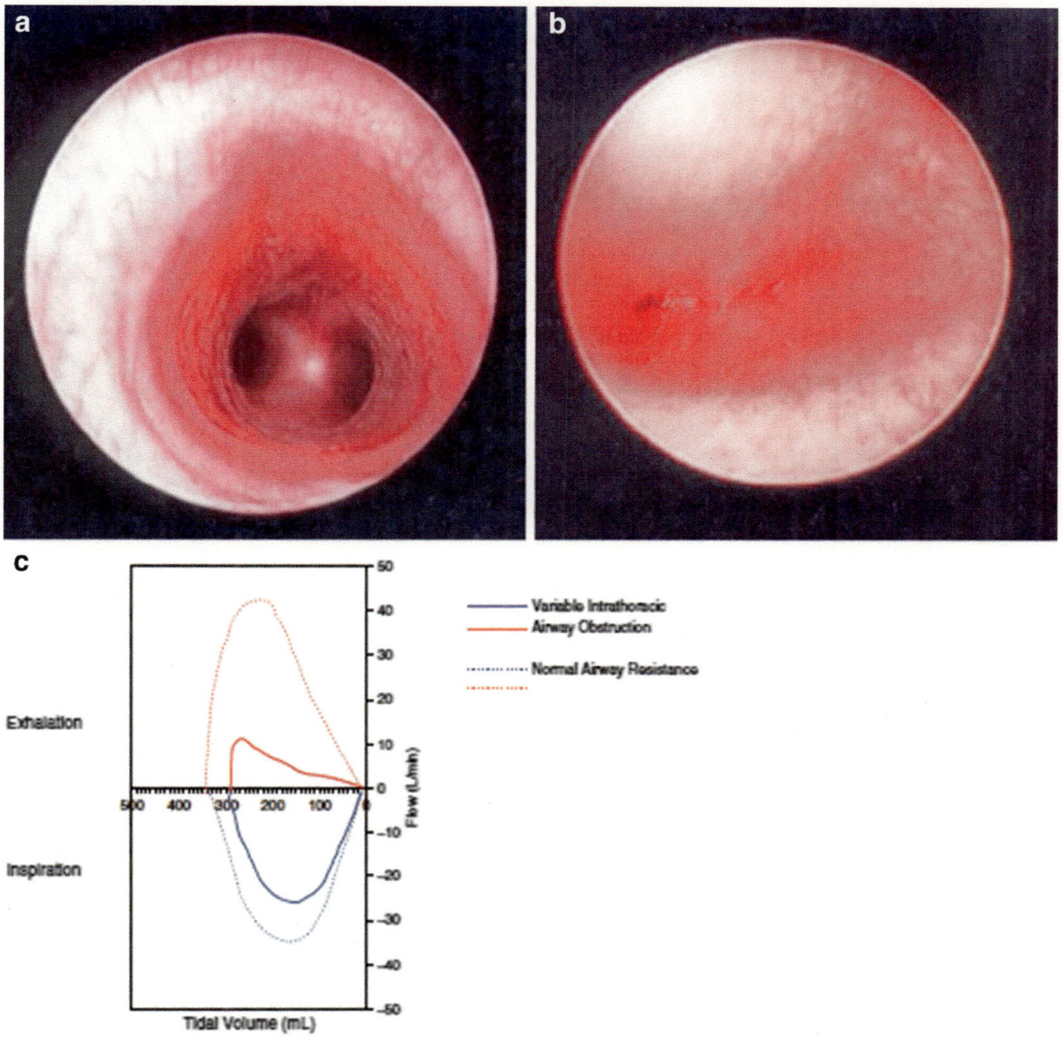

Fig. 9 Endoscopic appearance of the trachea in a patient with dynamic airway compression secondary to tracheomalacia. (**a**) Normal trachea. (**b**) Child with severe tracheomalacia demonstrating total collapse of the airway during inspiration. (**c**) Flow-volume loops further demonstrating evidence of worsening intrathoracic airway obstruction during expiration (Reprinted from Shanley et al. [66]. Copyright 2014 with permission from Springer)

passages, and less commonly, ventilator failures can result in morbidity and mortality, particularly after discharge. Prevention of these unexpected events depends on careful attention to discharge planning and caregiver education, assessment of the home environment and needed support structures, and proper equipment.

After decannulation, the tracheostomy site is routinely left to heal by secondary intent. This process can result in hypertrophic or depressed scars, at times necessitating tracheal scar revision. Perhaps the most common complication seen after decannulation is a persistent tracheocutaneous fistula (TCF), which is essentially a failure of the stoma to close (Fig. 11). Persistent TCF occurs in up to 50 % of patients after decannulation [14, 20, 23, 24]. The risk of TCF is inversely correlated with the age at cannulation and increases with the duration of cannulation. It is common practice to observe a TCF for 6–12 months before closing it surgically [25].

Timing of Tracheostomy

Very little research is available to guide decisions about the timing of tracheostomy placement in the neonate or infant. Existing data are universally retrospective and therefore reflect variations in surgical attitudes, rather than experimental approaches to determining best practice. There is a recent movement toward earlier tracheostomy in adult critical care. This is supported by data linking earlier tracheostomy (typically at 3–10 days) with improved outcomes including shorter durations of mechanical ventilation, intensive care, and hospitalization, and lower costs [26–28]. However, a 2012 Cochrane systematic review of randomized trials on this subject concludes that there is not sufficient evidence to support a decrease in mortality after early tracheostomy [29] Though the adult data are not conclusive, some authors are

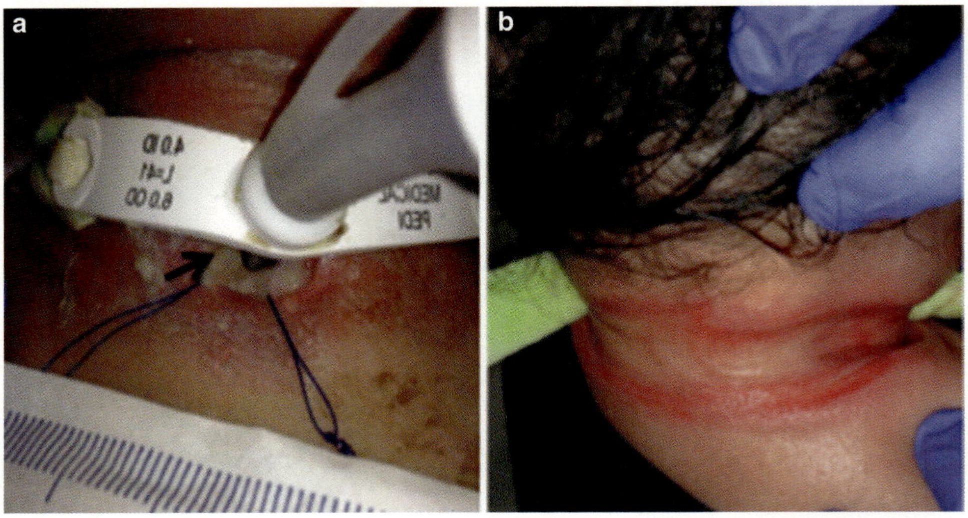

Fig. 10 Tracheostomy-associated infections. (**a**) stoma infection (*black arrow*). Surrounding erythema represents cellulitis. (**b**) Breakdown on the neck from tracheostomy ties. (Courtesy of Steve Sobol, CHOP Neonatal Airway Program)

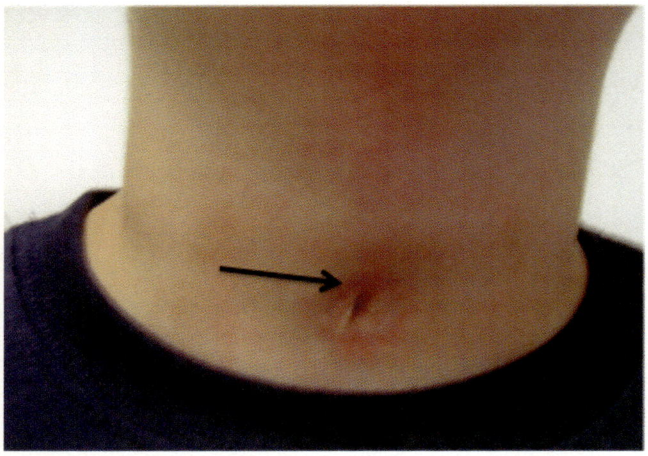

Fig. 11 Tracheocutaneous fistula (*black arrow*). (Courtesy of Steve Sobol, CHOP Neonatal Airway Program)

beginning to suggest that children or even infants might also benefit from earlier tracheostomy [5, 30, 31].

Two single-center studies have evaluated the relationship between timing of tracheostomy and outcomes. The first included 43 infants born before 36 weeks postmenstrual age (mean gestational age 27.9 weeks) [32]. The mean age at tracheostomy placement was 21.4 weeks, and the more preterm infants were more likely to be cannulated later in life. However, timing of cannulation did not correlate with successful weaning from mechanical ventilation, decannulation, or the timing of these events. The second included 127 infants with mean gestational age of 28 weeks [33]. Mean age at tracheostomy was similar at 45 weeks postmenstrual age. Twenty-one percent of the infants died and, after adjustment for gestational age and respiratory support, mortality was unrelated to the timing of tracheostomy. A large, multicenter study from the NICHD Neonatal Research Network reported the outcomes of 304 preterm infants (<30 weeks gestation) who underwent tracheostomy placement and were followed until 18–22 months of age. The study reported that the adjusted odds of death or developmental impairment at 18–22 months were significantly lower (adjusted odds ratio 0.5, 95 % CI 0.3–0.9) among infants who underwent tracheostomy before 120 days of life, as compared to those who underwent tracheostomy after 120 days of life. The authors were unable to report indication for tracheostomy, so it is possible that the patients who underwent later tracheostomy were a population with unmeasured risk factors for adverse outcome. Alternately, it is also possible that there is a developmental advantage to earlier tracheostomy in preterm infants [34].

Many factors other than postnatal age must be considered when determining the appropriate timing of tracheostomy. Sometimes the diagnosis or indication dictates the timing of tracheostomy. For instance, some anatomic anomalies (e.g., tracheal stenosis) cannot be managed without tracheostomy and the procedure must be performed urgently. However, in the majority of cases, the decision is less clear-cut. Some authors have suggested that infants, particularly preterm infants with chronic lung disease, undergo tracheostomy placement after a certain number of failed attempts at extubation. Sisk reported in 2006 that the median number of intubation events among a group ($n=18$) of very low-birth weight infants who eventually underwent tracheostomy was 11.5 (range 7–25) [14]. Pereira et al. reported an average of 5.2 failed extubations among tracheostomized infants with birth weight <1 kg and 3.2 failed extubations among infants with birth weight >1 kg [4]. The same author concluded in another report that "infants with gestational ages of 30 weeks and below, those with low-birth weights and chronic lung disease are unlikely to benefit from more than three trials of extubation despite minimal ventilatory requirements at that time"[35]. On the other hand, among infants who underwent tracheostomy after repair or palliation of congenital heart disease, numbers of extubations prior to tracheostomy ranged from 0 attempts in those who could not wean from mechanical ventilation to more than three attempts [36]. Finally, while (as discussed above) complications of tracheostomy are more common among smaller and younger infants, it remains unclear whether complication rates differ significantly when tracheostomy is performed at different times within the first year of life. At a minimum, recent data suggest that for preterm infants, later tracheostomy (beyond 16 or 20 weeks of age) is not associated with increased need for tracheal reconstruction [32]. This finding suggests that acquired subglottic stenosis is not more common when the procedure is delayed for a few months.

Why might infants benefit from earlier tracheostomy? One hypothesis is that earlier tracheostomy allows faster weaning of sedating medications and muscle relaxants and earlier institution of developmentally appropriate activities [32, 34]. Early developmental interventions improve cognitive outcomes and may improve motor outcomes for preterm infants [37]. With the more stable airway provided by the tracheostomy, infants who have suffered prolonged intubation can often begin to sit in chairs and swings, lay prone, and participate more actively in interactions with parents and caregivers. However, more studies are needed to confirm that earlier tracheostomy is the safest option for infants before this strategy could be recommended to practitioners.

Survival and Decannulation After Neonatal Tracheostomy

Historically, there has been a perception that tracheostomy in infants resulted in increased risk of death. Indeed, in reports of tracheostomy in infants less than 1 year of age, published mortality rates range from 6 to 35 %. However, more recent data indicate that survival rates after neonatal tracheostomy may be improving over time. For example, in 1989, Singer reported 29 % mortality in a population of 130 infants who underwent tracheostomy before 13 months of age [38]. In 2013, Overman reported 89 % 5-year survival of 165 infants with tracheostomies [5]. However, this report excluded infants with congenital heart disease, who constitute an important segment of the population with particularly high mortality. More recently, DeMauro reported 92 % survival to 18–22 months among 304 preterm infants who survived to 36 weeks and then underwent tracheostomy placement [34]. More detailed evaluation of the changing survival rates over time is hindered by the inclusion of *all* children, rather than just neonates and infants, in many reports, or only subgroups of infants in other reports. All cause mortality in a population

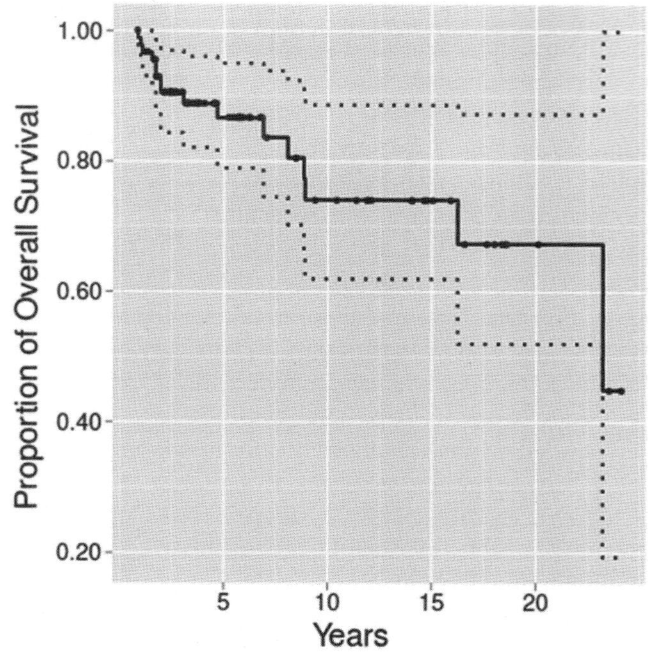

Fig. 12 Survival analysis of children treated with tracheostomy and positive-pressure ventilation at home: unadjusted Kaplan-Meier plot shows time of death with 95 % confidence band. (Reprinted from Com et al. [34]. Copyright 2014 with permission from Sage)

of 91 children who were discharged with tracheostomies has been described over a 20-year period [39] (Fig. 12).

Survival rates after tracheostomy depend heavily on the initial indication for the tracheostomy, progression of underlying medical conditions and comorbidities. For instance, survival is higher for potentially reversible conditions such as airway obstruction and respiratory failure: survival for children with bronchopulmonary dysplasia (BPD) is about 80–90 %. On the other hand, mortality is higher among children with irreversible conditions such as progressive neurologic impairment, complex congenital heart disease, and genetic syndromes: survival for infants who undergo tracheostomy after surgery for complex congenital heart disease is 50–70 % [39–44]. One explanation for these widely disparate outcomes is that higher mortality rates in some subgroups are likely related to mortality from the underlying condition rather than differences in rates of "tracheostomy accidents" by subgroup [3, 39]. Certainly, both complication and mortality rates are also linked to the number of comorbid conditions present [45]. Unfortunately, cause of death after neonatal tracheostomy is rarely reported in the existing literature. When all infants and children with tracheostomies are considered, overall mortality is about 12–20 %; however, only about 10–25 % of these children die secondary to complications of the tracheostomy [3, 46].

One critical factor in the decision by neonatologists to pursue tracheostomy in an infant is to enhance the likelihood that the child will be able to wean off respiratory support and undergo decannulation. Decannulation is a nearly a universal goal of pediatric otolaryngologists and neonatologists, as well as the parents and caregivers of infants who may require tracheostomy. Indeed, many children who have undergone tracheostomy before one year of age are subsequently decannulated, with rates that range from 30 to 75 %. The average duration of tracheostomy in these children ranges from 22 to 48 months. However, decannulation rates, like survival, depend on the underlying indication for tracheostomy placement. Five-year decannulation rates for children younger than 18 years who were discharged with tracheostomies vary from 0 % for those with neuromuscular disorders or spinal cord injury to 79 % for children with BPD but no central nervous system abnormalities [32, 39]. In one single-center study, the average age of decannulation for preterm infants (<36 weeks gestation) with tracheostomies was 27.9 months [32]. However, these same infants had been weaned from mechanical ventilation at an average age of 17.8 months.

While children who undergo tracheostomy for airway obstruction are more likely to ultimately achieve decannulation, many first require an airway surgical procedure. The need for open laryngotracheal reconstruction (LTR) prior to decannulation ranges from 4 to nearly 50 % in recent surveys. Children with a birthweight less than 1,000 g, while more likely in some studies to achieve decannulation, are more likely to require LTR, likely because more of these infants have acquired subglottic stenosis [18]. Overall, the key to successful decannulation is correction or resolution of the pathology that necessitated tracheostomy placement. The chances of success can be further improved by careful attention to protection of the surgical airway and prevention of and infection.

Developmental Outcomes After Neonatal Tracheostomy

Like survival, neurodevelopmental outcomes are also closely linked to the underlying indication for tracheostomy and to comorbid conditions. The first report of developmental outcomes of children who underwent tracheostomy placement before 2 years of age stated that "the children that were of school age were withdrawn in character and of poor academic and recreational standard"[47]. Interestingly, nearly all of these children underwent tracheostomy after acute infections, making them substantially different from the children who undergo tracheostomy today. In the 1980s, Singer reported that at least 27 % of children who underwent tracheostomy before 13 months of age survived with mental retardation or neurological handicap [38]. Of those not considered to be severely handicapped, intelligence testing at early school age revealed mostly low-normal scores and over half had behavioral or social problems. A 2013 single-center series reported that 64 % of 165 children who underwent tracheostomy placement in infancy had "some degree of developmental delay" [5]. Because no definition of developmental delay was provided, the utility of these data in clinical decision-making is limited.

In the largest study on this topic, DeMauro et al. reported the 18–22 month developmental outcomes of over 300 preterm children who underwent tracheostomy and were seen for follow-up in the NICHD Neonatal Research Network between 2001 and 2011 [34]. This study demonstrated that 81 % of children with tracheostomies had deafness, blindness, neurologic impairment/cerebral palsy, or severe developmental delay at 18–22 months. Importantly, 45 % had neurologic impairment, defined as Gross Motor Function Classification Scale level 2 or higher or moderate to severe cerebral palsy [48]. When compared to their peers, infants with tracheostomies also had higher rates of both expressive and receptive language delays and children with tracheostomies had higher risk for delays in social-emotional competence as measured by the Brief Infant/ Toddler Social and Emotional Assessment (Fig. 13). However, the authors were unable to separate these outcomes based on the indication for tracheostomy. As discussed above, both mortality and decannulation rates are strongly related to indication for tracheostomy. It is highly likely that the same is true for developmental outcomes. Future research will need to focus on clarifying the mechanisms behind the adverse developmental outcomes seen in this population and understanding the relationship between the underlying pathology and the long-term outcomes of infants with tracheostomies.

Functional Outcomes Following Neonatal Tracheostomy

Effects on Speech and Language

Tracheostomy placement in the neonatal period or the first year of life results in the presence of the tracheostomy cannula during the prelinguistic stage of language development. Evaluation of these children during and after cannulation suggests that many, if not all, experience some problems with speech and language [49–52]. Evaluation of the effect of tracheostomy on speech and language is often confounded by difficulty distinguishing the effects of tracheostomy from the effects of underlying comorbidities such as underlying syndromic or neurologic conditions. Recent studies have confirmed the high prevalence of speech delay in children who have undergone tracheostomy during the first year of life, including children without underlying conditions that would impair speech development in the absence of tracheostomy. Many studies suggest that the presence of a tracheostomy in infancy can result in impaired expressive language in school-age

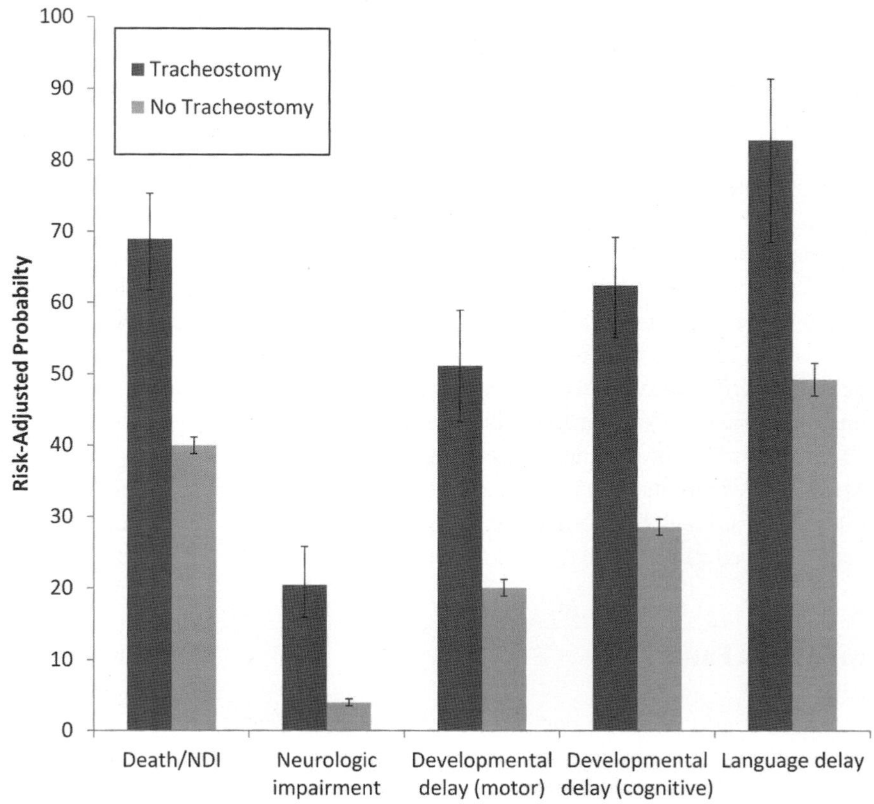

Fig. 13 Risk-adjusted probabilities of components of NDI and Bayley Scales of Infant Development (II or III), by tracheostomy. Error bars represent 95 % CIs for risk-adjusted probabilities. Language delay is defined as <85 (i.e., >1 SD below the expected mean score of 100, on the language scale of Bayley-III). Neurologic delay is defined as moderate to severe cerebral palsy with Gross Motor Function Classification Scale level of ≥2. Reprinted from DeMauro et al. [34]. Copyright 2014 with permission from Elsevier

children of normal intelligence. Possible reasons for these effects are varied. In addition to underlying pathology, long-term and frequent hospitalizations can contribute to speech delay. In addition, restriction of vocalization by the tracheostomy and the resultant loss of auditory and oral-motor feedback are thought to contribute. Speech pathologists have debated the importance of babbling for normal speech development, with some suggesting that this is a necessary step, while others show evidence that following decannulation, some children who underwent tracheostomy prior to babbling were able to begin vocalization shortly after removal of the tracheostomy [52].

Although some children remain aphonic for the duration of their tracheostomy, many do achieve some degree of vocalization with the tracheostomy tube in place, either in the course of normal breathing by moving air over the vocal cords around the tracheostomy tube or by plugging the tracheostomy during expiration. Some young children are able to tolerate expiratory speaking valves that direct air over the vocal cords, facilitating vocalization [53]. The ability to vocalize with a tracheostomy enhances communication between the child and caregivers, but even children who have opportunities to vocalize with a tracheostomy exhibit speech difficulties after decannulation. It is therefore crucial that evaluation and treatment by a speech therapist be part of care of these children during and after tracheostomy.

While expressive language development is affected more profoundly than receptive language, children with normal intelligence who have undergone tracheostomy as infants also exhibit receptive language delays. The etiology of the receptive delay is not clear, but may in some cases be due to decreased language stimulation by caregivers in the setting of an infant with no or decreased vocalization. Despite these concerns, by 5 years of age, many children who have had a tracheostomy as infants develop language skills commensurate with their nonverbal cognitive abilities [50].

Feeding and Swallowing

Similar to the effect on speech production, tracheostomy has been found to impair feeding and swallowing; in one study, up to 80 % of infants and toddlers with a tracheostomy exhibited some degree of dysphagia [54]. Problems were found in all three phases of swallowing: oral, pharyngeal, and esophageal. In patients with oral dysphagia, both oral-motor and oral-sensory problems were seen, with oral motor being more common. Pharyngeal phase disorders include delayed or absent swallow response, nasopharyngeal backflow, laryngeal penetration, and aspiration. The most common esophageal phase symptom is gastroesophageal reflux. The mechanism of pharyngeal dysphagia in this population is not entirely known. There has been speculation that anchoring of the larynx by the tracheostomy leads to reduced laryngeal elevation during swallowing. Other possible factors include decreased sensation of the larynx, resulting in decreased awareness of aspiration and impaired coordination of laryngeal closure. As with speech impairment, many infants with tracheostomies have underlying conditions, such as extreme prematurity, neurologic impairment, or craniofacial disorders, that place them at high risk for feeding and swallowing disorders independent of the presence of a tracheostomy tube. Feeding problems in infants with tracheostomies can have implications for long-term development of normal oral feeding skills. Difficulty with feeding can impair normal mealtime interaction and socialization, and cause increased stress for caregivers. The involvement of speech therapists that have experience with infants and toddlers with tracheostomy tubes is therefore critical for normal long-term development of feeding as well as speech in these children.

Impact on Family

One major consideration for both physicians and parents when contemplating tracheostomy is a concern for the impact tracheostomy will have on the family. Several recent studies have begun to address and quantify this concern, as well as to explore strategies for reducing the burden to caregivers of infants and children with tracheostomies [55, 56]. These studies suggest that tracheostomy does pose a significant burden to caregivers, and has a substantial impact on the quality of life. This burden increases with increasing severity of the child's illness. The imposed burdens can be physical, economic, psychological, and emotional in nature. Physical demands include increased home care responsibilities and disruption of sleep. Economic burdens result not only from the costs associated with medical care, supplies, and follow-up, but reflect decreased family income that results from diminished ability to work at a paying job. The physical and mental health status of adult caretakers of children with tracheostomies has been found to be reduced, with mental health status being more significantly affected than physical health. In addition to lack of sleep, caretakers express anxiety about their child's psychological well-being, and about the impact on relationships and family life. Many caretakers feel isolated, and report an increased incidence of broken marriages, which often result from the inability of one partner to deal with the day-to-day demands of care for a child with a tracheostomy. While some families prefer to care for their children without outside nursing help, the majority feel that they do not receive optimal/adequate nursing support. These studies suggest that adequate counseling prior to tracheostomy and adequate nursing and respite support could reduce much of the burden of the care of a child with a tracheostomy after discharge.

Discharge Planning Following Tracheostomy

Tracheostomy is a highly demanding intervention that tasks the families' emotional well-being and financial resources. Anticipatory guidance to prepare the family for assuming responsibility of caring for the tracheostomy is critical during the period of hospitalization. Well-established programs will prepare the family for coping with the demands of taking their child with tracheostomy home. Frequently, a 4–6 week schedule of discharge planning is mandatory to prepare a family for caring for a child with tracheostomy at home. At minimum, a multidisciplinary team consists of pediatric otolaryngology airway surgeons, critical care pulmonary physicians, pediatric intensive care physicians, pediatricians, nurse practitioners, nurses, respiratory therapists, occupational therapist, physical therapist, speech therapist, child life therapist, dietitian, social worker, case managers with discharge coordinator, and lastly the home care company.

All training requires extensive teaching and hands-on demonstration of equipment and procedures to ensure the caregivers are adept and comfortable at recognizing difficulties with the tracheostomy and responding appropriately. Teaching should begin on the day of the surgery and should include at least two caregivers. Preparation for discharge culminates in "transition care" whereby the caregivers provide tracheostomy care for an entire day and night without supervision from the medical staff. Prior to discharge, the caregivers should become adept at suctioning the tracheostomy tube, tracheostomy skin care, tracheostomy tie change, be able to recognize signs of respiratory distress, should be able to prevent or remove mucus plugs, recognize and rectify accidental dislodgement of the tracheostomy tube, and quickly replace the original tube with a smaller size tracheostomy tube. If needed, the family is taught how to a administer collar mist and must have a fully stocked emergency bag (with extra tracheostomy tube with ties already secured, self-inflating bag with face mask, lubricant, suctioning machine and catheters) handy at all times. In addition, the family should have a list of telephone numbers including home care equipment company, local police, fire, closest physician, pulmonary and ENT nurse practitioner, social workers and case managers. Many Children's Hospitals offering tracheostomy to infants, especially those with fetal surgery departments, have formal educational programs for families as described above.

Figures 14–21 below are examples of educational materials used to prepare families to take their children home with tracheostomies. (Cincinnati Tracheostomy Manual—figures below Courtesy of Michael Rutter, Cincinnati Children's Hospital) (Figs. 14, 15, 16, 17, 18, 19, 20 and 21).

Fig. 14 Parent "Learning List" for the care of an infant with a tracheostomy. Adapted from the Cincinnati Tracheostomy Manual, 2012. Permission from Michael Rutter

LEARNING LIST FOR THE CARE OF YOUR CHILD WITH A TRACHEOTOMY

Before your child goes home, you and a co-caregiver need to learn the following care. Any person staying with your child will also need to learn all of this information.

	Caregiver	Co-Caregiver
1. Why your child needs a tracheotomy tube	☐ ☐ ☐	☐ ☐ ☐
2. Type, size and length of your child's tracheotomy tube	☐ ☐ ☐	☐ ☐ ☐
3. Why, when and how to suction the tracheotomy tube	☐ ☐ ☐	☐ ☐ ☐
4. Why, when and how to clean the skin around the tracheotomy tube	☐ ☐ ☐	☐ ☐ ☐
5. Why, when and how to change the tracheotomy ties	☐ ☐ ☐	☐ ☐ ☐
6. Why, when and how to change the tracheotomy tube	☐ ☐ ☐	☐ ☐ ☐
7. Humidification	☐ ☐ ☐	☐ ☐ ☐
8. Supplies to have with your child at all times	☐ ☐ ☐	☐ ☐ ☐
9. Potential emergencies and how to help your child	☐ ☐ ☐	☐ ☐ ☐
10. The signs of respiratory distress and how to help your child	☐ ☐ ☐	☐ ☐ ☐
11. How to give oxygen through the tracheotomy tube	☐ ☐ ☐	☐ ☐ ☐
12. The signs of infection	☐ ☐ ☐	☐ ☐ ☐
13. Activities your child can do and activities to avoid	☐ ☐ ☐	☐ ☐ ☐
14. How to give medications, aerosols if needed	☐ ☐ ☐	☐ ☐ ☐
15. The use of necessary equipment and monitors	☐ ☐ ☐	☐ ☐ ☐
16. Use of home equipment ____________(date of set up/education)	☐ ☐ ☐	☐ ☐ ☐
17.How to do rescue breathing and cardiopulmonary resuscitation (CPR)	☐ ☐ ☐	☐ ☐ ☐
18. 24-hour transitional care completed	☐	☐
19. Other ________________________________	☐ ☐ ☐	☐ ☐ ☐

When you and your co-caregiver have shown success three different times for each item above, place a check in the box and the date it was completed above the box.

We have read and understand what we must learn to give tracheotomy care. We understand these items must be learned before ________________________ is discharged to home under our care.

Caregiver ________________________ **Co-caregiver** ________________________

Future Directions

Pediatric otorhinolaryngology (ears, nose, and throat) has come of age as a specialty with extensive expertise with the neonatal neck and airway. Concurrently, complications associated with tracheostomy have declined over the years.

The diagnosis and management of diseases of the airway continue to evolve [57]. Diagnoses of airway anomalies are often aided with prenatal ultrasounds and magnetic resonance imaging. This allows adequate time for planned delivery in hospitals with the capability to support the airway and provide the appropriate level of care. Such infants might require ex-utero intrapartum treatment (EXIT) at delivery to secure the airway [8]. Video-assisted intubation with flexible direct laryngoscopy is supplanting emergency tracheostomy in newborns with obstructive lesions of the airway. The use of noninvasive positive-pressure ventilation has been utilized successfully as an alternative to tracheostomy and in the management of infants with obstructive sleep apnea [12]. Fiber-optic intubation, laryngeal mask airway, and intubation through supraglottic devices are alternatives to emergency tracheostomy.

Mandibular distraction osteogenesis is a promising therapy in newborn infants with upper airway anomalies [6]. It is used increasingly in managing infants with Pierre-Robin sequence and has largely supplanted tracheostomy as the preferred surgery [58]. However, for infants with multiple congenital anomalies, a tracheostomy may be unavoidable.

Supraglottoplasty is used increasingly to remove extra tissue from around the larynx as an alternative to tracheostomy

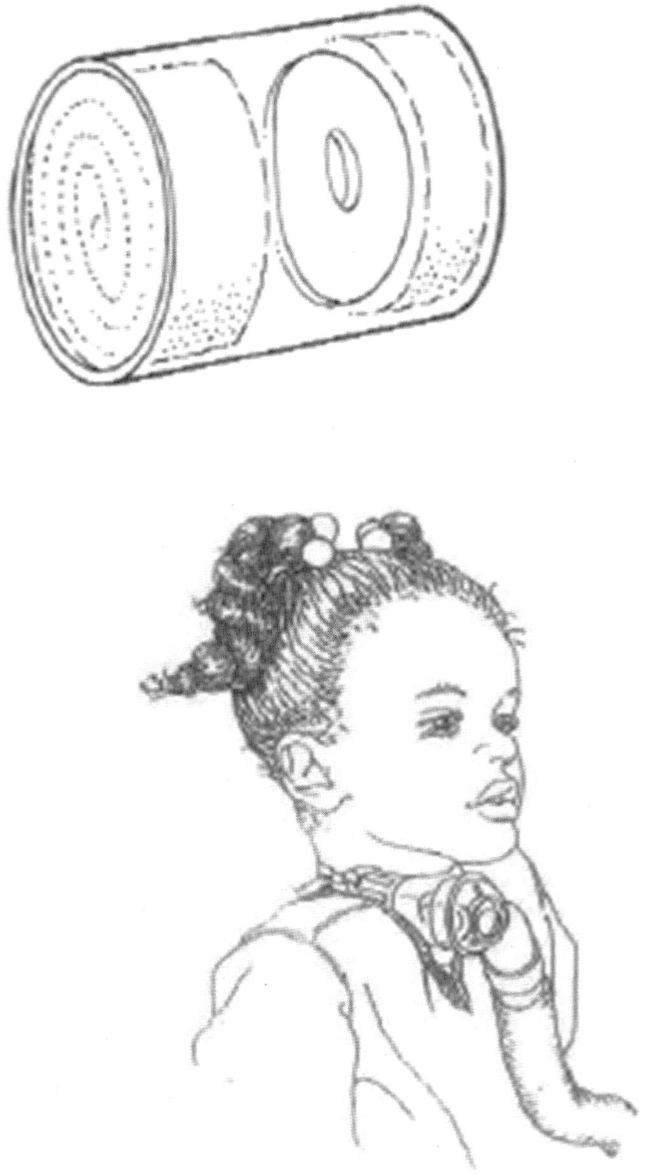

Fig. 15 Mist collar with a humidified moisture exchanger (HME), used for periods of disconnection from mechanical ventilation. Adapted from the Cincinnati Tracheostomy Manual, 2012. Permission from Michael Rutter

[59]. This shortens postoperative recovery time and length of hospital stay in carefully selected candidates with obstructive sleep apnea from laryngomalacia or from other causes.

Propranolol therapy has been proposed for treating congenital laryngotracheal hemangiomas [60]. Propranolol has gained currency as the treatment of choice for deforming hemangiomas or when the lesions compress vital organs. For non-life-threatening airway obstruction, propranolol remains a therapeutic option. Intralesional or systemic steroids in combination with CO_2 laser followed by intubation has also been used as an alternative to tracheostomy in infants with supraglottic hemangiomas.

Maturing the stoma to minimize complications of tracheostomy such as accidental decannulation is increasingly used [61, 62]. Maturation is achieved either by the use of traction sutures to pull the trachea up to the skin edge (anchor the trachea to the stoma) or by tethering the skin to the trachea. This process eliminates the complications of inserting the tracheostomy tube to a fresh stoma, reducing the risk of creating a false passage.

Finally, novel tracheostomy tube materials that minimize colonization of the cannula are addressing complications related to infections. Concern about the potential adverse effects of leachable materials from the plasticizer components of tracheostomy tubes is being addressed with replacement with DEHP- and PVC-free materials. However, this is an expensive endeavor. Research into how best to sterilize and safely recycle tracheostomy tubes is an area of current research.

Survival of extremely low birth weight infants and infants with congenital anomalies continues to increase. This population is at high risk for requiring tracheostomy. Therefore, continued research into best practices with regard to timing of tracheostomy, care of infants with tracheostomies, and outcomes of these patients is warranted. In the future, it will also be critical to continue developing novel surgical and medical approaches to avoid need for tracheostomy in the newborn and infant population.

Fig. 16 Correct positioning during planned tracheostomy change in an infant. Adapted from the Cincinnati Tracheostomy Manual, 2012. Permission from Michael Rutter

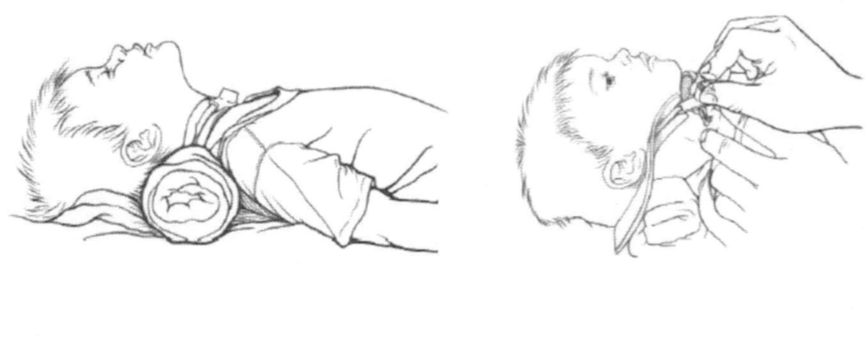

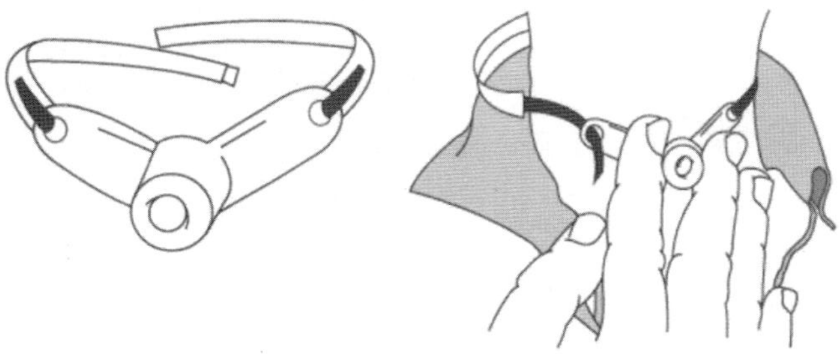

Fig. 17 Securing the tracheostomy at the stoma site. Adapted from the Cincinnati Tracheostomy Manual, 2012. Permission from Michael Rutter

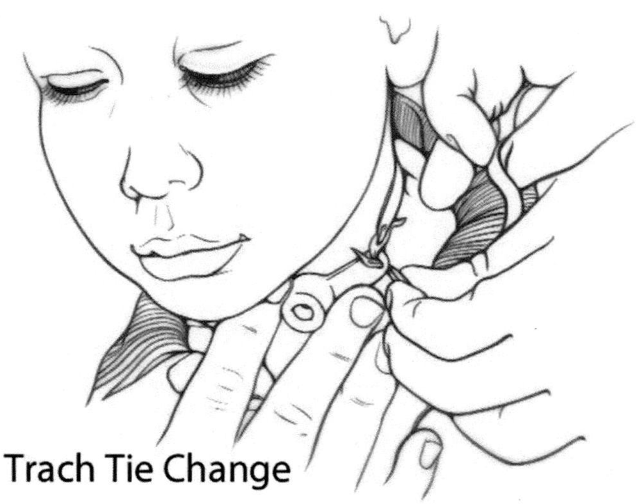

Fig. 18 Proper tracheostomy tie string changing procedure. Adapted from the Cincinnati Tracheostomy Manual, 2012. Permission from Michael Rutter

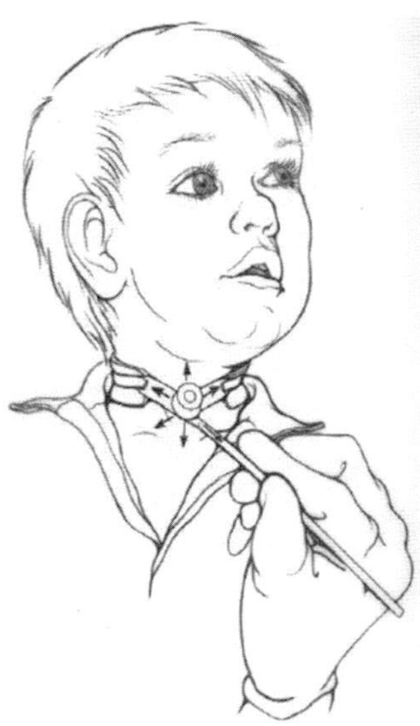

Fig. 19 Proper cleaning of the tracheostomy stoma with sterile water and Q tip applicator. Adapted from the Cincinnati Tracheostomy Manual, 2012. Permission from Michael Rutter

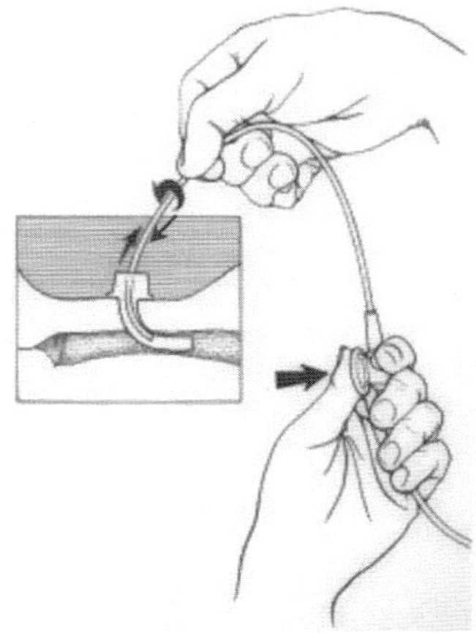

Fig. 20 Proper suction technique. Adapted from the Cincinnati Tracheostomy Manual, 2012. Permission from Michael Rutter

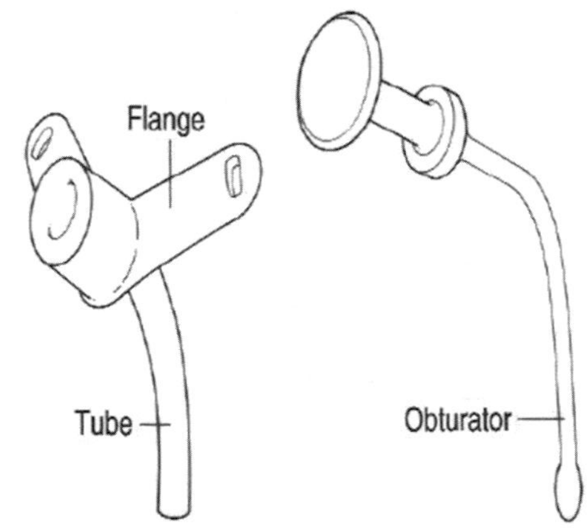

Fig. 21 The use of an obturator during a tracheostomy change. Adapted from the Cincinnati Tracheostomy Manual, 2012. Permission from Michael Rutter

References

1. Lewis CW, Carron JD, Perkins JA, Sie KC, Feudtner C. Tracheotomy in pediatric patients: a national perspective. Arch Otolaryngol Head Neck Surg. 2003;129(5):523–9. PubMed PMID: 12759264. Epub 2003/05/22.
2. Dursun O, Ozel D. Early and long-term outcome after tracheostomy in children. Pediatr Int. 2011;53(2):202–6. PubMed PMID: 20667029. Epub 2010/07/30. eng.
3. Perez-Ruiz E, Caro P, Perez-Frias J, Cols M, Barrio I, Torrent A, et al. Paediatric patients with a tracheostomy: a multicentre epidemiological study. Eur Respir J. 2012;40(6):1502–7. PubMed PMID: 22496314. Epub 2012/04/13. eng.
4. Pereira KD, MacGregor AR, McDuffie CM, Mitchell RB. Tracheostomy in preterm infants: current trends. Arch Otolaryngol Head Neck Surg. 2003;129(12):1268–71. PubMed PMID: 14676150. Epub 2003/12/17.
5. Overman AE, Liu M, Kurachek SC, Shreve MR, Maynard RC, Mammel MC, et al. Tracheostomy for infants requiring prolonged mechanical ventilation: 10 years' experience. Pediatrics. 2013;8. PubMed PMID: 23569088. Epub 2013/04/10. Eng.
6. Mackay DR. Controversies in the diagnosis and management of the Robin sequence. J Craniofac Surg. 2011;22(2):415–20. PubMed PMID: 21403570. Epub 2011/03/16. eng.

7. Hedrick MH, Ferro MM, Filly RA, Flake AW, Harrison MR, Adzick NS. Congenital high airway obstruction syndrome (CHAOS): a potential for perinatal intervention. J Pediatr Surg. 1994;29(2):271–4. PubMed PMID: 8176604.
8. Liechty KW. Ex-utero intrapartum therapy. Semin Fetal Neonatal Med. 2010;15(1):34–9. PubMed PMID: 19683972. Epub 2009/08/18. eng.
9. Donn SM, Sinha SK. Can mechanical ventilation strategies reduce chronic lung disease? Semin Neonatol. 2003;8(6):441–8. PubMed PMID: 15001116. Epub 2004/03/06. eng.
10. Zenk J, Fyrmpas G, Zimmermann T, Koch M, Constantinidis J, Iro H. Tracheostomy in young patients: indications and long-term outcome. Eur Arch Otorhinolaryngol. 2009;266(5):705–11. PubMed PMID: 18766359. Epub 2008/09/04. eng.
11. Kremer B, Botos-Kremer AI, Eckel HE, Schlondorff G. Indications, complications, and surgical techniques for pediatric tracheostomies—an update. J Pediatr Surg. 2002;37(11):1556–62. PubMed PMID: 12407539. Epub 2002/10/31. eng.
12. Wormald R, Naude A, Rowley H. Non-invasive ventilation in children with upper airway obstruction. Int J Pediatr Otorhinolaryngol. 2009;73(4):551–4. PubMed PMID: 19144413. Epub 2009/01/16. eng.
13. Kenna MA, Reilly JS, Stool SE. Tracheotomy in the preterm infant. Ann Otol Rhinol Laryngol. 1987;96(1 Pt 1):68–71. PubMed PMID: 3813388. Epub 1987/01/01. eng.
14. Sisk EA, Kim TB, Schumacher R, Dechert R, Driver L, Ramsey AM, et al. Tracheotomy in very low birth weight neonates: indications and outcomes. Laryngoscope. 2006;116(6):928–33. PubMed PMID: 16735883. Epub 2006/06/01.
15. Pereira KD, MacGregor AR, Mitchell RB. Complications of neonatal tracheostomy: a 5-year review. Otolaryngol Head Neck Surg. 2004;131(6):810–3.
16. Murthy K, Savani RC, Lagatta JM, Zaniletti I, Wadhawan R, Truog W, et al. Predicting death or tracheostomy placement in infants with severe bronchopulmonary dysplasia. J Perinatol. 2014;34:543–8. PubMed PMID: 24651732.
17. Mandy G, Malkar M, Welty SE, Brown R, Shepherd E, Gardner W, et al. Tracheostomy placement in infants with bronchopulmonary dysplasia: safety and outcomes. Pediatr Pulmonol. 2013;48(3):245–9. PubMed PMID: 22570313. Epub 2012/05/10.
18. Overman AE, Liu M, Kurachek SC, Shreve MR, Maynard RC, Mammel MC, et al. Tracheostomy for infants requiring prolonged mechanical ventilation: 10 years' experience. Pediatrics. 2013;131(5):e1491–6. PubMed PMID: 23569088. Epub 2013/04/10.
19. Schlessel JS, Harper RG, Rappa H, Kenigsberg K, Khanna S. Tracheostomy: acute and long-term mortality and morbidity in very low birth weight premature infants. J Pediatr Surg. 1993;28(7):873–6. PubMed PMID: 8229557. Epub 1993/07/01.
20. Wootten CT, French LC, Thomas RG, Neblett 3rd WW, Werkhaven JA, Cofer SA. Tracheotomy in the first year of life: outcomes in term infants, the Vanderbilt experience. Otolaryngol Head Neck Surg. 2006;134(3):365–9.
21. Carr MM, Poje CP, Kingston L, Kielma D, Heard C. Complications in pediatric tracheostomies. Laryngoscope. 2001;111(11 Pt 1):1925–8. PubMed PMID: 11801971. Epub 2002/01/22.
22. Cardone G, Lepe M. Tracheostomy: complications in fresh postoperative and late postoperative settings. Clin Pediatr Emerg Med. 2010;11(2):122–30.
23. Mahadevan M, Barber C, Salkeld L, Douglas G, Mills N. Pediatric tracheotomy: 17 year review. Int J Pediatr Otorhinolaryngol. 2007;71(12):1829–35. PubMed PMID: 17953995. Epub 2007/10/24.
24. Parrilla C, Scarano E, Guidi ML, Galli J, Paludetti G. Current trends in paediatric tracheostomies. Int J Pediatr Otorhinolaryngol. 2007;71(10):1563–7. PubMed PMID: 17628704. Epub 2007/07/14.
25. Tasca RA, Clarke RW. Tracheocutaneous fistula following paediatric tracheostomy—a 14-year experience at Alder Hey Children's Hospital. Int J Pediatr Otorhinolaryngol. 2010;74(6):711–2. PubMed PMID: 20394992. Epub 2010/04/17.
26. Tong CC, Kleinberger AJ, Paolino J, Altman KW. Tracheotomy timing and outcomes in the critically ill. Otolaryngol Head Neck Surg. 2012;147(1):44–51. PubMed PMID: 22412177. Epub 2012/03/14. eng.
27. Zheng Y, Sui F, Chen XK, Zhang GC, Wang XW, Zhao S, et al. Early versus late percutaneous dilational tracheostomy in critically ill patients anticipated requiring prolonged mechanical ventilation. Chin Med J (Engl). 2012;125(11):1925–30. PubMed PMID: 22884055. Epub 2012/08/14. eng.
28. Brook AD, Sherman G, Malen J, Kollef MH. Early versus late tracheostomy in patients who require prolonged mechanical ventilation. Am J Crit Care. 2000;9(5):352–9. PubMed PMID: 10976359. Epub 2000/09/08. eng.
29. Gomes Silva BN, Andriolo RB, Saconato H, Atallah AN, Valente O. Early versus late tracheostomy for critically ill patients. Cochrane Database Syst Rev. 2012;3, CD007271. PubMed PMID: 22419322. Epub 2012/03/16. eng.
30. Mok Q. Tracheostomies in paediatric intensive care: evolving indications and changing expectations. Arch Dis Child. 2012;97(10):858–9. PubMed PMID: 22894799. Epub 2012/08/17. eng.
31. Scales DC, Thiruchelvam D, Kiss A, Redelmeier DA. The effect of tracheostomy timing during critical illness on long-term survival. Crit Care Med. 2008;36(9):2547–57. PubMed PMID: 18679113. Epub 2008/08/06. eng.
32. Cheng J, Lioy J, Sobol S. Effect of tracheostomy timing in premature infants. Int J Pediatr Otorhinolaryngol. 2013;77:1873–6. PubMed PMID: 24035735. Epub 2013/09/17. Eng.
33. Rane S, Bathula S, Thomas RL, Natarajan G. Outcomes of tracheostomy in the neonatal intensive care unit: is there an optimal time? J Matern Fetal Neonatal Med. 2014;27(12):1257–61. PubMed PMID: 24215607. Epub 2013/11/13. Eng.
34. Demauro SB, D'Agostino JA, Bann C, Bernbaum J, Gerdes M, Bell EF, et al. Developmental outcomes of very preterm infants with tracheostomies. J Pediatr. 2014;164:1303–10. PubMed PMID: 24472229.
35. Pereira KD, Smith SL, Henry M. Failed extubation in the neonatal intensive care unit. Int J Pediatr Otorhinolaryngol. 2007;71(11):1763–6. PubMed PMID: 17850890. Epub 2007/09/14. eng.
36. Hoskote A, Cohen G, Goldman A, Shekerdemian L. Tracheostomy in infants and children after cardiothoracic surgery: indications, associated risk factors, and timing. J Thorac Cardiovasc Surg. 2005;130(4):1086–93. PubMed PMID: 16214524. Epub 2005/10/11. eng.
37. Spittle A, Orton J, Anderson P, Boyd R, Doyle LW. Early developmental intervention programmes post-hospital discharge to prevent motor and cognitive impairments in preterm infants. Cochrane Database Syst Rev. 2012;12, CD005495. PubMed PMID: 23235624. Epub 2012/12/14. eng.
38. Singer LT, Kercsmar C, Legris G, Orlowski JP, Hill BP, Doershuk C. Developmental sequelae of long-term infant tracheostomy. Dev Med Child Neurol. 1989;31:224–30.
39. Com G, Kuo DZ, Bauer ML, Lenker CV, Melguizo-Castro MM, Nick TG, et al. Outcomes of children treated with tracheostomy and positive-pressure ventilation at home. Clin Pediatr (Phila). 2013;52(1):54–61. PubMed PMID: 23155195. Epub 2012/11/17. eng.
40. Cristea AI, Carroll AE, Davis SD, Swigonski NL, Ackerman VL. Outcomes of children with severe bronchopulmonary dysplasia who were ventilator dependent at home. Pediatrics. 2013;132(3):e727–34. PubMed PMID: 23918888. Epub 2013/08/07. Eng.

41. Cotts T, Hirsch J, Thorne M, Gajarski R. Tracheostomy after pediatric cardiac surgery: frequency, indications, and outcomes. J Thorac Cardiovasc Surg. 2011;141(2):413–8. PubMed PMID: 20638080. Epub 2010/07/20. eng.
42. Edwards JD, Kun SS, Keens TG, Khemani RG, Moromisato DY. Children with corrected or palliated congenital heart disease on home mechanical ventilation. Pediatr Pulmonol. 2010;45(7):645–9. PubMed PMID: 20575088. Epub 2010/06/25. eng.
43. Berry JG, Graham DA, Graham RJ, Zhou J, Putney HL, O'Brien JE, et al. Predictors of clinical outcomes and hospital resource use of children after tracheotomy. Pediatrics. 2009;124(2):563–72. PubMed PMID: 19596736. Pubmed Central PMCID: 3614342.
44. Challapudi G, Natarajan G, Aggarwal S. Single-center experience of outcomes of tracheostomy in children with congenital heart disease. Congenit Heart Dis. 2013;8:556–60. PubMed PMID: 23510243. Epub 2013/03/21.
45. Gianoli GJ, Miller RH, Guarisco JL. Tracheotomy in the first year of life. Ann Otol Rhinol Laryngol. 1990;99(11):896–901. PubMed PMID: 2241016. Epub 1990/11/01. eng.
46. Edwards JD, Kun SS, Keens TG. Outcomes and causes of death in children on home mechanical ventilation via tracheostomy: an institutional and literature review. J Pediatr. 2010;157(6):955–9. e2. PubMed PMID: 20713294. Epub 2010/08/18.
47. Freeland AP, Wright JL, Ardran GM. Developmental influences of infant tracheostomy. J Laryngol Otol. 1974;88(10):927–36. PubMed PMID: 4470580. Epub 1974/10/01. eng.
48. Palisano R, Rosenbaum P, Walter S, Russell D, Wood E, Galuppi B. Development and reliability of a system to classify gross motor function in children with cerebral palsy. Dev Med Child Neurol. 1997;39(4):214–23. PubMed PMID: 9183258. Epub 1997/04/01. eng.
49. Hill BP, Singer LT. Speech and language development after infant tracheostomy. J Speech Hear Disord. 1990;55(1):15–20. PubMed PMID: 2299831. Epub 1990/02/01.
50. Jiang D, Morrison GA. The influence of long-term tracheostomy on speech and language development in children. Int J Pediatr Otorhinolaryngol. 2003;67 Suppl 1:S217–20. PubMed PMID: 14662199. Epub 2003/12/10.
51. Kaslon KW, Stein RE. Chronic pediatric tracheotomy: assessment and implications for habilitation of voice, speech and language in young children. Int J Pediatr Otorhinolaryngol. 1985;9(2):165–71. PubMed PMID: 4030238.Epub 1985/07/01.
52. Ross GS. Language functioning and speech development of six children receiving tracheotomy in infancy. J Commun Disord. 1982;15(2):95–111. PubMed PMID: 7096617. Epub 1982/03/01.
53. Hull EM, Dumas HM, Crowley RA, Kharasch VS. Tracheostomy speaking valves for children: tolerance and clinical benefits. Pediatr Rehabil. 2005;8(3):214–9. PubMed PMID: 16087556. Epub 2005/08/10.
54. Norman V, Louw B, Kritzinger A. Incidence and description of dysphagia in infants and toddlers with tracheostomies: a retrospective review. Int J Pediatr Otorhinolaryngol. 2007;71(7):1087–92. PubMed PMID: 17482279. Epub 2007/05/08.
55. Hartnick CJ, Bissell C, Parsons SK. The impact of pediatric tracheotomy on parental caregiver burden and health status. Arch Otolaryngol Head Neck Surg. 2003;129(10):1065–9. PubMed PMID: 14568788. Epub 2003/10/22.
56. Hopkins C, Whetstone S, Foster T, Blaney S, Morrison G. The impact of paediatric tracheostomy on both patient and parent. Int J Pediatr Otorhinolaryngol. 2009;73(1):15–20. PubMed PMID: 19019462. Epub 2008/11/21.
57. Daniel SJ. The upper airway: congenital malformations. Paediatr Respir Rev. 2006;7 Suppl 1:S260–3. PubMed PMID: 16798587. Epub 2006/06/27. eng.
58. Murage KP, Tholpady SS, Friel M, Havlik RJ, Flores RL. Outcomes analysis of mandibular distraction osteogenesis for the treatment of Pierre Robin sequence. Plast Reconstr Surg. 2013;132(2):419–21. PubMed PMID: 23897339. Epub 2013/07/31. eng.
59. White DR. Is supraglottoplasty underutilized? Laryngoscope. 2012;122 Suppl 4:S91–2. PubMed PMID: 23254618. Epub 2013/01/04. eng.
60. Truong MT, Chang KW, Berk DR, Heerema-McKenney A, Bruckner AL. Propranolol for the treatment of a life-threatening subglottic and mediastinal infantile hemangioma. J Pediatr. 2010;156(2):335–8. PubMed PMID: 20105647. Epub 2010/01/29. eng.
61. Colman KL, Mandell DL, Simons JP. Impact of stoma maturation on pediatric tracheostomy-related complications. Arch Otolaryngol Head Neck Surg. 2010;136(5):471–4. PubMed PMID: 20479378. Epub 2010/05/19. eng.
62. Park JY, Suskind DL, Prater D, Muntz HR, Lusk RP. Maturation of the pediatric tracheostomy stoma: effect on complications. Ann Otol Rhinol Laryngol. 1999;108(12):1115–9. PubMed PMID: 10605914. Epub 1999/12/22. eng.
63. Wetmore RF. Pediatric otolaryngology: the requisites in pediatrics. 1st ed. Philadelphia: Mosby; 2007. p. 237. xii.
64. Cincinnati Tracheostomy Manual. (Courtesy of Michael Rutter, M.D., pediatric otolaryngologist, University of Cincinnati Medical Center).
65. Corbett HJ, Mann KS, Mitra I, Jesudason EC, Losty PD, Clarke RW. Tracheostomy--a 10-year experience from a UK pediatric surgical center. Journal of pediatric surgery. 2007;42(7):1251–4.
66. Wheeler et al. Life Threatening Disorders of the Respiratory Track: Pediatric Critical Care Medicine: Volume 2: Respiratory, Cardiovascular and Central Nervous Systems. Shanley, et al, eds. 2nd ed. Springer 2014.

Gastroesophageal Reflux and the Neonatal Airway

Thane Blinman

Introduction

Confusion surrounds the clinical implications of the phenomena in which gastric contents travel backward into the esophagus, mouth, or parts of the airway. In no small part, this confusion seems to arise first in the imprecise manner in which terms are used in discussions and published literature. In particular, failure to distinguish explicitly between "GER" and "GERD" confuses both clinicians and parents, and apparently leads to overuse of medications in children who do not actually have "disease" associated with their reflux [1]. Similarly, the terms "reflux" and "emesis" are used interchangeably, even though these are quite different processes. Meanwhile, it is not clear that many of the apparent manifestations traditionally ascribed to "GERD"—arching, emesis, coughing, irritability, or apneic episodes—are caused by reflux. Because *reflux* is nearly universal in infants while *reflux disease* is rare, some clinicians caring for infants have even gone so far as to label declare as "myth" the proposition that gastroesophageal reflux may be pathologic in infants [2]. Finally, care of children can be confused by biases left over from experience with adults, e.g., that when we talk about "reflux" we mostly mean "acid reflux," or that "reflux disease" is primarily a disease of the stomach. This is not what we mean in children.

This chapter attempts to clear up this murky topic of reflux disease in sick neonates with particular emphasis on the effects of reflux on the airway. It describes what we think are the essential contributors to neonatal gastroesophageal reflux disease (GERD); what is believed about the detrimental effects on the airway; aspects of nonsurgical and surgical amelioration; and how to manage postoperative feeds and common complications in order to obtain the best surgical result.

To begin with, let us state the first premise: gastroesophageal reflux (GER) disease is not a problem of the stomach or even the esophagus, but a problem of the *foregut*, or what some call the aerodigestive tract.

To be more explicit, consider these terms:

Foregut: the cephalic portion of the embryonic alimentary canal. Foregut consists of endoderm, and gives rise to the pharynx, esophagus, stomach, liver, pancreas, most of the small intestine, and respiratory ducts [3]. While some have questioned whether the lungs and airways are actually embryologically foregut, the innervation of both proximal gut and airways by the vagus nerve displays these structures' functional unity: the lungs and gut are "wired" together.

GER: the passive flow of gastric contents retrogrades through the lower esophageal sphincter complex (LES) into the esophagus or higher, typically during transient LES relaxations (TLESRs). When GER reaches beyond the esophagus, it is common in the otolaryngology literature to see it referred to as "laryngopharyngeal reflux" (LPR) [4].

Refluxate: the material that moves in a retrograde fashion from stomach to esophagus during reflux symptoms.

GERD: GER, plus some detrimental effect attributed to GER e.g., growth failure, abnormal oxygen requirement, esophageal or tracheal stricture, aspiration pneumonia, pneumonitis, pulmonary hypertension, chronic otitis, etc. As with GER and LPR, a subset of GERD produced by refluxate reaching above the esophagus is sometimes called "larygopharyngeal reflux disease" (LPRD) [4]. It is these "extra-esophageal" manifestations of GER that we are interested in treating, and what most general pediatric surgeons and neonatologists mean when they talk about "GERD." As with GER and LPR, in this chapter, "GERD" and "LPRD" are lumped together as "GERD."

T. Blinman, M.D., F.A.C.S. (✉)
Division of General, Thoracic, and Fetal Surgery, The Children's Hospital of Philadelphia, 34th Street and Civic Center Boulevard, Philadelphia, PA 19104-4399, USA

University of Pennsylvania, Perelman School of Medicine, Philadelphia, PA, USA
e-mail: BLINMAN@email.chop.edu

J. Lioy and S.E. Sobol (eds.), *Disorders of the Neonatal Airway: Fundamentals for Practice*, DOI 10.1007/978-1-4939-1610-8_26, © Springer Science+Business Media New York 2015

Emesis: an active motor program originating in the vagal nuclei and mediated by the vagal nerve, producing retrograde gastric peristalis and forceful expelling of gastric contents through the LES. Observe that while "reflux" and "emesis" both involve retrograde movement of gastric contents into the esophagus, reflux is essentially a *passive* process stemming from decreased motor activity, whereas emesis is essentially an *active* process stemming from increased motor activity. These terms are often confused, in no small part because of the "reflux-->retch-->regurgitate" phenomenon, when refluxate stimulates the vagus nerve triggering the emesis motor program.

Fundoplasty v. fundoplication: Both terms refer to operations to attenuate reflux. The more commonly used *fundoplication* comes from Latin *plicare,* "to fold." Others prefer *fundoplasty*, from the Greek *plasso* "I fold" or *plastikos* "able to be shaped or molded." Either is correct, but it is interesting to note that neither means "to wrap". As will be seen the actual mechanisms by which anti-reflux operations work involves a reshaping of the lower esophageal sphincter region, with the "wrap" performing only one part of the work. Interestingly, the root of both words, *fundus*, comes from the Latin for "bottom" or "base" a curious choice of naming for a portion of the stomach that is at the uppermost part. So while both terms are a bit upside down, *fundoplication* is more etymologically pure (all Latin roots), while *fundoplasty* more correctly describes the operation. In modern English usage, these terms are interchangeable.

Pathophysiology

Reflux is a function of fluid, pressure, viscosity, and the mechanisms of the so-called LES. More than simply a circular muscle that maintains tonic constriction while opening when required physiologically, the LES is really part of a greater "LES complex" that includes the diaphragmatic crura and the Angle of His. The function of the LES is imperfectly understood, even with sophisticated mathematical models [5]. But it is probably not oversimplifying the case too much to say that the LES is a control point between chest and abdominal cavities, a valve with *asymmetric resistance*: Resistance is relatively low for swallowing (antegrade flow), and relatively high for reflux and emesis (retrograde flow). The anatomical mechanisms that allow this asymmetric resistance are complex.

The lower 2/3 of the esophagus is not under voluntary control. It automatically propagates a peristaltic wave initiated by a swallow, and the last few centimeters of the esophagus normally hold intrinsic tone that relaxes in response to these swallows. But the lower esophageal tone is also lost in events known as *transient lower esophageal sphincter relaxations* (TLESR's). Transient LES relaxation appears to be the chief physiologic antecedent of GER in children [6].

But other mechanical effects contribute. In particular, there must be a *pressure gradient* from abdomen to chest (or, more particularly, between stomach and lower esophagus), a gradient that is magnified during, for example, pregnancy. Importantly for infants, a full stomach also translates to greater intragastric pressure. Meanwhile, the *viscosity* of the gastric contents also plays a part. The *radius* and *length* of the LES are also important. The general relationship of these mechanical factors is seen in the "reflux equation," which is really just a version of Hagen–Poiseuille equation [7]:

$$Flow \propto \frac{\left(P_g - P_e\right) \cdot R^4}{c \cdot L \cdot \eta}$$

where

$P_g - P_e$ = the pressure gradient between stomach and lower esophagus

R = the radius of the esophagus

L = the length of the LES (essentially, the distance from crura to GE junction)

η = the fluid viscosity

As a model of flow through the LES, this equation is wrong, but useful. The flow through the LES is not laminar, the tube is not rigid, and none of the parameters is constant. Still, the relationship given in the equation does reveal what constrains the mechanics of the LES as a valve. Several elements of the LES work together to create its asymmetric resistance [8]. All of these physiological elements (and all successful treatments for GERD) work through at least one element of this equation. The functional elements of the LES include:

1. Crus muscle: When contracted, the diaphragmatic crura shorten and pinch the esophagus. This decreases the radius R, blocking reflux. It also contributes to the pressure gradient ΔP blocking GER by increasing P_e.
2. Intrinsic tone (or elastance) of the distal esophagus: most reflux occurs during "transient lower esophageal relaxations" (TLESRs), or brief episodes when the LES relaxes [6]. In contrast, the elastance of the LES inhibits reflux by reducing R and by creating higher pressure P_e in the LES than in the stomach.
3. Intra-abdominal esophageal length: the length of the esophagus inferior to the diaphragmatic crus (L). A "negative" length here would be a hiatal hernia, where the gastroesophageal junction (GEJ) sits superior to the crura. In the newborn, the intra-abdominal esophagus may be less than 1 cm, but is reported to be 3 cm at 3 months of age [8]. Perhaps this anatomical development (as well as other effects) explains in part how infants tend to "grow out of" reflux problems.

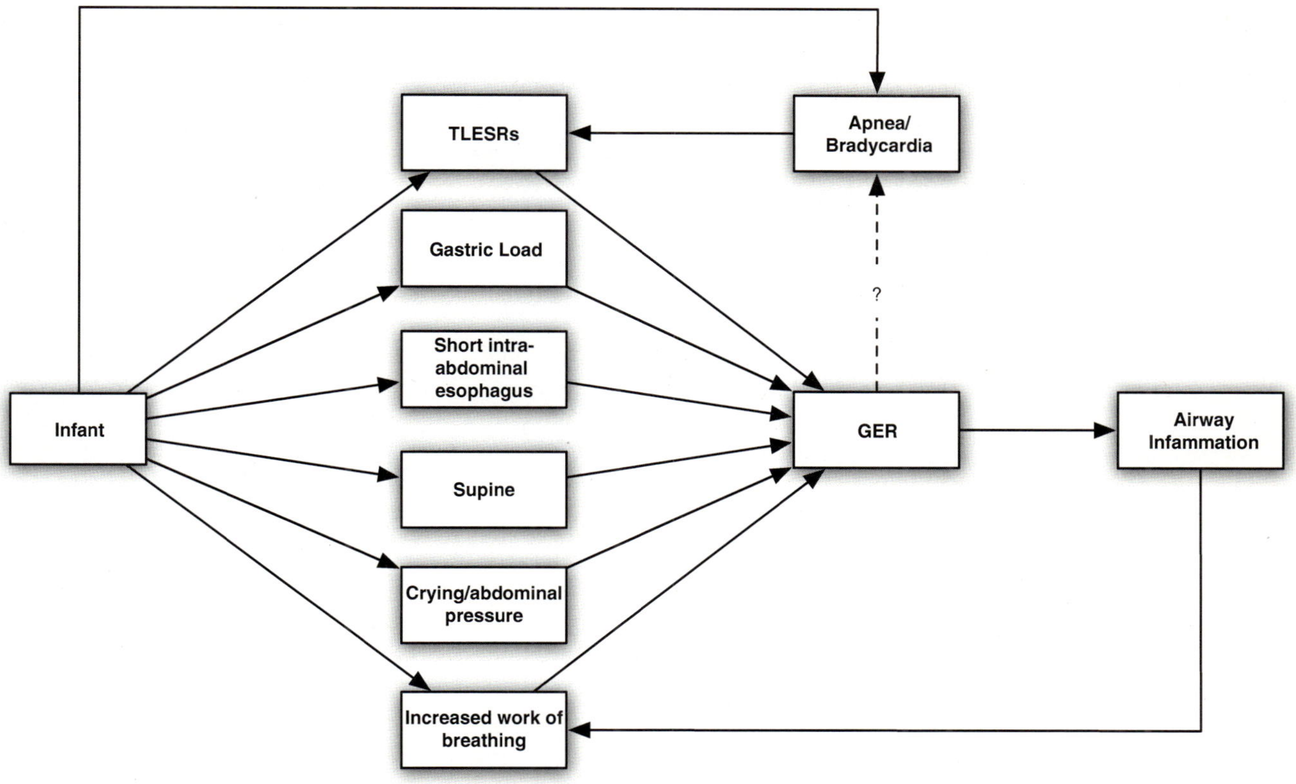

Fig. 1 Multiple mechanisms are likely to contribute to GER in infants, but GER only becomes GERD when the airway and lungs become damaged. The connection between GER and apnea is less clear. At least two positive feedback loops may exist here, where the effects of reflux potentiate factors that contribute to reflux

4. The cardiac angle: Also known as the "Angle of His." It is believed that an acute angle protects against reflux because a filling fundus will tend to close the LES if the angle is acute, but tends to open the LES if the angle is obtuse. When functioning properly, this mechanism should both reduce R and produce a restrictive pressure gradient between stomach and LES.

All of these are weaker in small children, increasing the propensity to have GER events. But even if the LES was functioning well, it bears repeating that it is not a perfect one-way valve. As most pregnant women can attest, a strong enough pressure gradient from abdominal to throracic cavities can overcome the resistance in the LES. Infants have extra mechanisms that similarly increase the tendency to overcome the LES:

Scaling: Mismatch between gastric scaling and energy scaling means that the stomach of an infant carries a larger burden than an adult's. While the capacity of the stomach scales with body mass *linearly* (a reasonable heuristic is around 22 mL/kg), energy scales *nonlinearly*, roughly according to an inverse power law [9, 10]. For example, a 3 kg infant will require around 128 kcal/kg/day but his 80 kg father uses just 34 kcal/kg/day. However, both have similar gastric capacity relative to body mass. It is this mismatch that explains why infants need to eat every 3 h, and why they are so "spitty": To ingest 128 kcal/kg/day of breast milk (~20 kcal/30 mL) requires drinking 576 mL/day, or 72 mL every 3 h, or 24 mL/kg/feed—right at the limit of gastric capacity. A constantly "loaded" stomach increases opportunities for reflux events.

Relatively slower gastric emptying: It appears that infants (especially premature infants) have relatively slow emptying of gastric volumes compared to adults, a problem easily made worse by various medications administered to neonates [11, 12]. This longer dwell time probably contributes to GER by increasing the probability of refluxate with a given TLESR.

Work of breathing: Breathing requires energy, and is associated with cyclical pressure gradients between abdominal cavity and chest cavity. Here again we see a mismatch between linear and nonlinear physiological scaling [13]. The disproportionally greater energy requirements ($\dot{V}_{O_2}$) and carbon dioxide production ($\dot{V}_{CO_2}$) plus the linear tidal volume (~7–8 mL/kg/breath) translate necessarily into a higher respiratory rate. For a given airway impedance, work is a function of this rate. Of course, several diseases greatly increase impedance per breath, compounding increases of WOB in sick infants.

These mechanisms explain why babies universally have some GER (Fig. 1). Moreover, "some GER" may be quite a lot, with around 70 GER events/day recorded in normal newborns [14, 15]. But nothing here explains why some infants cross a threshold into GERD. It is reasonable to assert that GERD appears whenever the amount of airway soiling exceeds some capacity of the airways to recover. It follows that GERD will become manifest whenever the *amount of refluxate* in GER is very high (e.g., hiatal hernia, increased frequency of TLESRs, etc), the *ability to protect* the airway from refluxate is inhibited (e.g., neurological degradation, tracheomalacia, etc.), *pulmonary repair* mechanisms are degraded (e.g., bronchopulmonary dysplasia (BPD), pulmonary hypertension, cystic fibrosis, etc.), or the *character of the refluxate* is particularly toxic (e.g., acid, bile acids, pepsins, bacteria).

Several surgical diseases in the neonate also come accompanied by GERD. Patients with diaphragmatic hernia, tracheoesophageal fistula, and gastroschisis commonly exhibit difficulties with enteric feeds, and resort to surgical control of reflux is common here. In all of these, a specific failure of the LES can be posited. For instance, in CDH, the diaphragmatic crus is typically dysfunctional and GERD is common [16–18]. In TEF, the distal esophagus has decreased tone and motility [19]. In gastroschisis, hiatal hernia is common [20], and intra-abdominal pressure can be elevated for weeks while downstream small bowel motility [21] (and therefore gastric emptying) can be slowed for months (or longer).

Regardless of etiology, lungs are damaged by large amounts of debris (milk proteins and fats); acid, bile acids, bacteria, and digestive enzymes. Of these, it seems that acid, while plainly damaging to the respiratory epithelium, is the least problematic in infants. Certainly acid in the esophagus produces a noxious feeling that can lead to arching, pain, and reduced oral intake ("food fear"). But babies tend to have weakly acidic refluxate [15]. As a result, in neonates there may not be enough acid reaching the airway to provoke the intense inflammatory reaction seen in GERD both clinically and experimentally.

The same cannot be said about the effects of digestive enzymes, particularly the pepsins. This family of proteases (particularly Pepsin 3) is manufactured only in the stomach. While pH-dependent, the enzyme remains active at relatively high pH (i.e., pH 5) and does not denature until pH > 7.2. Once aspirated into the airways, these enzymes spark intense inflammation [22]. These inflammatory changes degrade the ability of pulmonary epithelium to clear debris and aspirated organisms. Probably, the lungs become more vulnerable as their "clearance capacity" is overwhelmed by large amounts of aspirate, and later even relatively small amounts of aspirated refluxate may provoke inflammation, wheeze, cough and elevated work of breathing. These inflammatory changes are posited to exacerbate BPD, pulmonary hypertension, and prolonged oxygen requirements in infants. However, despite a great deal of opinion and investigation, this causal chain has not been established. Still, in documented refluxers, damage to the airway may sometimes be demonstrated on inspection (see Fig. 2).

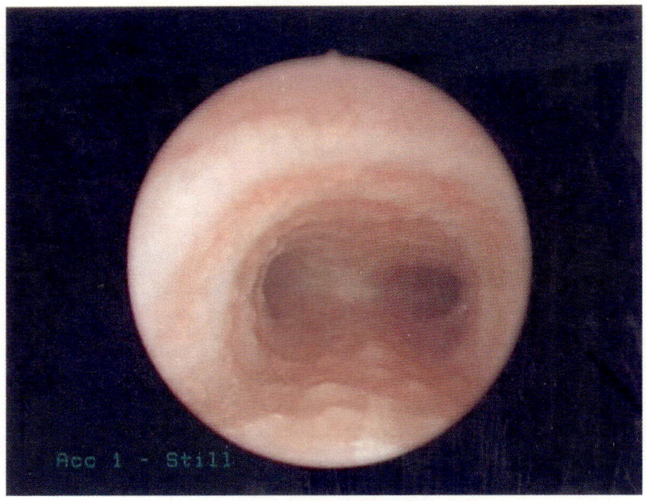

Fig. 2 A bronchoscopic view of the trachea and carina in an infant with GERD. Observe the "cobblestone" eruptions along the epithelium attributed to constant microaspiration of gastric contents

At this point, one may notice that the elements of this list could comprise a harmful positive feedback loop between lung damage and reflux. As reflux damages the lung parenchyma, work of breathing and inspiratory pressure may rise. As these rise, energy needs for growth increase, further increasing the filling pressure on the stomach while the inspiratory pressure steepens the pressure gradient between abdominal and thoracic cavities. Meanwhile, apneic spells may not always be caused by GER as commonly believed, but may not be effective but *cause*, contributing to TLESRs [23]. All of these effects must increase refluxate, leading to further lung damage. Treatment, then, should be aimed at interrupting this positive feedback loop.

Diagnosis

Diagnostic interventions seek to determine whether GER may be the cause of pulmonary manifestations or failure to thrive. There is no single best test for "GERD" in infants. Instead, the clinician must combine specific testing with clinical context of a given patient. Several diagnostic tests are available.

pH-probe/impedance probe: probes introduce an esophageal tube with multiple side ports each able to detect pH or electrical impedance or both. For pH probes, a falling pH at a certain detector site in the esophagus is a proxy for gastric contents, presumably with low pH. Similarly, a decline in impedance suggests fluid at the detector. With multiple channels, these devices reliably detect GER (and its character—acidic, weakly acidic, or alkaline), and give an indication of its severity: how far up the esophagus refluxate travels, how often refluxate appears, and how fast it is cleared [24]. pH/impedance is often referred to as the "gold standard" for diagnosis of GER.

It cannot however provide sole evidence that GER is actually GERD, nor can it reveal problems with gastric emptying or altered anatomy (like malrotation or hiatal hernia).

Fluoroscopy: To reveal anatomical problems that may present as GER, esophagosocopy and upper gastrointestinal (UGI) series are helpful. While insensitive to GER (reported sensitivity is under 50 %) [25], the images are far more specific in revealing hiatal hernia, H-type tracheoesophageal fistula, microgastria, esophageal stricture, and malrotation. Some surgeons insist on UGI before fundoplasty in order to plan the operation, for example to allow for the need to perform a Ladd's procedure concomittantly [26] or even *instead of* fundoplication [27]. Data suggests that at least 4 % of patients being considered for fundoplasty will be found to have a surgically important abnormality [28]. But this value alone does not give the value of information from the UGI. For example it is reasonable to place premium value on decreased uncertainty about malrotation; that is, to assert that avoiding one missed malrotation is worth more than the cost of 24 negative studies. Value judgments of this kind resist standard calculus.

Manometry: this method uses a series of pressure sensors in the esophagus to describe esophageal pressure waves. Critical for diagnosis of motility disorders like achalasia in older children and adults, manometry contributes little to the workup of GERD in infants.

Esophagoscopy: Regarded as a mandatory diagnostic step by some, esophagoscopy is critical for diagnosis of esophageal metaplasia, ulcers, eosiniphilic esophagitis, conditions rarely encountered in newborns. Like manometry, esophagoscopy is not routinely used in newborns for workup of GERD.

Bronchoscopy: Bronchoscopy may provide compelling evidence of reflux with aspiration (see Fig. 2) but is not a front line tool in initial workup. On the other hand, patients who appear to have severe "reflux" may require interrogation of the airway to identify other structural problems that can mimic GERD, e.g., laryngeal cleft, H-type tracheoesophageal fistula, or tracheomalacia.

Nuclear scintigraphy: Radionuclide scintigraphy is attractive because it is noninvasive, carries no X-ray exposure, and can purportedly detect GER and microaspiration while quantifying gastric emptying. When compared to pH monitoring, the sensitivity of radionuclide scintigraphy is reported to be between 75 and 100 %, and specificity between 81.2 and 100 % [29]. But the usefulness of these "milk scans" in practice is less clear. Milk scans confirm that reflux is common in preterm infants, but it turns out that "positive scintigraphy has no correlation with symptoms" [30]. In that study, the authors found no discrimination at all in detection of GER between symptomatic babies and asymptomatic babies. Others report that the scans do not offer any information that guides whether pyloroplasty is indicated along with fundoplasty (Pyloroplasty is very rarely indicated in any case, and its routine use with fundoplication is condemned) [31]. Most likely, these scans are of little value in infants in the NICU: virtually always "positive" (even in children who have intact and working fundoplasty), their specificity appears considerably lower than reported for other populations. At the same time, the sensitivity to detect aspiration also appears in daily practice to be far below reported levels. In other words, in infants, they merely confirm reflux that is nearly universal, while failing to detect the "disease" in GERD.

Biomarkers: In patients undergoing bronchoscopy, who are intubated, or have a tracheostomy, bronchoalveolar lavage allows examination of the fluid in the airways. While traditional diagnosis relied on the presence of "lipid-laden macrophages" as a proxy for lung soilage, this finding appears to lack specificity [32]. Others have used the presence of pepsin [22, 33], measured according to various assays, to indicate GERD. This method seems to have promise, but lack of guidelines regarding interpretation of results, lack of standard methods for measurement, limited availability of the tests and restriction to patients with some tube in the airway all prevent widespread use for now.

N-of-one trials: While this method has the least published evidence, it is arguably the method to which experienced neonatal clinicians resort the most. N-of-1 trials are single-patient trials with "multiple-period crossover experiments comparing two or more treatments within individual patients" [34]. In detecting GERD, the clinician will observe the patient while being fed normally (orally or by tube) into the stomach. Frequency of apneas, oxygen requirement, discomfort, and other signs of symptomatic reflux are noted. Then feeds are withheld, with nutrition supported either by nasojejunal enteral feedings or parenteral nutrition. If GER is really GERD, improvement in respiratory and other symptoms will manifest within 2 or 3 days (sometimes less). Return to gastric feeds will reproduce the symptoms, and a second period of non-gastric nutrition relieves them. Each "block" of these trials is about 1 week long. While this method does not rule out laryngeal cleft or other anomalies in orally fed children, these confounders can be controlled by restricting enteral nutrition to tube feeding. While evidence is scant regarding this method, and criticisms are plain (jejunal feeds are imperfect protection against reflux; trials take a long time; etc.), this pragmatic method may yield the highest individual validity.

Medical Treatment

Traditionally, the mainstay of control of GERD has been drugs which fall into two categories: motility agents and acid blockers.

From the discussion above on pathophysiology, the usefulness of acid blockade on the control of GERD manifestations should seem suspect. Nothing in the function of the LES depends on pH; acid is weak in infants already; and decreased pH creates an important "deflector screen" against enteric organisms migrating from the stomach back into the airway. It is plausible that reliable acid control could act to deactivate pepsin and other digestive enzymes, but this has not been shown. At the same time, while improvements in pediatric asthma have been shown in the past, more recent trials show no benefit, and even harm in asthmatic children [35]. Meanwhile, there is increasing skepticism about acid blockade in infants. Proton-pump inhibitors (PPIs) carry serious risks and little effect on GERD symptoms [36], and even H2 blockers were recently associated with serious, even fatal, problems in infants [37]. While these medications have their place in gastritis with bleeding, or GERD manifesting largely as oral resistance and discomfort, it is plain that they are over-prescribed [1] and undereffective.

Motility agents fare little better. Metoclopramide (Reglan), bethanechol, cisapride, and erythromycin have all been tried as frontline treatments for GERD. In theory, increasing "motility" (i.e., decreasing gastric emptying time, decreasing intestinal transit time) should decrease GER events associated with TLESRs by reducing the dwell time of feeds in the stomach.

These posited effects have not been demonstrated practice. Reglan has no measurable effect on GERD in infants but carries a high risk of dystonic reactions [38]. Cisapride was shown to be effective, but was removed from the US market after several patients developed cardiac dysrythmias attributed to it [39]. Bethanechol, a parasympathomimetic, was posited to aid GERD by increasing intestinal motility, but trials have failed to demonstrated effectiveness (for example [40]). Erythromycin, a motilin agonist, certainly increases gastric emptying, but has not been shown to be an effective treatment for GERD, perhaps because of its strong tendency toward tachyphylaxis [39, 41]. At one time, it was common to place almost every baby in the NICU on "R&R" (reglan and ranitidine), a practice now, unsurprisingly, out of favor.

The reflux equation described above illustrates why other therapies that seem reasonable have unclear power to attenuate GER. Chief among these is the practice of "thickening" feeds. In this practice, a thickening agent (rice cereal, guar gum, cornstarch) is added to milk or infant formula. This "thickening" is actually a change in viscosity, η. From the equation, it is apparent that in order to halve GER, one would need to double the viscosity. The viscosity of human breast milk is around 3 cP (pumped, untreated), but addition of a commercial thickener (Nestle ThickenUp®, a preparation of cornstarch) demonstrated a large increase in measured viscosity: "In relation to untreated pumped human milk without thickener, we observed that the addition of 7 % of the thickener increased the viscosity up to ninefold" [42]. So far so good. But this improvement comes at a cost—delayed gastric emptying. There are other costs: infants have diminished alpha-amylase and thus diminished ability to digest cornstarch which can produce diarrhea [43] Increasing viscosity delays gastric emptying [44]. With contrary effects and varied effects of different thickeners plus the confounder of varied viscosity of human infant milk formulas, mixed results with use of thickeners is unsurprising. Pectin, another thickening agent, appears to delay gastric emptying [45] but a trial in neurologically injured children showed improvement in GERD [46]. In sum, no reliable evidence exists to support or decry use of thickeners as GER treatment in infants. A Cochrane review in 2002 concluded "There is no evidence from randomised controlled trials to support or refute the efficacy of feed thickeners in newborn infants with [GER]" [47]. In a more recent study, the results are, again, mixed: "A formula thickened with amylopectin did not reduce the number of apnea of prematurity or GER-related apneas. It reduced acid GER features but had no effect on non-acid GER indexes" [48].

Others have turned to "elemental" formulas in order to treat GERD. There is nothing in these formulas that can be expected to improve the function of the LES or to increase gastric emptying. Rather the opposite is true—all of these formulas share one counterproductive characteristic, relatively high osmolarity. While breast milk has an osmolarity similar to serum (~290 mOsm/L), elemental formulas are much higher (e.g., Alimentum™, 370 mOsm/L when prepared at 20 kcal/30 mL). The stomach responds to elevated osmolarity by holding the fluid longer and diluting, since the small bowel does not tolerate high osmolarity fluid well (producing cramping, flushing, and diarrhea recognized as dumping syndrome). Changing a baby to an elemental formula may certainly be the right intervention for many diseases (protein hypersensitivity, malabsorption, etc.). But pathophysiologically, if a change to an elemental formula does ameliorate some observed manifestation of "feeding intolerance," it is unlikely that the cause was GERD.

Surgical Treatment

Surgical control of GER aims to restore normal functioning of the LES. "Normal" function does not include the inability to vomit, the inability to burp, or total elimination of reflux. Instead, surgery aims to re-establish or reinforce the mechanical functions that the LES normally employs [8]. To review:

1. The "pinch cock" effect of the crus muscle.
2. Adequate intra-abdominal esophageal length.
3. An acute angle at the cardia (Angle of His).
4. Decreased compliance (increased elastance) at the lowest portion of the esophagus, i.e., "tone".

Table 1 Common types of fundoplasty for reflux control

Complete wrap (360°)	–	Nissen
		Nissen–Rossetti
		Collis–Nissen
		Floppy Nissen
Partial wrap	Anterior	Dor (180°)
		Thal (240°)
		Boix Ochoa (240°)
		Belsey Mark IV (240°)
	Posterior	Toupet (270°)
No wrap	–	Hill gastropexy

An additional surgical objective is *removal of barriers to gastric emptying* (e.g., malrotation, overdistended stomach, etc.). The underlying objective is to attain these results without creating unwanted problems like dysphagia.

All surgical fundoplasties achieve these mechanical objectives. It may surprise readers familiar only with the "Nissen" fundoplication, but surgical control of GERD does not begin and end with the Nissen. Instead, there are several approaches (Table 1).

While all these procedures have an eponym, rarely does the modern application of various procedures conform to the original description. This chapter confines discussion to the three most common fundoplasty types performed in North America:

Nissen: the modern Nissen is sometimes called a "floppy Nissen" to distinguish it from its original namesake, or even its modified form the "Nissen–Rossetti." The modern Nissen creates as 360° wrap looser and shorter (e.g., 2 cm) than originally described, and involves division of the short-gastric vessels between spleen and the greater curvature. Unlike the variant called a "Collis-Nissen," the modern Nissen places the wrap entirely above the GEJ (Fig. 3).

Toupet: Observe the spelling, distinguishing this wrap named after French surgeon Andre Toupet from the hairpiece (a toupee') which some have imagined that this wrap might somehow resemble. It does not. Instead, the modern version is a posterior 270° wrap that cushions the esophagus. Essentially an open and longer form of the Nissen, the Toupet resembles a hot dog (esophagus) in a bun (the sides of the wrap) (Fig. 4).

Thal: More popular in the 1980s, the Thal has become rare in the laparoscopic era. This is an anterior 240° wrap that also differs from other fundoplasties in the direction of the wrap. While both the Nissen and Toupet (and Dor) pull the fundus across the esophagus laterally, the Thal creates a kind of "hood" by pulling the anterior portion of the stomach from inferior to superior (Fig. 5).

All of these procedures may be done in infants via an open or laparoscopic approach. Experienced pediatric surgeons increasingly favor a laparoscopic approach because of the demonstrated superiority in surgical comorbidities (pain, time to feeds, adhesions, abdominal wall scarring, etc.) as well as opportunities for improved visualization and surgical precision [49]. For patients who are candidates, laparoscopic fundoplasty yields results at least as good as open approaches.

Moreover, it has been repeatedly shown that no particular fundoplasty type is superior to any other. All are expected to provide clinical improvement in manifestations of GERD in at least 85 % of patients [50], and to provide similar protection [51–54]. This equivalence may seem counterintuitive, but is only surprising if one believes that a fundoplasty must be "tight" to be effective. This is untrue. Instead, an effective fundoplasty must reinforce the normal physiological mechanisms of the LES without creating dysphagia. That is, an ideal fundoplasty must increase retrograde resistance without increasing antegrade resistance. The Nissen, Toupet, and Thal all restore the crus, increase intra-abdominal esophageal length, restore an acute angle of His, increase the elastance of the LES (i.e., reduce TLESRs) and probably increase gastric emptying. When these mechanisms are understood, it is clear that a "tight" fundoplasty is beside the point.

Moreover, surgical amelioration of reflux, regardless of particular type of fundoplasty, appears to provide powerful protection to the lungs. Rothenberg et al. demonstrated that pulmonary function was improved by Nissen fundoplication in children with asthma in a large cohort [55]. Oxygen requirement appears to be lower and ventilator weaning appears to be aided [56]. In pediatric patients with severe reactive airway disease, fundoplication reduces symptoms and medications (including steroids) [57]. However, there is no convincing evidence in the literature to demonstrate that fundoplication effectively treats apneic spells in premature or full-term neonates. This is unsurprising given the unclear causal relationship between apnea and GER [23].

Where these variations on fundoplasty differ is in mechanical complications. While the rate of "slipped" or failed fundoplasty appears to be independent of type, excessive dissection of the hiatus certainly shortens the expected lifetime of a working fundoplasty [58]. Fundoplication is expected to continue to provide reflux protection to 90 % of patients who had initial improvement at 5 years [59]. However, both the Thal and Toupet have markedly better results in terms of dysphagia, bloat, and inability to burp or vomit (e.g., [53]). In order to overcome these problems, surgeons work to make Nissens very "floppy," and a good "floppy Nissen" yields results very much like the partial fundoplasties.

Nevertheless, there is no consensus regarding the choice of one procedure over another. Most surgeons in North America are most familiar with the Nissen, and this procedure is

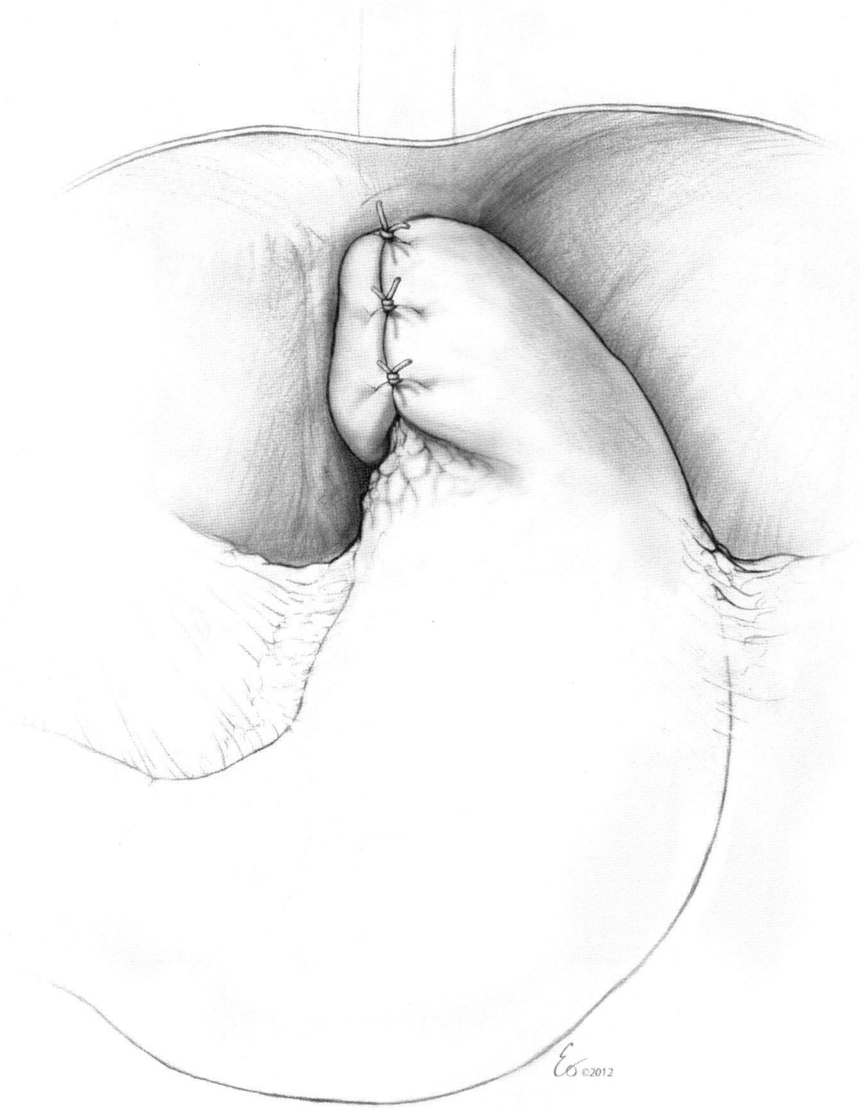

Fig. 3 The modern Nissen fundoplication is a 360°, loose wrap located between the diaphragm and gastroesophageal junction (GEJ)

arguably easier to complete laparoscopically than the others (for example, the Nissen may be completed with as few as four sutures, but the Toupet requires at least seven). Still, in special circumstances, a Nissen may be the wrong choice. For example, in babies with poor esophageal motility (e.g., esophageal atresia), a Toupet may be a better choice. Similarly, some babies can be better served by a Thal which can be performed in the setting of a small gastric fundus whereas a Nissen would be forced. Surgical pragmatism works where evidence is scant.

Respiratory Support as Adjunct Treatment

From the discussion above, it follows that any intervention that decreases work of breathing may aid reflux. In particular, use of positive airway pressure (or other means, e.g., plication of a paralyzed hemidiaphragm) to improve functional residual capacity and chest mechanics may decrease the tendency to defeat the LES. These interventions, including even surgical tracheostomy in some patients, may improve lung mechanics and reduce the effects of GERD by interrupting the cycle on the ventilatory part.

But this effect may not only depend on chest mechanics. Any brake on oxygen delivery will be borne heavily by the gut. Mild hypoxia combined with heavy work load to the gut is likely to produce some gut dysfunction, especially, dysmotility. This failure of downstream flow in the gut can easily manifest as signs that look like reflux (or other kinds of intolerance). In more severe circumstances, mismatch between oxygen delivery and demand in the gut may lead to "cleaving" of the villi at the tips where the countercurrent vascular system leaves the tip most vulnerable [60]. The result is a marked reduction in gut surface area, and setup of another potential destructive positive feedback loop as the same absorptive work must be done with less absorptive

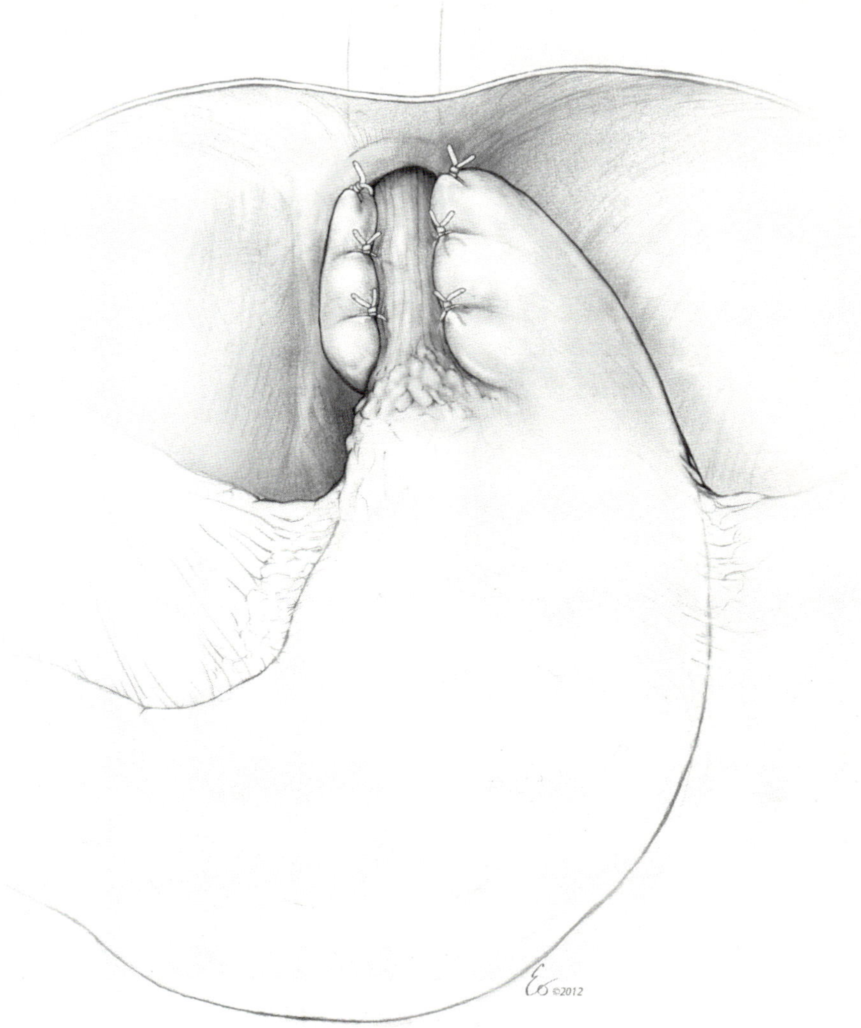

Fig. 4 The modern Toupet fundoplasty is a posterior, 240–270° wrap. Slightly longer than the Nissen, this wrap also is located above the GEJ

surface area. What the clinician may see is a child who is "stooling out," with loose watery stools. Alternatively, the clinician may see gut slowing, delayed gastric emptying, high gastric residuals, and retching.

When surgeons say that the purpose of the lungs is to perfuse the gut, they seem to know what they are talking about. More seriously, however, these interrelationships between intestinal and airway function belie the notion that functional divisions neatly separate these organ systems.

Care of the Post-fundoplasty Patient: The Missing Manual

In general, fundoplasty is extremely successful at alleviating symptoms of GERD, with a relatively low rate of complications. Nevertheless, significant problems are seen after fundoplasty, and these can be exacerbated by a clinician unaware of the risk or of the altered state of the stomach after fundoplasty. Fundoplasty may be hugely successful in improving the nutrition and lungs of the child with bad GERD, but the surgeon who cedes all postoperative management to others does his patients a disservice. As with other surgical diseases like imperforate anus, many patients require ongoing gentle attention from a clinician who understands the mechanical constraints imposed by the operation.

Feeding

While actual volumetric measurements of the human stomach are elusive, a heuristic estimate is that the normal human stomach holds around 20–25 cm^3/kg of body weight. After fundoplasty, tube-fed babies usually can handle bolus feeds of only about 15 (±2) cm^3/kg. This is certainly adequate for growth, but ignoring this limit is one of the prime causes of retching (see below) postoperatively. In general, feeds can be started within 12 h of fundoplasty (the delay allows anesthetics

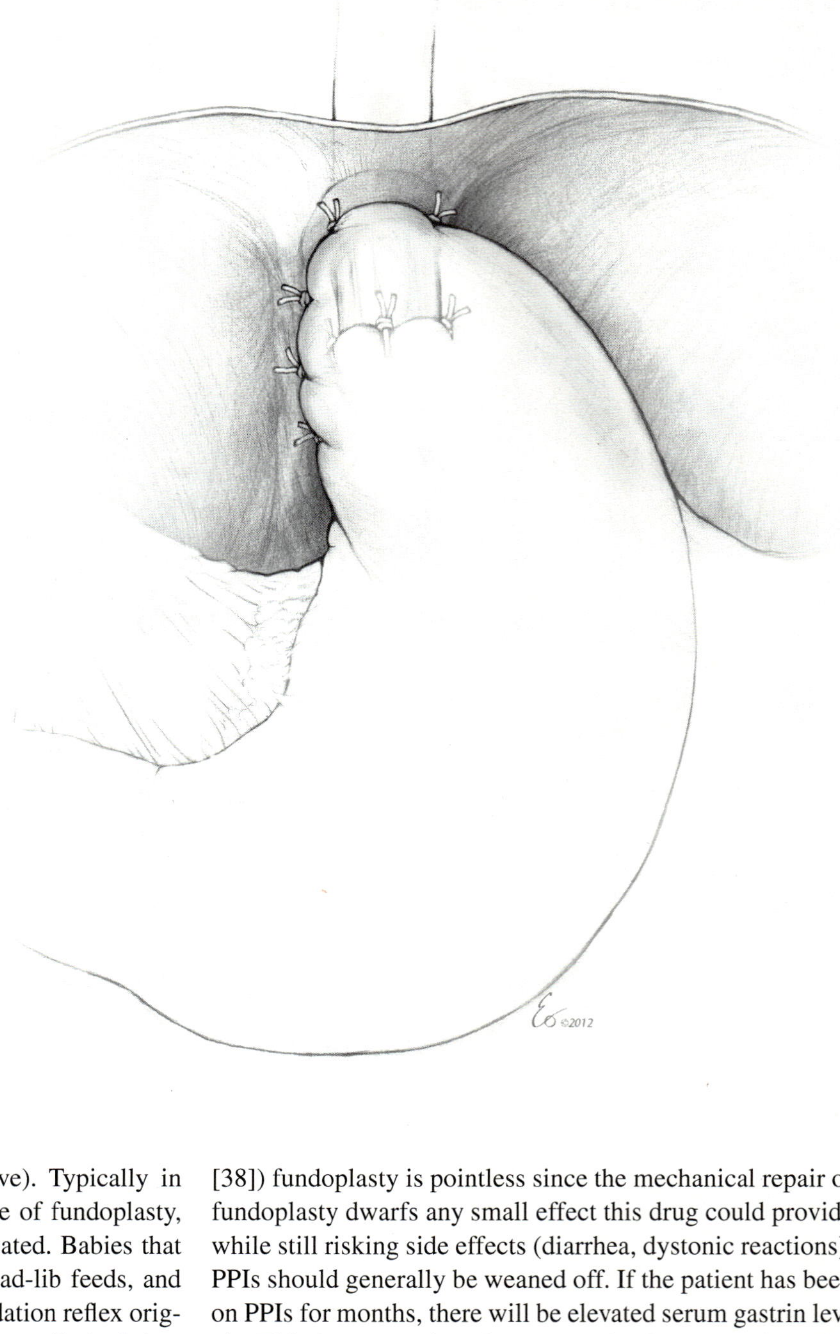

Fig. 5 The Thal fundoplasty is another partial wrap. Unlike the Toupet, the Thal brings stomach anterior to the esophagus to complete a 240° wrap. The inner layer of gastroesophageal sutures are revealed in the ghosted image

and anesthetic-associated nausea to resolve). Typically in infants, a gastrostomy is placed at the time of fundoplasty, and can be used for feeds as soon as indicated. Babies that are *orally* fed can be rapidly advanced to ad-lib feeds, and because of the vagally-mediated accommodation reflex originating in the pharynx, tend to be less volume-limited than gastrostomy fed babies. There is no evidence to support the practice of using all continuous feeds for the immediate postoperative fundoplasty patient, but different surgeons have strong opinions here.

Medications

Once the fundoplasty is completed, anti-reflux medications can be stopped. Ranitidine has no rebound associated with it, and continuing metoclopramide after (and indeed before [38]) fundoplasty is pointless since the mechanical repair of fundoplasty dwarfs any small effect this drug could provide while still risking side effects (diarrhea, dystonic reactions). PPIs should generally be weaned off. If the patient has been on PPIs for months, there will be elevated serum gastrin levels. This hypergastrinemia can persist for up to 6 weeks, raising the risk of hypersecretion of acid in the stomach with subsequent erosive gastritis [61–63]. Empirically, this problem can be ameliorated if PPIs are weaned off over 2–4 weeks. In cases where acid blockade is indicated for some other reason (e.g., to protect the esophageal atresia or laryngoplasty repair, or to guard against steroid-induced gastritis), PPIs should be continued after fundoplication. In other words, PPIs should be continued in any patient for whom they are indicated for mucosal protection or healing. Without an indication, these PPIs offer only complications (fungal overgrowth, hypocalcemia, etc.).

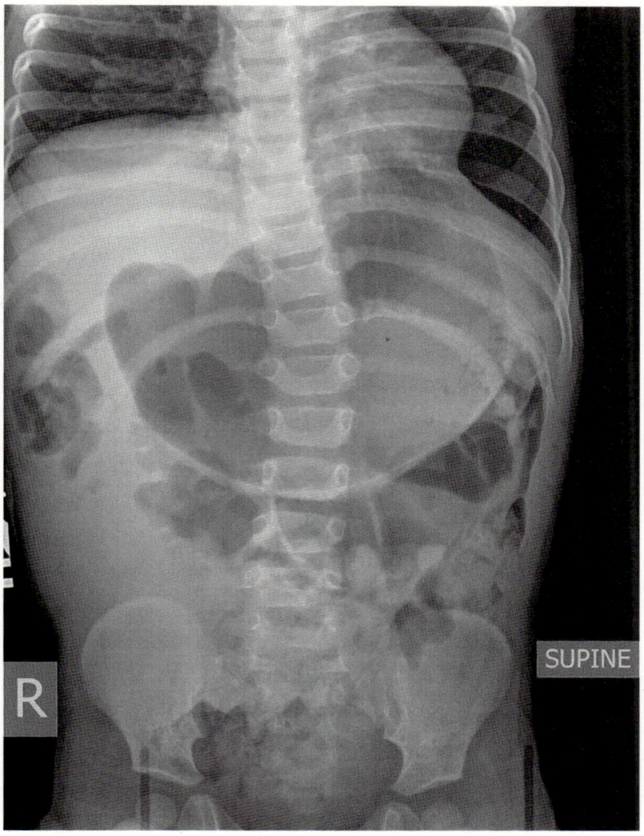

Fig. 6 Gas bloat syndrome. The X-ray shows a massively distended stomach in a baby unable to burp after Nissen fundoplication

Gas Bloat

Gas bloat syndrome is a somewhat-poorly defined "syndrome" in which air introduced into the GI tract either from the tube or via swallowing (aerophagia) is trapped in the stomach by the wrap. Instead of burping, the child can only handle the air two ways: by venting via the gastrostomy, or by passing the air through the anus. The resulting distension, cramping, and pain are the manifestations labeled as "colic" and the irritated child may cry inconsolably or retch. The best way to treat gas bloat is good venting. Some favor the use of a Farrell valve (™), but this long thin tube tends to have uneven performance in small babies in whom the Farrell valve is not the path of least resistance for ingested air. Often, better results are obtained by use of "chimney" venting. Other adjuncts include the use of simethicone, "tummy time," and avoidance of fiber or other feedings that promote gas formation in the colon (Fig. 6).

Dumping

When clinicians talk about "dumping" they really refer to two distinct phenomena after gastric surgery. The first is "early dumping" syndrome, in which relatively high osmotic foods enter the small bowel and induce a period of intestinal hypermotility. The exact pathogenesis is not known, but links to GLP-1, renin-angiotensin, VIP, cholesystokinin, and other mediators have been demonstrated or proposed. The manifestations include pain, cramps, flushing, tachycardia, and watery diarrhea in response to a bolus feed. Of the two syndromes labeled as dumping, this is more rarely seen in practice. Treatment consists of changing to lower osmotic feeds, slowing the rate of delivery, and in intractable cases, very cautious administration of octreotide. Meanwhile, because of the risk of this syndrome, rarely (if ever) should a pyloroplasty be done at the same time as a fundoplasty. The second type of dumping, "late dumping," is better understood as postprandial hypoglycemia (PPHG).

Postprandial Hypoglycemia

PPHG can occur after any gastric procedure, but as a practical matter it is encountered virtually exclusively after fundoplasty in children. Because the reactive hypoglycemia can be severe, this complication is arguably the most dangerous complication of fundoplasty. Because it may be asymptomatic, the method and criteria of diagnosis is in doubt, and awareness is poor, estimates of its prevalence range widely, from 2 to 30 %. PPHG appears to be essentially an overshoot feedback-and-control failure, with a spike in blood glucose leading to an "overshoot" of insulin secretion mediated by the incretin GLP-1. This insulin overshoot then produces hypoglycemia [64].

In practice, we screen every patient after fundoplication for PPHG by checking a series (30, 60, 90, and 120 min) of postprandial glucose levels (d-sticks) once the children are at full feeds, or anytime they exhibit unexplained lethargy, somnolence, irritability or retching. A very high (>180 mg/dL) followed by a very low (<50 mg/dL) sugar is diagnostic. Some premies will exhibit low sugars after feeds without a spike; this is not true PPHG, and more likely represents relatively poor hepatic sugar mobilization.

Treatment of PPHG is aimed at decreasing the rate and magnitude of the rise in glucose after a feed. Obviously, continuous feeding will avoid cyclic blood glucose levels, but also ties the child to a pump, and can exacerbate bloating and retching. Other options include use of any combination of acarbose (which blocks intestinal alpha glucosidase to slow absorption of intraluminal polysaccharides), uncooked cornstarch, microlipid, or even a simple change from formulas containing "corn-syrup solids" (pure glucose) to those containing maltodextrin (variable length short polymers of glucose) or other more complex sugars. Whatever strategy is employed, ongoing home monitoring of post-feed sugars is essential to safe management (and eventual weaning of the interventions used).

Retching

Of all of the complications after fundoplasty, retching is one of the most distressing to parents. Clinicians often mistake retching for evidence of new reflux after fundoplasty, and restart anti-reflux medications to treat this mistaken diagnosis. But wrap failure is actually a very unlikely cause of retching. Retching is not reflux; it is frustrated emesis. Any noxious stimulus that provokes emesis in a baby can cause retching when an intact wrap prevents this active retrograde flow. While mechanical problems such as a herniated wrap or esophageal obstruction certainly can cause retching, more commonly retching is actually evidence that the wrap is intact!

The approach to treating retching is to remove the noxious stimuli. For example, one of the most common causes of retching is over-large feeding boluses. Dropping feeding boluses below 15 cm^3/kg/bolus usually removes this stimulus. Meanwhile, high osmolarity either of feeds (such as elemental formulas) or drugs (especially KCl) decrease emptying while also appearing to directly stimulate vagal afferents in the stomach and duodenum. It is also important to look beyond the stomach. For example, some children retch because they cannot handle their postnasal drip, or because they have an acute exacerbation of pulmonary hypertension, or because they have an occult infection, or because they have unstable blood sugar. In general, a "whole-patient" approach to retching may be required to solve post-fundoplasty feeding intolerance. To solve retching, the doctor must find and eliminate the triggers of nausea, intestinal irritability, and vomiting that are the real sources of retching [65].

Dysphagia

Dysphagia (and odynophagia) occurs more often after Nissen than the partial fundoplications, but in patients of all ages is reported after any type of wrap in around 1 in 20 patients [53, 66]. However, these reports probably fail to capture the mild dysphagia often seen in the immediate postoperative period. While a surgeon can make a proper loose wrap over a large guide, he cannot control inflammation, edema, and related esophageal dysmotility after surgical manipulation. As a result, patients may have a transient (usually no more than 2 weeks, but some as long as 6 months) period of dysphagia. For this reason, for older patients most surgeons recommend a soft diet free of hard-to-swallow meats or breads initially, advice that is moot in the neonate. In some cases of persistent dysphagia, surgeons have tried a short burst of solumedrol or other corticosteroids to relieve the swelling but this has not been studied. Others patients may require gentle dilatation. Dysphagia that persists requires further workup (endoscopy, manometry) to determine if the wrap needs to be revised, or if actually there was another diagnosis (achalasia, eosinophilic esophagitis, etc.) that was mimicking GERD.

Essential Points

- GER is not the same as GERD. While virtually all infants exhibit GER, pulmonary manifestations are the hallmark of GERD.
- Pathological reflux is a mechanical disease that benefits from a mechanical (that is, a surgical) solution. Acid blockade appears to be ineffective or even dangerous for routine use in infants.
- There is no single best test for GERD.
- Surgical fundoplasty is highly effective in properly selected patients, and the effectiveness of the operation is enhanced by proper postoperative feeding strategies.

References

1. Scherer LD, et al. Influence of "GERD" label on parents' decision to medicate infants. Pediatrics. 2013;131(5):839–45.
2. Poets CF, Brockmann PE. Myth: gastroesophageal reflux is a pathological entity in the preterm infant. Semin Fetal Neonatal Med. 2011;16(5):259–63.
3. Mosby. Mosby's medical dictionary. 8th ed. St. Louis: Mosby; 2009. p. 312.
4. Venkatesan NN, Pine HS, Underbrink M. Laryngopharyngeal reflux disease in children. Pediatr Clin North Am. 2013;60(4): 865–78.
5. Ghosh SK, Kahrilas PJ, Brasseur JG. Liquid in the gastroesophageal segment promotes reflux, but compliance does not: a mathematical modeling study. Am J Physiol Gastrointest Liver Physiol. 2008;295(5):G920–33.
6. Kawahara H, Dent J, Davidson G. Mechanisms responsible for gastroesophageal reflux in children. Gastroenterology. 1997;113(2): 399–408.
7. Pandolfino JE, et al. Esophagogastric junction distensibility: a factor contributing to sphincter incompetence. Am J Physiol Gastrointest Liver Physiol. 2002;282(6):G1052–8.
8. Spitz L, McLeod E. Gastroesophageal reflux. Semin Pediatr Surg. 2003;12(4):237–40.
9. Popovic ZB, et al. Differences in left ventricular long-axis function from mice to humans follow allometric scaling to ventricular size. J Physiol. 2005;568(Pt 1):255–65.
10. Muller MJ, et al. Effect of constitution on mass of individual organs and their association with metabolic rate in humans—a detailed view on allometric scaling. PLoS One. 2011;6(7):e22732.
11. Gounaris A, et al. Gastric emptying of preterm neonates receiving domperidone. Neonatology. 2010;97(1):56–60.
12. Gounaris A, et al. Theophylline and gastric emptying in very low birthweight neonates: a randomised controlled trial. Arch Dis Child Fetal Neonatal Ed. 2004;89(4):F297–9.
13. Savage VM, Deeds EJ, Fontana W. Sizing up allometric scaling theory. PLoS Comput Biol. 2008;4(9):e1000171.
14. Vandenplas Y, et al. Gastroesophageal reflux, as measured by 24-hour pH monitoring, in 509 healthy infants screened for risk of sudden infant death syndrome. Pediatrics. 1991;88(4):834–40.
15. Lopez-Alonso M, et al. Twenty-four-hour esophageal impedance-pH monitoring in healthy preterm neonates: rate and characteristics

of acid, weakly acidic, and weakly alkaline gastroesophageal reflux. Pediatrics. 2006;118(2):e299–308.
16. Kamiyama M, et al. Gastroesophageal reflux after repair of congenital diaphragmatic hernia. J Pediatr Surg. 2002;37(12):1681–4.
17. Kawahara H, et al. Physiological and clinical characteristics of gastroesophageal reflux after congenital diaphragmatic hernia repair. J Pediatr Surg. 2010;45(12):2346–50.
18. Sigalet DL, et al. Gastroesophageal reflux associated with large diaphragmatic hernias. J Pediatr Surg. 1994;29(9):1262–5.
19. Pederiva F, et al. Intrinsic esophageal innervation in esophageal atresia without fistula. Pediatr Surg Int. 2008;24(1):95–100.
20. Tsai J, Blinman TA, Collins JL, Laje P, Hedrick HL, Adzick NS, Flake AW. The contribution of hiatal hernia to severe gastroesophageal reflux disease in patients with gastroschisis. J Pediatr Surg. 2014;49(3):395–8.
21. Santos MM, Tannuri U, Maksoud JG. Alterations of enteric nerve plexus in experimental gastroschisis: is there a delay in the maturation? J Pediatr Surg. 2003;38(10):1506–11.
22. Bardhan KD, Strugala V, Dettmar PW. Reflux revisited: advancing the role of pepsin. Int J Otolaryngol. 2012;2012:646901.
23. Abu Jawdeh EG, Martin RJ. Neonatal apnea and gastroesophageal reflux (GER): is there a problem? Early Hum Dev. 2013;89 Suppl 1:S14–6.
24. Dettmar PW, et al. Review article: reflux and its consequences - the laryngeal, pulmonary and oesophageal manifestations. Conference held in conjunction with the 9th International Symposium on Human Pepsin (ISHP) Kingston-upon-Hull, UK, 21-23 April 2010. Aliment Pharmacol Ther. 2011;33:1–71.
25. Macharia EW. Comparison of upper gastrointestinal contrast studies and pH/impedance tests for the diagnosis of childhood gastro-oesophageal reflux. Pediatr Radiol. 2012;42(8):946–51.
26. Chung C, et al. Simultaneous correction of malrotation and gastroesophageal reflux in infants. Am Surg. 1996;62(10):800–2.
27. Tiboni SG, et al. Management of gastroesophageal reflux associated with malrotation in children. J Pediatr Surg. 2011;46(2):289–91.
28. Valusek PA, et al. Does an upper gastrointestinal study change operative management for gastroesophageal reflux? J Pediatr Surg. 2010;45(6):1169–72.
29. Kashyap R, et al. Evaluation of radionuclide gastroesophagography as a suitable screening test for detection of gastroesophageal reflux. Indian Pediatr. 1993;30(5):625–8.
30. Morigeri C, et al. Radionuclide scintigraphy in the evaluation of gastroesophageal reflux in symptomatic and asymptomatic preterm infants. Eur J Nucl Med Mol Imaging. 2008;35(9):1659–65.
31. Johnson DG, et al. Are scintiscans accurate in the selection of reflux patients for pyloroplasty? J Pediatr Surg. 1998;33(4):573–9.
32. Rosen R, et al. Lipid-laden macrophage index is not an indicator of gastroesophageal reflux-related respiratory disease in children. Pediatrics. 2008;121(4):e879–84.
33. Njere I, Stanton M, Davenport M. Identification of pepsin in bronchoalveolar fluid (BAL) as a new test for the detection of pulmonary aspiration associated with gastroesophageal reflux. J Pediatr Surg. 2006;41(10):1787; author reply 1787–8.
34. Duan N, Kravitz RL, Schmid CH. Single-patient (n-of-1) trials: a pragmatic clinical decision methodology for patient-centered comparative effectiveness research. J Clin Epidemiol. 2013;66(8 Suppl):S21–8.
35. Holbrook JT, et al. Lansoprazole for children with poorly controlled asthma: a randomized controlled trial. JAMA. 2012;307(4): 373–81.
36. van der Pol RJ, et al. Efficacy of proton-pump inhibitors in children with gastroesophageal reflux disease: a systematic review. Pediatrics. 2011;127(5):925–35.
37. Terrin G, et al. Ranitidine is associated with infections, necrotizing enterocolitis, and fatal outcome in newborns. Pediatrics. 2012; 129(1):e40–5.
38. Hibbs AM, Lorch SA. Metoclopramide for the treatment of gastroesophageal reflux disease in infants: a systematic review. Pediatrics. 2006;118(2):746–52.
39. Corvaglia L, et al. Pharmacological therapy of gastroesophageal reflux in preterm infants. Gastroenterol Res Pract. 2013;2013: 714564.
40. Levi P, et al. Bethanechol versus antiacids in the treatment of gastroesophageal reflux. Helv Paediatr Acta. 1985;40(5):349–59.
41. Lamian V, et al. Characterization of agonist-induced motilin receptor trafficking and its implications for tachyphylaxis. Mol Pharmacol. 2006;69(1):109–18.
42. Almeida MB, et al. Adequacy of human milk viscosity to respond to infants with dysphagia: experimental study. J Appl Oral Sci. 2011;19(6):554–9.
43. Sevenhuysen GP, Holodinsky C, Dawes C. Development of salivary alpha-amylase in infants from birth to 5 months. Am J Clin Nutr. 1984;39(4):584–8.
44. Zhu Y, Hsu WH, Hollis JH. The impact of food viscosity on eating rate, subjective appetite, glycemic response and gastric emptying rate. PLoS One. 2013;8(6):e67482.
45. Sanaka M, et al. Effects of agar and pectin on gastric emptying and post-prandial glycaemic profiles in healthy human volunteers. Clin Exp Pharmacol Physiol. 2007;34(11):1151–5.
46. Miyazawa R, et al. Effects of pectin liquid on gastroesophageal reflux disease in children with cerebral palsy. BMC Gastroenterol. 2008;8:11.
47. Huang RC, Forbes DA, Davies MW. Feed thickener for newborn infants with gastro-oesophageal reflux. Cochrane Database Syst Rev. 2002;(3):CD003211.
48. Corvaglia L, et al. A thickened formula does not reduce apneas related to gastroesophageal reflux in preterm infants. Neonatology. 2013;103(2):98–102.
49. Rothenberg SS. The first decade's experience with laparoscopic Nissen fundoplication in infants and children. J Pediatr Surg. 2005;40(1):142–6; discussion 147.
50. Rothenberg SS. Two decades of experience with laparoscopic nissen fundoplication in infants and children: a critical evaluation of indications, technique, and results. J Laparoendosc Adv Surg Tech A. 2013;23(9):791–4.
51. Broeders JA, et al. Objective outcomes 14 years after laparoscopic anterior 180-degree partial versus nissen fundoplication: results from a randomized trial. Ann Surg. 2013;258(2):233–9.
52. Broeders JA, et al. Laparoscopic anterior versus posterior fundoplication for gastroesophageal reflux disease: systematic review and meta-analysis of randomized clinical trials. Ann Surg. 2011; 254(1):39–47.
53. Broeders JA, et al. Laparoscopic anterior 180-degree versus nissen fundoplication for gastroesophageal reflux disease: systematic review and meta-analysis of randomized clinical trials. Ann Surg. 2013;257(5):850–9.
54. Broeders JA, et al. Five-year outcome after laparoscopic anterior partial versus Nissen fundoplication: four randomized trials. Ann Surg. 2012;255(4):637–42.
55. Rothenberg SS, Bratton D. The effects of laparoscopic Nissen fundoplication to enhance pulmonary function in the treatment of a patient with severe asthma and gastroesophageal reflux disease. J Allergy Clin Immunol. 2008;121(4):1069–70.
56. Macharia EW, et al. Fundoplication in ventilator-dependent infants with gastro-oesophageal reflux. Eur J Pediatr Surg. 2012;22(1): 91–6.
57. Rothenberg SS, et al. Laparoscopic fundoplication to enhance pulmonary function in children with severe reactive airway disease and gastroesophageal reflux disease. Surg Endosc. 1997;11(11):1088–90.
58. St Peter SD, et al. Minimal vs extensive esophageal mobilization during laparoscopic fundoplication: a prospective randomized trial. J Pediatr Surg. 2012;46(1):163–8.

59. Ngerncham M, et al. Risk factors for recurrent gastroesophageal reflux disease after fundoplication in pediatric patients: a case-control study. J Pediatr Surg. 2007;42(9):1478–85.
60. Osborne MP, et al. Rotavirus-induced changes in the microcirculation of intestinal villi of neonatal mice in relation to the induction and persistence of diarrhea. J Pediatr Gastroenterol Nutr. 1991;12(1):111–20.
61. Fossmark R, et al. Rebound acid hypersecretion after long-term inhibition of gastric acid secretion. Aliment Pharmacol Ther. 2005;21(2):149–54.
62. Fossmark R, Waldum H. Rebound acid hypersecretion. Aliment Pharmacol Ther. 2007;25(8):999–1000; author reply 1000.
63. Waldum HL, et al. Rebound acid hypersecretion from a physiological, pathophysiological and clinical viewpoint. Scand J Gastroenterol. 2010;45(4):389–94.
64. Calabria AC, et al. Postoperative surveillance and detection of postprandial hypoglycemia after fundoplasty in children. J Pediatr. 2011;159(4):597–601.e1.
65. Cook R, Blinman T. The case of the wretched retcher. ICAN. 2009;1(2):94–7.
66. Ashcraft KW, et al. Thal fundoplication: a simple and safe operative treatment for gastroesophageal reflux. J Pediatr Surg. 1978;13(6D):643–7.

Part III

Education, Simulation and Quality Improvement

Airway Emergencies in the Neonate: Preparedness at the Bedside

Janet Lioy, J. Thomas Paliga, and Hitesh Deshmuhk

Overview

Bag mask ventilation has traditionally been used as the mainstay in neonatal resuscitation. The NRP guidelines maintain that positive pressure ventilation is the most important step in newborn resuscitation [13, 39, 62]. However, the recommended use of simple bag mask ventilation can be particularly difficult and, often times, ineffective in newborn infants. In a study of bag mask ventilation of almost 60 very preterm infants under 1 kg, 48 % demonstrated significant mask leak which could only be corrected with repositioning. Inappropriate positioning caused significant airway obstruction 25 % of the time [49]. In another study using colorimetric detectors, airway obstruction occurred in a majority of low birth weight infants receiving bag mask ventilation during resuscitation [13]. Consequently, a well-prepared neonatal unit will have a well-defined process for addressing airway emergencies far beyond the use of bag mask ventilation.

J. Lioy, M.D. (✉)
Attending Neonatologist, Director Neonatal Outreach, Medical Director, Neonatal Airway Program, The Children's Hospital of Philadelphia, Associate Professor of Clinical Pediatrics, The University of Pennsylvania Perelman School of Medicine, Philadelphia, PA 19104, USA
e-mail: lioy@email.chop.edu

J.T. Paliga
Division of Plastic Surgery, Department of Surgery, The Children's Hospital of Philadelphia, Philadelphia, PA, USA

Duke University School of Medicine, Philadelphia and Durham, PA & NC, USA

H. Deshmuhk, M.D.
Division of Neonatology, Pulmonary Biology, Cincinnati Children's Hospital Medical Center, Cincinnati, OH, USA

University of Cincinnati School of Medicine, Cincinnati, OH, USA

Neonatal Specific Algorithms

Traditionally, there was no need for algorithms. As the patients have become more complex and varied, neonatologists have developed specific algorithms for our heterogeneous population of neonates and infants that we have refined, used, and taught for more than 10 years now. Due to the major increase in births of infants with congenital anomalies such as oropharyngeal teratomas, CHAOS, severe micrognathia and similarly complex airway disorders being born at our institution, this became a necessary part of overall preparation for airway emergencies (Fig. 1a–c).

Implementation of Strategy: Mobilizing the Airway Team

While unnerving, dealing with a critical airway in a small neonate can be managed with five easy steps. When possible, anticipation, identification, preparation, mobilization, and execution should be the immediate steps that are set forth by the neonatal care team during an airway emergency (Fig. 2).

Anticipation

It is never a good idea to extubate or manipulate an unstable airway without alerting another skilled airway person. In the neonatal unit, emergency department, or in transport of an infant with a critical airway, alert another physician, anesthetist, or advanced practitioner. Making nurses and respiratory therapists aware of the plan to manipulate the endotracheal tube should be included in the first step of the process as well, so the entire care team can anticipate the clinical course.

J. Lioy and S.E. Sobol (eds.), *Disorders of the Neonatal Airway: Fundamentals for Practice*,
DOI 10.1007/978-1-4939-1610-8_27, © Springer Science+Business Media New York 2015

Identification

All caretakers should be made aware of the airway status of the neonatal patient. Furthermore, diagnoses and comorbidities need to be carefully evaluated for issues that would confound an airway emergency. Becoming familiar with the numerous and varied diagnoses causing acute airway obstruction (refer to Fig. 11 of chapter "Challenges of the Neonatal Airway"), is a good starting point. Additionally, measures should be taken so that patients with a history of a difficult or critical airway are readily available and recognized as such.

Preparation

A solid airway emergency plan includes equipment that is both ready for use and well known to those who will use it. A simple tackle box with laryngoscopes, multiple sized endotracheal tubes, stylettes, laryngeal mask airways, oral and nasal airways, and facemasks is all one needs to have at the bedside. Another option in a busy airway center is a dedicated mobile cart that has all the necessary equipment in labeled drawers. Additionally, more specialized ENT equipment, such as halogen light sources with fiberoptic bronchoscopes, specialized laryngoscopes, videolaryngoscopy and even a large display monitor should be available in large center neonatal-infant ICUs with large airway pathology volume [19, 27, 28].

Mobilization

Recruitment of the airway team in an instant is essential to any successful airway emergency process. Specialized reliable paging systems should be able to quickly alert trained personnel (physicians, respiratory therapists, nurses, clerks) for quick activation and mobilization of the team.

Execution

With a well-organized team, equipment available at the bedside, and roles clearly established, the final step in the process is addressing the critical airway. The exact techniques

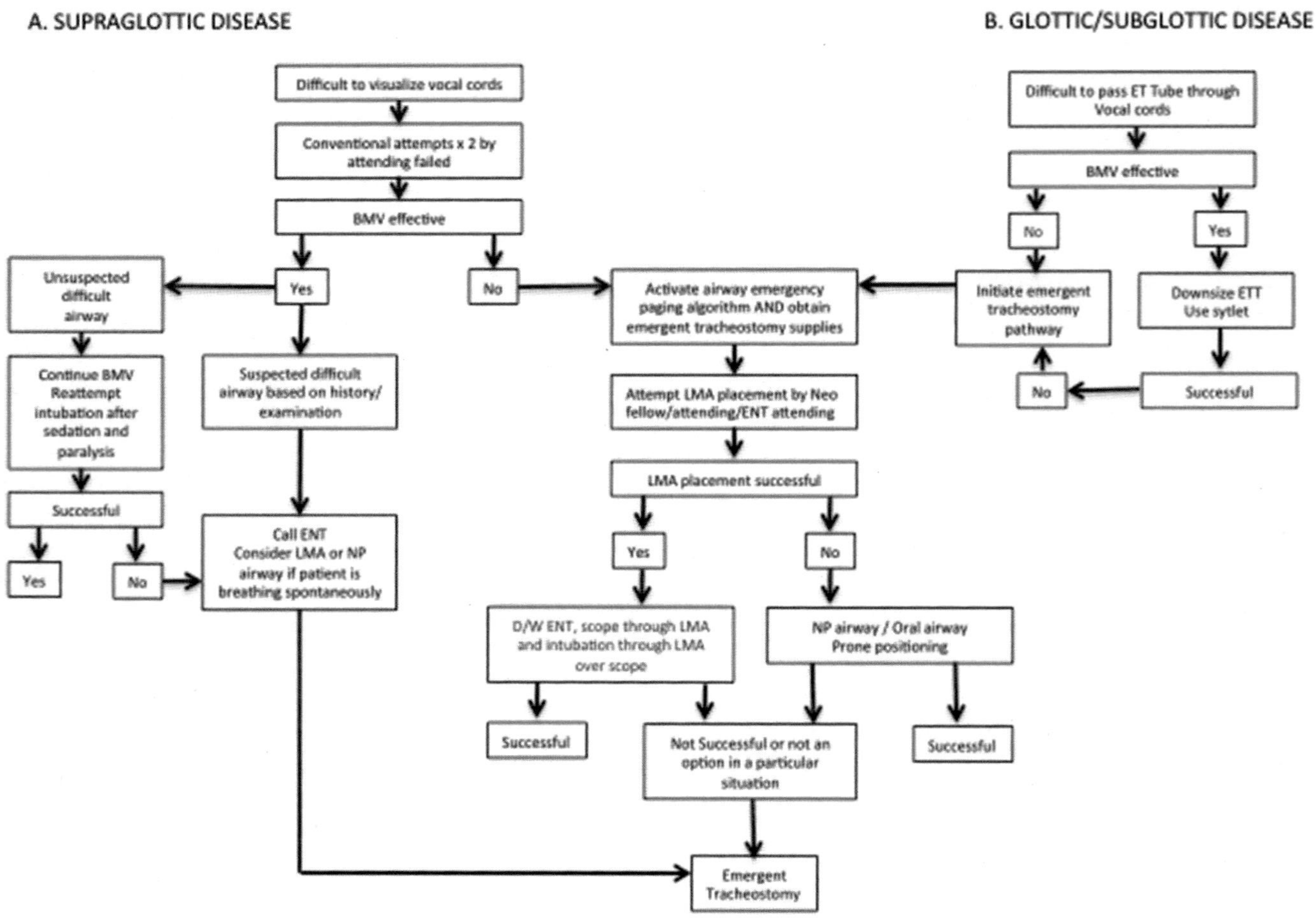

Fig. 1 Emergency Airway Management Algorithm for Difficult-Critical Airways. Note the differences and similarities between neonatal emergency algorithms and pediatric algorithms. (**a**) Neonatal algorithm (*courtesy of The Neonatal Airway Program-CHOP*). (**b**) algorithm, (adapted from Wheeler and Shanley, et al. eds. Resuscitaiton and Stabilization of the Critically Ill Child. Springer, 2009

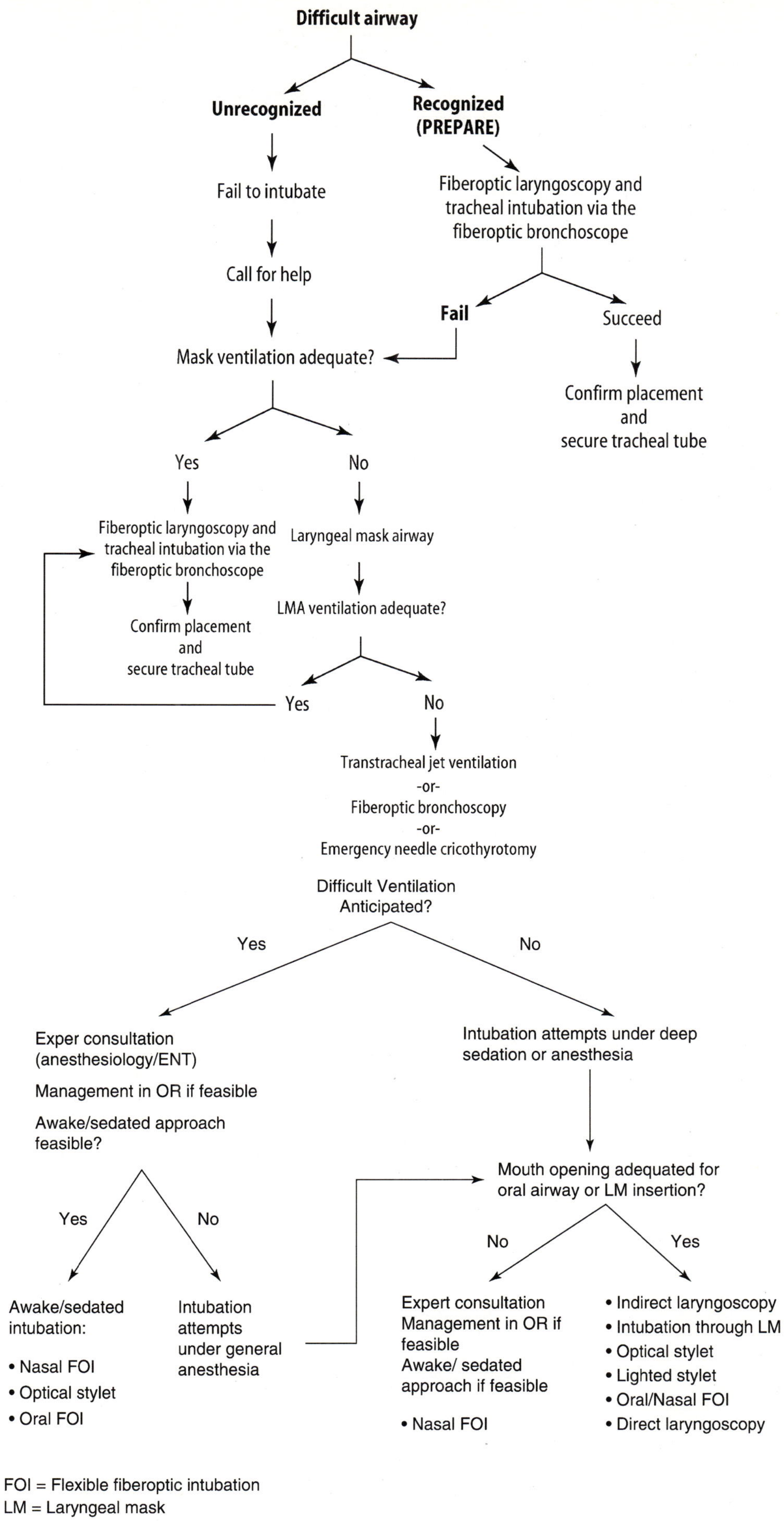

Fig. 1 (continued)

for establishing an airway are going to be specific for the individual patient. As attempts are made to rectify the obstruction, the team will work up the hierarchy of equipment and personnel available until the problem is resolved.

Education/Simulation Drills

Integral to being prepared is education and simulation. Education has to be global, widespread, and include all caregivers. An essential component of this education is frequent updates about equipment, new personnel, and newly established algorithms. There also must be an insurance of competency for all members of the team. The way to validate this competency is via simulated clinical scenarios. This is a relatively novel approach to training and should be utilized frequently, especially for procedures that do not occur often. Simulation should include key team members and key scenarios such as unplanned extubation, difficult airway conditions, critical airway conditions, and unplanned delivery of an infant with a critical airway.

Software and mannequins that allow for simulated reality are integral support components for training. These technologies allow for immediate feedback during procedures via changes in vital signs, respiratory distress symptoms, etc. These simulations should occur on a regular basis, at least once a week, and in a variety of different environments where these emergencies may occur. Debriefing and feedback should be a regular part of concluding simulated training and education sessions [62].

Activating Airway Emergency Response Team (Fig. 3)

Necessary Equipment for Airway Emergency Preparedness in the Neonate and Infant

Noninvasive Equipment

Bag Mask Ventilation

Bag mask ventilation is the cornerstone of neonatal resuscitation and is always attempted first. As mentioned previously in one study in premature infants, it can be difficult to adequately seal the facemask during bag mask ventilation thereby underestimating the delivered tidal volume [13].

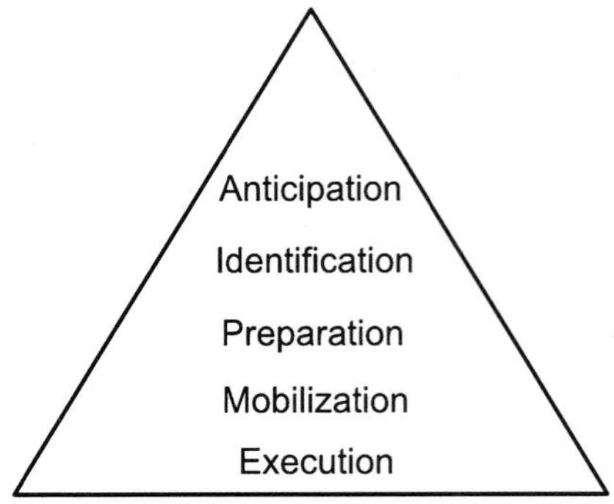

Fig. 2 "Pyramid of Action." Useful for quick thinking on step-by-step decision tree

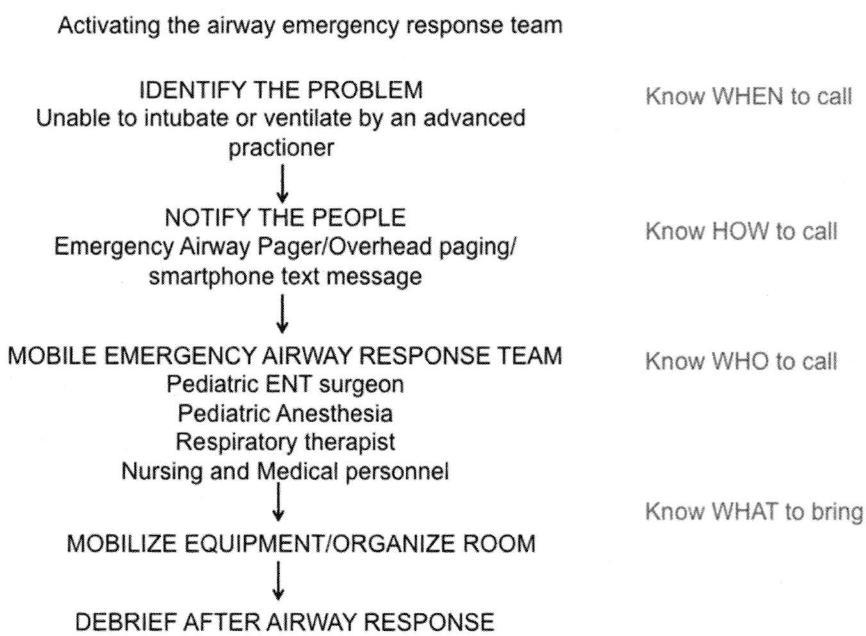

Fig. 3 "Algorithm of Action." Useful for actionable steps to mobilize team members

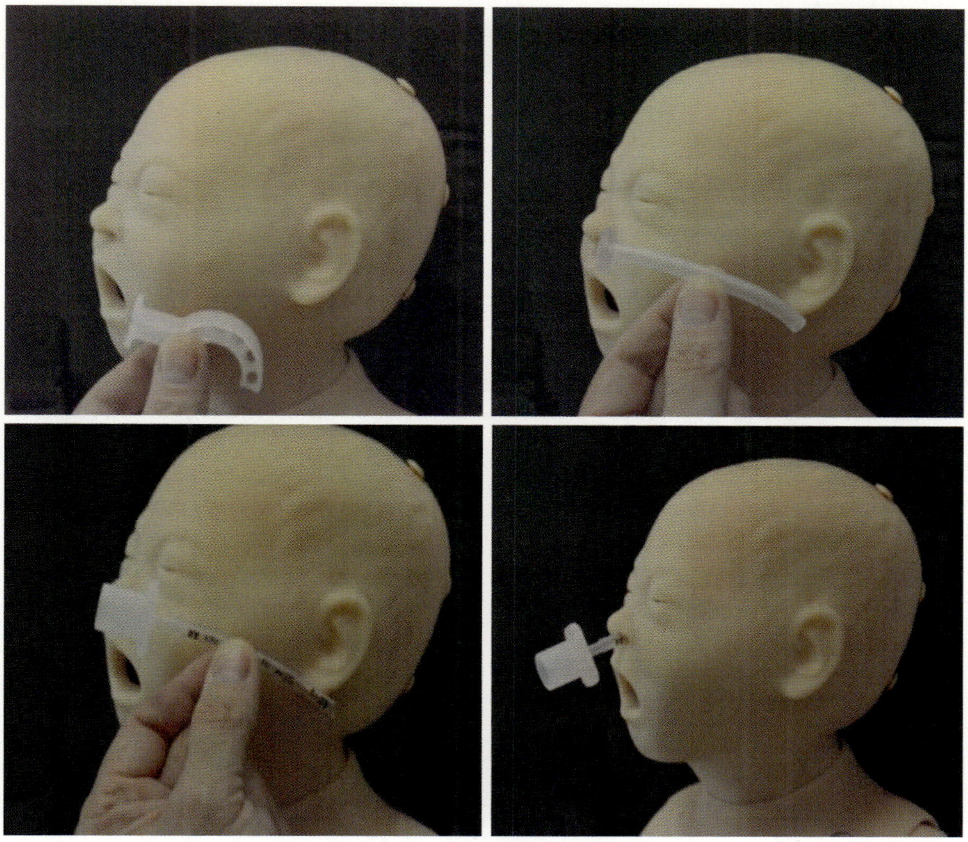

Fig. 4 Nasal Pharyngeal Airways. Guide to insertion, placement depth and stabilization of NP airways in life threatening oral obstruction. Note the nasal ETT is useful due to ease of bagging with connector

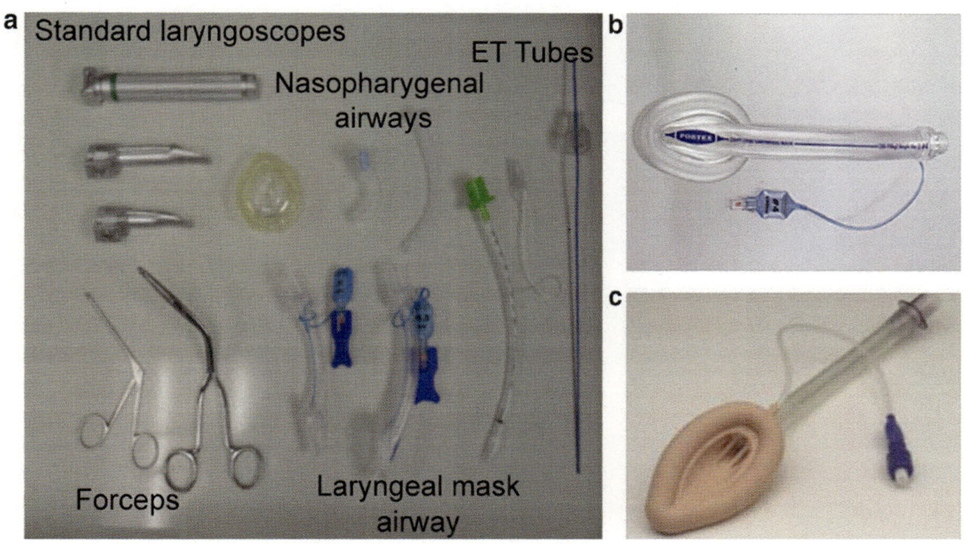

Fig. 5 Picture of essential intubation equipment-laryngoscopes, masks, LMAs, intubating nasal forceps

Oral Airway/Nasal Trumpet/Endotracheal Tube

Oral airways, nasal trumpets and nasal endotracheal tubes are often overlooked as a quick method to bypass tongue-based obstruction. These tools can provide a nasopharyngeal airway that can be used for hand ventilation and suctioning during emergencies (Figs. 4 and 5).

Laryngeal Mask Airway (LMA)

Also often overlooked are laryngeal mask airways. The LMA is a simple, easy to place device that can provide immediate access to the airway. Recently, LMA has been added to the tool set for noninvasive neonatal resuscitation. In a study evaluating newborns requiring positive pressure

Fig. 6 Springloading a bronchoscope-LMA with an ETT. A useful skill to allow rapid intubation over a bronchoscope during intubation of critical airway

ETT	Bronchoscope	Laryngeal Mask Airway	Spring load Scope
2.5	None	1/1.5	No
3.0	2.2	1/1/5	Yes
3.5	2.2./2.8	1/1/5	Yes

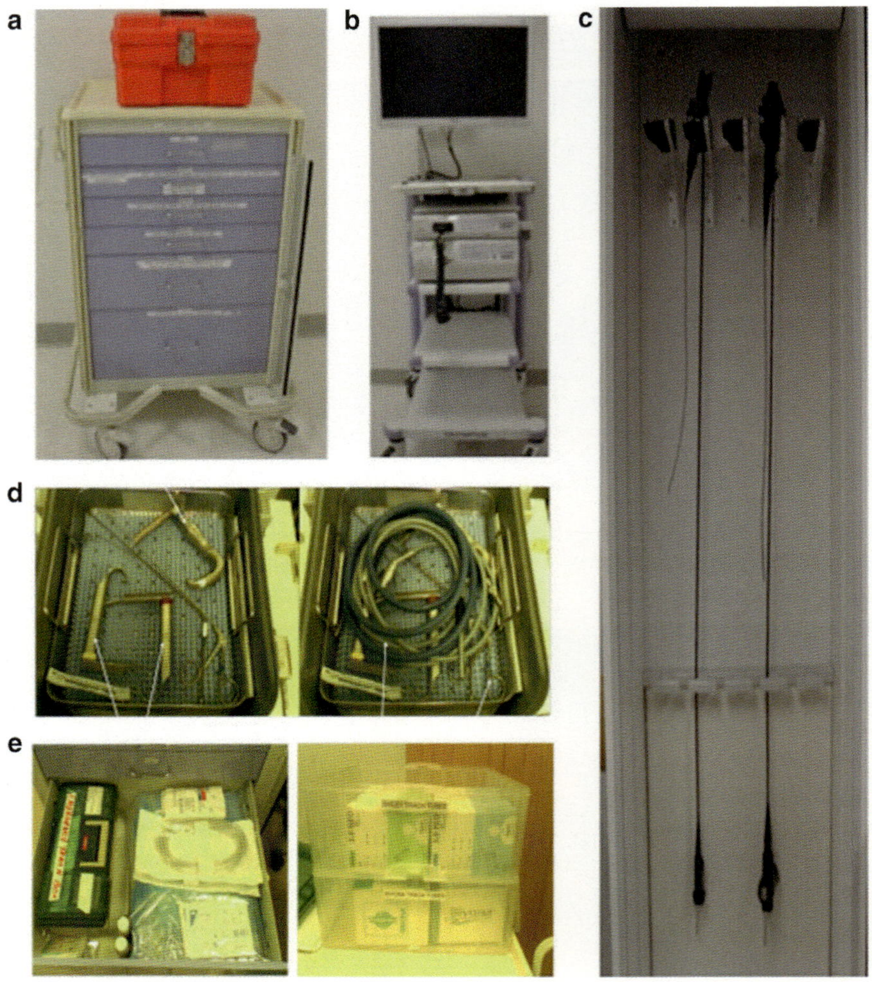

Fig. 7 AirwayCart and equipment: (**a**) airway cart, (**b**) Olympus Monitor-video recorder, (**c**) bronchoscopes, (**d**) special laryngoscopes—high intensity light source, (**e**) Tracheostomy equipment

ventilation, the LMA was successfully inserted on the first attempt and provided an airway with no complications recorded [39]. Intubating through an LMA is also possible when the proper equipment is mobilized beforehand. A bronchoscope spring-loaded with an endotracheal tube can be threaded through the LMA to intubate the trachea [27, 39, 56] (Figs. 6 and 7a–e).

Having a well-equipped, sturdy, and mobile cart containing all the necessary equipment is a top priority in an effective response to an airway emergency. The cart should have 6–7 drawers that are clearly labeled with basic airway equipment. Scopes, tubes, and masks should be kept in the upper drawers for easiest access. Larger equipment (fiber optic equipment and light sources, tracheostomy surgical trays) should be kept in the bottom drawers. Basic emergency equipment should also be kept in a medium-sized box kept atop the cart for rapid deployment to remote areas.

Direct/Indirect Laryngoscopy Equipment

Fiber Optic

Fiber optic laryngoscopy is frequently used for neonatal airway emergencies, particularly in sizes 2.2 and 2.8. Due to the size of the neonatal airway and limitations on the endotracheal tube, these are the only scopes that can be used. These

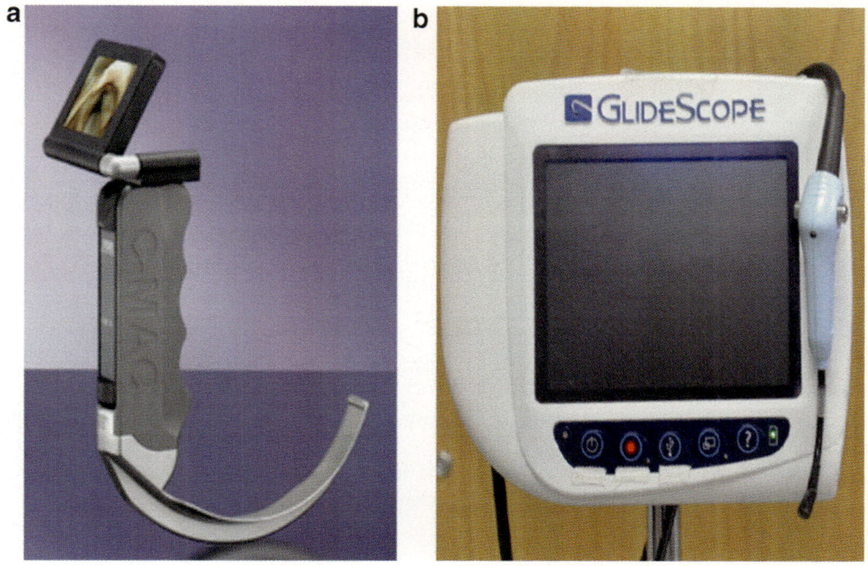

Fig. 8 Videolaryngoscopy: Glidescope and Storz CMAC-PM

scopes are equipped with xenon gas light source to provide optimal visualization of structures. As mentioned previously these, can be spring-loaded and used through an LMA. Furthermore, visualization with these scopes ranges from the nares to the carina, making them incredibly versatile. These are often specially handled and sterilized through very stringent procedures.

Fiber Optic Monitor/Light Source

Necessarily supporting fiber optic scopes is a cart combining both the Xenon source and a large HD flat-screen monitor with recording capabilities. This cart is mobile as to allow for rapid access to the bedside.

Direct

Traditional Neonatal Laryngoscope

The most commonly used laryngoscopes. These come in sizes 00 to 1-blade and should be available in all emergency airway carts.

Specialized Neonatal Laryngoscopes

More sophisticated scopes should be available for higher-level airway personnel (i.e., ENT and Anesthesia). These scopes require a portable halogen light source for illumination of the airway [61].

Indirect

Indirect video laryngoscopy has gained immense popularity for use in airway emergencies in neonatal units due to adoption of appropriate sizes for the smallest of infants. There are a few products on the market that can be used in neonates. The learning curve for these technologies is a bit steeper than some the traditional techniques. Practice and frequent use are the mainstays for efficacy (Fig. 8a, b).

A Last Resort: Cricothyroidotomy?

Cricothyroidotomies are not recommended in children less than 10 years of age as complication rates as high as 40 % have been reported, however recent discussion in pediatric critical care using large bore angiocatheter and transtracheal jet ventilation has been proposed as a life saving measure [63]. Due to the small almost nonexistent cricothyroid membrane in the infant and child needle cricothyrotomy is difficult to accomplish and not routinely recommended [27, 28, 56, 63].

Summary

Neonatal airway emergencies arise at any time and knowledge of the variety of levels of obstruction, quick thinking to act rapidly and available specialized equipment is essential. Team work and preparation is key in avoiding unwanted consequences in this population who lack reserve. Review of algorithms and maintenance of equipment is vital to comfort in response to neonatal airway emergencies.

References

1. Altman KW, Wetmore RF, Marsh RR. Congenital airway abnormalities in patients requiring hospitalization. Arch Otolaryngol Head Neck Surg. 1999;125(5):525–8. PubMed PMID: 10326809.
2. Arensman R. Surgical intervention for respiratory distress and airway management. In: Goldsmith J, Karotkin E, editors. Assisted ventilation of the neonate. 5th ed. Philadelphia, PA: Elsevier Saunders; 2011.
3. Bergeson PS, Shaw JC. Are infants really obligatory nasal breathers? Clin Pediatr (Pa). 2001;40(10):567–9. PubMed PMID: 11681824.
4. Bull P. Evaluation of the pediatric airway by rigid endoscopy. In: Mayer C, Cotton R, editors. Practical pediatric otolaryngology. Philadelphia, PA: Lippincott Williams & Wilkins; 1996.

5. Carrelton S, Brown C. Bag mask ventilation. In: Walls R, Murphy M, editors. Manual of emergency airway management. Philadelphia, PA: Lippincott, Williams and Wilkins; 2012.
6. Cotton R, Prescott, CA. Congenital anomalies of the larynx. In: Cotton R, Mayer C, editor. Philadelphia, PA: Lippincott Williams & Wilkins; 1996.
7. Desai B, Beattie L, Ryan MF, Falgiani M. Visual diagnosis: pediatric airway emergency. Case Rep Emerg Med. 2012;2012:495363. PubMed PMID: 23326717. Pubmed Central PMCID: 3542885.
8. Dickison AE. The normal and abnormal pediatric upper airway. Recognition and management of obstruction. Clin Chest Med. 1987;8(4):583–96. PubMed PMID: 3322644.
9. Dieckmann R. Pediatric assessment. In: Gausche-Hill MFS, Yamamoto L, editors. APLS: the pediatric emergency medicine. 4th ed. Burlington: Jones and Bartlett; 2004.
10. Drummond GB. Keep a clear airway. Br J Anaesth. 1991;66(2):153–6. PubMed PMID: 1817613.
11. Fearon B, Whalen JS. Tracheal dimensions in the living infant (preliminary report). Ann Otol Rhinol Laryngol. 1967;76(5):965–74. PubMed PMID: 6074243.
12. Fiascone J, Vreeland P. Neonatal lung disease and respiratory care. In: Burton G, Hodgkin J, Ward J, editors. Respiratory care: a guide to clinical practice, vol. 4. Philadelphia, PA: Lippincott Williams and Wilkins; 1997.
13. Finer NN, Rich W, Wang C, Leone T. Airway obstruction during mask ventilation of very low birth weight infants during neonatal resuscitation. Pediatrics. 2009;123(3):865–9. PubMed PMID: 19255015.
14. Gerber M, Dunham ME, Holinger LD. Stidor, aspiration and cough. In: Byron J, editor. Bailey's head & neck surgery—otolaryngology. Philadelphia, PA: Lippincott Williams & Wilkins; 2001.
15. Gibson S. Aerodigestive tract foreign bodies. In: Cotton R, Mayer C, editors. Practical pediatric otolaryngology. Philadelphia, PA: Lippincott Williams & Wilkins; 1996.
16. Hess D, Susan P. Neonatal lung disease and respiratory care. In: Burton J, Hodgkin M, Ward J, editors. Respiratory care: a guide to clinical practice. 4th ed. Philadelphia, PA: Lippincott Williams & Wilkins; 1997.
17. Hobolth N, Buchmann G, Sandberg LE. Congenital choanal atresia. Acta Paediatr Scand. 1967;56(3):286–94. PubMed PMID: 5340416.
18. Hudgel DW, Hendricks C. Palate and hypopharynx—sites of inspiratory narrowing of the upper airway during sleep. Am Rev Respir Dis. 1988;138(6):1542–7. PubMed PMID: 3202504.
19. Jacobs I. Bronchoscopy. In: Mattei P, editor. Fundamentals of pediatric surgery. New York: Springer; 2011.
20. John S, Swischuk LE. Airway imaging in children. In: Johnson J, Newlands S, Bailey B, editors. Byron J Bailey's head & neck surgery—otolaryngology. Philadelphia, PA: Lippincott Williams & Wilkins; 2001.
21. Karlovich G, Goldsmith J, Karotkin E. Resusication. In: Goldsmith J, Karotkin K, editors. Assisted ventilation of the neonate. 5th ed. New York: Elsevier Saunders; 2011.
22. Keller JL, Kacker A. Choanal atresia, CHARGE association, and congenital nasal stenosis. Otolaryngol Clin North Am. 2000;33(6):1343–51, viii. PubMed PMID: 11449791.
23. Keller R, Farmer D. Surgical disorders of chest and airways. In: Tauesch E, Gleason M, Devaskar S, editors. Avery's diseases of the newborn. New York: Elsevier Saunders; 2010.
24. Kurth CD, LeBard SE. Association of postoperative apnea, airway obstruction, and hypoxemia in former premature infants. Anesthesiology. 1991;75(1):22–6. PubMed PMID: 2064055.
25. Litman RS, Weissend EE, Shibata D, Westesson PL. Developmental changes of laryngeal dimensions in unparalyzed, sedated children. Anesthesiology. 2003;98(1):41–5. PubMed PMID: 12502977.
26. Lowinger D, Ohlms L. Otolaryngology: head and neck surgery. In: Hansen A, Pudler M, editors. Manual of neonatal surgical intensive care. 2nd ed. Shelton: People's Medical Publishing House; 2009. p. 70–118.
27. Luten R, Kissoon N. Approach to the pediatric airway. In: Walls R, Murphy MF, Luten RC, editors. Manual of emergency airway management. Philadelphia, PA: Lippincott, Williams and Wilkins; 2004. p. 263–81.
28. Luten R, Mick N. Differentiating aspects of pediatric airway. In: Walls R, Murphy M, editors. Manual of emergency airway management. 4th ed. Philadelphia, PA: Lippincott, Williams and Wilkins; 2012.
29. Mace SE, Khan N. Needle cricothyrotomy. Emerg Med Clin North Am. 2008;26((4)):1085–101, xi. PubMed PMID: 19059102.
30. Maniglia AJ, Goodwin Jr WJ. Congenital choanal atresia. Otolaryngol Clin North Am. 1981;14(1):167–73. PubMed PMID: 7254838.
31. Mehta R, Hariprakash S, Cox P, Wheeler D. Diseases of upper respiratory tract. In: Wheeler D, Wong H, Shanley T, editors. The respiratory tract in pediatric critical illness and injury. New York: Springer; 2009.
32. Miller MJ, Carlo WA, Strohl KP, Fanaroff AA, Martin RJ. Effect of maturation on oral breathing in sleeping premature infants. J Pediatr. 1986;109(3):515–9. PubMed PMID: 3746545.
33. Morley C. Continuous distending pressure. Arch Dis Child Fetal Neonatal Ed. 1999;81(2):F152–6. PubMed PMID: 10448188. Pubmed Central PMCID: 1720991.
34. Moss I. Physiologic considerations. In: McMillian J, Feigin RD, DeAngelis CD, editors. Oski's Pedaitrics. Philadelphia, PA: Lippencott Williams & Wilkins; 2006. p. 300–5.
35. Myer 3rd CM, O'Connor DM, Cotton RT. Proposed grading system for subglottic stenosis based on endotracheal tube sizes. Ann Otol Rhinol Laryngol. 1994;103(4 Pt 1):319–23. PubMed PMID: 8154776.
36. Myers C. Inflammatory diseases of the pediatric airway. In: Cotton R, Mayer C, editors. Practical pediatric otolaryngology. Philadelphia, PA: Lippincott Williams and Wilkins; 1996.
37. Nandi PR, Charlesworth CH, Taylor SJ, Nunn JF, Dore CJ. Effect of general anaesthesia on the pharynx. Br J Anaesth. 1991;66(2):157–62. PubMed PMID: 1817614.
38. Othetrsen H, Andre H. Choanal atresia, intraoral obstructions, laryngeal obstructions, laryngomalacia, webs, atresia, laryngoceles, lyphangiomas and hemangiomas papilloma. ashcraft and holder: pediatric surgery. New York: W.B. Saunders; 1993.
39. Paterson SJ, Byrne PJ, Molesky MG, Seal RF, Finucane BT. Neonatal resuscitation using the laryngeal mask airway. Anesthesiology. 1994;80((6)):1248—53;discussion 27A. PubMed PMID: 8010471.
40. Polgar G. Airway resistance in the newborn infant. Preliminary communication. J Pediatr. 1961;59:915–21. PubMed PMID: 14487521.
41. Polgar G, Kong GP. The nasal resistance of newborn infants. J Pediatr. 1965;67(4):557–67. PubMed PMID: 5833190.
42. Pudler M. Cleft lip/palate and robin sequence. In: Hansen A, Pudler M, editors. Otolaryngology: head and neck surgery. 2nd ed. Shelton: People's Medical Publishing House; 2009.
43. Rennie J. Neonatal resusication. In: Donn S, Sinha S, editors. Manual of neonatal respiratory care. New York: Springer; 2012.
44. Rutter M. Congenital airway and respiratory tract anomalies. In: Wheeler D, Wong H, Shanley T, editors. The respiratory tract in pediatric critical illness and injury. New York: Springer; 2009. p. 163–93.
45. Santillanes G, Gausche-Hill M. Pediatric airway management. Emerg Med Clin North Am. 2008;26((4)):961–75, ix. PubMed PMID: 19059095.
46. Sarnaik A, Heidemann SM. Respiratory pathophysiology and regulation. In: Kleigman R, Rehrman RE, Jenson HB, editors. Nelson's textbook of pediatrics. 18th ed. Philadelphia, PA: Saunders; 2007.

47. Scanlon C, Spearman C, Sheldon R. Neonatal and pediatric respiartory care. In: Kacmarek R, Stoller J, Heuer A, editors. Egan's fundamentals of respiratory care. 10th ed. New York: Springer; 1995.
48. Schaffer T, Wolfson M. Upper airway: structure, function and development. In: Abman S, Polin R, Fox W, editors. Fetal and neonatal physiology. 4th ed. Philadelphia, PA: Elsevier Saunders; 2011.
49. Schmolzer GM, Dawson JA, Kamlin CO, O'Donnell CP, Morley CJ, Davis PG. Airway obstruction and gas leak during mask ventilation of preterm infants in the delivery room. Arch Dis Child Fetal Neonatal Ed. 2011;96(4):F254–7. PubMed PMID: 21081593.
50. Stern Y, Cotton RT. Evaluation of the noisy infant. In: Cotton R, Charles M, editors. Practical pediatric otolaryngology. Philadelphia, PA: Lippincott Williams and Wilkins; 2001.
51. Vauthy P. Evaluation of the pediatric airway by flexible endoscopy. In: Cotton R, Mayer C, editors. Practical pediatric otolaryngology. Philadelphia, PA: Lippincott, Williams and Wilkins; 1999.
52. Walner D, Cotton RT. Acquired anomalies of the larynx and trachea. In: Cotton R, Mayer C, editors. Practical pediatric otolaryngology. Philadelphia, PA: Lippincott Williams & Wilkins; 1996.
53. Wetmore R. Management of acute airway obstruction. In: Wetmore R, Muntz HR, McGill TJ, editors. Pediatric otolaryngology: principles and practice pathways. New York: Thieme; 2000.
54. Wetmore R. Tracheotomy. In: Wetmore R, Muntz HR, McGill TJ, editors. Pediatric otolaryngology. Philadelphia, PA: Springer; 2003.
55. Wetmore RF, Marsh RR, Thompson ME, Tom LW. Pediatric tracheostomy: a changing procedure? Ann Otol Rhinol Laryngol. 1999;108(7 Pt 1):695–9. PubMed PMID: 10435931.
56. Wheeler D, Spaeth J, Mehta R, Hariprakash S, Cox P. Pediatric Critical Care Medicine: Ed. Shanley, Wheeler, Wong: Volume 1: Care of the Critically Ill or Injured ChildChapter 28. Pediatric Difficult Airway. Assessment and management of pediatric airway. In: Wheeler D, Wong H, Shanley T, editor. New York: Springer; 2009.
57. Whitaker K. Assessment of the neonatal and pediatric patient. In: Whitaker K, editor. Comprehensive perinatal & pediatric respiratory care. 3rd ed. New York: Delmar; 2001.
58. Wilson TG. Stridor in infancy. J Laryngol Otol. 1952;66(9):437–51. PubMed PMID: 12990908.
59. Wiseman K, Donn S. Laryngoscopy and endotracheal intubation. In: Donn S, Sinha S, editors. Manual of neonatal respiratory care. 3rd ed. New York: Springer; 2012.
60. Wittenborg MH, Gyepes MT, Crocker D. Tracheal dynamics in infants with respiratory distress, stridor, and collapsing trachea. Radiology. 1967;88(4):653–62. PubMed PMID: 6020927.
61. Wood R. Bronchoscopy in pediatric intesnive care unit. In: Wheeler D, Wong H, Shanley T, editors. The respiratory tract in pediatric critical illness and injury. New York: Springer; 2009.
62. Wycoff M, McGowan J, Coby C, Fairchild K, Henry L, Steven R. Textbook of neonatal resuscitation. In: McGowan J, editor. 6th ed. Elkgrove: American Academy of Pediatrics and American Heart Association; 2012.
63. Zur K. The critical airway. In: Mattei P, editor. Fundamentals of pediatric surgery. New York: Springer; 2011.

Unanticipated Airway Emergencies: Resuscitation in the Delivery Room and Emergency Department

Saima Aftab, Nathan W. Mick, and Joshua Nagler

Section 1: Resuscitation in the Delivery Room

Saima Aftab

Preparation for a Routine Delivery

In general, in order to adequately resuscitate and stabilize a newborn with anticipated difficulties, the delivery room should be prepared adequately. To do this effectively the most important basic questions that need to be answered are

1. What is the gestational age?
2. Is the fluid clear?
3. How many babies are expected?
4. Are there any additional risk factors?

Importance of Gestational age

Preterm newborns at high risk of primary apnea are more likely to need higher levels of resuscitation and establishing an airway is also more challenging. If time allows ensuring an advanced airway skills person such as a neonatologist, pediatrician, anesthesiologist be present at the delivery is helpful. In addition for resuscitation of the preterm neonate, additional equipment may be needed to ensure thermoregulation and establishing vascular access in the delivery room. Moreover and if possible, a preterm infant with suspected or confirmed airway anomalies with an anticipated difficult or critical airway should preferably have a pediatric ENT in attendance.

S. Aftab, M.D. (✉)
Division of Neonatology, Floating Hospital for Children, Tufts University School of Medicine, Boston, MA, USA
e-mail: saima.aftabmd@gmail.com

N.W. Mick, M.D., F.A.C.E.P.
Associate Chief, Department of Emergency Medicine, Associate Professor, Tufts University School of Medicine Director, Clinical Operations Maine Medical Center, Portland, MA, USA
e-mail: mickn@mmc.org

J. Nagler, M.D. M.H.P.Ed.
Department of Pediatrics, Harvard Medical School, Fellowship Director, Division of Emergency Medicine, Boston Children's Hospital, Boston, MA, USA

Significance of Meconium at the Delivery

Meconium-stained amniotic fluid may be a sign of fetal distress, newborns born through meconium-stained amniotic fluid are at risk for aspirating it after birth. The current NRP guidelines recommend that if a baby is delivered through meconium-stained amniotic fluid, a quick assessment of the baby's well being of vigor should be made. Vigor implies a baby who is not exhibiting signs of distress namely a HR >100, good tone and strong breathing or crying. If the baby is not vigorous i.e. missing any one of the above then it is recommended to intubate the baby for deep tracheal suctioning. Tracheal suctioning is done to prevent aspiration of meconium into the lungs. If meconium is recovered the first time the provider may repeat tracheal suctioning provided the baby remains stable. If no meconium is recovered or the baby becomes unstable at any given point, one must immediately abandon intubation attempts and start resuscitation from the very top of the NRP algorithm.

Multiple Births

Multiple Gestation delivery babies may need more resuscitation and always need more equipment and personnel. Often, there can be comorbidities that exist such as discordancy, twin-to-twin transfusion syndrome, and entrapment of one twin due to malposition.

J. Lioy and S.E. Sobol (eds.), *Disorders of the Neonatal Airway: Fundamentals for Practice*,
DOI 10.1007/978-1-4939-1610-8_28, © Springer Science+Business Media New York 2015

Other Risk Factors

Any significant findings in the history that could affect resuscitation causing airway difficulties such as polyhydramnios, suspected birth defects of the neck, trachea, esophagus, chromosome abnormality with severe micrognathia, and other craniofacial anomalies such as hemifacial microsomia can cause a serious situation for an unprepared team.

Evaluation of the Newborn at Delivery

After the delivery of the baby, answering three questions will determine the need for the initial steps at the radiant heat warmer
Is the newborn term?
Is the newborn breathing or crying?
Does the newborn have good muscle tone?

If the answer is NO to any question start NRP.

Currently the 6th *Edition of the Neonatal Resuscitation Program is considered the standard of care in neonatal resuscitation. We have described steps of neonatal resuscitation in detail in the following sections based on the NRP guidelines* (Please see 6th Ed. NRP manual for details).

Initial Steps

The NRP algorithm recommends starting with warming and drying any newborn in need for resuscitation. This will stimulate the baby to breathe, and a majority of newborns will just require this in order to start breathing. If the baby shows signs of airway obstruction oral and nasal suctioning can aid with stabilizing the airway.

At many large high volume obstetrical hospitals with academic connections, airway algorithms are available for staff review and preparation:

Administering Positive Pressure Ventilation

Positive Pressure ventilation may need to be administered according to the NRP algorithm after the initial steps or warming, drying, and stimulating the baby if the baby is apneic or gasping or has a heart rate of <100 beats per minute, persistent central cyanosis or desaturations despite increasing the FiO_2 to 100 %.

The two systems used for this purpose are a flow-inflating bag, self-inflating bag, or a T-piece resuscitator. When PPV is administered ensure there is a manometer in line to avoid barotraumas. The PPV is administered at a rate of about 30 breaths per minute.

Ensure adequate chest rise and air entry to assess effectiveness of PPV. The most consistent response to effective PPV will be an improvement in the HR and saturations.

Priority in Neonatal Resuscitation always remains establishing effective ventilation.

If the baby does not respond to the initial 30 s of PPV NRP recommends all providers to go through a series of ventilation corrective steps to ensure that PPV is in fact effective. The pneumonic is
M: Adjust Mask in the face
R: Reposition the head to open airway
S: Suction mouth and then nose
O: Open mouth and lift jaw forward
P: Gradually increase Pressure every few breaths until visible chest rise is noted

If this does not lead to improvement in heart rate, an Artificial Airway (ETT or LMA) should be considered.

Intubation and Use of a Laryngeal Mask Airway or LMA

An LMA may be indicated as an alternative to intubation when facial or upper airway malformations render bag-mask ventilations ineffective or PPV not effective and intubation is not possible.

Pulse Oximetry and Evaluation of Color

Pulse oximetry is an important tool to gauge the saturations of a baby in distress. It should be used if:
1. Resuscitation is anticipated
2. PPV is required for more than a few breaths
3. Central cyanosis is persistent
4. To confirm your perception of central cyanosis
5. Whenever supplemental oxygen is administered

In general, term infants may be resuscitated with 21 % O_2. Preterm infants may begin with a somewhat higher oxygen concentration. When using pulse oximetry pulse Ox probe on right hand or wrist as it measures the pre-ductal saturation.

Of note one must place on patient before connecting to Pox machine to achieve the fastest readings. Supplemental oxygen concentration should be adjusted gradually to achieve pre-ductal Saturations summarized in the NRP diagram below (Both Term & Preterm).

Chest Compressions

Chest compressions may need to be initiated per the NRP algorithm if the HR <60 bpm despite effective ventilation. One must coordinate chest compressions with ventilations for at least 45–60 s before stopping briefly to assess heart rate.

Compress 1/3 diameter of chest with 90 compressions to 30 ventilations/min (120 events). A good way to coordinate the compressions with ventilations is to call out One & two & three & breathe & One & two & three & breathe &....

Other things to remember are to increase FiO_2 to 100 % once you begin compressions. Pox may not work while newborn is receiving chest compressions.

Intubation is strongly recommended when compressions begin.

Umblical Venous Catheter UVC Placement and Epinephrine

Consider placement of UVC once compressions are initiated or if extended resuscitation is anticipated. Continue chest compressions by moving around to head of bed to allow room for MD to place UVC. Epinephrine is indicated when heart rate remains <60 despite 30 s of effective ventilations and at least another 45–60 s of coordinated compressions and ventilations.

Epinephrine

The ETT route has an unreliable absorption, which renders it less effective, but if it may be readily available so may be given while attempting to establish a UVC.

The UVC route is the preferred method for administering epinephrine; however, it requires a skilled person to place immediately. The IV epinephrine may be given as soon as the line is placed even after just giving via ETT. Doses of epinephrine are based upon the different concentrations used for different routes of administrations.

Post-resuscitation Care

There are two levels of post-resuscitation care:

Routine Care, which is for vigorous term infants with no risk factors or babies who required but responded to initial steps. These babies now can stay with their mothers and skin-to-skin contact recommended.

Extended Care is for babies with depressed breathing or activity such as those requiring supplemental oxygen &/or ongoing nursing care and those with high-risk factors requiring frequent evaluation may need to be evaluated in an ICU setting. These babies may possibly then transfer to routine care after a period of stability.

Role of T-Piece Resuscitator (TPR)

Effective positive pressure ventilation can be vital to neonatal resuscitation, in addition it is also important for uniform and effective surfactant distribution. A T-piece resuscitator TPR or the traditional flow bag valve mask apparatus can deliver this positive pressure. The TPR provides pressure-controlled, flow-delivered positive pressure ventilation. The positive end expiratory pressure (PEEP) valve can be rotated to modify the PEEP provided, and occlusion of the valve by the operator delivers peak inspiratory pressure (PIP). Its main purported advantages are the delivery of consistent pressures, the ability to adjust inspiratory time, and the control of PIP and PEEP. There is a wide variability in the use of T-piece resuscitator in neonatal resuscitations.

TPR users should also be aware of certain limitations of the device. Resuscitation is a dynamic process where the resuscitator needs to adapt to the response or non-response of the newborn. TPR users are not as good at detecting changes in compliance as users of the Self or Flow-inflating bags. TPR users also need more time to change the inflating pressures during resuscitation, compared to users of the SIB or FIB. Mask leak is greater with the TPR than with other devices.

TPRs are also the most technically difficult of the three devices to prepare for use. Operators who do not frequently use the device, and are not receiving regular training in its setup, forget how to prepare the device for use. Instructors should be aware that increases in gas flow before, or during resuscitation could result in significant increases in pressures unless the operator adjusts the dials accordingly.

Until evidence of clinical benefit is available, we recommend that healthcare providers are appropriately and regularly trained in the use of whatever device being used in their clinical practice, and are aware of the particular limitations of that device.

Identification and Evaluation of High-Risk Neonate with Difficult/Critical Airway

Neonatal airway obstruction, a frequent cause of respiratory distress, is a common indication for NICU admission. Ventilation is the cornerstone of neonatal resuscitation and when airway obstruction presents in the delivery room, it poses a unique challenge to transition the neonate. Presence of airway obstruction in the delivery room may be unexpected and may escalate to life-threatening situations or present at facilities that do not routinely cater to high-risk population.

Prenatal history and findings may give the neonatal provider valuable clues towards making the diagnoses. However, the same may not always be available or known prenatally. Thus, the delivery room may serve as the first opportunity or site for the presentation and detection of neonatal obstruction. Ventilation is the cornerstone of neonatal resuscitation and when airway obstruction presents in the delivery room, it poses a unique challenge to transition the neonate. Thus it is of utmost importance for the neonatal provide to review all available prenatal information when available that maybe pertinent for the neonate's delivery room needs.

Table 1 Epinephrine administration guidelines for resuscitation

• Concentration 1:10,000 (0.1 mg/mL)
• ETT dose is 0.5–1 mL/kg
• UVC/IV dose is 0.1–0.3 mL/kg
• Follow with a 0.5–1 mL flush NS
• Re-check heart rate after 1 min of compressions and ventilations
• Repeat dose every 3–5 min

Table 2 Special considerations for preterm neonates

1.	Increase temperature of the delivery room to approx. 25–26°C (77–79°F)
2.	Polyethylene plastic wrap
3.	Place portable warming pad under the layers of
4.	Towels at the radiant heat warmer
5.	Use blended O_2
6.	Consider CPAP for good heart rate but an increased work of breathing
7.	May need to administer surfactant for preterm infants intubated for respiratory distress syndrome or RDS

Table 3 Prenatal ultrasound finding associated with neonatal airway obstruction. Congenital high airway obstruction, (CHAOS)

Non-immune Hydrops—severe neck edema
Polyhydramnios with tracheal atresia
Severe Micrognathia-craniofacial/genetic syndromes
Large echogenic fetal lungs-upper airway obstruction
Dilated airways with stenosis
Cervical lymphangiomas/teratomas
Neuromuscular condition with arthrogryposis and jaw immobility

Table 4 Common causes of neonatal airway that may present in the delivery room setting

Conditions associated with extrinsic compression of the airway
1. Cervical lymphatic malformation (cystic hygroma)
2. Cervical teratoma
3. Associated with mandibular hypoplasia:
(a) Pierre Robin sequence (Stickler syndrome)
(b) Nager Syndrome
(c) Treacher Collins Syndrome
(d) Bilateral hemifacial microsomia—Goldenhars Syndrome
4. Associated with macroglossia
(a) Down's Syndrome
(b) Beckwith Weidmann Syndrome
(c) Lymphangioma
Conditions associated with intrinsic airway compression
1. Lingual thyroid
2. Vallecular cyst
3. Others, such as Nasal encephalocele, ranula, glioma, dermoids, etc.
Intrinsic airway obstruction
1. Choanal atresia/stenosis
2. Tracheal agenesis/stenosis
3. Laryngeal agenesis/stenosis
4. Congenital high airway obstruction sequence (CHAOS)
5. Vocal cord palsy (primary condition, associated with hydrocephalus)
6. Laryngeal web
7. Tracheomalacia/Laryngomalacia

Prenatal Diagnoses and Fetal surveillance

Ultrasound remains the first and main diagnostic modality for fetal assessment [1]. Anatomic fetal surveillance is usually performed at 18–22 weeks gestation. In high-risk case, fetal MRI has been employed with significant benefit. Fetal MRI does have technical challenges but gives a level of anatomic detail that may have substantial prognostic and therapeutic implications [2, 3]. Table 1 lists the most common prenatal imaging and clinical findings that raise the possibility of neonatal or fetal airway obstruction [4]. Many neonates are now born in centers with "fetal therapy programs" and delivery units within specialized Children's Hospitals. However, many of these neonates must be born in larger maternity hospitals due to maternal reasons: (severe preeclampsia; HELLP syndrome; acute bleeding; maternal cardiac disorders). These are the infants that will be delivered in a perinatal center and those with airway issues will be the challenge for the team at resuscitation:

It is important to note that while actual anatomical details such as cervical neck masses give a direct clue towards the likely airway obstruction, other findings maybe more indirect and thus evade an easy association. These indirect clues may arise as a consequence of airway obstruction, such as hydrops or polyhydramnios. They may also be part of a syndrome of which airway obstruction is a feature. A good example of this is coexistence of structural heart anomalies and coloboma in a fetus may alert the provider to the possibility of choanal atresia as part of the CHARGE syndrome (previously thought to be an association). As such existence of major congenital anomalies should raise the index of suspicion for airway anomalies as part of a global pathology. Other syndromes such as Treacher Collins, Goldenhars and Pierre Robin syndromes can also present with significant airway obstruction due to the severe micrognathia. Common diagnoses associated with neonatal airway obstruction that may present in the delivery room are listed in Tables 2, 3 and 4.

However, during intubation, conditions affecting the supra, glottic and subglottic area may only then become obvious and hinder the neonatologist from routine intubation. Conditions such as subglottic stenosis, masses, vocal cord paralysis, or atresia can be uncovered in the delivery room.

Airway Emergencies in the Delivery Room

Specific airway-related diagnoses, such as listed above likely mandate a customized approach to neonatal resuscitation. Another group of conditions that deserves a special mention here, comprise conditions that are not directly associated

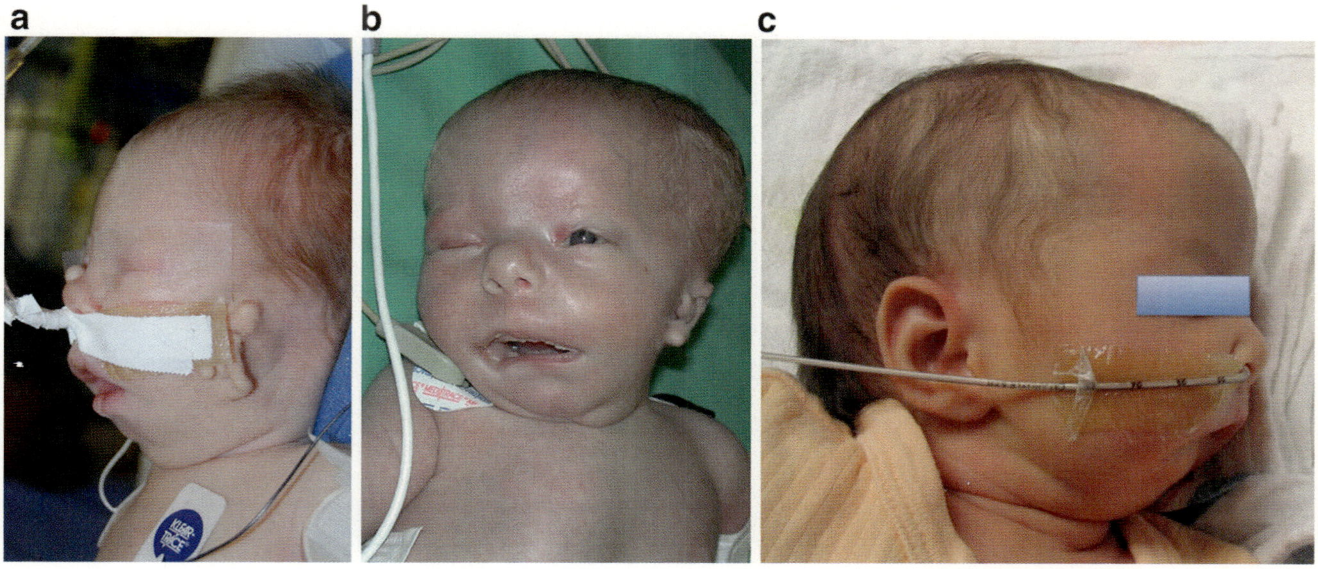

Fig. 1 (**a**–**c**) Goldenhars Syndrome with severe micrognathia and airway obstruction requiring specialized airway management in immediate birth period

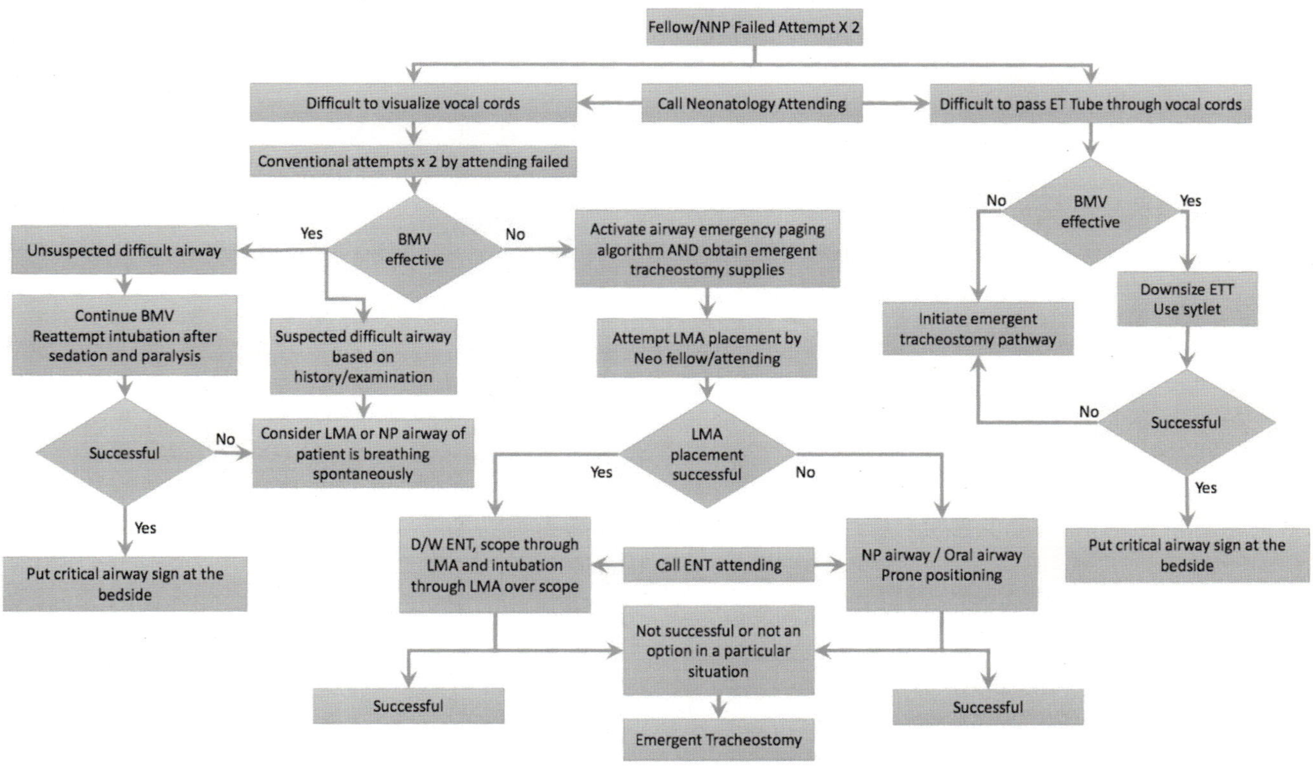

Fig. 2 Delivery room airway emergency algorithm:**Courtesy of Michael Posencheg, MD, medical director of the Hospital of the University of Pennsylvania neonatal unit. **

with a specific airway diagnoses, nevertheless have implications for airway management in the delivery room. These mainly include conditions wherein the role of bag-mask ventilation is limited and prompt orotracheal intubation is recommended for example, esophageal atresia, and congenital diaphragmatic hernia.

Once an airway obstruction has been identified, the fetus needs to be evaluated for other possible coexisting conditions. The airway obstructions maybe an isolated finding or part of a global/syndromic condition. The latter raises serious ethical questions as more neonates with severe birth defects are now being born at Children's Hospitals with immediate access to

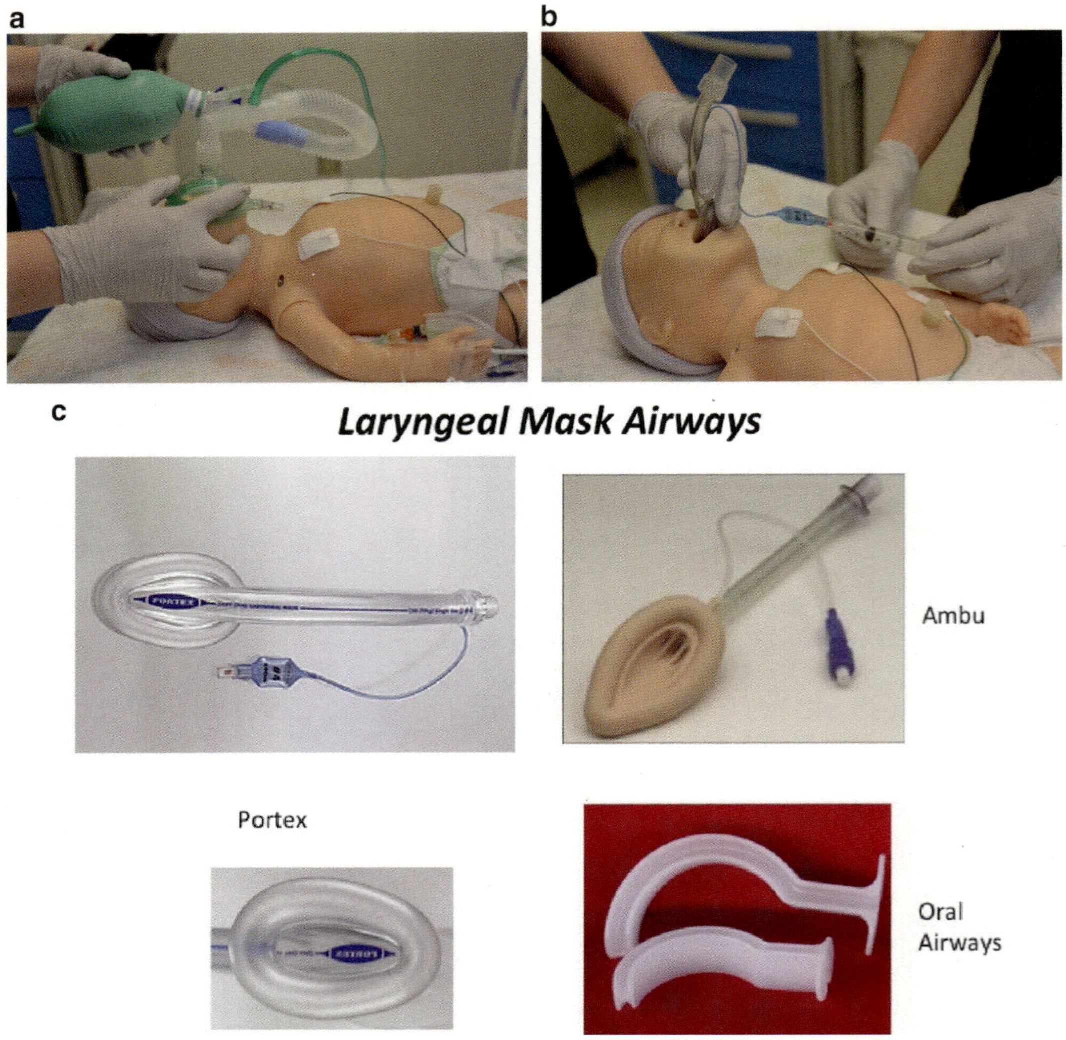

Fig. 3 (**a**) BMV placement in a neonate. (**b**) LMA Placement in a neonate. (**c**) Different LMA types

subspecialty services Figs. 1, 2, 3 and 4. show how organization and practice can prepare for an airway emergency.

Timing and Mode of Delivery

Understandably, the identification of fetal airway obstruction has significant implications for the plans surrounding the delivery. As with many other complex congenital anomalies, cases with suspected fetal airway obstruction should be referred for further evaluation to a tertiary center. Ideally such a referral center should have dedicated, multidisciplinary teams with advanced neonatal, otorhinolaryngology and pediatric surgery services with experience in fetal/neonatal airway issues. The course based on the diagnoses may comprise minimal noninvasive support to requiring EXIT delivery [5]. (Discussed in Chapters "Prenatal Assessment and Perinatal Management of Suspected Airway Compromise in the Fetus and Neonate" and "Operative Surgical Management of Fetuses with CHAOS, (Congenital High Airway Obstruction Syndrome): Management at Delivery"). The timing and choice of delivery will also be influenced by fetal and maternal health, particularly in cases of fetal hydrops and/or maternal "mirror syndrome" [6]. The most important thing when there is time to prepare is having experienced pediatric ENT present with full service tracheostomy tray and set up. Everyone should be prepared Figs. 5, 6, 7, 8 and 9.

Postnatal Diagnoses

In situations where the diagnoses of airway obstruction are not available or suggested prenatally, the clinician can get valuable information from the delivery room experience.

Respiratory distress, especially when unresponsive to routine resuscitative measures, is always an obvious presenting complaint of significant airway obstruction. Externally visible masses and dysmorphic features suggestive of micrognathia and/or retrognathia [7] can be important clues.

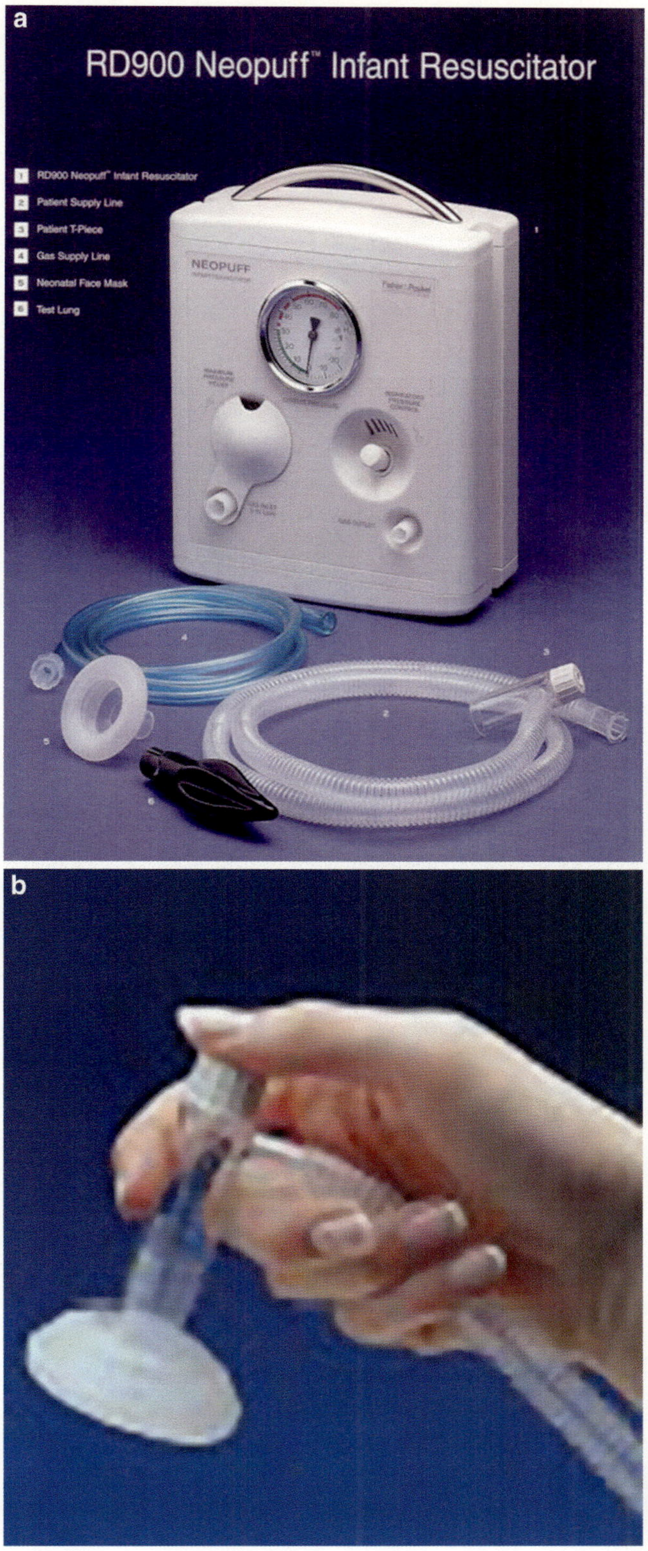

Fig. 4 (**a**) The Fisher Paykel NEOPUFF RD 900 Neopuff™ Infant Resuscitator. (**b**) Use of the mouthpiece with the Neopuff™ Infant Resuscitator

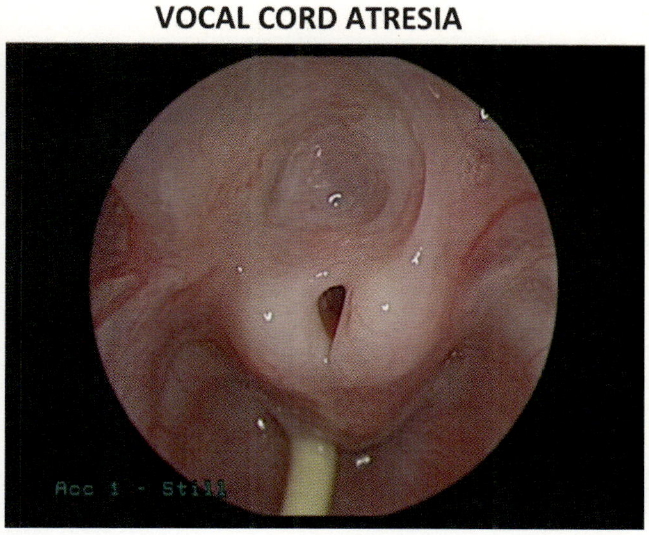

Fig. 5 Vocal Cord atresia causing airway obstruction during intubation

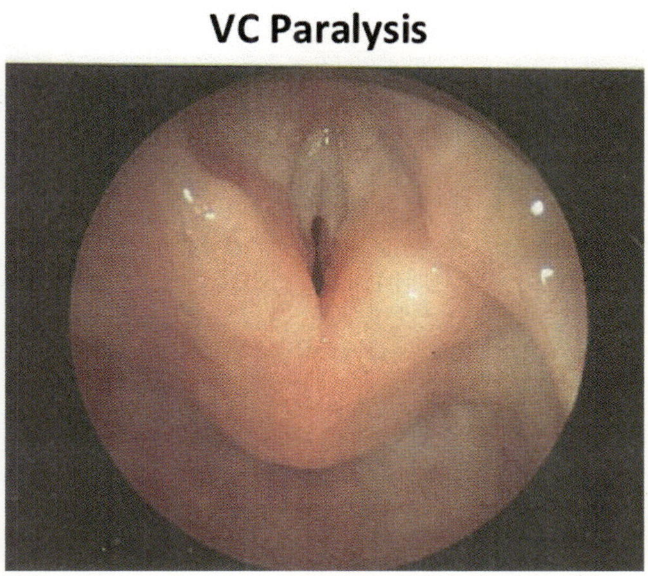

Fig. 6 Vocal Cord paralysis causing airway obstruction at delivery

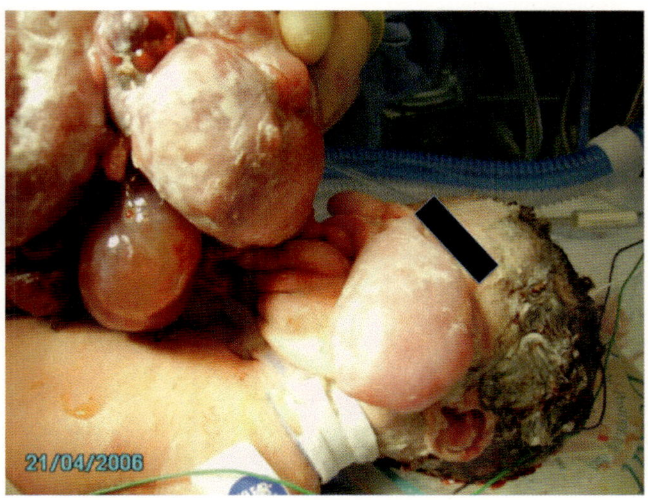

Fig. 7 Epulis/Epignathus causing acute oral obstruction and an airway emergency at birth Tracheostomy may be the only treatment for these types of obstructions

Other such symptoms may include excessive secretions, stridor, and inability to pass suction catheters through one or both nostrils Figs. 10, 11, 12, 13 and 14.

Birth Trauma

Finally, the possibility of birth trauma causing airway obstruction or impairment should be considered. This is especially true for macrosomic neonates with history of prolonged shoulder dystocia. While, such delivery circumstances may result in perinatal asphyxia, the clinician should still be cognizant of the possibility of airway trauma. Cases of tracheal or laryngeal tears are rare but have been reported in the literature [8, 9].

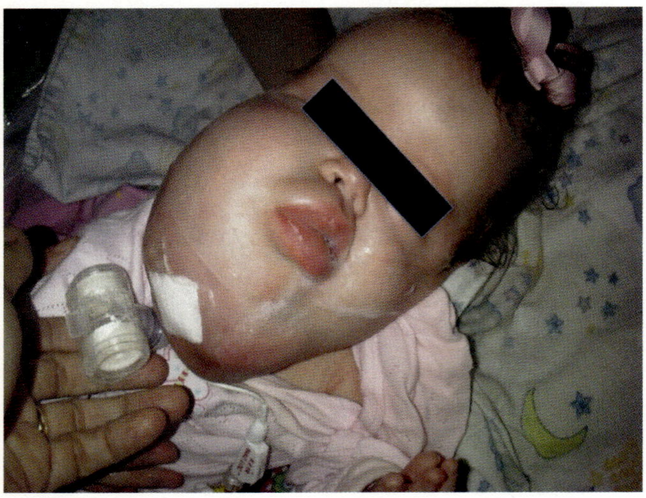

Fig. 8 Giant lymphangiomas causing acute oral obstruction and an airway emergency at birth Tracheostomy may be the only treatment for these types of obstructions

Summary of Delivery Room Management

Benefits exist in standardizing the care patients receive. We have discussed how things should be done in the delivery room regarding thermoregulation, oxygen titration, and respiratory support. However, the infrastructure to perform these interventions including who should perform which tasks requires some more detail. Understanding that we are trying to provide the best medical care, while training residents and fellows. We recommend the following guidelines to establish roles and responsibilities:

1. Establish a team leader—this person is usually a fellow for attending.
2. Airway—experienced personnel, usually a senior front line clinician, fellow for attending.
3. Umbilical Lines—should have an experienced person assisting residents to balance efficiency with training.
4. Nursing—at least one for baby (thermoregulation) and one recording. If possible, an additional medication nurse is optimal.
5. Respiratory Therapy—Need a dedicated person to manage CPAP nasal interface and oxygen titration. Surfactant administration if applicable.

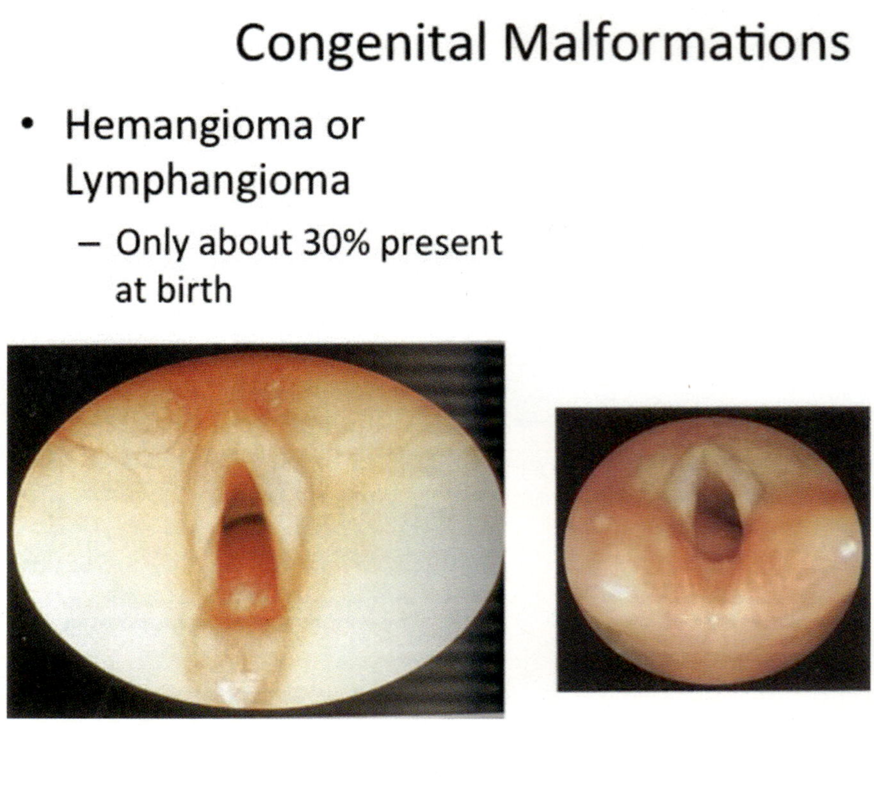

Fig. 9 Laryngeal Hemangioma or Lymphangioma can easily obstruct the entrance to the glottis and only be found upon intubation in a neonate with respiratory distress

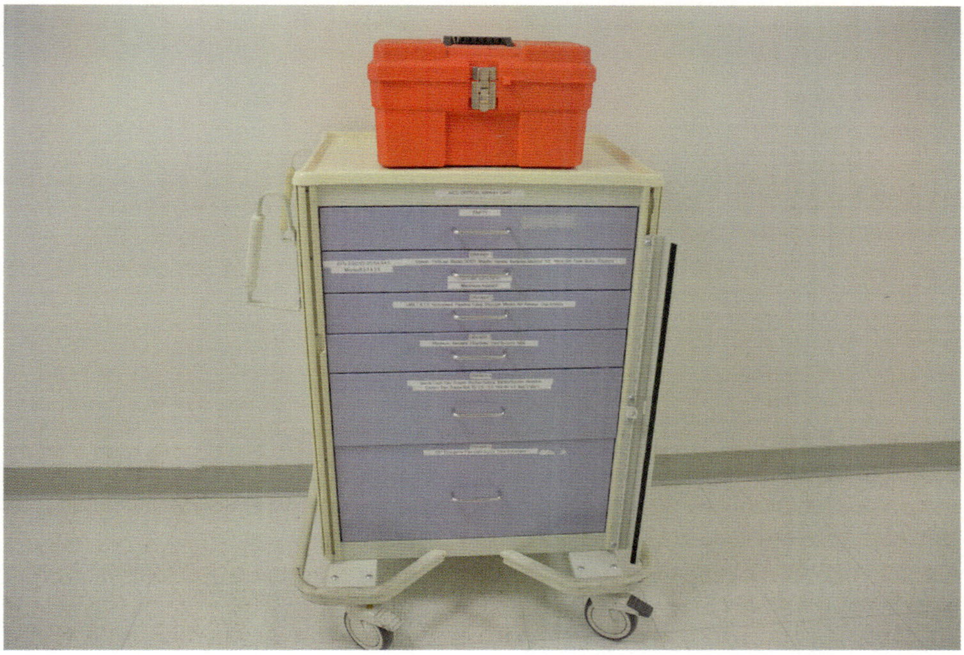

Fig. 10 Standard type neonatal delivery room critical airway cart

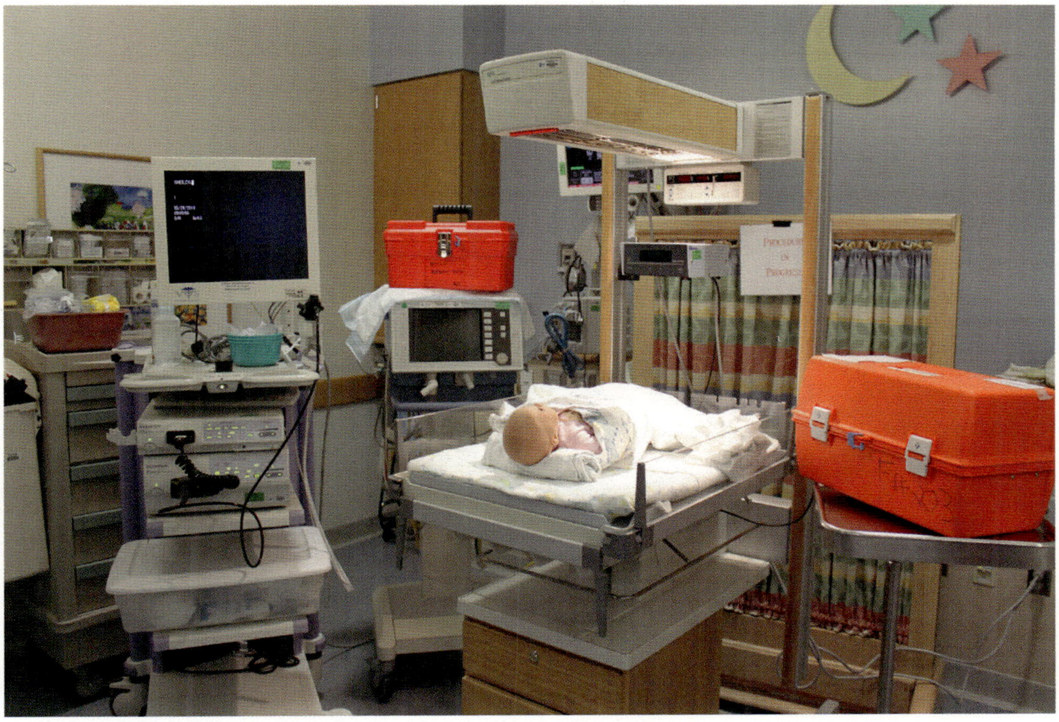

Fig. 11 Emergency set up of delivery room resuscitation

6. Limit traffic—personnel without roles should leave the room, with rare exception. Attempt to keep doors closed to maintain room temperature.
7. Be prepared to handle unexpected situations arising out of unanticipated airway emergencies. Simple cues on physical exam and history maybe very important to direct management.
8. In cases of unexpected airway emergencies, understand your resources and involve specialists in a time-sensitive manner. Other teamwork guidelines apply with more focused communication and heightened sense of urgency.

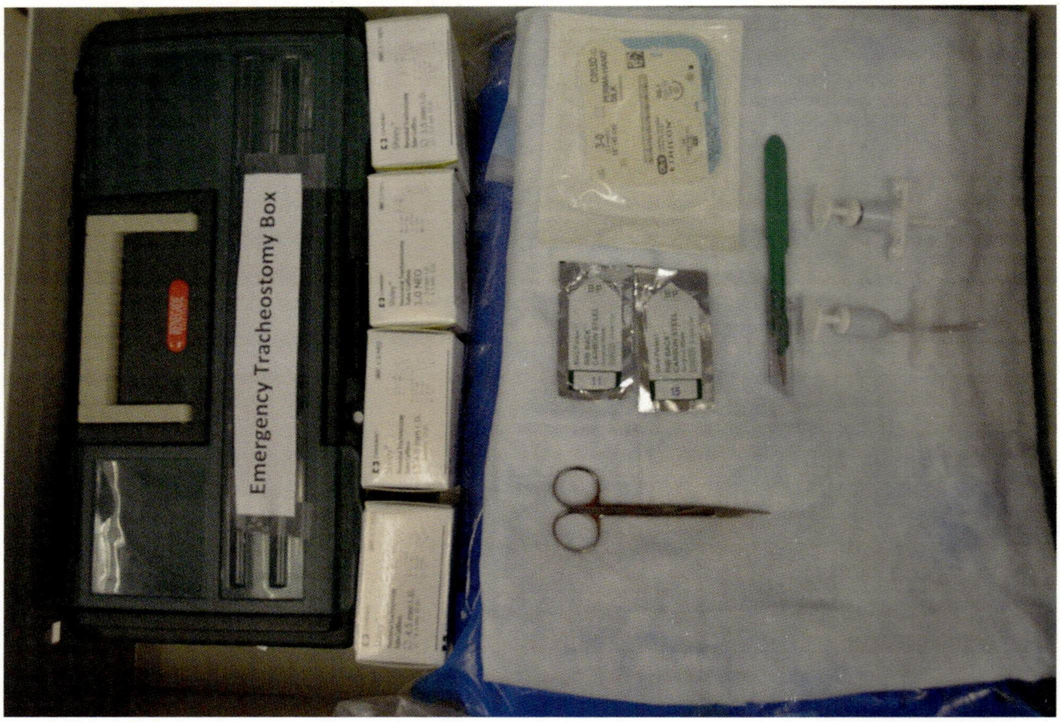

Fig. 12 Emergency tracheostomy set up

Fig. 13 Essential basic delivery room airway equipment: LED laryngoscope handles and blades, LMAs, ETTs, masks, ETTs, and stylettes

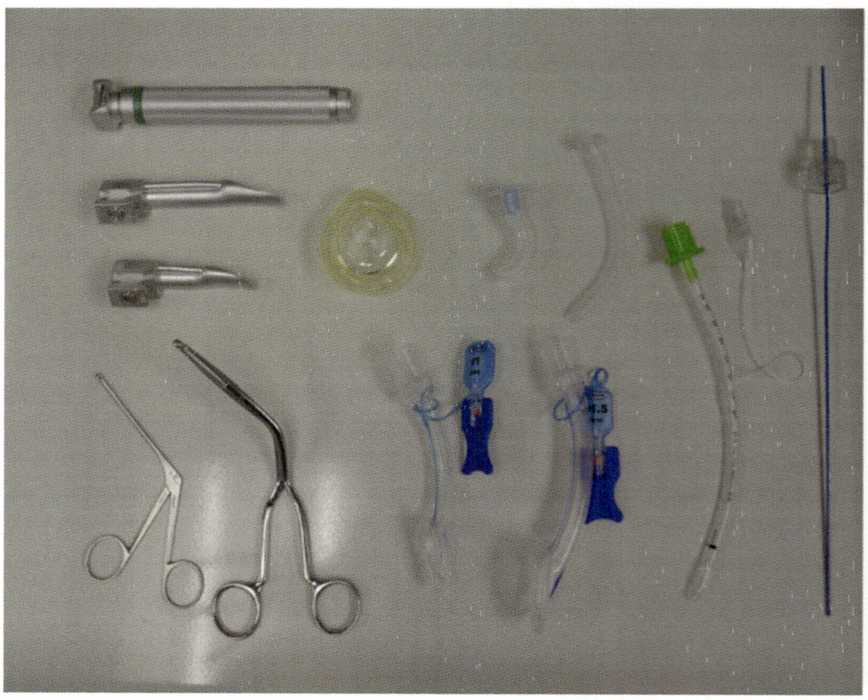

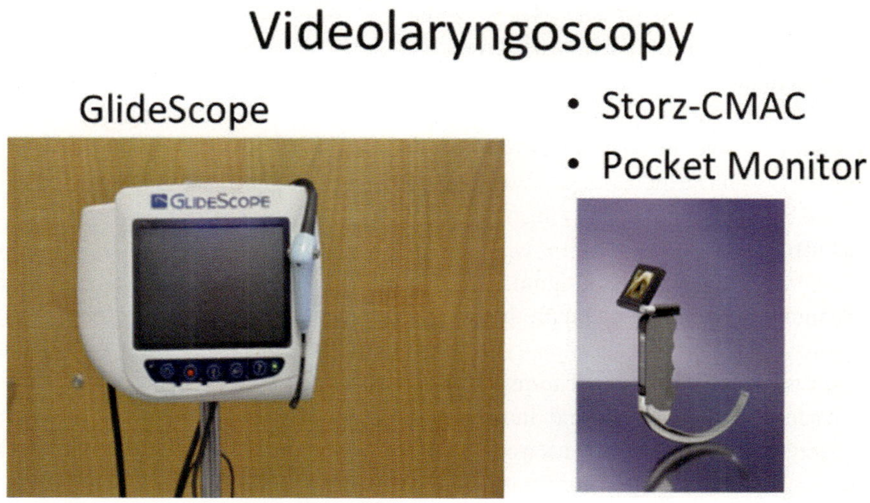

Fig. 14 Videolaryngoscopy: Glidescope and Storz CMAC now available for neonatal patients with size 0 and 1 blades

Section 2: Resuscitation in the Emergency Department

Nathan W. Mick and Joshua Nagler

Background

Neonatal airway management in the Emergency Department (ED) is an infrequent but critically important skill for emergency medicine providers. The psychomotor skills required to perform laryngoscopy and intubation in a neonate are similar to those utilized in the care of an older child or adult. However, there are key anatomic and physiologic differences between these disparately aged patient populations, which are most pronounced in neonates who are at the youngest end of the pediatric age spectrum. These differences impact the indications for airway management and necessitate modifications in approach.

Emergency medicine providers are further challenged by a relative inexperience in caring for critically ill neonates. Those with fellowship training in pediatric emergency medicine may have some additional experience from their neonatal and pediatric intensive care rotations as well as scheduled training in the operating room setting. However, the vast majority of neonatal intubations in EDs occur outside of a tertiary care children's hospital by providers with limited and often remote pediatric training. Nonetheless, neonatal and pediatric "readiness" is an essential component of general ED operations. Fortunately, most emergency medicine providers will have comfort in recognizing critical illness and responding quickly; however, there are a myriad of cognitive barriers (e.g., appropriate equipment sizes, drug doses) that make emergency airway management in neonates and children a source of significant anxiety.

Utilizing a systematic approach to airway management in young infants is paramount to success. This includes: (1) recognizing and addressing the predictable anatomic and physiologic differences in neonatal airway management, and (2) consistently applying an approach to airway management that identifies and addresses potential difficulties. In this chapter, we will review the most common presentations of neonatal patients requiring airway management in the ED, as well as provide a methodical approach to addressing both anticipated and unanticipated challenges that may occur.

Epidemiology and Experience

Opportunities to perform direct laryngoscopy and intubation are much less common in the pediatric than the adult population. It is estimated that airway management is required in 1–3 patients per 1,000 pediatric visits in the average ED compared with 6–10 intubations per 1,000 adult visits [10–12]. This number is further diluted when looking specifically at the care of young infants. The distribution of ages of patients requiring endotracheal intubation at a single tertiary care center for a 1-year period suggests that only a fraction of the pediatric population requiring airway management are neonates or young infants (Fig. 15). Given that the average ED physician will be unlikely to encounter opportunities for a significant number of pediatric airway procedures during typical clinical practice, skill acquisition, and retention can be difficult. Pediatric intubation success rates vary quite dramatically with experience. Studies performed in the operating room with anesthesia providers suggest that the success rate for endotracheal intubation after ten airways is less than 50 % while greater than 50 intubation attempts are required before success reaches 90 % [13, 14]. Therefore for emergency medicine providers with lim-

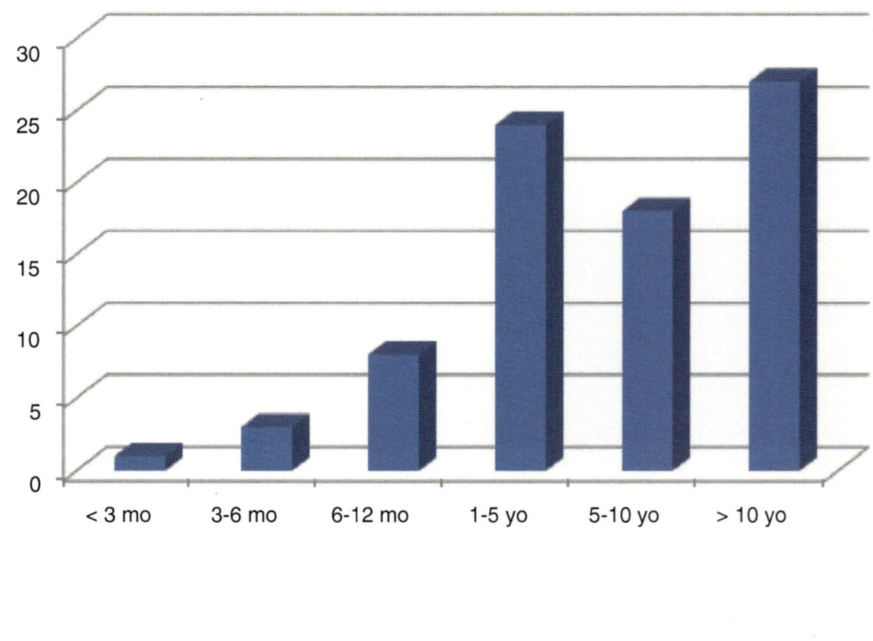

Fig. 15 Frequency of endotracheal intubation stratified by age

ited in situ clinical opportunities, the required number of intubations to attain "mastery" may therefore necessitate dedicated time in the operating room or augmentation of skills in a simulated environment [15].

Pathophysiology

There are many unique anatomic and physiologic features that impact emergent neonatal airway management. These differences are predictable, and therefore can be anticipated and addressed to optimize early success and mitigate adverse events.

Anatomic differences in neonates compared to larger children or adults include relatively large occiputs compared with body size, a superior and anterior larynx, a large tongue relative to the oral cavity, a weaker hyoepiglottic ligament, and a large floppy epiglottis. The impact of each of these unique features on airway management, as well as the strategies to accommodate them is reviewed in Table 5.

Physiologically, the most striking difference between neonates and their older pediatric and adult counterparts is the tendency toward rapid desaturation. This occurs as a result of increased oxygen consumption secondary to higher metabolic rates combined with decreased oxygen reservoirs reflecting relatively smaller functional residual capacities [16]. Also notable in neonates is increased vagal tone. This translates into a higher likelihood of bradycardia secondary to hypoxia, pharyngeal manipulation during laryngoscopy, or select medications (i.e., succinylcholine).

Table 5 Addressing anatomic differences in children

Anatomic difference	Effect	Approach to management
Large occiput	• Head flexion causes airway obstruction and limits glottic view	• Shoulder or neck roll to open airway and help align airway axes
Superior/anterior larynx	• May limit glottic view • Makes endotracheal tube delivery and passage difficult	• Look up during laryngoscopy • Apply external laryngeal pressure • Create acute angle to styletted endotracheal tube
Large tongue	• Falls onto posterior pharyngeal wall when supine obstructing airway • May impede laryngoscopy	• Airway maneuvers or oral or nasal airway to open upper airway • Sweep the tongue when obstructing glottic view
Weak hyoepiglottic ligament	• Limits elevation of epiglottis through vallecular pressure	• Use straight laryngoscope blades • Place the blade tip beneath the epiglottis and lift directly
Large epiglottis	• May fold on itself with placement of extragottic devices (EGD) • Obscures view during laryngoscopy	• Rotational technique for EGD insertion • Direct elevation of epiglottis with straight blade

Clinical Presentation

Indications for neonatal airway management in the ED are vastly different than those in the delivery room, and have only limited overlap with the Neonatal Intensive Care Unit (NICU) setting. Neonates returning after hospital discharge no longer have issues related to difficult transitions to extrauterine life, and are rarely in need of suctioning of meconium or delivery of surfactant. Instead, most indications for airway management in the ED are related to acute illness or injury, though the cohort of neonates with underlying conditions (i.e., chronic lung disease) may be at increased risk for decompensation from superimposed acute insults. Respiratory embarrassment and apnea are most common. Depressed mental status from sepsis, head injury, seizure, or shock with resultant failure to maintain or protect the airway are also relatively frequent indications to secure a child's airway (Fig. 16). Data suggest that the number of intubations performed on trauma and non-trauma patients on children in the ED is approximately equal, though this distribution may differ when looking exclusively at neonates or young infants [11, 17].

General Algorithm

Consistently utilizing a systematic approach to airway management in patients of all ages is a sound strategy to reduce error, improve provider comfort, and minimize the "cognitive burden" inherent in pediatric procedures. Cognitive burden here refers to the mental load that is required to identify the correct drug dosing and equipment sizes across the age spectrum. There are several commercially available resuscitation aids (e.g., The Broselow–Luten System) that seek to minimize the challenge of addressing size or weight-based variables that occur in pediatric resuscitation (Fig. 17). These guides provide a means to identify the correct medication doses and equipment sizes for a pediatric patient based on weight or length with minimal or no reliance on mathematic calculations.

All patients who undergo intubation in the ED should have a pre-procedure airway assessment. Rapid sequence intubation (RSI) is the procedure of choice for emergency intubation in patients in whom difficulty is not anticipated. The LEMON© mnemonic can be used as a quick, reliable method to screen for the difficulty prior to laryngoscopy (Table 6) [18]. The LEMON© mnemonic can be summarized as follows:

L—Look externally: This is the gestalt "feel" of the patient and the airway and involves assessing for evidence of anatomic disruption as well as specific findings such as micrognathia (Fig. 18).

E—Evaluate 3-3-2: This step involves assessment of mouth opening, the length of the mandible, and the position of the glottis in relation to the base of the tongue (Fig. 19).

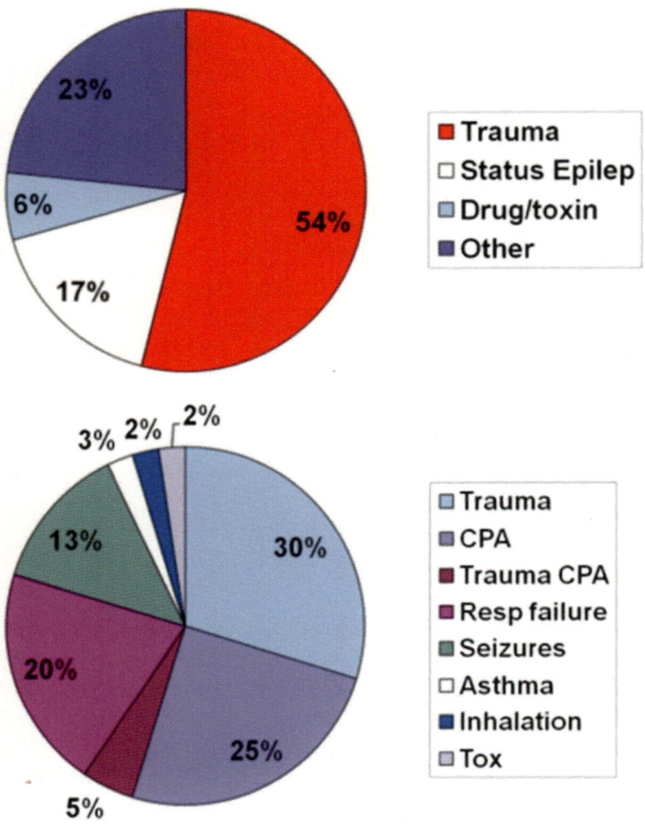

Fig. 16 Indications for intubation of pediatric patients in the Emergency Department. *Panel A*: Data from the National Emergency Airway Registry. *Panel B*: Data from Children's Hospital of Philadelphia

M—Mallampati score: This involves assessing how much of the posterior oropharynx is visible with the mouth open and the tongue protruded (Fig. 20). A modified version in children involves the use of a tongue depressor rather than reliance on voluntary protrusion of the tongue.

O—Obstruction or obesity: Evidence of upper airway obstruction, either by foreign body or swelling (i.e., croup or epiglottis may make laryngoscopy difficult. Obesity ought not be an issue in neonates but has been associated with airway management difficulty.

N—Neck mobility: Conditions that affect cervical spine mobility are very rare in neonates (either congenital or acquired). In the trauma setting, cervical spine immobilization with a cervical collar may impact laryngoscopic success.

Aspects of difficulty identified during application of the LEMON© mnemonic can be helpful in prompting emergency providers to alter their approach or recruit additional equipment or personnel prior to proceeding. Figure 18 shows an infant with Pierre Robin who would be identified as a potentially difficult airway based on the "Look" and "Evaluate" components of this screening strategy.

Once an airway assessment has been performed and intubation is felt to be indicated, RSI is the recommended approach. Prior to intubation, there are several preparatory considerations that will increase the likelihood of a smooth, successful procedure. As stated earlier, neonates have a high metabolic rate and are prone to rapid desaturation with apnea. Preoxygenation with a non-rebreather mask or BVM is critical if time allows. Neonates have a large occiput with respect to their bodies so proper positioning is important to allow for alignment of the oral, pharyngeal, and laryngeal axes. For these patients, a towel roll placed under the shoulders will elevate the body in relation to the head and put the patient in the proper position for laryngoscopy. The BURP (backward, upward, rightward pressure) maneuver can be helpful for glottic visualization, particularly in patients in whom cervical spine immobilization is in place.

EQUIPMENT		
E.T. Tube (mm)	**3.5 uncff**	**3.5 uncff**
Lip-Tip distance	**10.5**	**10.5**
Suction	**8F**	**8F**
Laryngoscope blade	**1 straight**	**1 straight**
Stylet	**6F**	**6F**
Oral airway	**50 MM**	**50 MM**
Nasopharyngeal Airway	**14F**	**14F**
BVM	**INFANT**	**INFANT**
VENTILATION**		
Tidal volume	**60-100 mL**	**75-125 mL**
Frequency (bpm)	**20-25**	**20-25**

Fig. 17 An example of the Broselow–Luten system for length-based estimation of equipment size and drug dosing

Table 6 Key features in applying the LEMON assessment in children

Look	• *Gestalt* is most important predictor • Dysmorphic features associated with abnormal airways
Evaluate (3:3:2)	• Not tested in children, difficult with "pudgy" necks • If attempted, use child's fingers
Mallampati	• Cooperation may be an issue • Mixed data in children
Obstruction	• Common indication for airway management in children • Focused disease history is key • Obesity is growing concern in children
Neck	• Limited positioning secondary to trauma similar to adults • Intrinsic congenital or acquired anomalies are rare

Used with permission from Walls RM and Murphy MF: Manual of Emergency Airway Management, 4th Edition, Philadelphia, Walters Kluwer, 2012

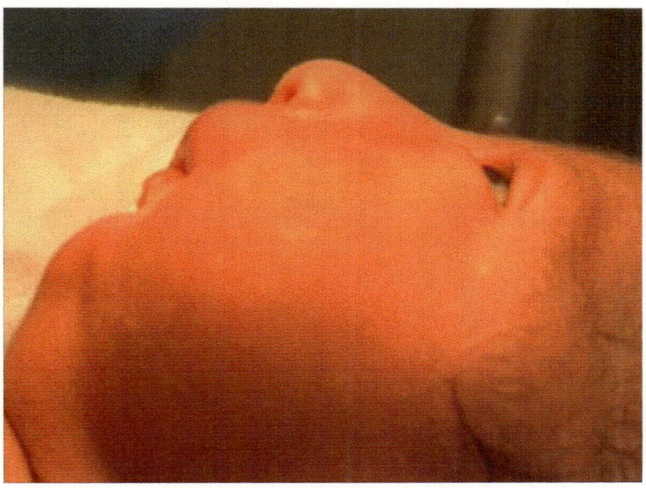

Fig. 18 Micrognathia in the Pierre Robin sequence

Ideal equipment for intubation in neonates consists of a straight (i.e., Miller) laryngoscope blade and a styletted, cuffed endotracheal tube. Young children have large epiglottises that are most amenable to manipulation with a straight blade. Stylets can be safely used in pediatric patients and have benefits in both direct and video laryngoscopy to direct the tip of the tube through the cords. Although uncuffed endotracheal tubes have been traditionally used in airway management in the ED, there are many situations where a cuffed tube may be beneficial. The admonition to "never use a cuffed tube" in pediatric patients is a historical argument arising from a time when large cuffs would necessitate use of significantly smaller diameter tubes, and cuff pressures could not be reliably monitored. High cuff pressures placed the patient at risk for tracheal ischemia and resulting subglottic

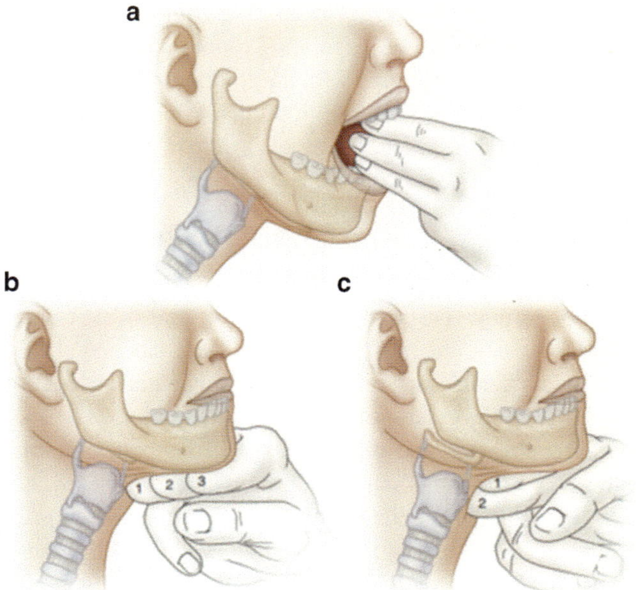

Fig. 19 (**a–c**) Show key features of the 3-3-2 rule to assess for likely anatomic difficulty aligning the oral, pharyngeal, and laryngeal axes for intubation. Used with permission from Walls RM and Murphy MF: Manual of Emergency Airway Management, 4th Edition, Philadelphia, Walters Kluwer, 2012

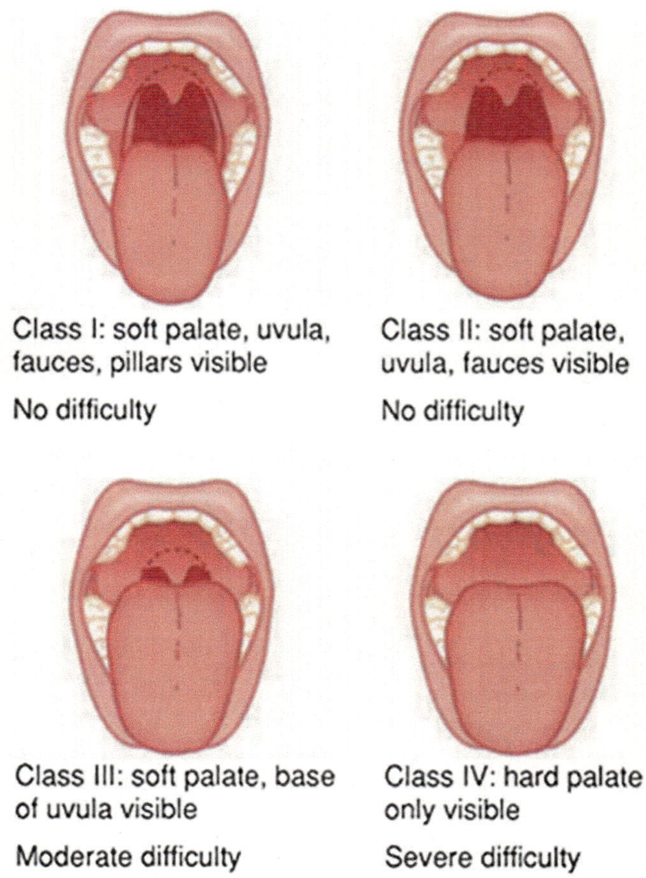

Fig. 20 The Mallampati scale used to predict difficult laryngoscopy based on the extent of the posterior oropharynx visible with the mouth open and tongue protruding. Used with permission from Walls RM and Murphy MF: Manual of Emergency Airway Management, 4th Edition, Philadelphia, Walters Kluwer, 2012

stenosis. Recently, there has been increasing use of cuffed tubes in the ED, ICU, and operating room owing to modern tubes that are manufactured with the ability to more carefully monitor cuff pressures. In addition, increasing cuff inflation may be useful to prevent air leak in cases where high airway pressures are necessary or changing lung compliance is likely (i.e., ARDS, reactive airway disease).

Correct endotracheal tube placement should be confirmed using either quantitative or qualitative end-tidal carbon dioxide monitoring. Disposable qualitative end-tidal carbon dioxide devices are most frequently used. They typically come in an "adult" and "pediatric" size. The pediatric-sized devices are appropriate for use in neonates (as low as 1 kg body weight) and have the advantage of a smaller internal volume and lower resistance to flow. There is concern that applying an adult qualitative device to an intubated neonate will result in a false "negative" reading even when the endotracheal tube is correctly placed due to the low tidal volumes circulating through the device. Similar concerns have been raised about using the pediatric size for extremely low birth weight infants. However, for patients large enough to have been discharged from the NICU, these colorimetric capographs have been deemed to be reliable.

Post-intubation management of the neonate intubated in the ED revolves around careful attention to patient movement to prevent tube dislodgement and appropriate sedation. Multiple different methods of securing the endotracheal tube have been shown to be effective. These include taping to the mouth/upper lip, tape around the neck, and commercially available tube holders.

Young age has been shown to be an independent risk factor for ETT dislodgement [19]. Appropriate sedation can limit this risk. Post-intubation sedation is best achieved in the ED with intermittent boluses of a sedative such as midazolam or lorazepam. Continuous infusions of propofol, a staple in adult airway management post-intubation, is to be avoided due to the risk of propofol infusion syndrome.

Rapid Sequence Intubation

The immediacy of need for neonatal resuscitation in the delivery room means that airway management often occurs prior to vascular access. As such, both bag-mask ventilation and endotracheal intubation in this setting almost always occur without premedication. In the NICU, however, the utilization of premedication for intubation is becoming more common, particularly in non-emergent cases; a practice supported by AAP issued guidelines [20–22].

In the Emergency Department, the vast majority of patients, regardless of age, are intubated using RSI. Based on the systematic approach described above, any neonate who is deemed to require intubation and is not immediately identified as a crash airway should be screened for difficulty. If no risk factors for difficulty are identified, these patients should undergo RSI.

By definition, RSI involves the delivery of premedications, sedatives, and neuromuscular blocking drugs for the purpose of decreasing awareness, pain, and movement (including protective airway reflexes) to facilitate emergent endotracheal intubation and to minimize the risk of aspiration. Given the certainty of apnea in this approach, preoxygenation is vital to reduce the likelihood of clinically significant hypoxemia. There is no single combination of medications that is optimal in all circumstances. Instead, selection will vary based on hospital protocols, clinical context, and provider familiarity and comfort. However, an overview of commonly used medications follows below.

Given the propensity for bradycardia from increased vagal tone in this young population, premedication with atropine is recommended. Although the data to support the ability of atropine to diminish the occurrence or severity of bradycardia is limited, its use is supported by anecdotal experience as well as biological plausibility. In addition, as a medication with very little cost or downside, the potential benefit outweighs the relatively low risk of harm. Atropine may also be helpful in drying secretions though this effect does not occur for 15–20 min after administration which will often be well after the patient has been intubated.

The safety profile and efficacy of various sedatives and analgesics in neonates continues to emerge. In addition, hospital protocols will guide which medications are available for use in EDs. However, there are certain mainstays within the pharmacopeia that should be familiar to emergency medicine practitioners. Opioids have the advantage of combining a potent analgesic effect with sedative properties. Although morphine can be used, fentanyl has a pharmacokinetic profile that is much better suited for RSI, with onset of action within 30 s and peaking in just a few minutes. Remifentanil is used in many NICUs, though it is not commonly used in EDs. Midazolam is commonly used in combination with fentanyl to provide additional sedative as well as amnestic qualities. When using this drug combination, careful attention for compromise in spontaneous respiratory effort and hypotension is warranted. Data regarding isolated midazolam use in preterm infants shows a high rate of peri-intubation decompensations, though this has not been similarly demonstrated in term infants and therefore is not an issue for ED management [23]. Etomidate is a favorite sedative for RSI in pediatrics given its predictable efficacy and stable hemodynamic profile. Ketamine has the advantage of analgesic and amnestic effects, hemodynamic support, and bronchodilatory effects. It has been demonstrated to be effective and safe for use in the neonatal age group, and concerns related to neurodegenerative effects in neonatal animal models have not been shown to translate into use in human infants or older children [24].

Propofol induction is a favorite of anesthesiologists, and is becoming more commonly used in EDs. It has been shown to be both safe and effective for RSI with extremely rapid and predictable effects. There are, however, three relevant precautions regarding the use of propofol: (1) prolonged infusions should be avoided given the risk of propofol infusion syndrome, (2) optimal dosing for RSI has not been well established in young infants, and (3) hypotension is a relatively common effect and should be anticipated.

Use of neuromuscular blocking drugs is commonplace for older children and adults; however, many providers are more reluctant to do the same when attempting neonatal intubation in the ED. One reason for this is that it is relatively easy to overcome the limited strength of neonates and perform laryngoscopy and endotracheal intubation without pharmacologic assistance. A second reason is that providers may have reluctance to deliberately compromise spontaneous respiratory effort based on fear that they may have difficulty successfully intubating the child. Nonetheless, studies have demonstrated that intubation success rates of newborns in the NICU as well as pediatric patients in the ER favors the use of neuromuscular blocking drugs [17, 25]. Succinylcholine has the advantage of rapid onset and offset, and predictable pharmacokinetics whether given intravenously or intramuscularly. It should not be used in patients with hyperkalemia, or patients known or suspected to have any type of neuromuscular disorder. Although an FDA Black Box warning exists for succinylcholine use in children, it includes the qualifier that is "should be reserved for emergency intubation or instances where immediate securing of the airway is necessary." This justifies its common use in the ED setting. Rocuronium is the other neuromuscular blocking drug frequently used in neonatal and pediatric intubation in the ED. Initial dosing at 0.6 mg/kg resulted in a longer time to intubating conditions. However, currently supported dosing at 1.2 mg/kg has been shown to reach intubating conditions in an equivalent time frame as succinylcholine. Rocuronium has the advantage of safe use in patients in whom hyperkalemia or neuromuscular disease exists, or simply is not known. However at the higher dosing schedule, it also has a much longer duration of action than succinylcholine. This needs to be considered in a patient in whom difficulty with intubation is possible, or in patients in whom a neurological examination or a return to spontaneous respiration is needed quickly.

Videolaryngoscopy

If a patient has clinical features that suggest airway management may be difficult (e.g., LEMON screen is positive), then alternative approaches should be considered. Videolaryngoscopy has emerged as a favored approach in these clinical circumstances. Given that neonates are likely to have the most anterior and superior larynx, the wider viewing angle offered by these devices may afford improved visualization, even in those not anticipated to be "difficult." Therefore, many emergency medicine providers will use videolaryngoscopy as a primary approach even for routine neonatal intubations as well.

Numerous studies demonstrate that videolaryngoscopy offers improved views over conventional direct laryngoscopy in children. The benefit of "seeing around the corner" of the airway rather than needing to line up the oral, pharyngeal, and laryngeal axes to provide a direct line of site has been clearly described [26]. In addition, data suggest that videolaryngoscopy has a relatively shorter learning curve than traditional direct laryngoscopy for less experienced laryngoscopists, which is likely to be true for most emergency medicine providers caring for neonates. Finally, although more of a secondary benefit, the shared view during videolaryngoscopy also provides an educational opportunity for more experienced providers to teach or guide this critical procedure.

Although a number of video-assisted devices exist for the management of pediatric patients, only a few currently include a complete range of sizes that would allow for their use in a child as small as a neonate. Glidescope has blades sizes for use down to preterm infants, Storz C-MAC has a Miller 0 blade, and Airtraq has a size 0 device that accommodates endotracheal tubes down to size 2.5 mm. Different options exist for disposability versus reusable blades, proceduralist viewfinder versus video screen display, and recording abilities. Importantly, differences in construction and blade angle require somewhat different technique for each, and therefore separate training and experience is required for any given device to be used.

Clinical data support the successful use of videolaryngoscopy in the ED; however, pediatric-specific data in this context is limited. The majority of reported experience using videolaryngoscopy in children comes from anesthesia literature, with several case series demonstrating successful use specifically in neonatal airway management, both routine and difficult [27–29] Therefore, given emergency medicine providers comfort and familiarity with videolaryngoscopy with demonstrated benefit in the ED setting, coupled with data demonstrating feasibility and safety in neonates, this approach is becoming increasingly common in the emergency management of critical neonatal airways.

Extraglottic Devices

Another available approach to the management of critical neonatal airways in the ED is the use of extraglottic devices (EGD). Case series and observational trials as well as randomized controlled trials support laryngeal mask airways as a feasible and safe modality for neonatal resuscitation [30]. EGD may be helpful as the primary approach for patients anticipated to have difficult airway management or as a rescue device in circumstances of unexpected inability to intubate.

Bag-mask ventilation, as described above, is the most fundamental and immediately available approach to supporting a child's respiratory effort emergently. However, the ability to maintain an adequate mask seal and patency of the airway requires ongoing effort. This may consume personnel resources and requires persistent, deliberate attention to the task, which can easily wane in the chaotic environment of the ED. In addition, mask ventilation, even when using appropriately limited pressures can easily lead to gastric insufflation as positive pressure breaths travel from the hypopharynx down the esophagus as well as into the trachea, unless gentle cricoid pressure is maintained. An appropriately placed EGD allows for similar ventilation pressures without the need for a continuous mask seal. The risk of gastric inflation is lower, and some devices now have a channel through which to pass a nasogastric tube to allow gastric decompression. Nonetheless, an EGD is not considered a "secure" airway, and the patient remains at risk of aspiration were secretions or gastric contents to pass the glottis.

The first clinical circumstance where an EGD might be used in the ED is in a child anticipated to have an anatomically difficult airway. In this circumstance, proceeding to RSI and relinquishing spontaneous ventilation may be risky. Primary placement of an EGD provides a relatively secure means to support oxygenation and ventilation. Awake patients will not tolerate an EGD, therefore this strategy is only effective in patients who have a depressed level of consciousness secondary to their underlying illness or injury, or secondary to pharmacologic sedation.

A more commonly recognized use of EGDs in the ED is as a rescue device following failed airway interventions. That is, for patients requiring respiratory support but in whom laryngoscopy and endotracheal intubation is not successful, an EGD can be placed as an alternative management strategy.

First pass success rates for placement of EGDs is very high, even by less experienced providers [30]. For young children, placement using a rotational technique may be advantageous to insure that epiglottis does not fold on itself and block the glottic opening following placement [31]. Once placed, the EGD may serve as the primary means of oxygenation and ventilation until a patient no longer requires respiratory support, or may serve as a bridge until endotracheal intubation can be performed by an experienced provider. In addition to serving as a temporizing approach, select EGDs can be used as conduits for endotracheal intubation, most safely accomplished with a flexible bronchoscope. Although many EGDs have aperture bars that preclude the passage of a scope or an endotracheal tube, newer generation devices use alternative designs with no obstructing features allowing easy passage of a tube through the EGD into the glottic opening.

Surgical Devices

The incidence of truly difficult pediatric intubations is estimated to be much less than 1 %. Airway difficulty may be encountered in the rare case of a previously undiagnosed congenital midface abnormality or in acquired conditions such as upper airway infection (i.e., tracheitis) or trauma. In the rare case of a neonate who cannot be intubated orotracheally and in whom ventilation via BVM or EGD is not possible (can't intubate, can't ventilate CICV), a surgical approach to airway management is indicated. In the CICV scenario in a neonate, surgical cricothyrotomy is exceedingly difficult due to the small size of the cricothyroid membrane and its position high in the neck. In small infants, needle cricothyrotomy (or more aptly named needle tracheostomy) is indicated. Needle tracheostomy has its basis in early animal studies using dogs, during which oxygenation was accomplished through a percutaneous catheter in the neck [32]. Using this technique, oxygenation was maintained for up to 1 h which conceivably could allow for additional orotracheal attempts as well as summoning additional resources to the bedside to aid in definitive airway management.

Diagnosis

The clinical conditions most commonly associated with the need for ED endotracheal intubation in the neonate are respiratory emergencies such as bronchiolitis, sepsis, and trauma.

Bronchiolitis

Neonates with bronchiolitis frequently require airway management due to centrally occurring apnea as well as respiratory fatigue from secretions and increased work of breathing. Nasal continuous positive airway pressure has been shown to improve respiratory outcomes in neonates with bronchiolitis and may be considered prior to intubation in select infants [33, 34]. If intubation is indicated and no difficult airway predictors are present, RSI is the procedure of choice. Preoxygenation will potentially be very difficult due to lower respiratory tract congestion. Atropine (0.02 mg/kg, minimum 0.1 mg) should be a strong consideration due to age. Induction with either etomidate (0.3 mg/kg) or ketamine (1–2 mg/kg) followed by paralysis with either succinylcholine (2 mg/kg) or rocuronium (1.2 mg/kg) would be reasonable choices.

Sepsis

Neonatal sepsis can present with fever or hypothermia or more protean manifestation such as increased sleepiness, poor perfusion, or poor feeding. Intubation may be indicated in situations in which the child's oxygenation is poor due to a pulmonary source of infection (i.e., pneumonia, viral causes) or the infant's work of breathing is leading to respiratory failure and fatigue. In the poorly perfused infant with sepsis, pretreatment with aggressive IVF (60 cc/kg over the first hour of resuscitation in 20 cc/kg aliquots) and consideration of vasopressor support can be critical to ensure that circulatory collapse does not occur peri-intubation. Atropine should again be strongly considered. Etomidate is somewhat controversial in the setting of sepsis due to concerns about cortisol insufficiency in critical illness [35, 36]. It is known that etomidate reversibly suppresses adrenal hormone production but it has not been shown to conclusively affect mortality. If etomidate is felt to be contraindicated, ketamine is a reasonable alternative for induction with either succinylcholine or rocuronium given for paralysis.

Trauma

In the setting of trauma, airway management may be indicated due to failure of oxygenation or ventilation or depressed mental status with the inability to protect the airway. Many of these neonates may be in a cervical collar which will make it difficult to optimally position these children. This difficulty can be overcome by removing the front of the cervical collar and holding manual in-line stabilization during direct laryngoscopy and employing videolaryngoscopy (if available) which allows for better visualization of the glottis. In the hemodynamically unstable trauma patient, induction with etomidate, which has a stable cardiovascular profile, or ketamine is preferable. There is a growing body of literature suggesting ketamine is safe, even in cases of neurotrauma, particularly when the patient is hemodynamically compromised [37, 38].

Multidisciplinary Considerations

Advanced airway management in the neonatal population is a rare procedure for many practicing emergency providers. RSI should only be performed by practitioners skilled in the practice. In cases where no practitioner who has trained in intubation is present, ventilation with BVM or an EGD can be lifesaving. When feasible, it may be helpful to consider consultation with a neonatal intensivist, ENT surgeon, or pediatric anesthesiologist and approach airway management in a multidisciplinary fashion.

References

1. American Institute of Ultrasound in M. AIUM practice guideline for the performance of obstetric ultrasound examinations. J Ultrasound Med. 2010;29(1):157–66.
2. Coleman AM, Merrow AC, Elluru RG, Polzin WJ, Lim FY. Tracheal agenesis with tracheoesophageal fistulae: fetal MRI diagnosis with confirmation by ultrasound during an ex utero intrapartum therapy (EXIT) delivery and postdelivery MRI. Pediatr Radiol. 2013;43(10): 1385–90.
3. Courtier J, Poder L, Wang ZJ, Westphalen AC, Yeh BM, Coakley FV. Fetal tracheolaryngeal airway obstruction: prenatal evaluation by sonography and MRI. Pediatr Radiol. 2010;40(11):1800–5.
4. Mong A, Johnson AM, Kramer SS, Coleman BG, Hedrick HL, Kreiger P, et al. Congenital high airway obstruction syndrome: MR/US findings, effect on management, and outcome. Pediatr Radiol. 2008;38(11):1171–9.
5. Lim FY, Crombleholme TM, Hedrick HL, Flake AW, Johnson MP, Howell LJ, et al. Congenital high airway obstruction syndrome: natural history and management. J Pediatr Surg. 2003;38(6):940–5.
6. Braun T, Brauer M, Fuchs I, Czernik C, Dudenhausen JW, Henrich W, et al. Mirror syndrome: a systematic review of fetal associated conditions, maternal presentation and perinatal outcome. Fetal Diagn Ther. 2010;27(4):191–203.
7. Bookman LB, Melton KR, Pan BS, Bender PL, Chini BA, Greenberg JM, et al. Neonates with tongue-based airway obstruction: a systematic review. Otolaryngol Head Neck Surg. 2012;146(1):8–18.
8. Mahieu HF, de Bree R, Ekkelkamp S, Sibarani-Ponsen RD, Haasnoot K. Tracheal and laryngeal rupture in neonates: complication of delivery or of intubation? Ann Otol Rhinol Laryngol. 2004;113(10):786–92.
9. Ammari AN, Jen A, Towers H, Haddad Jr J, Wung JT, Berdon WE. Subcutaneous emphysema and pneumomediastinum as presenting manifestations of neonatal tracheal injury. J Perinatol. 2002;22(6):499–501.
10. Levitan RM, Everett WW, Ochroch EA. Limitations of difficult airway prediction in patients intubated in the emergency department. Ann Emerg Med. 2004;44:307–13.
11. Losek JD, Olson LR, Dobson JV, Glaeser PW. Tracheal intubation practice and maintaining skill competency: survey of pediatric emergency department medical directors. Pediatr Emerg Care. 2008;24:294–9.
12. Sakles JC, Laurin EG, Rantapaa AA, Panacek EA. Airway management in the emergency department: a one-year study of 610 tracheal intubations. Ann Emerg Med. 1998;31:325–32.
13. Konrad C, Schupfer G, Wietlisbach M, Gerber H. Learning manual skills in anesthesiology: is there a recommended number of cases for anesthetic procedures? Anesth Analg. 1998;86:635–9.
14. Mulcaster JT, Mills J, Hung OR, et al. Laryngoscopic intubation: learning and performance. Anesthesiology. 2003;98:23–7.
15. Kennedy CC, Cannon EK, Warner DO, Cook DA. Advanced airway management simulation training in medical education: a systematic review and meta-analysis. Crit Care Med. 2014;42: 169–78.
16. Lindahl SG. Oxygen consumption and carbon dioxide elimination in infants and children during anaesthesia and surgery. Br J Anaesth. 1989;62:70–6.
17. Sagarin MJ, Chiang V, Sakles JC, et al. Rapid sequence intubation for pediatric emergency airway management. Pediatr Emerg Care. 2002;18:417–23.
18. Reed MJ, Dunn MJ, McKeown DW. Can an airway assessment score predict difficulty at intubation in the emergency department? Emerg Med J. 2005;22:99–102.

19. Kupas DF, Kauffman KF, Wang HE. Effect of airway-securing method on prehospital endotracheal tube dislodgment. Prehosp Emerg Care. 2010;14:26–30.
20. Sarkar S, Schumacher RE, Baumgart S, Donn SM. Are newborns receiving premedication before elective intubation? J Perinatol. 2006;26:286–9.
21. Chaudhary R, Chonat S, Gowda H, Clarke P, Curley A. Use of premedication for intubation in tertiary neonatal units in the United Kingdom. Paediatr Anaesth. 2009;19:653–8.
22. Kumar P, Denson SE, Mancuso TJ, Committee on Fetus and Newborn, Section on Anesthesiology and Pain Medicine. Premedication for nonemergency endotracheal intubation in the neonate Pediatrics. Pediatrics. 2010;125:608–15.
23. Attardi DM, Paul DA, Tuttle DJ, Greenspan JS. Premedication for intubation in neonates. Arch Dis Child Fetal Neonatal Ed. 2000;83:F161.
24. Barois J, Tourneux P. Ketamine and atropine decrease pain for preterm newborn tracheal intubation in the delivery room: an observational pilot study. Acta Paediatr. 2013;102(12):e534–8.
25. Feltman DM, Weiss MG, Nicoski P, Sinacore J. Rocuronium for nonemergent intubation of term and preterm infants. J Perinatol. 2011;31:38–43.
26. Kaplan MB, Ward D, Hagberg CA, Berci G, Hagiike M. Seeing is believing: the importance of video laryngoscopy in teaching and in managing the difficult airway. Surg Endosc. 2006;20 Suppl 2:S479–83.
27. Trevisanuto D, Fornaro E, Verghese C. The GlideScope video laryngoscope: initial experience in five neonates. Can J Anaesth. 2006;53:423–4.
28. Vlatten A, Aucoin S, Litz S, Macmanus B, Soder C. A comparison of the STORZ video laryngoscope and standard direct laryngoscopy for intubation in the Pediatric airway—a randomized clinical trial. Paediatr Anaesth. 2009;19:1102–7.
29. Xue FS, Tian M, Liao X, Xu YC. Safe and successful intubation using a Storz video laryngoscope in management of pediatric difficult airways. Paediatr Anaesth. 2008;18:1251–2.
30. Trevisanuto D, Doglioni N, Gottardi G, Nardo D, Micaglio M, Parotto M. Laryngeal mask: beyond neonatal upper airway malformations. Arch Dis Child Fetal Neonatal Ed. 2013;98:F185–6.
31. Ghai B, Makkar JK, Bhardwaj N, Wig J. Laryngeal mask airway insertion in children: comparison between rotational, lateral and standard technique. Paediatr Anaesth. 2008;18:308–12.
32. Cote CJ, Eavey RD, Todres ID, Jones DE. Cricothyroid membrane puncture: oxygenation and ventilation in a dog model using an intravenous catheter. Crit Care Med. 1988;16:615–9.
33. Cambonie G, Milesi C, Jaber S, et al. Nasal continuous positive airway pressure decreases respiratory muscles overload in young infants with severe acute viral bronchiolitis. Intensive Care Med. 2008;34:1865–72.
34. Thia LP, McKenzie SA, Blyth TP, Minasian CC, Kozlowska WJ, Carr SB. Randomised controlled trial of nasal continuous positive airways pressure (CPAP) in bronchiolitis. Arch Dis Child. 2008;93:45–7.
35. Dmello D, Taylor S, O'Brien J, Matuschak GM. Outcomes of etomidate in severe sepsis and septic shock. Chest. 2010; 138:1327–32.
36. Hohl CM, Kelly-Smith CH, Yeung TC, Sweet DD, Doyle-Waters MM, Schulzer M. The effect of a bolus dose of etomidate on cortisol levels, mortality, and health services utilization: a systematic review. Ann Emerg Med. 2010;56:105–13e5.
37. Himmelseher S, Durieux ME. Revising a dogma: ketamine for patients with neurological injury? Anesth Analg. 2005;101:524–34; table of contents.
38. Schreiber MA, Aoki N, Scott BG, Beck JR. Determinants of mortality in patients with severe blunt head injury. Arch Surg. 2002;137:285–90.

Transport of the Neonate with a Difficult/Critical Airway

Elliott M. Weiss and Nicholas Tsarouhas

Part I. Overview of Transport Systems, Models, and Regulations

Introduction

The safe transport of the neonate is the culmination of well-trained, highly skilled hospital teams working in well-organized transport systems. These programs function best when adhering to institutional, regional, and nationally accepted safety and quality standards. There are multiple successful transport team models, with no one model being universally acknowledged at "the gold standard." Each institution must maximize its available staff and resources to optimize their ability to safely retrieve patients.

The Section on Transport Medicine of the American Academy of Pediatrics conducted a National Consensus Conference on pediatric and neonatal transport in 2011. This conference, and subsequent panels and forums led to the publication of a "State of Transport" Consensus document [1]. The document outlined current transport models, discussed best practices, reviewed regulations, and gave recommendations for optimal transport systems, as well as future direction of the field. For transport programs to optimally meet the needs of the patient populations, institutions, and communities which they serve, their infrastructures must be solid, their protocols clear, and all must be cognizant of the rules which govern interfacility transport.

E.M. Weiss, M.D.
Division of Neonatology, The Children's Hospital of Philadelphia, Philadelphia, PA, USA

Department of Medical Ethics & Health Policy, University of Pennsylvania, Philadelphia, PA, USA

N. Tsarouhas, M.D. (✉)
Department of Pediatrics, The Children's Hospital of Philadelphia, University of Pennsylvania, Perelman School of Medicine, Philadelphia, PA, USA
e-mail: tsarouhas@email.chop.edu

EMTALA and the Principles of Transporting Patients

The Emergency Medical Treatment and Active Labor Act (EMTALA), passed in 1986 as part of the Consolidated Omnibus Budget Reconciliation Act (COBRA), is the cornerstone of transport law [2]. These federal acts were established to prevent inappropriate transfers and prohibit any transfer decision based on financial considerations. While the EMTALA obligations technically end when a patient becomes an inpatient, other regulatory statutes, medical–legal implications, and medical ethics have guided many to embrace these transport principles as best practices for safe and high-quality patient management across the continuum of care.

One such principle revolves around patient stabilization. EMTALA mandates that a patient presenting to an Emergency Department receive a medical screening examination by a qualified person to ascertain if an emergency medical condition exists [3]. An emergency medical condition is one with acute symptoms of sufficient severity in which the absence of immediate medical attention could seriously jeopardize patient health, or health of an unborn child [4]. If none exists, the EMTALA obligation ends. If an emergency medical condition exists, the hospital must admit, stabilize, or transfer. If the hospital cannot provide necessary patient care, then transfer is warranted.

Importantly, stability is not a prerequisite for transport. EMTALA defines "stabilized" to mean that no deterioration is likely to result from, or occur during transfer. The referring institution is required to stabilize the patient to the best of their institutional capabilities [5]. For example, a neonate with a critical airway might optimally be stabilized with a surgical airway. However, if the referring institution does not have those capabilities, they must secure the airway to the best of their abilities, and enact the transfer.

Once the transfer decision is made, the transferring physician must obtain acceptance from a receiving physician. For non-inpatients, a receiving hospital must accept a transfer request if it can provide specialized care not available at the

J. Lioy and S.E. Sobol (eds.), *Disorders of the Neonatal Airway: Fundamentals for Practice*,
DOI 10.1007/978-1-4939-1610-8_29, © Springer Science+Business Media New York 2015

referring facility if it has the capacity to do so [6]. Even if the receiving hospital believes that a transfer is not warranted, it is highly suspect to refuse. The receiving hospital should avoid judgment about referring hospital capabilities. For cases in which the team feels that transport may not be warranted, a complaint should be filed with the Centers for Medicare and Medicaid Services (CMS). For inpatients not under the EMTALA umbrella, it should always be kept in mind that a "refusal to accept patients" is subject to intense scrutiny from moral, as well as legal, standpoints.

Pre-Hospital Decision-Making

Decision-making responsibilities of the referring versus the accepting physician is frequently misunderstood and improperly interpreted. In short, the referring physician is the ultimate decision-maker. This is true for all decisions, including mode of transfer (air vs. ground), transport team composition, and clinical management. For example, the neonatologist may not mandate that a neonate be intubated prior to transport. While the receiving neonatologist is an "obligate consultant," the referring physician is not obligated to follow the receiving physician's advice. Moreover, transfer acceptance should never be contingent on the referring physician carrying out diagnostic or therapeutic recommendations. Of course, ideally, collaboration and collegiality should be the rule for both the receiving and accepting physicians.

Team Composition

While the composition of the transport team is ultimately the decision of the referring physician, the accepting physician should advise the referring physician on this important decision. A crucial axiom espoused by the "State of Transport" Consensus document [1] was that "the goal of critical care transport is to take services to the patient and begin advanced care rapidly." This goal dispels the notion that medical transport is merely transferring patients between institutions.

Many neonatal transports are performed by general transport teams without specific pediatric or neonatal training. Research has shown that critically ill children can be transferred most safely using a dedicated pediatric transport teams [7]. Even with very experienced groups, technical skills in general adult transport do not necessarily translate into adequate technical skills to manage smaller patients [8]. There is growing momentum in favor of such teams; this may be especially important when considering the transport of the neonate with a critical airway [9].

It is important to remember that there are several common models of transport teams across the country. Dedicated pediatric transport teams are free-standing teams whose primary responsibility is to transport patients. These teams routinely take on no non-transport patient assignments, though often assist throughout the hospital during "downtime." Most dedicated teams transport neonatal as well as "pediatric" patients, although some teams are exclusively "neonatal transport teams." Another model is the "unit-based" team. These teams mobilize team members from clinical units when a transport request is made. For example, a neonatal nurse is pulled from a patient assignment to go retrieve a patient for the NICU. Finally, there are some programs that utilize hybrid models of the above.

Personnel composition of each specific team also varies widely from center to center. A recent study reported the most common model for neonatal transport teams is one registered nurse and a respiratory therapist [10]. The same study, however, found 26 different team configurations. The second most common model is two nurses, but other combinations add physicians (residents, fellows, or attendings), nurse practitioners, physician assistants, and paramedics. Most experts recommend at least two clinical members on each team, but some one-person teams still exist. Other teams routinely utilize three members. Transport-specific training and experience may be more important than the specific combination of professional individuals [11]. Simulated team training has become standard at most institutions, to augment both didactic and "hands-on" training (Fig. 1). Of course, there should be someone with advanced neonatal airway skills on all transports of neonates with known or potential critical airways.

Mode of Transport

The neonate with a critical airway is amongst the highest acuity patient. Consequently selection of the optimal transport mode—ground vs. air—is a crucial decision. In certain situations, critically ill neonates may be most appropriately transported by rotor-wing aircraft (helicopter). There are many variables which must be considered in this decision-making, and a well-designed, well-staffed "Transport Command Center" is often invaluable in these decisions.

Weather is often the initial determinant of whether air transport is feasible. Rain, snow, wind and fog may all preclude rotor-wing transport in most cases. It is important that the pilots of flight teams make their decision to fly without any knowledge of the degree of critical illness of the patient. This best practice prevents the acuity of the patient from compromising the safety of the crew—and patient.

Distance is also of obvious importance. Specific practice paradigms vary widely for "how far" or "how long" should prompt flight (versus ground) consideration, but many start considering flight near the 60 min ground transport time. Consequently, traffic patterns are also major factors. A premier Transport Command Center will have continual traffic

a b

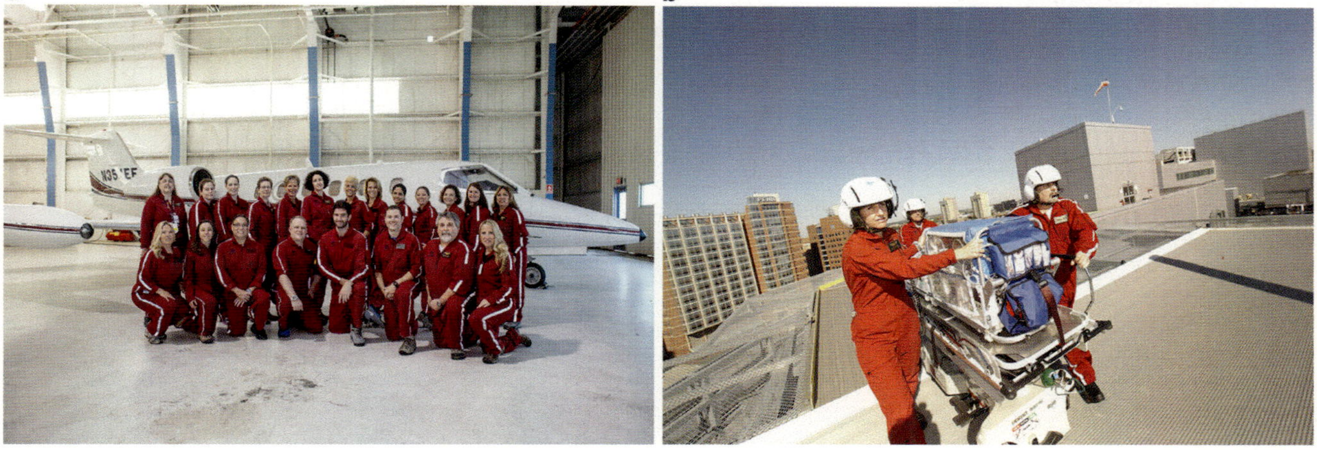

Fig. 1 (**a**) The Children's Hospital of Philadelphia Transport Team includes nurses, respiratory therapists, paramedics, EMTs, physician assistants, nurse practitioners, doctors, communications specialists, and other essential staff. (**b**) Members of the transport team participating in "Simulated Team Training" at the on-site helipad

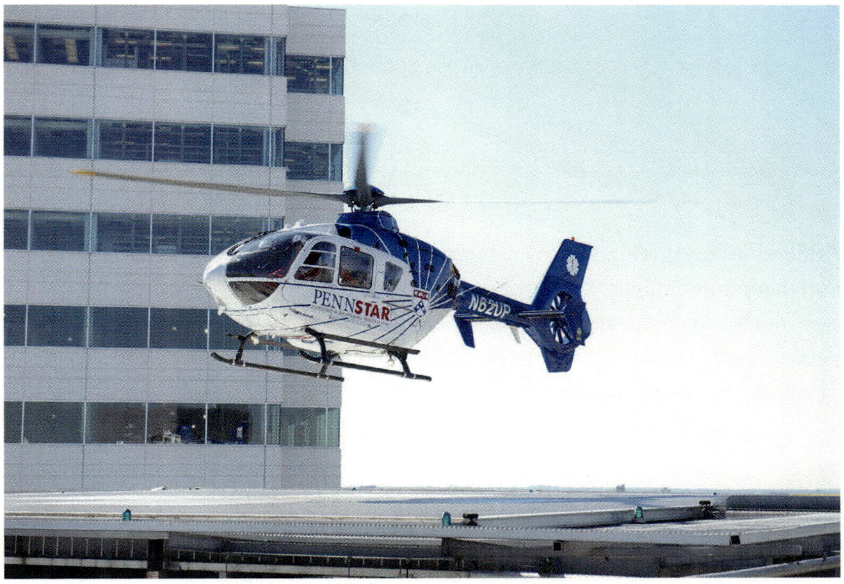

Fig. 2 Helicopter landing with a critical neonate at the on-site Children's Hospital of Philadelphia transport helipad

pattern monitoring to aid in decision-making. The presence or absence of an on-site helicopter landing zone is also crucial. An on-site helipad is highly preferable (Fig. 2). If the helicopter must land remotely, the patient must be transferred to a ground ambulance at the remote site; this may negate some of the benefits of air transport.

Of course, the acuity of the patient factors heavily into the decision-making. It often seems intuitive that "flight is better" for the very sick babies because it allows for more rapid transport; however, in some cases, the opposite may be true. A small, cramped cockpit restricts access to the critical neonate, so some life-saving interventions (e.g. endotracheal intubation) may be more difficult. Monitoring is also more challenging, from auscultation of breath sounds to pulse oximetry measuring. Some of these factors are discussed in more detail below.

Other variables to consider include team or mode availability (e.g., aircraft wait times), ability of the aircraft to accommodate equipment (e.g., isolettes), weights of staff (fuel requirements are heavily contingent on both air temperature and weight of aircraft), and request of parents to travel with their transported baby. Sometimes, a hybrid transport method, such as sending team via ground ambulance, with planned return via helicopter, may be the quickest and safest option available.

There has been much media, professional, and government attention directed at the safety of medical helicopter transports in recent years, with some high-profile tragedies [12]. One report noted the use of rotor-wing transport may be more dangerous than other methods and should only be utilized when medically necessary [13]. While there is

Table 1 Pros and cons of ground vs. helicopter vs. fixed-wing aircraft transports

	Ground	Helicopter	Fixed wing
Advantages	Availability Convenience (only two transfers of patient required: hospital to ambulance and ambulance to hospital) Ideal environment for "mobile ICU" Relative cost	Rapid transit time	Rapid transit time over extremely long distances
		Ability to reach inaccessible or remote areas	Able to fly above or around inclement weather
			Cabin size larger than helicopter cabin
			Cabin pressurization
Disadvantages	Not ideal for long distance transports	Adequate, unobstructed landing space required (field, helo pad, etc.)	Airport required
	Limitations of road and traffic conditions	Limitations of weather conditions (more prone to weather restrictions than ground transport)	Multiple transfers required (at least four transfers required: hospital to ambulance, ambulance to aircraft, aircraft to ambulance, ambulance to hospital)
		Multiple transfers may be required	Long distance from airport to either referring or referral hospital
		Limited range because of fuel capacity (compared with both ground and fixed wing)	Noise and vibration interfere with monitoring the patient
		Limited cabin space	Environment stresses of altitude
		Lack of cabin pressurization	High maintenance cost
		Noise and vibration interfere with monitoring of patient	Expensive
		High maintenance costs	
		Expensive	
		Safety?	

considerable disagreement over whether air transport is "more dangerous," it is not controversial that each time flight is considered, the risks and benefits should be carefully considered (Table 1) and the safety of the crew, patient, and family should not be compromised if there are any concerns from any team member.

Transfer of Responsibility

Regardless of how the team is to get there, after transfer acceptance, the referring facility must continue to manage the patient until the transport team arrives. The referring facility must keep the accepting facility updated on changes in the patient's condition, as well as important diagnostic study results. The accepting facility continues to serve as a consultant, but again, the ultimate decision-making lies in the hands of the referring physician.

Upon arrival at the referring institution, transferring clinicians should provide further clinical updates. The transport team should be congenial and professional, and avoid any insinuations of suboptimal management. While collaborative management is always paramount, as long as the transport team is in the referring hospital, ultimate responsibility rests with the referring physician. The transporting team assumes full control of medical decision-making when they leave the referring facility.

Medical Records and Consents

The referring institution must copy all records and include copies of all radiologic images. For patients subject to EMTALA, it is a violation to send only radiologic reports and not actual copies of the radiologic studies. Again, it is logical that all patients be transferred with radiologic studies which can be reviewed by the receiving institution.

The referring facility must also obtain consent for transfer [14]. Medical necessity and risks must be explained to the parent or legal guardian. This requirement may be waived if an emergent transfer is necessary.

Part II. Transport of the Neonate with a Critical Airway

Initial Triage

The transport starts with initial triage of the patient, with active involvement from both the referring and accepting medical teams. As detailed above, a dedicated transport communication center is crucially important. All calls from outside hospital providers should be on recorded lines for quality assurance and improvement purposes, as well as for medical–legal considerations. It is most helpful for a

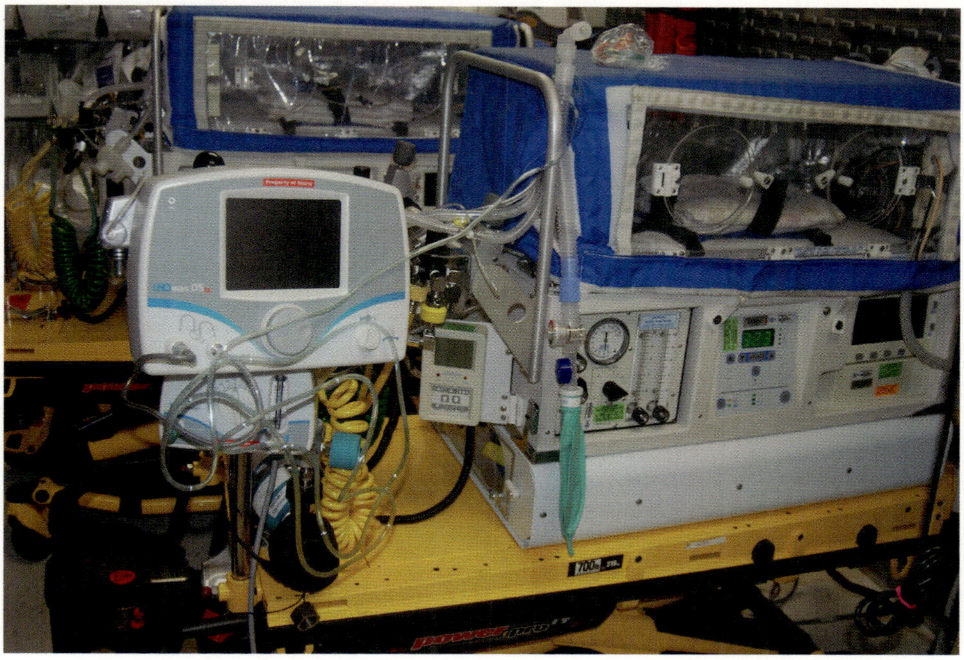

Fig. 3 Neonatal transport isolette with all standard equipment including a "built-in" neonatal ventilator, cardiopulmonary monitoring, inhaled nitric oxide all mounted on a sturdy sled

member of the communications center staff to be actively listening to conversations between the referring and accepting physicians. This allows for "real-time" decision-making between the two clinicians and the transport team. It also allows for optimal coordination with groups not otherwise privy to these discussions, such as inpatient nursing leadership, bed management, and security. It also has the benefits of keeping the medical record up to date in a timely fashion. Finally, the transport team staff will often ask additional questions which may not be obvious to the medical command physician, but essential for transport. Some examples include questions about patient weight, the security of current intravenous access, the presence of copied radiographic studies and completion of consents, and parental availability at the referring hospital.

The medical command physician must, of course, ascertain the current adequacy of the airway and determine if recommendations are warranted for alternative airway procurement. A focused, pertinent history must be obtained to assess for prior difficulties with intubation or anatomic anomalies that might increase the likelihood of a critical airway. The respiratory status must be evaluated, along with the current mode of ventilation. Hemodynamic stability and support should be reviewed, as well as the current state of intravenous access. Teams must consider if there is specific time sensitivity for potential treatment protocol (i.e., therapeutic hypothermia) or surgical procedures (i.e., volvulus reduction.)

Pre-dispatch Preparation

After the decision has been made to transport a patient, preparations must be made to dispatch the team. Once the team composition and mode are determined (see above) the medical command physician and transport team clinicians must determine the equipment necessary for safe transport. This might include, for example, assuring that the isolette is compatible with the chosen mode of transport, and if inhaled nitric oxide is being used, ensuring its requisite set-up is appropriate (Fig. 3). Transport-ready "go-bags" (Fig. 4) stocked with a consistent set of common medications and standard equipment (Tables 2) are a must. In some cases, additional medications or equipment might need to be obtained prior to departure.

The transport team must ensure that an adequate supply of oxygen is available for the duration of transport. This must factor in unexpected acute decompensations. The oxygen supply of each tank can be determined by the following formula:

Minutes of O2 flow = cylinder pressure x cylinder factor / flow of oxygen (in L/min).

Standard size tanks each have a coordinating cylinder factor: D (0.16), E (0.28), and H (3.14).

A pre-transport "Safety Checklist" is an invaluable tool for every transport team. This should be a comprehensive review of necessary equipment, medications, oxygen supply, essential demographic information, and other important

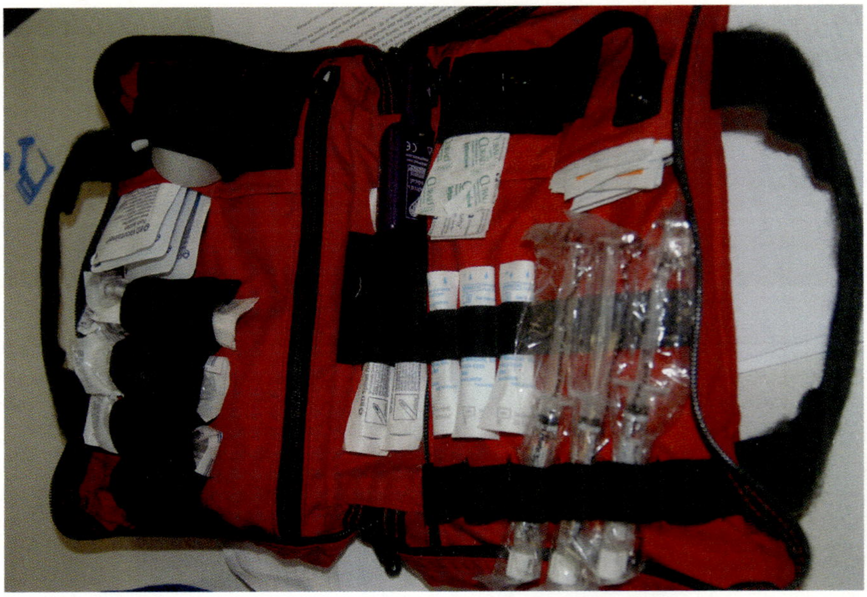

Fig. 4 Transport-ready "Go-bags" with all needed equipment and medications

Table 2 Basic equipment necessary for neonatal transport

Monitoring	Access	Point of care	Airway
Mapleson bag	IV catheters	I-Stat Cartridges	Laryngoscopes
Face masks	UV catheters	Capillary Tubes	Endotracheal tubes
Nasal cannulas	IO supplies	Finger/Heel Lancets	Styletes
Manometer with tubing	Tape	Glucometer	Magill forceps
	Flushes		Meconium aspirator
	Needles		Pedi-caps
	Syringes		Butterfly needles
Electrodes	T-connectors		Ventilator set-up
Oximeter probe	Stopcocks		Inhaled nitric oxide set-up
End-tidal CO_2 monitor	Alcohol/Betadine		
	Arm boards		
	Tegaderm dressing		
	Gauze		

reminders. All team members should participate in the completion of the safety checklist. This should be done for all modes of transport. A checklist should also be completed prior to departing for and from the referring institution. Fig. 5 depicts a sample checklist from The Children's Hospital of Philadelphia.

Considerations upon Arrival to Bedside

The arriving transport team should quickly perform an assessment to confirm clinical status. It is possible that the patient's condition may have changed and be significantly different than anticipated. The transport team should establish continuous monitoring and confirm placement of all support tubes and lines. Care should be taken to minimize tangling of lines, which can increase risk of dislodgement. It is extremely important to have unobstructed intravenous access and to have all lines carefully labeled for fluid boluses, re-administration of sedation, or in case resuscitation medications become necessary.

Special attention should be made to the pre-transport stabilization of any advanced airway and widely used non-invasive airways such as nasal CPAP. Importantly, the use of nasal CPAP has risen substantially over the last ten years, with many more infants now being transported on these devices (Fig. 6).

Before departing, recent radiographs should be reviewed to confirm endotracheal tube location and vascular access placement. A single-center study found that post-intubation chest radiographs resulted in endotracheal tube position change in nearly half of neonates awaiting transport. Not surprisingly, this was also associated with an increased time at referring hospital [15].

While all team members ideally should function in predetermined roles to streamline the process, it is also useful to have a team approach to ensure all duties at the outside hospital

The Children's Hospital of Philadelphia®

TRN 202 Rev. 9/12

PRE-TRANSPORT SAFETY CHECKLIST

For use with all Ground Ambulance, Rotor Wing and Fixed Wing Flights

REPORT / PLANNING

- ☐ Patient name (bracelet √ when applicable)
- ☐ Diagnosis
- ☐ Reason for transport
- ☐ Hospital name
- ☐ Hospital city & state
- ☐ Patient's unit location
- ☐ Transport plan of care discussed
- ☐ Team leader identified
- ☐ Team responsibilities defined – Routine
- ☐ Team responsibilities defined – Emergencies
- ☐ Destination airport: ____________________ ☐ NA
- ☐ Interim ground transport: ☐ ALS ☐ BLS ☐ SCTU ☐ NA

OXYGEN CALCULATION

Cylinder Oxygen:

$$\frac{\text{(gauge psi in tank - residual pressure) X cylinder constant}}{\text{Total Flow Rate in LPM}} = \text{Oxygen Duration (in minutes)}$$

Tank Size	Cylinder Constant	Residual Pressure (psi)
D	0.16	200
E	0.28	200
M	1.56	200
H	3.14	200

Liquid Oxygen:

$$\frac{\text{Total LPM x 60 x Duration of flight in hours}}{804} = \text{Amount of liquid oxygen needed}$$

EQUIPMENT NEEDED (check all that apply)

- ☐ Calculate oxygen requirements (2 times length of transport)
  - o Current oxygen requirement:__________ liters
  - o Emergency oxygen requirement:________ liters
- ☐ Air/Oxygen Requirement (Bring Compressor from CHOP and extra tanks for flight)
- ☐ Ambulance Inverter/Air Equipped
- ☐ Primary Transport Bag
- ☐ Secondary Transport Bag
- ☐ Rotor Flight Bag
- ☐ Red Medication Pouch (helo)
- ☐ Grey Box (fixed wing)
- ☐ 3% Saline
- ☐ Medfusion Pumps
- ☐ LTV Ventilator
- ☐ Nitric System (Nitric bag, Inomax, Tank)
- ☐ Pedimate
- ☐ Isolette
- ☐ Cardiac monitor
- ☐ Team Members' IDs, Passports, Licenses, Certifications, Money, Credit Cards, and Phones

PRE-DESTINATION DEPARTURE CHECKLIST

- ☐ All records copied including LABS
- ☐ Copies of all radiologic studies
- ☐ All Transport equipment retrieved
- ☐ Destination Unit
- ☐ Family informed of patient's destination
- ☐ Accompanying family/guardian with government-issued ID

Signatures of all CHOP personnel on transport:

Clinical Leader Signature	Printed Name	/ and/or Contact Number	Date	/ Time
Additional Staff Signature	Printed Name	/ and/or Contact Number	Date	/ Time
Additional Staff Signature	Printed Name	/ and/or Contact Number	Date	/ Time
Additional Staff Signature	Printed Name	/ and/or Contact Number	Date	/ Time

Fig. 5 Pre-Transport Safety Checklist used prior to departure

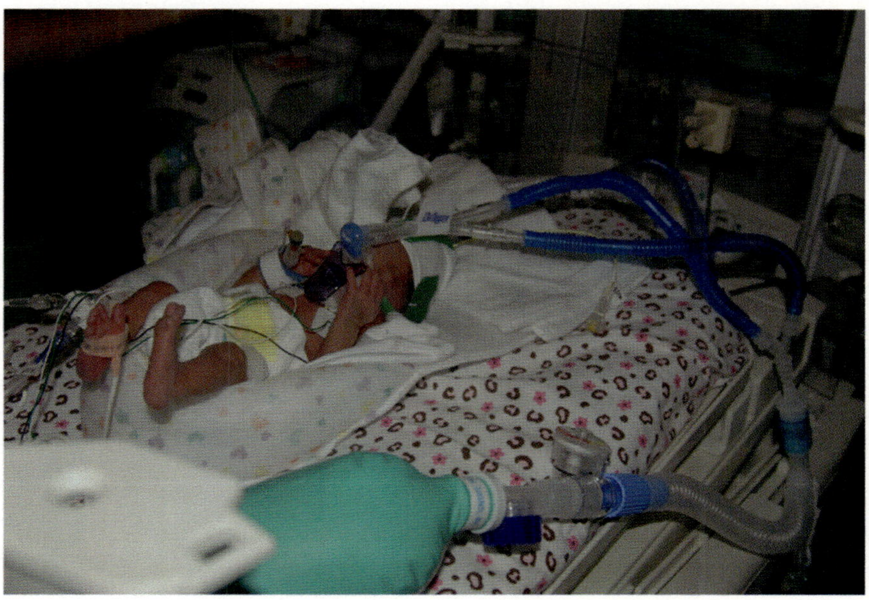

Fig. 6 Critical preterm neonate on nasal CPAP modified for transport

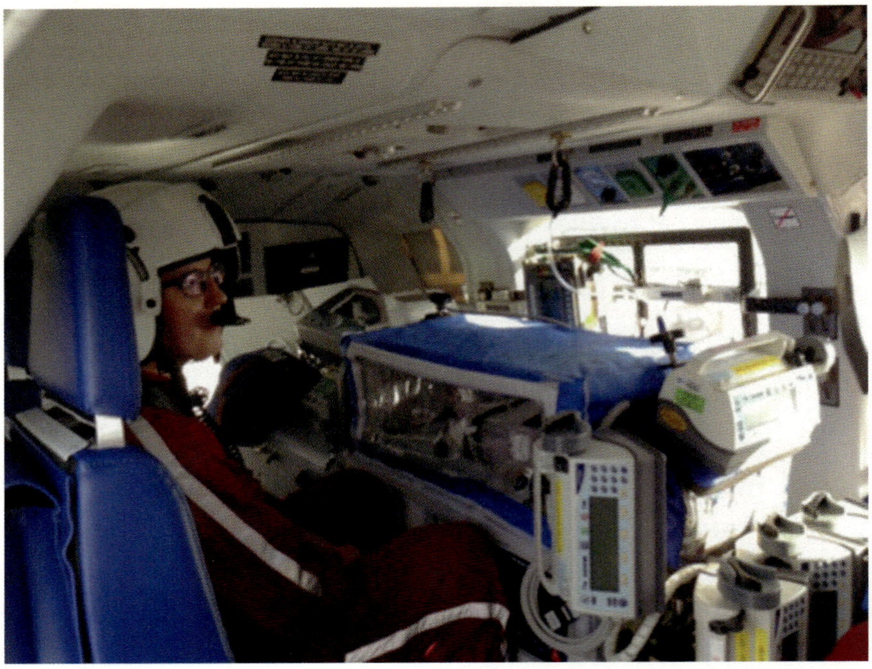

Fig. 7 Restrictive seating for Transport Staff inside Helicopter with loaded Isolette

are completed in a timely fashion. Constant communication is paramount, and frequent reevaluations are necessary.

Consent

As above, the responsibility for obtaining consent for transport is primarily the role of the transferring institution. However, it is always good practice for the transport team to review the risks and benefits of the transport with the family. When practical, one team member may leave the immediate bedside to have this discussion with the parents. The needs for transport and additional resources available at accepting institution should have been reviewed with the family by the transferring physician, but these topics may be reinforced. Parents should have the opportunities to ask questions. Many institutions hand out a "Welcome Pamphlet" with important information about the receiving institution. When practical, support, such as clergy, should be present if requested.

Transfer of the Patient in an Isolette

The physical transfer of the patient to the isolette may be the point of greatest vulnerability to the patient. The team member executing the transfer is responsible for assuring lines and equipment do not tether patient. Astute attention must be paid to vital signs and patient response to transfer, with a team member free to respond quickly if intervention is required. The transfer process should be performed while attached to the referring hospital's oxygen and medical air supply, thus reserving transport isolette resources for time out of hospital. Once the patient is in the transport isolette, a quick but thorough repeat assessment is performed of all support apparatuses before securing the patient into a neonate restraint system. After it is determined all necessary emergency equipment is accessible and belongings have been gathered, the last step is to disengage from referring hospital oxygen source, medical air, and electrical sources.

Prior to Departure from Referring Hospital

Once again, the team must review roles, discuss management plan, confirm what parameters will be targeted for return trip, and develop an emergency plan for unexpected acute decompensations. This plan should be carefully reviewed with the medical command physician. As a final check, the team should confirm that all appropriate documentation and copies of all radiographic studies are accompanying the patient.

Parental Accompaniment

At times, a parent will accompany the patient on transport. This is a best practice, when possible. On ground transport of sick neonates, the parent will often ride in the front of the ambulance,

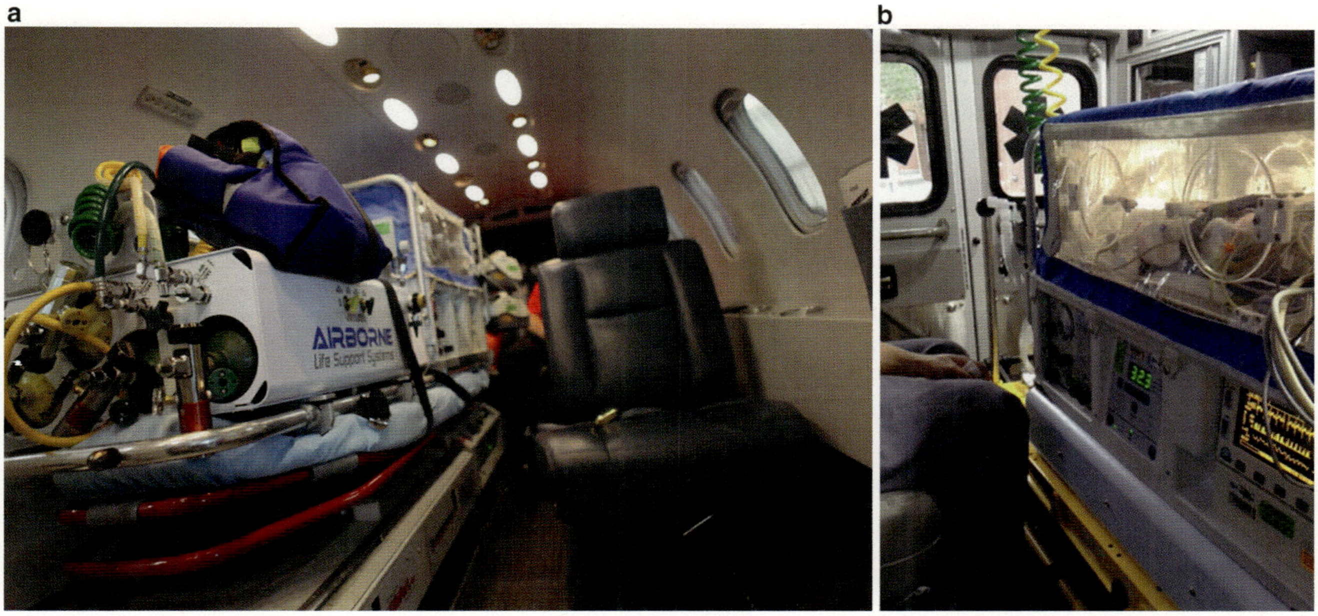

Fig. 8 (**a**, **b**) Limited seating inside a crowed fixed-wing jet and ambulance leaves little room for extra personnel

next to the driver, to ensure maximal contact and proximity of the transport clinical staff with the critical baby. Air transport is more challenging due to the limited weight and seating capacity. While helicopter seating is extremely restrictive (Fig. 7), even fixed-wing transport, seating is at a premium (Fig. 8a, b). Team members must be very mindful of their dialogue in front of the parents to prevent misunderstandings and to avoid unnecessarily frightening the family. If the parents will not be able to accompany the baby on the transport, they should be given time to say goodbye to their baby prior to the transport.

Transit to the Ambulance or Aircraft

Once in transit to ambulance, heliport, or tarmac, there should be one team member monitoring vital signs, while the remaining team members are managing isolette travel. As best as possible, trauma to the isolette should be minimized, as this could result in serious harm to the baby, such as interruption of continuous infusions, or dislodging of a piece of respiratory circuit tubing. Upon arrival to the ambulance or aircraft, the team must again work together to safely load the isolette (Figs. 9a, b). Great care must be taken for the safety of the patient, as well as the team members. There are several crush points to hands and fingers when loading an isolette. Serious lifting injuries may also occur. Situational awareness is paramount throughout the transport process.

Considerations during Ground Transport

Once the patient is safely loaded into ambulance, isolette resources must again be conserved by quickly converting to ambulance oxygen, medical air, and electricity. Note that with any change in air source, there is a risk of change in pressure delivery to patient; the knobs may have to be adjusted to keep delivery constant.

Prior to the departure, thought again should be given to all supplies, medicines, and equipment that may potentially be needed en route. It is important to realize that space is limited even with a ground ambulance (Fig. 10). Nevertheless, every attempt should be made to have everything needed within arm's reach and properly secured. Nothing that has potential to become a projectile in the event of a sudden stop, swerve, or collision, should be unsecured. Team members should make every attempt to not be unrestrained in a moving vehicle.

Developmental care and thermoregulation are especially challenging during this phase of transport, but remain important, particularly for the low birth-weight infant. Longer length of transports and temperature instability correlated with more severe transport physiological stability scores in a retrospective analysis of neonatal transports [16]. High levels of sound and vibration exposure in both ground and air transports have led some groups to recommend neonatal ear protection [17]. Nesting, minimal stimulation, and creating a calm environment are challenging, but can have tremendous positive effects.

a b

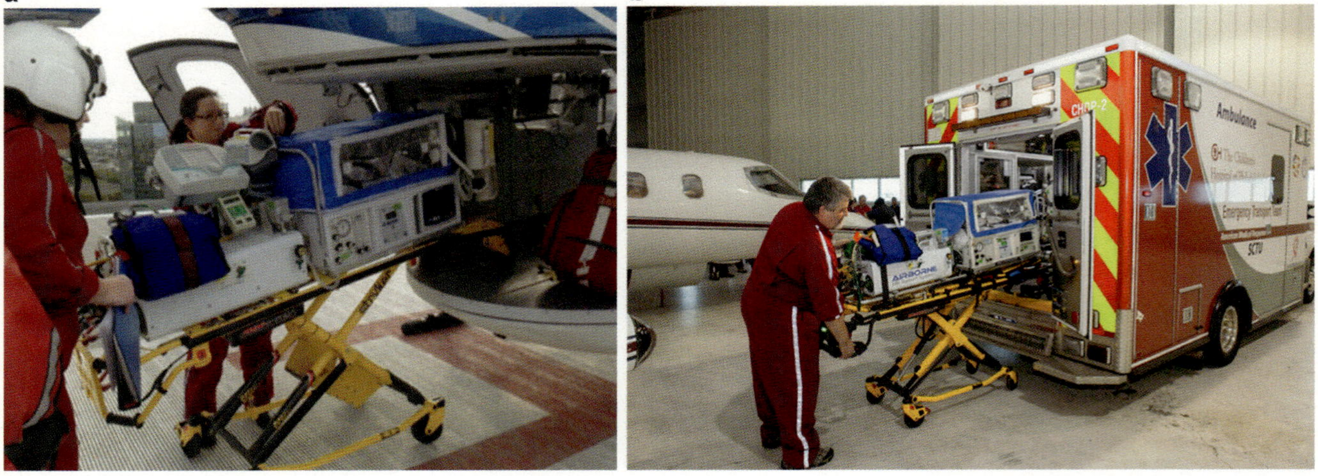

Fig. 9 Transport Team carefully loading the isolette with multiple mounted pieces of equipment into (**a**) the helicopter, and (**b**) the ground ambulance

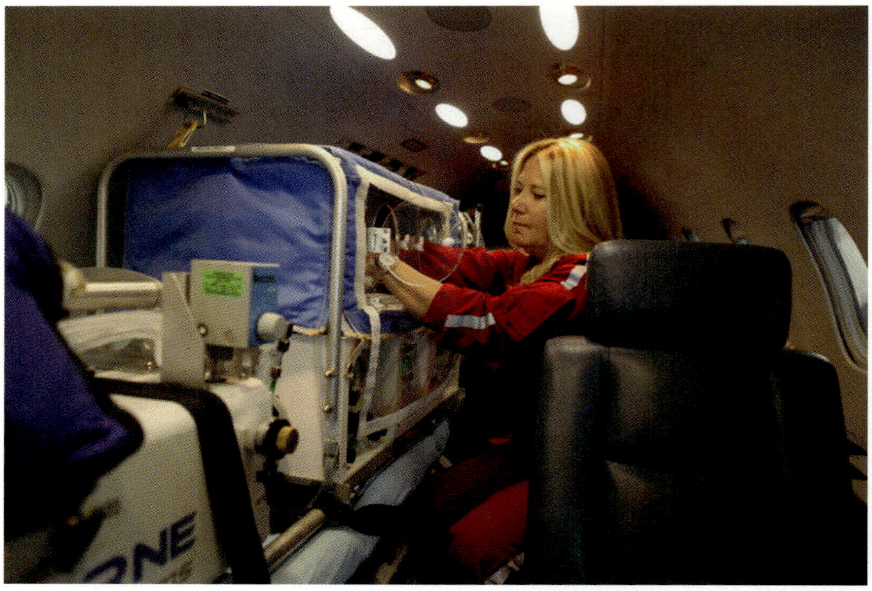

Fig. 10 Transport nurse working within limited space in a fixed-wing jet

Interestingly, ground ambulance transport has been associated with increased physiological stressors, as compared even with rotor-wing flight [18].

Once the team has arrived at the destination hospital, the same care used to load the patient into the ambulance should be used to off-load. Prior to disconnecting from ambulance resources, a careful assessment of the isolette should be performed to ensure adequate oxygen and medical air is available. If not, these can be brought to the ambulance bay prior to off-loading. Transport is not completed until the patient has been safely transferred from the transport isolette to the receiving radiant warmer bed or isolette. The same mindful process used to move the patient into the isolette is repeated in reverse order.

Special Considerations for Rotor-Wing Transport: Monitoring and Access

Situational awareness is never more critical than during a rotor-wing flight. All team members are now part of a medical flight crew, in addition to their roles as care providers to a critically ill patient. The safety of each crew member relies on those around them staying acutely aware of their surroundings. All members of the medical team should have undergone a helicopter orientation prior to embarking on their first rotor-wing flight. This should include a didactic session, as well as a helipad and helicopter session. The basics of safety are reviewed at such an orientation, including how to even approach the helicopter (i.e., never near

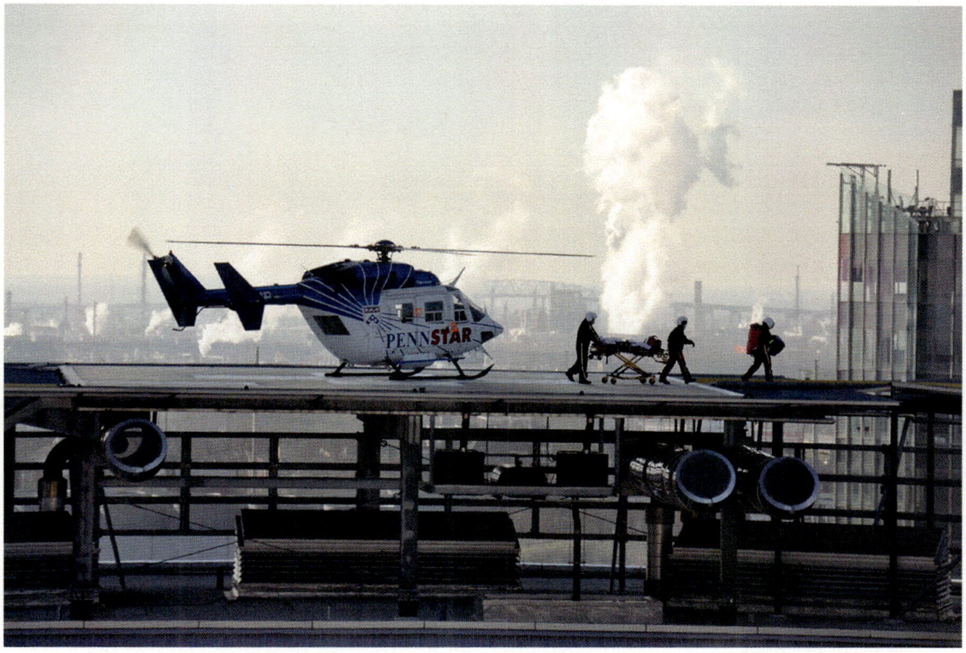

Fig. 11 The walk from the helicopter along a narrow path to the hospital

the tail wing!). Despite having to transport a sick neonate, a helicopter flight on a nice day can be a rewarding experience as the team is privileged to soar above the ground (Figs. 2 and 11).

Lift-off and landing are the most dangerous times in air travel. During this period, it is standard to have a "sterile cockpit," meaning no talking except for flight-safety issues. As possible, attention should be paid to potential air traffic, wire hazards, and migratory birds. Observing a sterile cockpit can create a significant challenge if the patient should decompensate and require active resuscitation. It is an option for the pilot to isolate the cabin microphones in such cases, but that should never be done without serious consideration and agreement of the entire crew, as the pilot will not be able to hear if a team member should need to alert them to a hazard. Of course, Communication with the accepting medical command physician is rarely feasible at this time.

In general, most helicopter flights do not impose significant flight physiology concerns. Flights over mountainous areas such as the Rockies, however, may present similar altitude concerns as with some fixed-wing transports. Altitude concerns and management adjustments are described in the fixed-wing section below.

The most common and important in-flight concerns on rotor-wing transports revolve around patient monitoring and physical access to perform care. While auscultation of breath sounds is difficult and highly inaccurate during ground ambulance transport, there is usually the option of safely pulling over to the side of the road. As this is obviously not possible for helicopter flights, it is important to realize that breath sound auscultation is essentially impossible during rotor-wing flight [19, 20] Heart sound auscultation has the same limitations. Moreover, for the neonate with the critical airway, there should be no realistic expectation that "upper airway sounds," such as stridor, will be audible during flight.

Pulse oximetry, usually reliable on ground transports, may be problematic on rotor-wing flights. Other noninvasive monitoring, such carbon dioxide monitoring, can be useful adjuncts. End-tidal CO_2 and transcutaneous CO_2 have been successfully employed for neonatal transport. However, some evidence suggests these methods are imperfect, and may not correlate well with arterial CO_2; their ability to reliably trend CO_2 is controversial [21, 22]. Nonetheless, noninvasive carbon dioxide monitoring may be a useful method to identify loss of an artificial airway on transport.

Limited access to the patient has been discussed above, but should again be emphasized. Simple things including checking the integrity of IV sites may become fraught with challenge. Staff, who should ideally be seat-belted at all times, must unbuckle themselves and sometimes maneuver toward the patient in awkward positions. Even essential clinical skills such as assessing for abrupt color changes (e.g., cyanosis, mottling, or pallor) can be problematic. Procedures, such as endotracheal intubation or intravenous line placement, are sometimes impossible.

Special Concerns for Fixed-Wing Transport: High Altitude

Fixed-wing transport can be utilized for transports of longer distances. Most of these aircraft are relatively compact jet

a b

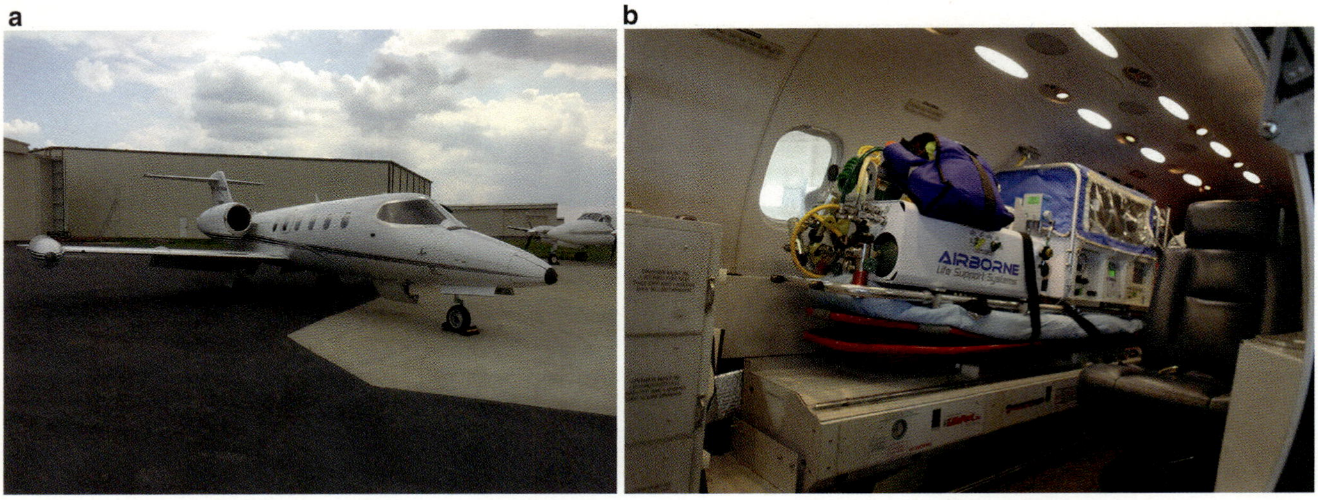

Fig. 12 (**a**, **b**) Compact fixed-wing jet used for medical transport with the isolette securely strapped to the anchoring sled

planes; some are used exclusively for medical flights (Fig. 12a). Again, each team has varying mileage range standards, geographic constraints, airport access variables, and flight vendor availability factors to consider. Additionally, due to rigid FAA restrictions, long flights may require an overnight stay due to mandated pilot "time out" rest. All equipment requires FAA approval for use during flight and everything must be secured to avoid injury (Fig. 12b). Once again, meticulous attention to limited oxygen, medical air, electricity, medical supplies, and medications is crucial. Communication with the medical command physician can be restricted during periods of flight, making advanced detailed planning especially important. Transfer of isolettes or stretchers into a fixed-wing cabin, like with rotor-wing, is challenging. The quarters within a fixed-wing aircraft, while not as restrictive as within a helicopter, are still space-limited. Extreme care to the physical stability of the isolette and to team safety to prevent injury is first and foremost.

Altitude considerations should be reviewed before each fixed-wing (and some rotor-wing) flights. As above, only high altitude flight significantly affects decision-making for helicopters, but it should always enter into fixed-wing discussions. Cabin pressurization (which must be discussed with the pilot in advanced) offsets some of the fixed-wing concerns, but does not eliminate them.

Fixed-wing flights require careful attention to the principles of flight physiology. At higher altitudes, there is an increase in size of enclosed air spaces, and a decrease in oxygen availability. The first concern relates to Boyle's law, which states that at constant temperatures, $P_1V_1 = P_2V_2$ (P = pressure; V = volume) for an enclosed volume of gas. At increased altitudes, there is a decrease in barometric pressure. Therefore, there is an increase in trapped gas volume at higher altitudes (Table 4). This is important to consider in infants with pulmonary, cardiac, and abdominal pathophysiologies. Additionally, monitoring with near-infrared spectroscopy suggests that clinically significant changes in cerebral oxygenation manifest at above 5,000 ft [35].

In neonates with air trapping physiology, most classically meconium aspiration syndrome, there will be an increased volume of trapped air compartments within the lung. This can result in worsening ventilation-perfusion mismatch, increased intrathoracic pressure (with decreased venous return to the heart), need for higher ventilation pressures, and increased risk of pneumothorax. A small air collection, such as a simple pneumothorax, can become clinically significant at higher altitudes.

Infants with known or suspected bowel obstruction also must very carefully scrutinized prior to transport for the presence of free air in the abdominal cavity. The increased volume of entrapped bowel air at higher elevations can become painful and increase abdominal competition on the lungs. Any draining devices (chest tubes, peritoneal drains, gastric tubes, ventricular drains) may require increased venting at higher altitudes. Care must be taken for any devices with entrapped air components, such as cuffed endotracheal tubes, tracheostomy tubes, Foley catheters, and even blood pressure cuffs. For example, to keep volume stable, the air in a cuffed endotracheal tube must be halved for a transport at an (unpressurized) altitude of 18,000 ft.

The second major concern related to altitude change is the decrease in oxygen availability. Dalton's law, $P_T = P_1 + P_2 + P_3 + P_4 \ldots$ states that the total pressure of a mix-

Table 3 Sedatives and paralytics commonly used for neonatal transport

Agent	Mechanism	Dose	Use	Onset	Recovery
Ketamine	NMDA antagonist	1–2 mg/kg IV	Dissociative agent	1–2 mins	5–10 mins
		3–4 mg/kg IM			
Propofol	From Wheeler & Wong—[36, 37]	2–4 mg/kg IV	Hypnotic, amnestic	30–60 secs	3–5 mins
Midazolam	GABA agonist	0.05–0.1 mg/kg IV/IM	Sedation, anxiolysis	3–5 mins	20–30 mins
		0.2–0.3 mg/kg IN			2–6 h (IM)
Lorazepam	GABA agonist	0.05–0.1 mg/kg IV	Sedation, anxiolysis	15–30 mins	Up to 8 h
Pentobarbitol	GABA agonist	2–3 mg/kg IV/IM	Sedation, anxiolysis	3–5 mins	15–45 mins
Fentanyl	μ-opioid agonist	1–2 μg/kg/ IV	Analgesia	30–60 secs	30–60 mins
Morphine	μ-opioid agonist	0.05–0.1 mg/kg IV	Analgesia	20 mins	3–5 hrs
Atracurium	NDNMB	0.25–0.4 mg/kg IV	Paralysis	2–3 mins	20–30 mins
Cisatracurium	NDNMB	0.1 mg/kg IV	Paralysis	2–3 mins	25–40 mins
Rocuronium	NDNMB	0.45–0.6 mg/kg IV	Paralysis	60 secs	25–35 mins
Vecuronium	NDNMB	0.1–0.2 mg/kg IV	Paralysis	1–2 mins	20–40 mins
Pancuronium	NDNMB	0.05–0.1 mg/kg IV	Paralysis	2–3 mins	45–120 mins

ture of gases is equal to the partial pressures of the gases within the mixture. Although the components of air remain stable at increased altitudes (i.e., oxygen 21 %, nitrogen 78 %), the decrease in barometric pressure means that air is less dense. Therefore, there is less oxygen available within a given volume of inhaled air. As altitude increases, there is a resultant alveolar hypoxemia, which can cause hypoxic pulmonary vasoconstriction leading to increased pulmonary vascular resistance. This can be combated by administering increased percentage of FiO_2 to keep oxygen availability stable at higher elevations during fixed-wing transport.

For example, there will be a similar PaO_2 attainable at 30,000 ft if given 100 % oxygen compared with the 21 % in room air on the ground. For patients who are hypoxemic on 100 % FiO_2 in hospital, the team must anticipate worsening hypoxia in-flight. Pressurization of cabins results in effective barometric pressures equivalent to altitudes of approximately 5,000–8,000 ft; as above, this will diminish, but not eliminate these problems. Increases in delivered pressure to the patient are typically not effective in reversing this problem. Finally, like oxygen, P_ACO_2 also decreases with altitude, because of hypoxic stimulation of the arterial chemoreceptors and subsequent increase in alveolar ventilation (Table 5).

Table 4 Effect of altitude on oxygenation

Altitude (ft)	Gas volume
Sea level, 0	1
5000	1.2
8000	1.3
10,000	1.5
15,000	1.8
18,000	2
20,000	2.2
25,000	2.7
30,000	3.4
35,000	4.2

Lower PaO_2s are seen with higher altitude due to the lower barometric pressures
P_B atmospheric pressure, PIO_2 partial pressure of O_2, $PACO_2$ partial pressure of CO_2, PAO_2 alveolar oxygen pressure, PaO_2 arterial oxygen pressure

Table 5 Effect of altitude on gas partial pressures

Altitude	P_B	PIO_2	$PACO_2$	PAO_2	PaO_2
Sea level 0 ft	760	150	40	110	105
Cleveland, OH 450 ft	747	147	40	107	120
Denver, CO 5280 ft	640	125	34	91	86
Pike's Peak, CO 14114 ft	450	85	30	55	52
Mount Everest 29028 ft	253	43	7.5	35	30

Sedation and Paralysis

The use of sedatives and paralytics (Tables 3) is an unresolved topic in neonatal medicine, and their use in transport is no different. Adverse consequences have been shown after exposure to untreated pain, as well as after administration of pharmacologic agents used to treat pain [23, 24]. The safety and long-term effects of opioids remain controversial, especially with preterm infants [25]. Benzodiazepines are often used as adjuncts for neonatal sedation, but also have potential adverse effects on the developing brain [26]. The neonate should be made as comfortable as possible on transport using non-pharmacological techniques such as swaddling and limiting unnecessary stimulation. However, clinicians must recognize that acute events which can usually be quickly and safely addressed in the hospital may be

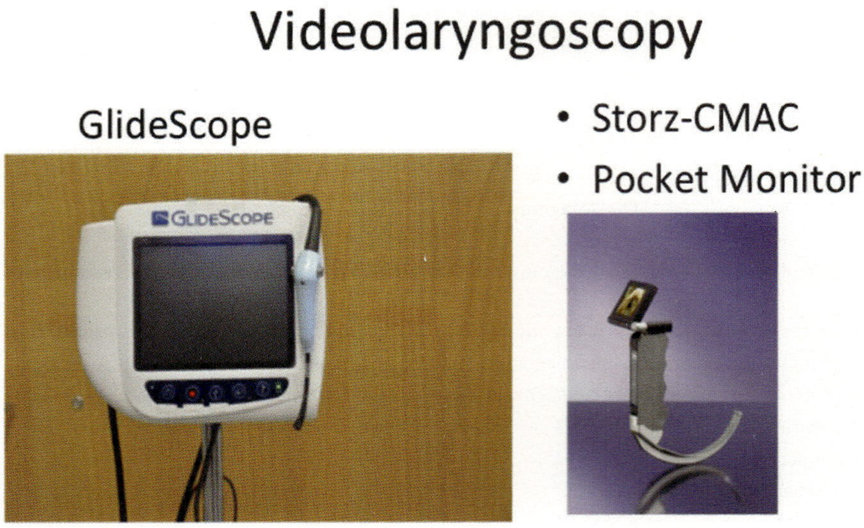

Fig. 13 Videolaryngoscopy used for intubation in critical or difficult neonatal airway emergencies. The Glidescope and Storz CMAC are the 2 "neonatal sized" videolaryngoscopes that are commonly used for transport

catastrophic on transport. Chief among these for the neonate with a critical airway is an accidental extubation or tracheostomy decannulation, which quickly become life-threatening events during transport. Sedation decreases the likelihood of unplanned extubations [27]. Therefore, a different calculus is required when assessing the risks and benefits of sedation and paralysis within the transport setting. The same level of sedation that would be acceptable in a neonatal intensive care unit may be inadequate for transport.

Similarly, there exists debate regarding the appropriate use of neuromuscular blocking agents in neonates. A systematic review of paralysis in neonates suggested a benefit in patients with asynchronous respiratory efforts [28]. Very limited neonatal literature is available, and the long-term safety profile and neurodevelopmental effects are unknown [29]. Paralysis can be a useful tool to maximize ventilation strategies and minimize risk of unplanned extubations during patient transport. Although each must be approached on a case-by-case basis, if the transport team and the medical command physician feel that the neonate's activity level increases the risk of life-threatening device dislodgment, then additional pharmacological sedation or paralysis is reasonable. Short-acting medications, with repeat doses en route as required, enable limited patient exposure, and minimize risk. It can be reasonable to consider longer-acting medications or infusions, especially in patients with previous opioid exposure.

Newer agents continue to be developed and applied to neonates. Dexmedetomidine, a G-protein coupled α_2-agonist, has been suggested as an alternative to opioid infusions, although the available data in neonates are limited [30]. This agent appears to have increased volume of distribution, decreased clearance, and increased half-life in infants, especially premature neonates [31]. Synthetic fentanyl derivatives such as remifentanil, sufentanil, and alfentanil are very short-acting opioids, but have very limited data available regarding neonatal use [32]. (See Table 3) The list is short for the more common sedatives and paralytics used for neonatal transports.

Advanced Airway and Ventilation of the Critical Neonate

As mentioned in other chapters, various advanced techniques for obtaining artificial airways are at the disposal of neonatologists treating patients with critical airways. Beyond endotracheal tubes and laryngeal mask airways are video laryngoscopy devices such as the C-MAC® and GlideScope®. If a difficult airway is anticipated, these can be brought with the transport team to the referring hospital. Of note, even commonly available devices may not be available in neonatal sizes at many hospitals; it is generally best to assume that the transport team will need to bring all necessary airway equipment (Fig. 13).

Ventilation support available on transport varies widely, but virtually all support that can be employed in the NICU can be provided by most transport teams. Nasal CPAP is a frequently employed method, but requires close attention on transport because of the risk of dislodgement from nares; this may require conversion to face-mask administration. Conventional ventilation can be provided in pressure control mode, rather than volume control, both because of device capability, and the difficulty to maintain pressure control ventilation with vibration and movement of transport.

High-frequency ventilation may be available to transport teams, including jet and percussive devices. Although very limited data are available, some centers have reported improved ventilation outcomes in extremely ill neonates requiring transport for surgical or ECMO evaluation [33, 34]. In babies with pulmonary hypertension, inhaled nitric oxide can be dramatically effective. Ideally, these advanced interventions and therapies should be trialed prior to team arrival, in order to allow for an appropriate period of assessment. However, in some circumstances, these interventions may be started immediately upon transport team arrival at the referring hospital. Once again, a period of observation as to adequacy of the trial is mandatory.

A few centers have the capability to perform surgical cannulation for ECMO upon arrival at a referral site, and/or the ability to transport a patient who has been started on ECMO at another center. The detailed of use of such modes of support is mentioned elsewhere in this book. The use or anticipated use of complex modes of ventilation support may require additional personnel on transport, such as respiratory therapy, additional nursing, or ECMO specialists. Physical space is often a constraining factor, especially in air transports.

Responding to Acute Decompensation

Within the inherently high-risk environment of neonatal transport, a relatively minor or moderate patient status change can have severe consequences. One of the most common and most feared events is an endotracheal extubation, with subsequent rapid decompensation of a neonate in respiratory failure. If this should occur in a moving ambulance, the driver should be asked to pull over so that team members can be safely unrestrained to assess the emergency. The patient should then be removed from the isolette to adequately perform a complete assessment and give better access for a potential reintubation. Such lifesaving procedures may lead to a loss of temperature control, so it is essential to replace the patient into the isolette as soon as possible Table 5.

If the infant's condition should deteriorate so profoundly such that the patient will not tolerate the time to reach the home facility, diversion may be necessary. Returning to the referring center, when practical due to proximity, is an excellent option, as they are already familiar with the patient. Diverting to any local hospital, however, is also reasonable, as it allows for patient stabilization under more controlled circumstances. Even an ambulatory urgent care center will have bright lights, solid ground, electricity, oxygen, and medical air. However, if it is clear that definitive care can only be provided by the destination/receiving facility, proceeding by ground may be the only viable option.

Every effort should be made to anticipate and prepare for decompensations in advance. Still, however, some changes cannot be predicted. An important option for ground transports, whether at the initial referring institution or at a diverted institution, is rotor-wing retrieval of the team and patient. Whether mode of transport needs to be altered due to patient changes (e.g., new pulmonary hemorrhage) or non-patient issues (e.g., weather, fuel, traffic), the medical command physician should be actively involved in the decision-making.

The Infant with an Unstable Tracheostomy

A special note should be made of infants with unstable tracheostomies who may require transport. Safe transport of this group of patients is often very tenuous. Prior to transfer to transport isolette, the stoma should be examined and the tube stability confirmed. There should be replacement tracheostomy tubes immediately available of the same size and one size smaller. These patients should be well sedated prior to and during transport in order to maximally protect their critical airways.

If the tracheostomy tube should be become dislodged, replacement should be primary goal (Figs. 14 and 15). If unable to immediately replace a tracheostomy tube through the stoma, oral endotracheal tube intubation or laryngeal mask placement may be life-saving options. If a patient with an open stoma is reintubated from above, care should be taken to cover the stoma with gauze and occlusive dressing to create an air-tight seal. Other emergency techniques that may be attempted in life-threatening situations include nasally inserted endotracheal tubes, and endotracheal tube insertion through the tracheostomy stoma. These critical airway techniques are also discussed elsewhere.

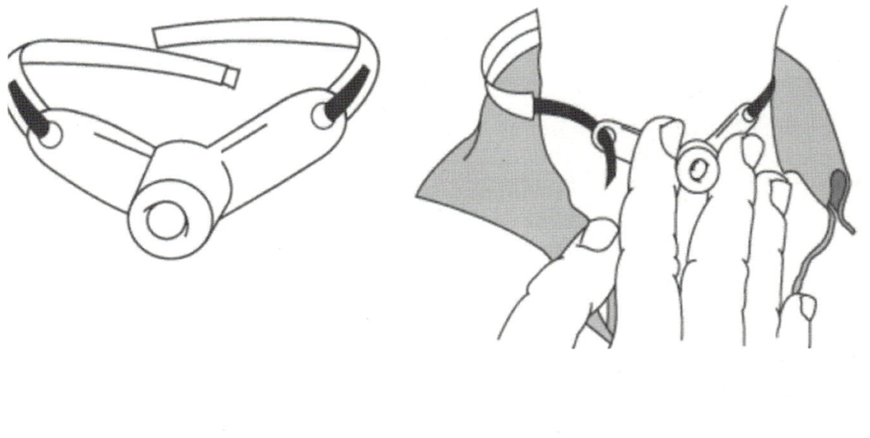

Fig. 14 Securing a tracheostomy during transport takes knowledge and skills learned during practice and simulation. (Courtesy of Michael Rutter, MD; Cincinnati Children's Hospital. Adapted from the CINCINNATI TRACH MANUAL)

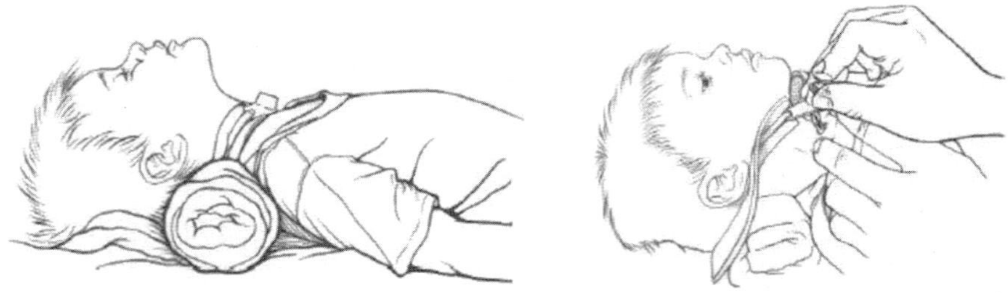

Fig. 15 Securing a tracheostomy during transport takes knowledge and skills learned during practice and simulation. (Courtesy of Michael Rutter, MD; Cincinnati Children's Hospital. Adapted from the CINCINNATI TRACH MANUAL)

Conclusion

This chapter has given the reader a solid background into the world of Transport Medicine as it relates to neonatal transport. Knowledge of interfacility transport laws, such as EMTALA, as well as decision-making responsibilities of the referring vs. the accepting physicians is imperative to ensure proper planning and outcomes. Because ground ambulance, rotor-wing, and fixed-wing transports all have their advantages and unique challenges, a thorough understanding of these modes of transport allows for maximal safety and optimal outcomes. The management on transport of this fragile population of neonates with critical airways must be swift and precise; a comprehensive understanding of the clinical factors and potential pitfalls cannot be overstated.

References

1. Stroud MH, Trautman MS, Meyer K, Moss MM, Schwartz HP, Bigham MT, Tsarouhas N, Price-Douglas W, Romito J, Hauft S, Meyer MT, Insoft R. Pediatric and neonatal interfacility transport: results from a national consensus conference. Pediatrics. 2013;132(2):359–66.
2. U.S. Code of Federal Regulations. U.S. Government Printing Office. EMTALA Statute. Title 42 USC 1395dd.
3. Testa PA, Gang M. Triage, EMTALA, consultations, and prehospital medical control. Emerg Med Clin North Am. 2009;27(4):627–40. Viii–ix.
4. Teshome G, Closson FT. Emergency Medical Treatment and Labor Act: the basics and other medicolegal concerns. Pediatr Clin North Am. 2006;53(1):139–55.
5. Glass DL, Rebstock J, Handberg E. Emergency Treatment and Labor Act (EMTALA). Avoiding the pitfalls. J Perinat Neonatal Nurs. 2004;18(2):103–16.
6. Glover RL. Hospital's duty to accept transfers under EMTALA. American Academy of Emergency Medicine; http://www.aaem.org/em-resources/regulatory-issues/emtala/transfer; 2012.
7. Orr RA, Felmet KA, Han Y, McCloskey KA, Dragotta MA, Bills DA, Kuch BA, Watson RS. Pediatric specialized transport teams are associated with improved outcomes. Pediatrics. 2009;124(1):40–8.
8. Woodward GA, Garrett AL, King BR, Baker MD. Emergency medical services and transport medicine. In: Fleisher GR, Ludwig S, editors. Textbook of pediatric emergency medicine. Philadelphia: Wolters Kluwer; 2010. p. 85–124.
9. Ajizian SJ, Kawagawa TA. Interfacility transport of the critically Ill pediatric patient. Chest. 2007;132(4):1361–7.
10. Karlsen KA, Trautman M, Price-Douglas W, Smith S. National survey of neonatal transport teams in the United States. Pediatrics. 2011;128(4):685–91.
11. Fenton AC, Leslie A. Who should staff neonatal transport teams? Early Hum Dev. 2009;85(8):487–90.
12. Association of Air Medical Services. Air medical accident/incident preparation, response, and recovery: lessons from crash survivors. 2012.
13. National Transportation Safety Board. Special Investigation Report on Emergency Medical Services Operations. Aviation Special Investigation Report. 2006; NTSB/SIR-06/01; PB2006-917001. Washington, DC.
14. Peth HA. The Emergency Medical Treatment and Active Labor Act (EMTALA): guidelines for compliance. Emerg Med Clin North Am. 2004;22(1):225–40.
15. Sanchez-Pinto N, Giuliano JS, Schwartz HP, Garrett L, Gothard MD, Kantak A, Bigham MT. The impact of postintubation chest radiograph during pediatric and neonatal critical care transport. Pediatr Crit Care Med. 2013;14(5):e213–7.
16. Arora P, Bajaj M, Natarajan G, Arora NP, Kalra VK, Zidan M, Shankaran S. Impact of interhospital transport on the physiologic status of very low-birth-weight infants. Am J Perinatol. 2014;31(3):237–44.
17. Karlsson BM, Lindkvist M, Lindkvist M, Karlsson M, Lundström R, Håkansson S, Wiklund U, van den Berg J. Sound and vibration: effects on Infants' heart rate and heart rate variability during neonatal transport. Acta Paediatr. 2012;101(2):148–54.
18. Bouchut JC, Van Lancker E, Chritin V, Gueugniaud PY. Physical stressors during neonatal transport: helicopter compared with ground ambulance. Air Med J. 2011;30(3):134–9.
19. Brown LH, Gough JE, Bryan-Berg DM, Hunt RC. Assessment of breath sounds during ambulance transport. Ann Emerg Med. 1997;29(2):228–31.
20. Hunt RC, Bryan DM, Brinkley VS, Whitley TW, Benson NH. Inability to assess breath sounds during Air medical transport by helicopter. JAMA. 1991;265(15):1982–4.
21. Tingay DG, Stewart MJ, Morley CJ. Monitoring of end tidal carbon dioxide and transcutaneous carbon dioxide during neonatal transport. Arch Dis Child Fetal Neonatal Ed. 2005;90(6):F523–6.
22. Bhende MS, Karr VA, Wiltsie DC, Orr RA. Evaluation of a portable infrared end-tidal carbon dioxide monitor during pediatric interhospital transport. Pediatrics. 1995;95:875–8.
23. Smith GC, Gutovich J, Smyser C, Pineda R, Newnham C, Tjoeng TH, Vavasseur C, Wallendorf M, Neil J, Inder T. Neonatal intensive care unit stress is associated with brain development in preterm infants. Ann Neurol. 2011;70:541–9.
24. Davidson A, Flick RP. Neurodevelopmental implications of the use of sedation and analgesia in neonates. Clin Perinatol. 2013;40(3):559–73.
25. McPherson C, Grunau RE. Neonatal pain control and neurologic effects of anesthetics and sedatives in preterm infants. Clin Perinatol. 2014;41(1):209–27.

26. Nelson MA, Bradshaw WT. Use of benzodiazepines as anxiolytics in neonates: are we there yet? Adv Neonatal Care. 2014;14(2):78–85.
27. Little LA, Koenig JC, Newth CJL. Factors affecting accidental extubations in neonatal and pediatric intensive care patients. Crit Care Med. 1990;18(2):163–5.
28. Cools F, Offringa M. Neuromuscular paralysis for newborn infants receiving mechanical ventilation. Cochrane Database Syst Rev. 2005;18(2), CD002773.
29. Honsel M, Giugni C, Brierley J. Limited professional guidance and literature are available to guide the safe use of neuromuscular block in infants. Acta Paediatr. 2014;103(9):e370–3.
30. O'Mara K, Gal P, Wimmer J, Ransom JL, Carlos RQ, Dimaguila MA, Davanzo CC, Smith M. Dexmedetomidine versus standard therapy with fentanyl for sedation in mechanically ventilated premature neonates. J Pediatr Pharmacol Ther. 2012;17(3):252–62.
31. Chrysostomou C, Schulman SR, Herrera Castellanos M, Cofer BE, Mitra S, da Rocha MG, Wisemandle WA, Gramlich L. A phase II/III, multicenter, safety, efficacy, and pharmacokinetic study of dexmedetomidine in preterm and term neonates. J Pediatr. 2014;164(2):276–82.
32. Allegaert K, Tibboel D, van den Anker J. Pharmacological treatment of neonatal pain: in search of a new equipoise. Semin Fetal Neonatal Med. 2013;18(1):42–7.
33. Mainali ES, Greene C, Rozycki HJ, Gutcher GR. Safety and efficacy of high-frequency jet ventilation in neonatal transport. J Perinatol. 2007;27(10):609–13.
34. Zhang Q, Macartney J, Sampaio L, O'Brien K. High frequency Jet ventilation during initial management, stabilization, and transport of newborn infants with congenital diaphragmatic hernia: a case series. Crit Care Res Pract. 2013;2013:937871.
35. Stroud MH, Gupta P, Prodhan P. Effect of altitude on cerebral oxygenation during pediatric interfacility transport. Pediatr Emerg Care. 2012;28(4):329–32.
36. Wheeler DS, Poss WB. Pediatric transport medicine. In: Wheeler DS, Wong HR, Shanley TP, editors. Resuscitation and stabilization of the critically ill child. London: Springer; 2009. p. 125–36.
37. Wheeler DS, Spaeth JP, Mehta R, Hariprakash SP, Cox PN. Assessment and management of the pediatric airway. In: Wheeler DS, Wong HR, Shanley TP, editors. Pediatric critical care medicine: basic science and clinical evidence. London: Springer; 2007. p. 223–52.

The Use of Simulation Training in Preparation for Neonatal and Infant Airway Emergencies

Megan Gray and Heather M. French

Abbreviations

AAR	After action review
ACGME	Accreditation Council for Graduate Medical Education
ANTS	Anesthesia nontechnical skills
BMV	Bag mask ventilation
CT	Computed tomography
DL	Direct laryngoscopy
ENT	Ear nose throat
EXIT	Ex utero intrapartum treatment
ICU	Intensive care unit
LMA	Laryngeal mask airway
NICU	Neonatal intensive care unit
NP	Nasopharyngeal
NRP	Neonatal resuscitation protocol
OP	Oropharyngeal
OR	Operating room
PPV	Positive pressure ventilation
SBML	Simulation-based mastery learning
TIAE	Tracheal intubation associated events

Introduction

Educating the next generation of medical professionals and refreshing the skills of current professionals around management of the difficult neonatal airway are of paramount importance. Infants with difficult-to-manage airways are at extremely high risk of adverse outcomes and long-term morbidity and mortality. Advanced prenatal imaging and heightened awareness of infants at risk in the Neonatal Intensive Care Unit (NICU) have led to better anticipation of difficult airway situations. However, infants with undiagnosed airway or head and neck malformations may deliver in community hospitals without pediatric subspecialty support, present in well baby nurseries, or come to medical attention in local emergency departments when a concurrent illness pushes them into distress. As such, the first medical provider who sees such an infant could be a nurse, nurse practitioner, physician assistant, pediatric resident, community hospital provider or outpatient clinician who may not have advanced training in management of infants who require artificial airways.

Every medical professional who will interact with neonates and infants needs to be trained to identify risk factors, signs, and symptoms of airway problems. Additionally, every provider should be competent with basic airway management skills necessary to stabilize these infants until they can be evaluated by personnel with advanced airway skills. The Pediatric Residency Review Committee requires that pediatric residents receive sufficient training with neonatal endotracheal intubation prior to independent practice, and in a survey of program directors, neonatal intubation and bag mask ventilation (BMV) rank as "extremely important" among procedures for trainees [1, 2]. In the past, airway education took place on the job, but the relative rarity of these events combined with limited exposure at the individual level has created a knowledge and skill gap that may put patients at risk.

Historically, physician training relied heavily on patient volume to ensure proficiency. Long hours, clinical focus on inpatient care, and limited in-house attending and subspecialty supervision on call meant that residents had multiple chances for hands-on exposure to patients with airway conditions requiring intervention. Training was predominantly with live patients in actual clinical settings, and the majority of patients with pulmonary pathology were intubated, making opportunities for intubation more plentiful. Over time, global clinician exposure to intubation and difficult airways

Electronic Supplementary Material: The online version of this chapter (doi: 10.1007/978-1-4939-1610-8_30) contains supplementary material. This video is also available to watch on http:/www.springerimages.com/videos/978-1-4939-1609-2.

M. Gray, M.D. (✉) • H.M. French, M.D.
Division of Neonatology, The Children's Hospital of Philadelphia, University of Pennsylvania, Perelman School of Medicine, 34th St and Civic Center Blvd, Philadelphia, PA 19104-4318, USA
e-mail: grayml@email.chop.edu; frenchh@email.chop.edu

DOI 10.1007/978-1-4939-1610-8_30,

has steadily decreased. For example, the Neonatal Resuscitation Program (NRP) no longer recommends that vigorous infants with meconium staining be intubated for tracheal suctioning [3]. Additionally, more patients are managed with noninvasive ventilation techniques, reducing the number of opportunities to use intubation skills [4].

Over the years, the traditional model of physician training has changed in many ways. Duty-hour restrictions have lead to greatly reduced patient care hours, thus decreasing the number of opportunities for procedural performance. Since the 1990s, intubation opportunities at some pediatric residencies have been reduced over 50 % to less than 20 chances per resident to attempt intubation [5]. As attempts are successful only about 20–30 % of the time in pediatric residents, a resident may graduate with less than six successful intubations and even fewer neonatal intubations [4, 5]. Studies done with anesthesia residents have shown that a trainee needs approximately 40 intubations in order to achieve an 80 % success rate [8]. This means that many, if not most, pediatric residents lack sufficient experience to perform neonatal intubations upon residency graduation. Additionally, neonatal resuscitation skills, including airway management, are difficult to master; despite NRP training, many residents still lack basic delivery room skills [9].

Along with the many changes to training, pediatric residencies are working to create tract systems that allow residents with specific interests to use their limited training time to focus their rotations on their chosen career paths. For residents pursuing a primary care career, this may mean as little as 2 months of time devoted to neonatal intensive care. To fill the gap in neonatal front line patient care created by duty-hour restrictions and tract systems for residents, most hospitals have switched to having non-resident front line clinicians. Front line clinicians may include nurse practitioners, physician assistants, clinical nurse specialists, and hospitalists. In addition to residents needing extra training to manage the difficult neonatal airway, a large group of front line clinicians also require the same education. In an age where fewer infants require advanced airway management and there are more clinicians to train and ensure proficiency, creative educational solutions are required.

With the known gaps in basic airway management skills, it is reasonable to assume that the majority of residents and front line clinicians lack adequate training and exposure to manage infants with normal airways, let alone those with difficult or abnormal airways. To fill these gaps, educators have many options including lecture, operating room training, and simulation. In a large meta-analysis, simulation was shown to be the superior training method for airway management [10]. Simulation training can first be used to elucidate knowledge gaps and identify areas for improved training. Subsequently, simulations can be designed to address these identified gaps in knowledge and performance.

Infant care providers require education in many areas of airway management. Even the most basic skill of bag mask ventilation requires training to perform properly. Procedures such as the use of laryngeal mask airway, oropharyngeal or nasopharyngeal airways, oral intubation, nasal intubation, and care of tracheostomy tubes all require education and practice to perform competently. Airway education programs can use manikins, animals, or live or deceased patients to practice important airway maneuvers. Manikin-based simulation provides an easily accessible and risk free means for many healthcare providers to obtain this valuable education.

Acceptance of and requirements for simulation-based education are expanding. Simulation and skills laboratories are required by the Accreditation Council for Graduate Medical Education (ACGME) for accredited general surgery programs [11]. Simulation has been recognized as such a valuable airway training tool in the field of Anesthesia that all attending anesthesiologists must participate in a simulation program, including difficult airway management, in order to satisfy their Maintenance of Certification requirements for the American Board of Anesthesiology [12]. Additionally, insurance premiums have been reduced for obstetricians and for general surgeons who have undergone simulation training [13]. Ziv et al. challenges physicians to consider that training using simulation, when available and appropriate, is an ethical imperative [14].

Models of Airway Training

Simulation training programs can span a wide range of options ranging from simple, supervised patient encounters to multidisciplinary simulations using highly realistic patient simulators [15]. Traditional medical training programs often used actual or standardized patients, providing trainees an opportunity to practice taking a medical history and performing a physical exam. This type of model has obvious significant limitations, both for infants and airway management. Live patients provide the most valuable learning experience but carry risks to patients and occur under unpredictable conditions. As such, new modalities were created to assist trainees to improve their airway management skills. These include live animal or human cadaveric models, airway task trainers, virtual models, and low- and high-technology patient manikins.

Airway models do not necessarily need to include the entire body or even the entire respiratory tract. Task trainers are models designed to replicate only the anatomic area necessary to practice a specific procedure. For example, an airway task trainer needs only to include the upper respiratory tract down to the trachea (Fig. 1). Task trainers can be used to practice bag mask ventilation, jaw thrust, oral and nasal endotracheal intubation, and the use of alternative airway devices.

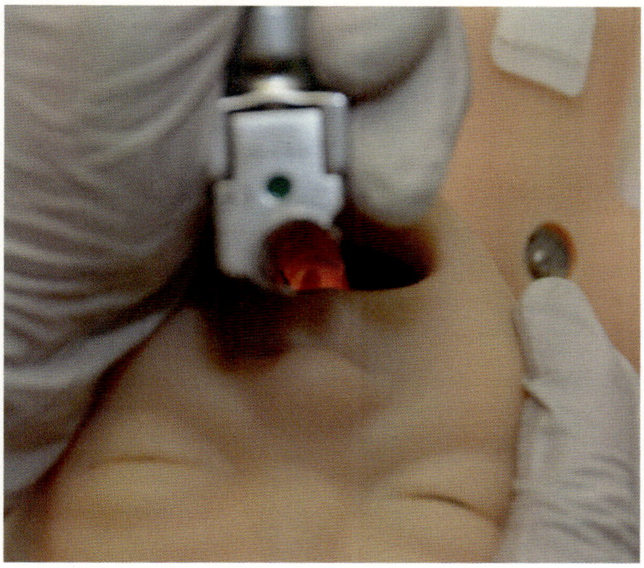

Fig. 1 Task trainer model of upper airway. This photo shows the view of the manikin's vocal cords as seen during intubation.

Task trainers are ideal for procedural training but have limited utility in practicing comprehensive emergency airway management. Educational objectives in broader airway management scenarios are often better achieved with manikins.

There are many options for simulation manikins available on the market that range in cost from a few hundred to several thousand dollars. The fidelity, or technological capability, of a manikin refers to how closely the model represents an actual patient. A high-fidelity patient simulator incorporates a manikin upon whom procedures such as intubation and chest tube placement can be performed, as well as physical exam findings that can be manipulated, and real time vital sign monitors that are controlled by computer software. The available software programs allow the simulation facilitator to change the manikin's physical exam findings and vital signs as the clinical scenario progresses. Centers with high-fidelity simulators often perform simulations in situ or have a space set up to resemble their unit's standard patient room or resuscitation room to add realism (Fig. 2).

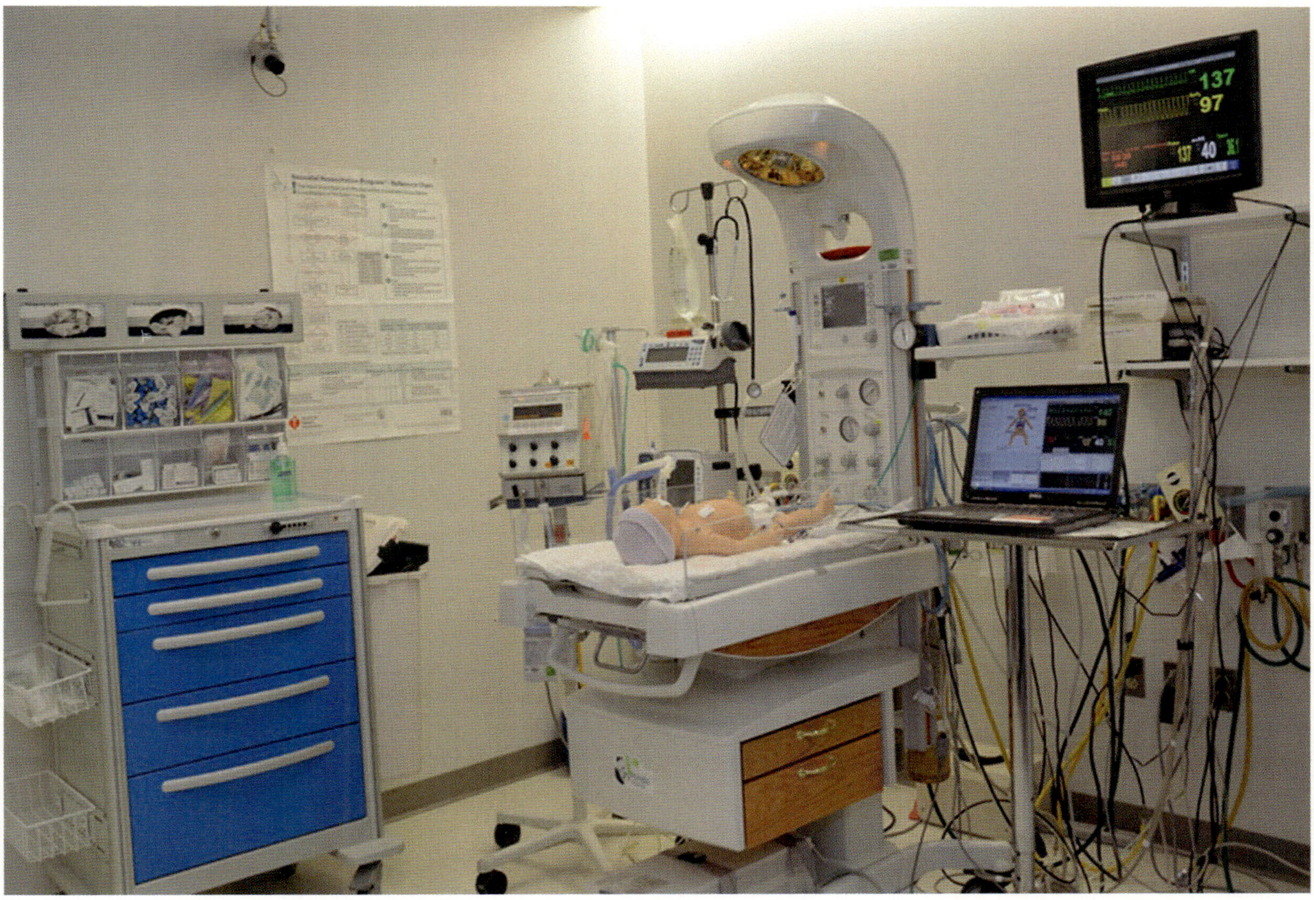

Fig. 2 High fidelity simulation center. This simulation center has a high-fidelity manikin connected to monitors and controlled by a laptop. The standard neonatal bed space includes a warmer bed, ventilator, IV poles and a bedside cart. In the upper left is a camera for recording simulation for later review

Table 1 Manikin modifications of difficult airways

Condition	Goal	Modification
Subglottic stenosis	Narrow airway below vocal cords	Apply external pressure to trachea with zip-tie or insert putty below vocal cords
Laryngospasm[a]	Narrow airway above vocal cords	Apply external pressure to airway above vocal cords
Macroglossia[a]	Provide an obstruction in the oral cavity	Overfill the manikin tongue or add volume to the outside of the tongue
Meconium in the airway or airway bleeding	Obstruct the view of the vocal cords with an opaque substance	Insert thinned paste dyed green or red into the oropharynx
Micrognathia or Pierre Robin[a]	Increase difficulty with jaw retraction and view of the vocal cords	Move manikin jaw posterior to standard position
Enlarged epiglottis	Obstruct the view of the vocal cords with the epiglottis	Apply putty to enlarge or elongate epiglottis
Unable to bag mask ventilate or intubate[a]	Force learner to perform cricothyroidotomy	Replace airway below vocal cords with disposable tubing/skin covering and/or use putty to fully obstruct airway
Cervical tumor/mass[a]	Obstruct the view of the vocal cords, restrict neck movement	Insert bean bag or firm mass under skin of manikin's neck, pushing on airway
Cervical spine immobility[a]	Restrict available movement of airway	Place cervical spine brace around manikin's neck
Spinal condition requiring side-lying position	Intubation in nonstandard position	Turn manikin on side
Tracheostomy tube obstruction[a]	Force learner to remove/replace tracheostomy tube	Occlude tracheostomy tube lumen

[a]Specific models or features commercially available

Low-fidelity simulators span a wider range of options but do not have integrated software or electronics. In its most basic form, a low-fidelity simulator may be a simple doll or homemade approximation of an airway. Low-fidelity options on the market range from manikin head task trainers to full body manikins with many interactive features for the learner such as inflatable lungs to simulate ventilation. Both the homemade and purchased manikins can be modified to create difficult airway models (Table 1). Both low- and high-fidelity manikins can also be used to practice intubation in nonstandard positions, such as might be needed for a patient with an open neural tube defect or after spinal surgery [16] or with conjoined twins (Figs. 3 and 4).

One high-technology option for simulation is virtual patients. Software can be used to model the human airway and adjust the view on screen depending on input from the user. The model can be created from 3D reconstructions of actual patient airways or built from scratch to demonstrate a particular condition. The user input can be obtained from a laryngoscope wired to sense the user's movements so that the screen view changes based on the accuracy of their movements. A virtual model constructed from 3D CT scan images has been shown to be as effective as a manikin for intubation training [17]. This technology permits educators to make airway models from CT scan images of real patients with difficult airways or airway malformations, allowing multiple trainees to get experience from one patient without risk to the actual patient.

Cadaver and animal airway models have high rates of satisfaction among learners, as they have been shown in small studies to improve patient level outcomes [10]. There are no reported studies of neonatal cadaveric models for intubation, but in adult models, fresh frozen cadavers have the highest rate of realism for intubation [18]. Animal model programs have reported using ferrets and piglets to simulate the neonatal airway. This technique is generally considered safe for the animals and adds a significant level of realism to the encounter without any risk to human patients. This method can be used to train clinicians in the intubation of patients with normal airways but is less useful in difficult airway management. Technology-based strategies can help to improve the learning experience using many different types of airway trainers.

Bag Mask and Alternative Airway Training

Infants with difficult and critical airway issues may not be able to be intubated at delivery or presentation to care, even by experienced airway personnel. For these fragile infants, provider proficiency with bag mask ventilation (BMV) and alternate airways can mean the difference between survival and death. During a 6-month period of neonatal training, one group of Australian residents had an average of 17 opportunities to provide BMV [17]. In the current American pediatric training model most residents will get only 2–3 months of

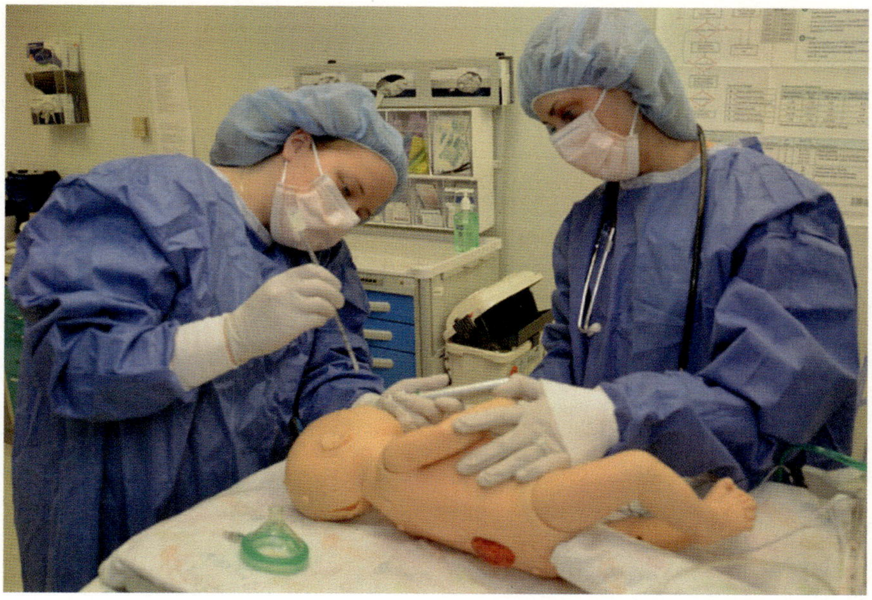

Fig. 3 Side-lying intubation. This manikin has been modified to have an open neural tube defect, forcing the learner to intubate in a nonstandard position

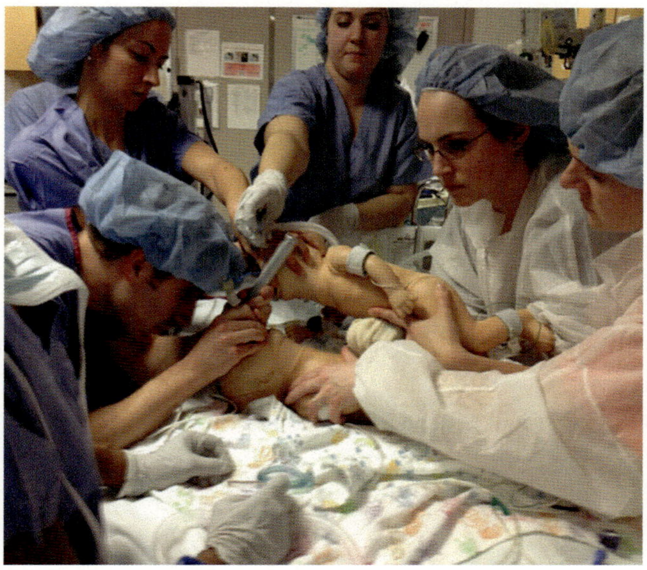

Fig. 4 Conjoined twin intubation. In this scenario two manikins were used to simulate the anticipated delivery of omphalopagus conjoined twins, allowing the team to practice airway management prior to delivery

training in neonatal care, potentially reducing their opportunities to learn and practice this life saving skill to less than ten instances throughout residency. Opportunities for use of alternative airways, such as a laryngeal mask airway (LMA), are even less frequent. As with other airway procedures and tools described in previous sections, lack of familiarity and infrequent use can result in poor performance of a task. In a study of the effectiveness of resident positive pressure ventilation (PPV) delivery to preterm infants, one quarter of the resuscitations demonstrated significant airway obstruction during PPV, and another quarter were noted to have significant mask leaks [18]. Simulation manikins can provide an important opportunity to practice these life saving skills. For experienced providers, manikin demonstration is more effective at decreasing mask leak during PPV then watching simple instructional videos [21].

BMV is a critical component of the NRP algorithm and the first step in resuscitating a depressed infant. Both low- and high-fidelity manikins can be used to practice BMV and LMA placement. Providing adequate BMV requires correct hand placement, correct mask position on the neonate's face, adequate jaw thrust, and appropriate pressure on the mask (Fig. 5). All of these tasks can be assessed on a manikin. High-fidelity manikins may also be able to record the volume or pressure of the delivered breaths to provide feedback regarding the effectiveness of the mask seal and delivered inspiratory pressures [22]. Providers must be able to troubleshoot mask air leaks and airway obstruction during BMV. Even in the hands of experienced providers, neonatal facemasks can still have significant air leaks that compromise ventilation [23]. The steps to resolve inadequate ventilation described in NRP follow the acronym "MR SOPA" and include: mask and patient repositioning, suctioning, opening the mouth, increasing pressure, and considering an alternative airway support device [3]. Manikins with articulating jaws and realistic upper airways can provide an important opportunity to practice these steps, including the use of alternative airways.

The LMA has been shown to be effective for establishing ventilation and resolving bradycardia in the delivery room [24]. LMAs are simple to insert and come in many sizes. A size 1

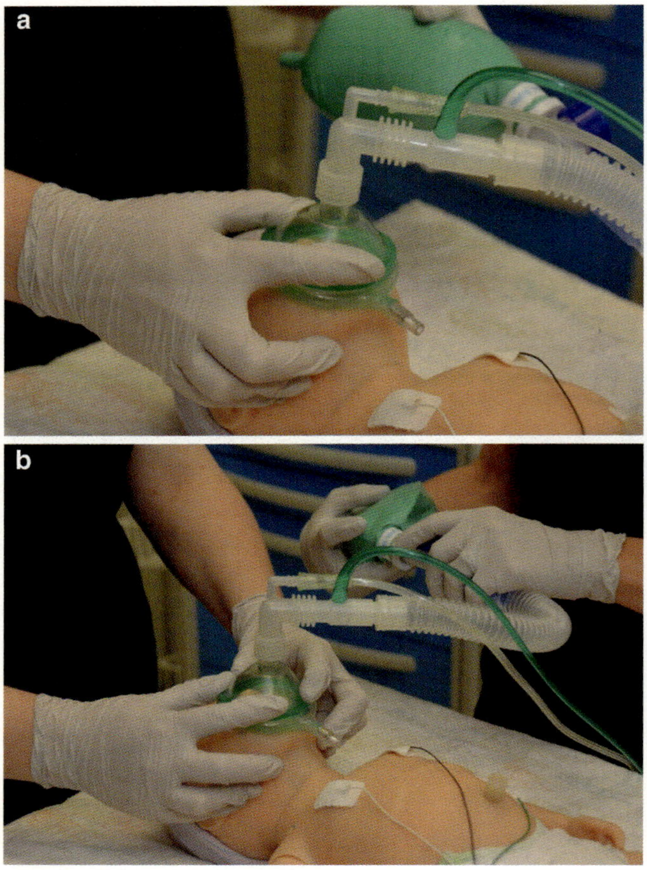

Fig. 5 Bag mask ventilation techniques. (**a**) One person BVM demonstrating correct hand and mask placement. (**b**) Two person BMV demonstrating correct hand and mask placement

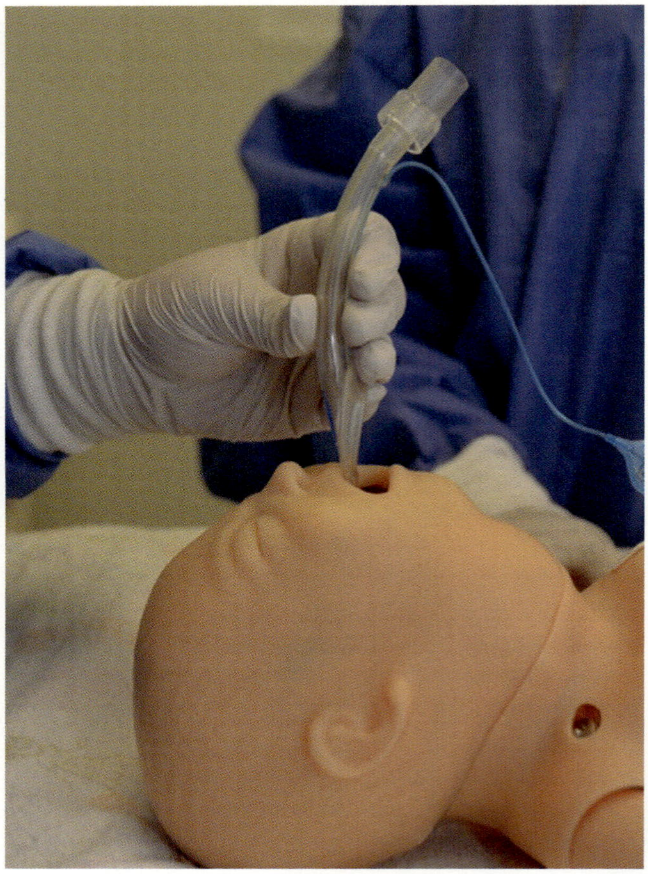

Fig. 6 LMA insertion. This manikin has been modified to have a difficult airway due to cervical neck mass requiring the learner to use an LMA

LMA is approved for use in infants less than 5 kg and there are reports of its successful use in premature infants as small as 1.1 kg [25]. As residents may be the only providers present at a delivery and have low reported success with endotracheal intubation, an LMA may provide a safe temporizing measure while advanced airway providers are called to the bedside. LMAs also have a major role in stabilizing infants with difficult or critical airway conditions, such as cervical neck masses (Fig. 6).

Nasopharyngeal and oropharyngeal airway insertion should also be included in airway training programs. Nasopharyngeal (NP) airways use a tube inserted in one nostril that opens a conduit between the nostril and the nasopharynx above the level of the epiglottis and can be used to bypass obstructions at the levels of the nose, nasopharynx, and base of the tongue. Oropharyngeal (OP) airways use a small piece of curved plastic inserted into the unconscious patient's mouth that bypasses obstructions at the base of the tongue. Both NP and OP airways can be inserted into term or near-term neonates and can be combined with BMV to achieve adequate ventilation when intubation is not possible. These devices are especially useful in infants with micrognathia, such as in Pierre Robin Syndrome, who may present unexpectedly at delivery. As both of these devices can be inserted quickly and easily, it is imperative that trainees be proficient in their use in case of an emergency. Most airway manikins can be used to practice NP and OP airway insertion, and all delivery room providers should practice their insertion regularly to maintain competence.

Intubation Training

Learning and maintaining proficiency for complex procedures like endotracheal intubation can be divided into two steps: a cognitive step and a psychomotor step [26]. The cognitive step is a period devoted to learning about the procedure and developing an understanding of the indications, contraindications, and motor actions involved. Cognitive steps about intubation should include a review of normal and abnormal anatomy, types of equipment needed, and the procedural steps. The important strategies of didactic learning include cognitive engagement, repetitions, feedback and variety [27]. Learners can be cognitively engaged by interactive

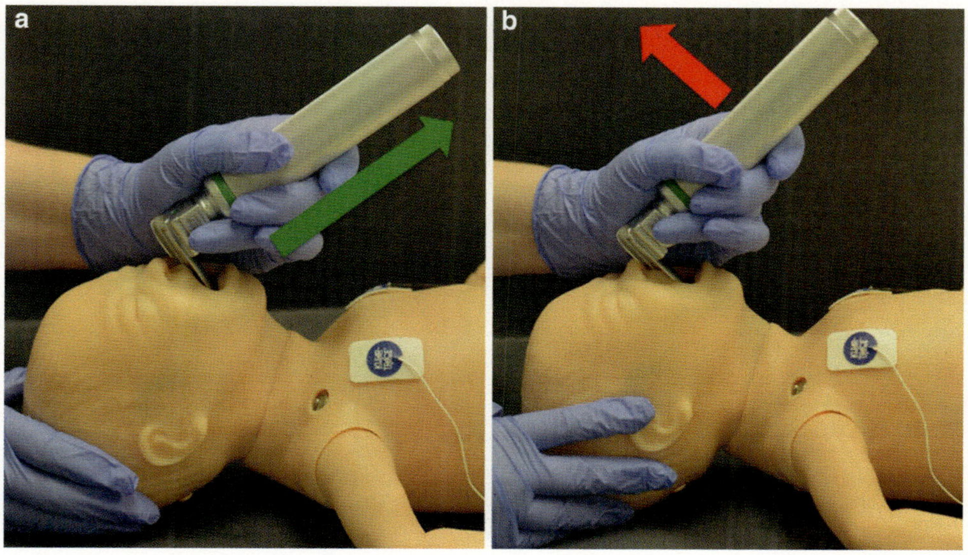

Fig. 7 Using a manikin to practice intubation. This airway manikin is being used to practice the physical skills of intubation. (**a**) Correct laryngoscope positioning, proper arm movement shown with *green arrow*. (**b**) Incorrect laryngoscope positioning restricting view of the airway, improper arm movement showing rocking of the laryngoscope shown with *red arrow*

teaching, such as walking through case examples, asking questions, and using videos or live demonstrations. Although didactic teaching alone is often insufficient for procedural training, a well-designed and executed class can add important layers to a provider's understanding of a process. For instance, knowing the names of anatomic landmarks aids communication during a difficult procedure, and understanding airway mechanics can aid in provider decision-making during emergencies. For these reasons, didactics should be integrated into simulation-based learning to maximize understanding.

The psychomotor step of procedural training involves practicing the procedure with correction and reinforcement. Allowing the trainee the opportunity for practice of the procedure in a safe learning environment using a partial task trainer, manikin, or virtual-reality training is known to be superior to traditional clinical medical education in achieving specific skill acquisition (Fig. 7) [27]. Instructional design features shown to improve simulation-based training can easily be incorporated into simulation training for endotracheal intubation. These include group practice, individualized learning, mastery level training, and variation in task complexity [27]. Repetition and instructor feedback remain crucial learning strategies, regardless of the training methodology.

Teamwork skills for intubation can occur in a multidisciplinary setting. During a standard intubation in the ICU there is a provider skilled in airway management, a bedside nurse, and a respiratory therapist. All of these people have individual roles that must integrate tightly together to successfully manage an airway emergency. A multidisciplinary intubation simulation could include a nurse who administers rapid sequence intubation medications and monitors vital signs, a respiratory therapist who prepares the equipment and secures the endotracheal tube, and a front line clinician who organizes the group and performs the procedure. By practicing these skills together, the team of care providers can improve communication, efficiency, and patient safety. Group practice can also be used to train a group of front line clinicians where each provider takes a turn in the different roles. This gives each person a chance to practice skills outside of his or her usual scope, which may be important as it provides perspective on communication and teamwork.

Individualized learning can take place both within the group practice model and in one-on-one instruction. Using this method, an individual learner's specific needs or deficiencies are identified, and the learner uses deliberate practice with facilitator input to improve his or her performance (Fig. 8). As defined by Ericsson, deliberate practice describes a regimen of effortful activity designed to optimize improvements in the acquisition of expert performance [29]. Deliberate practice with intubation simulations has been shown to improve resident success with intubation [29]. Deliberate practice can also be used to remediate individuals or provide additional experiences for learners that require additional training. For instance, if fellows in Neonatology programs identify the desire to have more practice with intubations, they can have individualized learning programs to practice intubation with different manikins and task trainers in both conventional and unconventional settings.

One critical component to intubation training is variation in procedural complexity. Once trainees have demonstrated

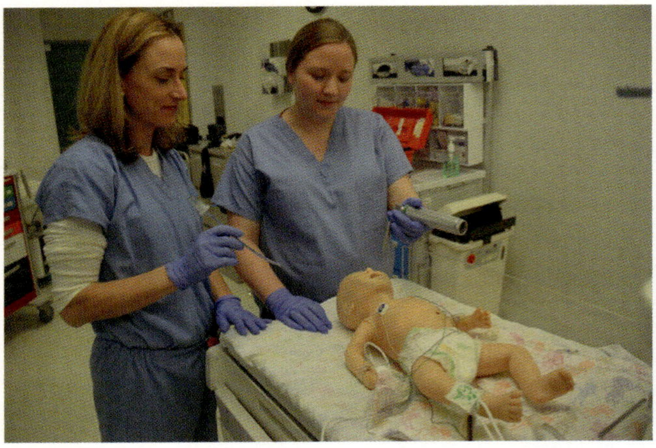

Fig. 8 Deliberate practice with facilitator. The facilitator provides instruction to help the trainee learn to intubate the manikin

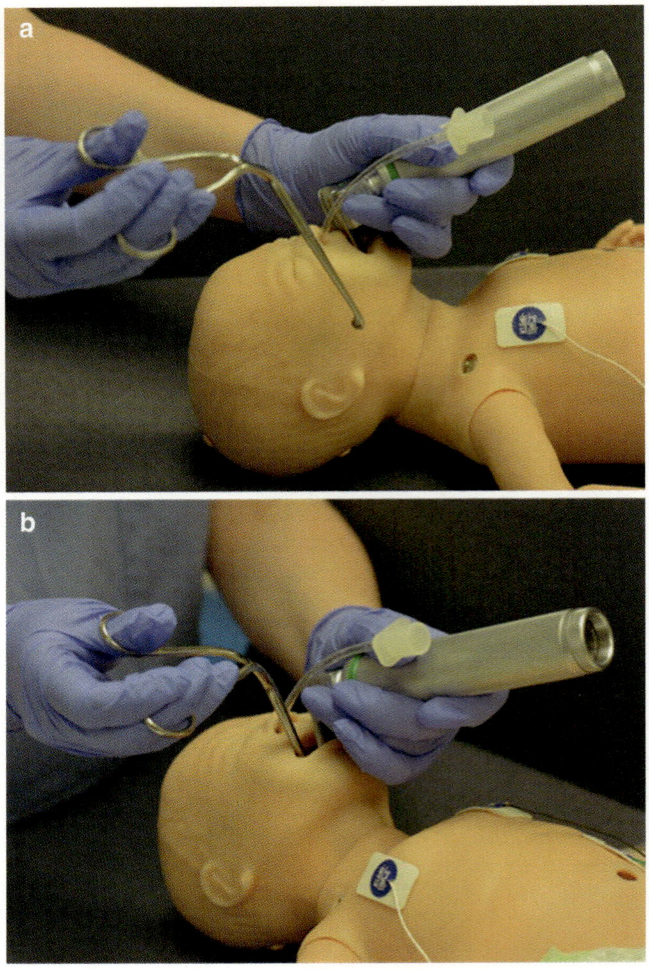

Fig. 9 Nasal intubation. (**a**) The provider prepares the manikin for nasal intubation by placing the endotracheal tube in the nare and obtaining a view of vocal cords using direct laryngoscopy. (**b**) The provider inserts the Magill forceps into the mouth, using them to guide the endotracheal tube through the vocal cords

proficiency at standard intubation, they should be challenged with increasingly complex scenarios to solidify their skills. Even intubation of the normal infant airway can be made more complex by varying the scenario to include different disease processes, different clinical environments, and a range of equipment availability. Specific intubation skills such as endotracheal tube replacement and nasal intubation should be rotated through the varied scenarios.

Endotracheal tube replacement can be used for upsizing the tube diameter or to remove a plugged tube. Patients requiring tube replacement may be too unstable to tolerate prolonged time without an artificial airway and so may not tolerate the time required for an existing endotracheal tube to be replaced. The procedure requires practice, because the timing element and coordination of steps can be difficult to manage. For example, in an endotracheal tube replacement scenario, the patient may be ventilating poorly due to a large air leak around a small endotracheal tube. The team would need to recognize that patient decompensation was due to improper tube size, choose an appropriate sized replacement tube, coordinate a secondary person to stabilize the existing tube, obtain an adequate view of the vocal cords, and coordinate the tube exchange while minimizing the length of time without ventilation. Multidisciplinary practice of this type of scenario is important, as it often requires a nurse or respiratory therapist to assist with the endotracheal tube replacement.

Another advanced airway skill amenable to simulation training is nasal intubation. Nasal intubation is ideal for patients with excessive oral secretions, surgical wounds in the mouth, older infants requiring prolonged intubation, and patients with facial malformations precluding proper oral tube securement. Some intensive care units may even use this as their primary method of endotracheal intubation. As such, all airway providers should be trained to perform nasal intubation. This procedure varies from traditional oral intubation in equipment and sequence of events. Magill forceps are unique to nasal intubation and unfamiliar to many providers. After inserting the endotracheal tube through a nare and advancing the tube down into the larynx, the provider uses a traditional laryngoscope to view the vocal cords while actively placing the endotracheal tube into the airway using Magill forceps (Fig. 9). Newer techniques using ENT "cupped ear" forceps allow easier instrumentation of the oral airway to facilitate nasal intubation in smaller infants. These forceps are jointed at the end of the device, limiting trauma to the epiglottis and other airway structures (Fig. 10). Many air-

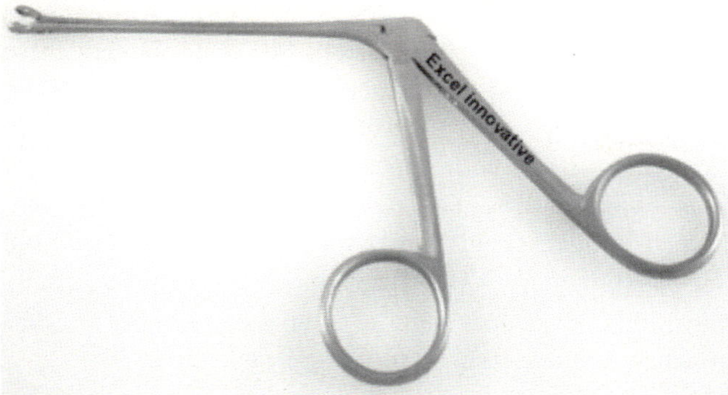

Fig. 10 Cupped ear forceps are more useful for nasal intubation for smaller neonates and infants than the larger MaGill-type forceps. Significantly small and longer with the movable joint at the tip allows for easy grab of the ETT

way task trainers and high-fidelity manikins have patent and anatomically correct nasal passages for use with nasal intubation, providing a valuable training experience for a rare intubation event.

Training programs often need to show that their graduates have adequate experience to practice independently and thus have designed procedure log systems to track both the frequency and success of trainee procedural attempts. As intubation experiences become increasingly rare, programs may need to find alternate ways to show regulatory agencies that they are producing clinicians who have mastered advanced airway management. One way to assess proficiency with procedures is through simulation-based mastery learning (SBML). SBML sets a predetermined minimal passing standard (e.g., "mastery level") and has several key characteristics which include practice that is focused on reaching mastery level performance, skill testing to assess achievement of mastery level performance, and continued practice, as needed, until the mastery level performance is achieved [31]. SBML can be used to verify proficiency with both commonly and uncommonly performed clinical and procedural skills. SBML augments deliberate practice through the addition of a clearly delineated level of performance that defines "mastery" with a given procedural skill and the requirement for continuous practice until mastery level performance is achieved [32]. Additionally, scenarios promoting mastery level skills should strive for realism; for intubation training this should include a realistic airway model, standard unit airway equipment, and airway personnel. Success metrics should include a time element and measures of communication, teamwork, and technical proficiency. A well-designed simulation program can be used to verify mastery level skills and can serve as evidence of proficiency for regulatory agencies.

Video Enhanced Laryngoscopy

The field of intubation has had many technologic advances. Using traditional direct laryngoscopy, only the user is able to see the airway; there may be delayed or no feedback regarding the success of the procedure, and there is no way to review the procedure after the event. New models of video or fiberoptically enhanced laryngoscopes allow more than one provider to see the airway. If the device has recording ability, it allows trainees to review their performance at a later time with supervisor feedback. In these devices a camera or fiberoptic scope sits near the light source on the laryngoscope blade and shows a magnified view on either a screen attached to the handle or a separate monitor. This method of intubation also improves awareness of procedural success since trainees have an enlarged view of the airway as the endotracheal tube is introduced. Furthermore, providers can receive feedback in real time about their skills. Even in experienced airway providers, fiberoptic and video laryngoscopes improve airway view grades [33] (See chapters "Anesthesia Challenges for the Difficult and Critical Neonatal Airway and Airway Emergencies in the Neonate: Preparedness at the Bedside" for full video laryngoscopy details).

Video and fiberoptic intubation devices can also be combined with patient manikins, both for task training and for use in larger airway emergency scenarios. This method of teaching advanced airway skills has been shown to be beneficial in the adult field. Anesthesia and Internal Medicine residents trained using a simulation manikin showed significantly better success in live patient intubation and time to intubation with a fiberoptic laryngoscope compared to residents trained via lecture from expert airway providers [34].

Identifying abnormal anatomy is an important step in the training of advanced airway providers such as anesthesiologists and intensivists but patients with these conditions are infrequently seen in standard practice. For rare airway anomalies, a video taken from within the airway, such as with a fiberoptic laryngoscope or flexible bronchoscope, allows multiple trainees and providers to learn how to recognize and manage the airway condition. Dynamic video recording can aid in the diagnosis of functional airway issues such as vocal cord paralysis or airway malacia [34]. This method is often employed in Otolaryngology training programs, where video recording of procedures is common but is rarely utilized by nonsurgical providers.

Tracheostomy Training

Infants with tracheostomies represent a very small proportion of the population but are frequently encountered in the intensive care units and operating rooms. They are a particularly vulnerable group of patients, as many have critical airway issues or severe lung disease. The National Audit Project of the Royal College of Anesthetists and the Difficult Airway Society emphasized the importance of tracheostomy care by stating: "displaced tracheostomy, and to a lesser extent displaced tracheal tubes, were the greatest cause of major morbidity and mortality in [the] ICU" [36]. To mitigate this risk, medical providers need to be familiar with the care and management of patients with tracheostomies, yet one-third of pediatric, non-otolaryngology healthcare providers rate their comfort with tracheostomy care as poor. Knowledge of tracheostomy tube management, even for advanced providers such as anesthesiologists, remains inadequate. In a series of questions regarding the care of tracheostomies, anesthesia residents scored only slightly higher than 50 % correct [37]. Fortunately, even one experience with changing a tracheostomy tube as a resident is correlated with a significant increase in comfort with the procedure [38]. Simulation provides a means to address these knowledge and skill deficiencies [39].

Many manikins can be modified or purchased to simulate an infant with a tracheostomy. Tracheostomy manikins can be used to practice technical skills such as tracheostomy tube changes or used in more elaborate simulation scenarios. Tracheostomy scenarios can include obstruction, dislodgement, or retrograde intubation depending on the discipline and level of the learner. Beginners may benefit from learning to provide PPV via a tracheostomy tube and performing a simple tracheostomy tube replacement. More advanced providers may benefit from practicing the management of a scenario in which a newly placed tracheostomy tube is dislodged and cannot be replaced.

Providers of all levels, from nurses to intensivists, should be familiar with simple tracheostomy tube care, making this an ideal topic for multidisciplinary simulation training. For example, a multidisciplinary scenario might start with a tracheostomy tube obstruction which progresses to bradycardia despite nursing efforts to suction and provide PPV via the tracheostomy. This scenario could require the resident or front line care provider to attempt a tracheostomy tube change and evolve to a full team code after the tracheostomy tube cannot be replaced through the stoma. Scenarios such as this happen infrequently in most institutions but carry a high risk of morbidity and mortality, especially in inexperienced hands.

Specially trained teams and protocols for how to manage emergency tracheostomy situations are starting to be used in institutions with high volumes of tracheostomy patients. Simple protocols regarding suctioning depth and pressure can improve patient safety [40]. Additionally, staff specially trained in tracheostomy care, such as nurse specialists or dedicated multidisciplinary teams can greatly improve outcomes in patients with tracheostomies with regards to complications and ICU admissions [40, 41]. Many of these care protocols and multidisciplinary teams are lead by Otolaryngology specialists who have the most experience in managing patients with critical airways. Once a protocol or team is created, disseminating the information can be accomplished through simulations with bedside nurses and front line care providers. As the care protocols and team assembly may rarely be needed, ongoing simulation provides a means to maintain a safe level of knowledge and skills.

Difficult Airway Management Simulation

Simulation allows for directed learning in an environment that is both safe for the learner and poses no threat to patient safety. Even a low-fidelity manikin can add realism to an airway emergency scenario. Appropriately designed simulations using high-fidelity simulators can come very close to the high pressures of a life-threatening emergency. In a large meta-analysis, simulation was found to be the superior method for teaching advanced airway management skills such as direct and fiberoptic intubation and surgical airways [10]. Manikins improve learner comfort with routine airway management and interventions, which can be translated to management of the difficult or malformed airway. For example, BMV, an essential skill for NRP algorithms, can be more challenging to perform effectively in an infant with severe micrognathia.

Each simulation scenario can be geared towards specific learning goals. A scenario may focus on procedures such as BMV, management of specific conditions such as subglottic stenosis, or on nontechnical skills of an airway code like teamwork and communication. Each type of scenario can also be tailored to different learner levels and disciplines (Table 2). During a scenario, if a learner is struggling with an objective, the facilitator can pause the scenario, provide immediate feedback, and then restart the simulation to allow the learner to improve upon his or her performance. Important advantages to simulation training include the ability to recreate a difficult or rare clinical presentation, allowing the trainee or team to redo the event with feedback, and for trainees to experience and practice the management of a rare event, especially if it has not been previously encountered during training.

Low-fidelity scenarios might use simple equipment such as a doll and a printed list of vital signs and events. The focus in this type of simulation may be on history taking, teamwork, or the cognitive exercise of decision-making. Low-fidelity simulation is low cost, portable, and does not require an experienced simulator operator. For example, a scenario involving an infant in the emergency department with respiratory

Table 2 Airway simulations for different levels of training

Trainee level	Example scenario	Goals	Objectives
Medical student	• Baby with small jaw presenting for a preoperative visit prior to hernia repair	• Identify risk • Anticipate issues • Teamwork	• Recognize significance of exam finding • Identify risk of airway obstruction • Anesthesia or ENT consult prior to OR
Nurse or respiratory therapist	• Infant with worsening stridor	• Recognize signs of respiratory distress • Use airway stabilizing maneuvers • Call for help at appropriate time	• Recognize stridor • Attempt airway repositioning • Use bag mask appropriately • Use code bell to get help
Resident/front line clinician	• Delivery of infant with prenatally diagnosed Down syndrome	• Prepare for delivery • Manage equipment • Recognize unstable patient	• Anticipate risk of airway issue • Prepare delivery room equipment • Use bag mask appropriately • Call for help when airway obstructs
Neonatal or ICU fellow	• Delivery of infant with prenatally diagnosed cervical mass	• Prepare team for resuscitation • Manage airway emergency • Use alternative airway	• Prep team/assign roles • Rapid assessment of airway status • Attempt intubation with DL • Use LMA when intubation unsuccessful
ENT resident or fellow	• Previously undiagnosed grade 4 subglottic stenosis, unplanned extubation	• Diagnose airway malformation • Use advanced intubation equipment • Emergency cricothyroidotomy	• Recognize subglottic stenosis on DL • Attempt intubation with fiberoptic scope • Preform emergency cricothyroidotomy
Advanced provider team	• EXIT procedure for a newborn with tracheal atresia requiring tracheostomy	• Organize large group resuscitation • Anticipate airway emergency • Use advanced airway equipment	• Assign team roles • Prep emergency equipment • Manage multi-organ system code • Use advanced equipment to establish airway

EXIT Ex Utero Intrapartum Treatment, *DL* Direct Laryngoscopy, *LMA* Laryngeal Mask Airway

distress may use only a facilitator and a non-mechanical doll where the trainee's goals are to elicit a history of airway symptoms and determine whether provided vital signs and exam findings are pathologic. This type of scenario may be ideal for beginner trainees who are encouraged to focus on simple history and physical exam techniques without the anxiety of a high-stakes situation. The main drawbacks are a lack of interactivity with the manikin and limitations to practicing procedures on some low-fidelity manikins. An exception to this is in learning to manipulate a laryngoscope or fiberoptic bronchoscope, in which the focus is on psychomotor dexterity. This type of low-fidelity simulation does not require the manikin to provide cues to learners or react to their manipulations. In comparing low-fidelity and high-fidelity simulation models for fiberoptic intubation, anesthesia residents seem to benefit equally from both models [43].

In contrast, high-fidelity simulation uses mechanical manikins, allowing the facilitator to pre-program responses or adjust the vital signs and manikin behaviors as the learner makes medical decisions. As the scenario plays out on the monitors and in the manikin's responses to interventions, the learner can stay within the moment, undistracted by interruptions in the flow of the scenario. This type of simulation is ideal for practicing physical exam skills, invasive procedures, and complex team-based scenarios. For example, a scenario involving a patient's extubation with subsequent stridor, where the goal is recognition of respiratory distress and reintubation, could be geared towards a team with clinicians, respiratory therapists, and nurses who would need to work together to accomplish goals to improve patient outcomes. High-fidelity manikins help the learner "suspend disbelief" by providing a more realistic experience (Fig. 11). The drawbacks of high-fidelity simulation are cost and the need for trained simulation facilitators and manikin operators. In some centers there are elaborate simulation facilities with mock delivery rooms and operating rooms, video recording, and full time simulation staff. However, these are not necessary to meet educational objectives.

As stated earlier, both homemade and purchased manikins can be modified to create difficult airway models (Table 1); (Video 1). Many modifications are simple and able to be added temporarily or permanently to existing airway manikins (Fig. 12). There are also commercially available difficult airway models that can be substituted for the standard manikin airway. Low- and high-fidelity manikins can also be used to practice intubation in nonstandard positions, such as might be needed for a patient with an open neural tube defect or after spinal surgery [16] or with conjoined twins. These difficult airway models can provide experience with the management of infants that many clinicians may rarely see in practice.

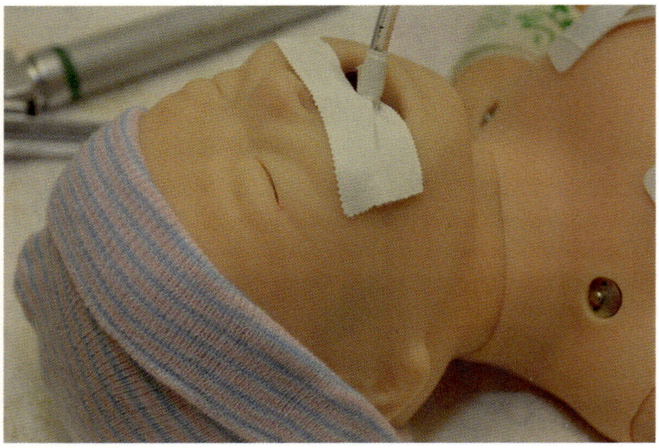

Fig. 11 High-fidelity manikin. This high-fidelity manikin has realistic facial features, responds to interventions and helps the learner "suspend disbelief"

Nontechnical Skills Training

Simulation plays a critical role in nontechnical skills training including teamwork, leadership, and crisis resource management. These skills are particularly important in the critical care, emergency, and surgical fields. The principles of good teamwork include situational awareness, communication, leadership, and shared mental models [44]. Teamwork has long been known to be an important factor in patient outcomes, and in a study of surgical outcomes, poor teamwork skills was highly associated with patient complications and death [45]. Due to this concerning finding, team skills have been identified as an important factor in patient safety [45]. Fortunately, simulation has been found to be an effective means for teaching team skills [44]. This focus on patient safety has lead to government sponsored training programs that include simulation of nontechnical skills, such as the TeamSTEPPS program, which showed significant improvement in communication, leadership, and team behaviors following structured simulation [47].

The principles of teamwork can be translated into measurable simulation outcomes. For instance, situational awareness, defined as the perception of the environment and

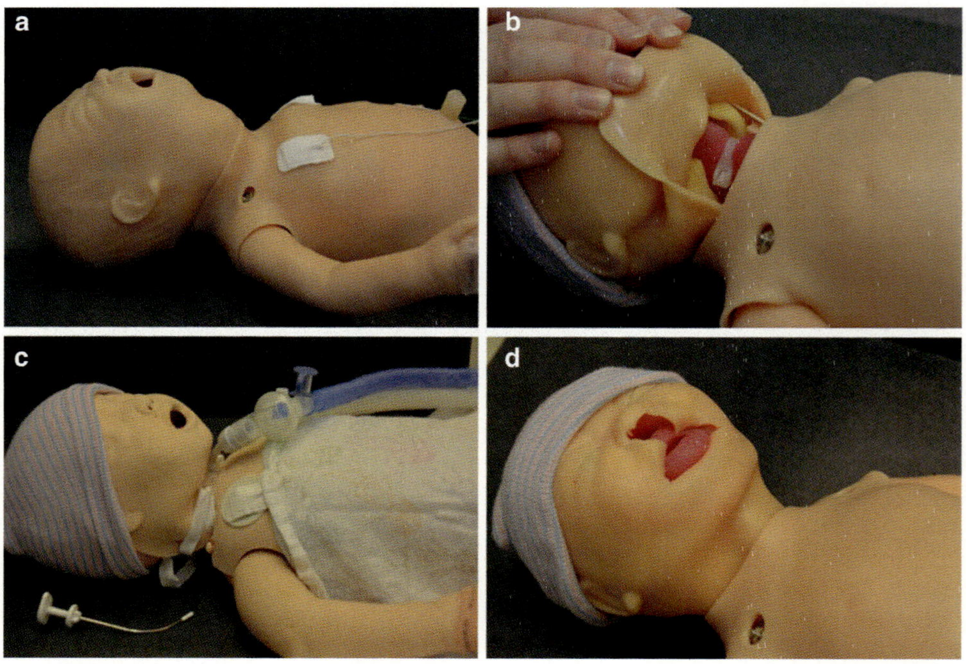

Fig. 12 Difficult airway manikin modifications. (**a**) A mass has been added under the neck skin to simulation a cervical teratoma. (**b**) A zip-tie has been placed around the subglottis to mimic subglottic stenosis. (**c**) A stoma was created in this manikin's neck to create a place for a tracheostomy tube. (**d**) The facial skin has been modified to simulate a cleft lip

anticipation of the situation's trajectory, can be measured by assessing how a learner collects necessary data and synthesizes it to formulate a plan and then adjusts that plan once new data is available. Communication measures can include the use of closed-loop feedback, clarity of speech, and subjective assessments of how well each team member worked together. The shared mental model is the idea that team performance improves if team members have a shared understanding of the necessary tasks and teamwork required to meet goals. This can be achieved by vocalizing clinical observations, patient information and a summary of the case and plans for management. A clear, unambiguous comment gives the rest of the team members an opportunity to reflect on the information and revise their situational awareness and their own mental model based upon new information. One method to measure non-procedural simulation performance is the Anesthesia Nontechnical Skills Scale (ANTS), which measures four main skill categories: situational awareness, team working, decision-making, and task management [48, 49]. Using a standard, validated measure allows for consistency in evaluating teamwork and provides a uniform way to report improvements in teamwork following a training session.

There are many models and theories of leadership, but some of the common themes are proactivity, flexibility, ability to delegate, openness, team management, and situational awareness. While some leadership skills are inborn or a product of early learning, many can be or must be specifically taught. Simulation provides a controlled arena for teaching leadership, since scenarios can be designed to involve high-tension situations, limited resources, and altered team dynamics. Leadership principles can be both the focus of a simulation or a secondary learning objective in group scenarios. For example, a scenario involving the delivery of an infant with an unanticipated critical airway can challenge the learner to take charge while testing his or her medical management skills. Alternatively, the scenario could be altered so that the focus is on managing a difficult team or family member rather than on the medical management. While research on leadership training programs has thus far been limited to learners' reactions to the experience, participants overwhelmingly report that training had a positive impact on their leadership skills [50].

Crisis resource management refers to how well a team uses its available equipment and personnel during an emergency. This can range from a scenario with a nonfunctioning bag and mask to an airway emergency with only a resident and bedside nurse present. These scenarios are especially important to incorporate into a simulation curriculum, as they are extremely rare and can result in significant morbidity and mortality for patients if the clinicians are unprepared to act quickly. Simulation has been shown to be effective for teaching crisis resource management with improvements in both transfer of learning to the workplace and in patient outcomes [51]. The focus of these scenarios should be on how well the learner or team is able to cope with the limiting factor and improvise alternative strategies.

Educational Venues

Airway management education can take place in multiple venues. Individual scenarios can be devised for use at an unoccupied patient bedside (in situ simulation) or in a space specially designated for simulation. A simulation center affords the opportunity to have a stable location with reusable equipment, while in situ simulation provides opportunities to learn in a true clinical environment. Depending on learning objectives, a given location may be preferable to another. For example, if a team is doing a simulation around the anticipated delivery of conjoined twins, the scenario is best acted out in the actual delivery suite so that the team can focus on their available resources, systems, and workflow. For skills that are more physical learning-based such as procedures, multiple simulations can be combined in one session as part of a skills fair in a simulation center. If time is limited, simulation "boot camps" can allow a group of providers to practice many scenarios in one day. Boot camps are especially useful for new provider orientation where a large group needs to learn about their specialty's or unit's practices quickly. Skills workshops or "skills boot camps" have been shown to increase resident confidence and competence with both common and rare procedures [52]. Both otolaryngology and neonatology boot camps have been previously described in the literature [52, 53].

Measuring Simulation Outcomes

For a simulation program to be successful, ideally, it should demonstrate measureable outcomes. Both qualitative and quantitative outcomes require creative outcome metrics. One classical model of assessing training is the Kirkpatrick model, in which there are four described levels of evaluating an educational program [55]. This model was originally developed for the non-medical field but has been adapted to medical training programs such as simulation [15]. Level one is "reaction," which refers to how a trainee reacts to the experience. Level two is "learning," in which the trainee demonstrates a quantitative improvement in his or her skills during simulation. Level three is "behavior," where a trainee is observed to have improvements in his or her performance with live patients. Level four is "results," where patient outcomes are measurably improved by a training program (Table 3).

The easiest qualitative outcome metrics to collect are surveys of learners' perceived competence and confidence.

Table 3 Examples of simulation evaluations using the Kirkpatrick model

Level		Example
1	Reaction	Trainee felt simulation was valuable and educational
2	Learning	Trainee shortens length of time to successful endotracheal intubation on manikin
3	Behavior	Trainee improves first-attempt intubation success on live patients
4	Results	Patients experience less Tracheal Intubation Associated Events (TIAE) and have fewer complications

These metrics are usually collected via simple self-report surveys given immediately following a simulation. Simulation is generally well liked and accepted by trainees, and pediatric trainees report improvements in self-confidence immediately following simulation experiences [9]. Unfortunately, improvements in self-confidence and clinical competence often degrade over time without continued reinforcement. Additionally, proficiency of rarely used skills tends to degrade over time. In a study of residents following their standard neonatal resuscitation training, simulation was able to demonstrate a time-dependent degradation of airway management and BMV skills within 3–5 months of their initial training [56]. The goal of simulation is to provide a means to maintain confidence and clinical competence over time. Data regarding the positive effect of repeated simulations have shown that on average, airway and resuscitation skills degrade within 12 months of training without continued practice [56, 57]. There are more studies looking at trainees than experienced providers, so more research is needed to determine the optimal frequency of simulation training to maintain proficiency [58, 59].

Subjective and objective measures of learner performance can be assessed in real-time by simulation facilitators or on video review using a checklist of tasks completed. For instance, reviewers can rank specific performance elements such as teamwork or length of time to complete time-sensitive tasks such as initiating chest compressions. Validated checklists exist in the adult and pediatric literature for both quality of teamwork and quality of overall airway emergency management [60–62]. High-fidelity manikins using simulation software can be particularly helpful, because the software can record time data and display physical measures of success, such as depth of chest compressions or effectiveness of BMV.

The ultimate goals of simulation are to improve individual and team performance in real life situations and positively impact patient outcomes. These metrics have been much harder to measure, but some small studies have been published. The majority of studies published on simulation and patient outcomes have been completed with paramedics and anesthesia trainees working with adult patients [64]. Simulation is known to improve compliance with airway protocols, such as emergency cricothyroidotomy, in adult airway providers [58]. Simulation is also reported to improve performance of airway management, including airway emergencies, by surgical residents when incorporated into traditional airway training programs [58]. Medical flight crews have demonstrated both improvements in intubation success and a decrease in tracheal intubation associated events (TIAE) following manikin training [65].

Pediatric airway management issues, such as intubation success, can be tracked prospectively, but linking this data to trainee participation in simulation can be challenging. Brief, refresher training just prior to an intubation attempt has not yet been shown to improve resident first-attempt success or decrease TIAEs in the pediatric ICU [66], but it has been shown to improve overall intubation success when multiple members of the ICU team are trained [67]. Tracking success with difficult airway management is even more challenging, given the rarity of these events. Scheduled events, such as the delivery of an infant with a known airway anomaly, provide a unique opportunity to simulate the encounter with the team participating in the delivery prior to the event (Figs. 3 and 4). This sort of goal-directed learning fits well with adult learning theory, emphasizing relevancy and practicality [69].

Debriefing

Debriefing is the process of reflective thinking following an event. For medical simulation training, this consists of reviewing the scenario and performance with the participants after the simulation using one of the many described debriefing frameworks in the literature. Fifty-one studies of high-fidelity simulation reported that debriefing was the single most important part of simulation training in a large meta-analysis [70]. The theory behind debriefing is that by actively reflecting on events group and individual performance, the learners can gain a deeper understanding of his own mental models. If a learner's mental model of a patient's airway anatomy and function is not correct, his or her resultant interventions will likely also not be correct. In order to effectively address why an intervention was incorrect, learners must dig into their mental models to discover their thought processes that led to the intervention. The debriefing facilitator can then help reframe incorrect thought processes by prompting the learners to reflect on their previous experiences with the current topic and compare their own mental models with the ideal mental model (Video 2). Ideal mental models and standards of practice can be explicitly offered by the facilitator if he or she is a content expert, or they can be "discovered" by the group through discussion [71]. The most effective time for debriefing appears to be immediately following the scenario, when memory is clearest and the learner is still engaged. Multiple studies comparing timing of debriefing have supported this as the optimal timing for reflective debriefing [72].

There are many different types of debriefing, including instructor-facilitated debriefing, video-assisted debriefing, and self-debriefing. Instructor-facilitated debriefing is the most commonly used debriefing technique. In this type of debriefing, an experienced facilitator asks open-ended questions and leads the learners through a review of their performance, reinforcing correct behaviors and actions as well as identifying areas for improvement. With video-assisted debriefing, the facilitator uses a recorded video of the simulation to help point out specific instances of superior and inferior performance by the learners. In contrast, self-debriefing uses a set of written questions to prompt the learners to review their own performances without the assistance of a facilitator. There are few studies directly comparing these methods, but in a small meta-analysis, video-assisted debriefing was found to be superior to standard facilitator-led debriefing [73].

For programs with significant budget limitations, self-debriefing may be an excellent method for guiding reflection without the need for additional trained staff. Furthermore, a program can use senior trainees as facilitators for junior trainees to reduce the need for faculty involvement. In one small study, emergency medicine residents were shown to be as effective at debriefing medical students as faculty [74]. Programs with trained facilitators have shown that even brief, focused facilitator-led debriefing can lead to significant improvements in lifesaving skills such as chest compressions [74]. In theory, an effective facilitator needs only to understand the ideal management of the clinical scenario being presented and be able to follow a framework for structured debriefing.

There are multiple frameworks described for simulation debriefing. One example of a debriefing framework is the modified U.S. Army's After Action Review (AAR) method, which has seven steps: define the rules of the debriefing, explain the learning objectives of the simulation, benchmark performance, review what was supposed to happen during the simulation, identify what actually happened, examine why events occurred the way they did, and formalize learning by reviewing with the group what went well, what did not go well, and what they would do differently if faced with a similar situation in real life [76]. Another published debriefing framework is the "3D" method of debriefing consisting of defusing, discovering and deepening [71]. Defusing allows the learners to discuss any emotions the scenario may have brought up and recap the events of the scenario. Discovering takes the learners through the events to reflect on their thinking at the time and offer alternative mental models for the events. Deepening guides the learners to connect the scenario to real life instances that may occur in clinical practice to cement their newfound knowledge. While these are just two frameworks for structured debriefing, there are many more described in the literature. Studies are still required to determine the optimal debriefing framework. For now, a framework should be chosen that matches the needs of a program's learners.

Given the high-stakes nature of airway management, the debriefing process may bring up issues from previous clinical experiences, such as emotionally significant events, positive and negative role models, and relationships with patients [76]. Discussing these types of topics can be valuable in creating an environment of open communication. Facilitators need to be prepared to recognize and address emotions and anxieties that come up during the scenario and debriefing. Uncovering emotions and experiences with previous clinical encounters, patients, and supervising physicians can help learners grow and build empathy. One study using standardized patient simulation was shown to improve measures of empathy in medical students [76]. Empathy and communication skills are critical to both patient care and long-term provider health.

In addition to debriefing after simulations, debriefing after a real airway emergency can be an invaluable learning opportunity. Video cameras can be mounted above resuscitation tables in the delivery and trauma rooms. Ideally, a video would be focused on the patient but also include a view of the team, have audio recording, and be time-stamped. When the video is reviewed by the team, they can observe the timeliness and skillfulness of interventions and identify areas for clinical improvement [78]. Teamwork and other nontechnical skills can also be reviewed. Video recording has the added benefit of being able to be reviewed by experts or supervisors. Resuscitations and airway emergencies may happen at unpredictable hours when advanced providers are not available to provide feedback. If there is a video of the event, advanced providers can review the team's performance and give valuable feedback at a later time.

Conclusions

Airway emergencies in neonates and infants are high risk and increasingly rare. As such, all pediatric trainees and providers working with this population need education on the basic skills required to stabilize the airways of these patients. Simulation-based medical education provides an excellent way to impart instruction and maintain skills in a safe learning environment. Simulation can be used to teach technical skills such as BMV, use of alternative airways, oral and nasal intubation, fiberoptic or video laryngoscopy, and care of tracheostomies as well as nontechnical skills such as teamwork, leadership, and communication. These skills benefit both the large number of infants with anatomically normal airways who require respiratory assistance and the small number of infants with difficult or critical airway diseases.

References

1. Gaies MG, Landrigan CP, Hafler JP, Sandora TJ. Assessing procedural skills training in pediatric residency programs. Pediatrics. 2007;120(4):715–22.
2. Education ACfGM. Revisions to the Pediatrics Program Requirements http://www.acgme.org/acgmeweb/2013.
3. American Academy of Pediatrics. Neonatal resuscitation textbook. 6th ed. Elk Grove Village: American Academy of Pediatrics; 2011.
4. Garg S, Sinha S. Non-invasive ventilation in premature infants: based on evidence or habit. J Clin Neonatol. 2013;2(4):155–9.
5. Leone TA, Rich W, Finer NN. Neonatal intubation: success of pediatric trainees. J Pediatr. 2005;146(5):638–41.
6. Sanders Jr RC, Giuliano Jr JS, Sullivan JE, Brown 3rd CA, Walls RM, Nadkarni V, et al. Level of trainee and tracheal intubation outcomes. Pediatrics. 2013;131(3):e821–8.
7. Haubner LY, Barry JS, Johnston LC, Soghier L, Tatum PM, Kessler D, et al. Neonatal intubation performance: room for improvement in tertiary neonatal intensive care units. Resuscitation. 2013;84(10):1359–64.
8. Konrad C, Schupfer G, Wietlisbach M, Gerber H. Learning manual skills in anesthesiology: is there a recommended number of cases for anesthetic procedures? Anesth Analg. 1998;86(3):635–9.
9. Cordero L, Hart BJ, Hardin R, Mahan JD, Giannone PJ, Nankervis CA. Pediatrics residents' preparedness for neonatal resuscitation assessed using high-fidelity simulation. J Grad Med Educ. 2013;5(3):399–404.
10. Kennedy CC, Cannon EK, Warner DO, Cook DA. Advanced airway management simulation training in medical education: a systematic review and meta-analysis. Crit Care Med. 2014;42(1):169–78.
11. ACGME Program Requirements for Graduate Medical Education in General Surgery https://http://www.acgme.org/acgmeweb/tabid/150/ProgramandInstitutionalAccreditation/SurgicalSpecialties/Surgery.aspx: ACGME; 2007.
12. Anesthesiology TABo. Maintenance of Certification in Anesthesiology Part IV: PPAI—simulation education courses. http://www.theABA.org.
13. Hanscom R. Medical simulation from an insurer's perspective. Acad Emerg Med. 2008;15(11):984–7.
14. Ziv A, Wolpe PR, Small SD, Glick S. Simulation-based medical education: an ethical imperative. Simul Healthc. 2006;1(4):252–6.
15. Javia L, Deutsch ES. A systematic review of simulators in otolaryngology. Otolaryngol Head Neck Surg. 2012;147(6):999–1011.
16. Van Zundert TC, Van Zundert AA. Tracheal intubation of patients in non-standard positions requires training. Minerva Anestesiol. 2013;79(6):679–82.
17. Lee DH, Kim JG, Kim CW, Lee CH, Lim JH. The usefulness of 3-dimensional virtual simulation using haptics in training orotracheal intubation. Biomed Res Int. 2013;2013:534097.
18. Yang JH, Kim YM, Chung HS, Cho J, Lee HM, Kang GH, et al. Comparison of four manikins and fresh frozen cadaver models for direct laryngoscopic orotracheal intubation training. Emerg Med J. 2010;27(1):13–6.
19. Ang H, Veldman A, Lewis A, Carse E, Wong FY. Procedural training opportunities for basic pediatric trainees during a 6-month rotation in a level III perinatal centre in Australia. J Matern Fetal Neonatal Med. 2012;25(11):2428–31.
20. Schmolzer GM, Dawson JA, Kamlin CO, O'Donnell CP, Morley CJ, Davis PG. Airway obstruction and gas leak during mask ventilation of preterm infants in the delivery room. Arch Dis Child Fetal Neonatal Ed. 2011;96(4):F254–7.
21. Wood FE, Morley CJ, Dawson JA, Kamlin CO, Owen LS, Donath S, et al. Improved techniques reduce face mask leak during simulated neonatal resuscitation: study 2. Arch Dis Child Fetal Neonatal Ed. 2008;93(3):F230–4.
22. O'Donnell CP, Kamlin CO, Davis PG, Morley CJ. Neonatal resuscitation 1: a model to measure inspired and expired tidal volumes and assess leakage at the face mask. Arch Dis Child Fetal Neonatal Ed. 2005;90(5):F388–91.
23. O'Donnell CP, Davis PG, Lau R, Dargaville PA, Doyle LW, Morley CJ. Neonatal resuscitation 2: an evaluation of manual ventilation devices and face masks. Arch Dis Child Fetal Neonatal Ed. 2005;90(5):F392–6.
24. Caldwell P, Srinivasjois R, Earley J. Use of laryngeal mask airway in near-term and term neonates during resuscitation: is it effective and safe? J Paediatr Child Health. 2011;47(10):753–6.
25. Velankar P, Joshi M, Sahu P. Use of laryngeal mask airway in premature infant. Indian J Anaesth. 2013;57(6):634–5.
26. Kovacs G. Procedural skills in medicine: linking theory to practice. J Emerg Med. 1997;15(3):387–91.
27. Cook DA, Hamstra SJ, Brydges R, Zendejas B, Szostek JH, Wang AT, et al. Comparative effectiveness of instructional design features in simulation-based education: systematic review and meta-analysis. Med Teach. 2013;35(1):e867–98.
28. McGaghie WC, Issenberg SB, Cohen ER, Barsuk JH, Wayne DB. Does simulation-based medical education with deliberate practice yield better results than traditional clinical education? A meta-analytic comparative review of the evidence. Acad Med. 2011;86(6):706–11.
29. Ericsson KA. Deliberate practice and the acquisition and maintenance of expert performance in medicine and related domains. Acad Med. 2004;79(10 Suppl):S70–81.
30. Sawyer T, Sierocka-Castaneda A, Chan D, Berg B, Lustik M, Thompson M. Deliberate practice using simulation improves neonatal resuscitation performance. Simul Healthc. 2011;6(6):327–36.
31. McGaghie WC, Issenberg SB, Petrusa ER, Scalese RJ. A critical review of simulation-based medical education research: 2003–2009. Med Educ. 2010;44(1):50–63.
32. McGaghie WC, Issenberg SB, Cohen ER, Barsuk JH, Wayne DB. Medical education featuring mastery learning with deliberate practice can lead to better health for individuals and populations. Acad Med. 2011;86(11):e8–9.
33. Yun BJ, Brown CA, Grazioso CJ, Pozner CN, Raja AS. Comparison of video, optical, and direct laryngoscopy by experienced tactical paramedics. Prehosp Emerg Care. 2014;18(3):442–5.
34. Naik VN, Matsumoto ED, Houston PL, Hamstra SJ, Yeung RY, Mallon JS, et al. Fiberoptic orotracheal intubation on anesthetized patients: do manipulation skills learned on a simple model transfer into the operating room? Anesthesiology. 2001;95(2):343–8.
35. Vanderhal AL, Berci G, Simmons Jr CF, Hagiike M. A videolaryngoscopy technique for the intubation of the newborn: preliminary report. Pediatrics. 2009;124(2):e339–46.
36. Cook TM, Woodall N, Frerk C. Major complications of airway management in the UK: results of the Fourth National Audit Project of the Royal College of Anaesthetists and the difficult airway society. Part 1: anaesthesia. Br J Anaesth. 2011;106(5):617–31.
37. Taylor C, Barrass L, Drewery H. Training for tracheostomy. Br J Anaesth. 2013;111(5):842–3.
38. Al Sharhan S, Sohail M, Ahmad K, Siddiqui MI. Self-reported comfort with tracheostomy tube care. Cross-sectional survey of non-ear, nose and throat health care professionals. Saudi Med J. 2014;35(1):63–6.
39. Dorton LH, Lintzenich CR, Evans AK. Simulation model for tracheotomy education for primary health-care providers. Ann Otol Rhinol Laryngol. 2014;123(1):11–8.
40. Ireton J. Tracheostomy suction: a protocol for practice. Paediatr Nurs. 2007;19(10):14–8.

41. Sodhi K, Shrivastava A, Singla MK. Implications of dedicated tracheostomy care nurse program on outcomes. J Anesth. 2013; 28(3):374–80.
42. de Mestral C, Iqbal S, Fong N, LeBlanc J, Fata P, Razek T, et al. Impact of a specialized multidisciplinary tracheostomy team on tracheostomy care in critically ill patients. Can J Surg. 2011;54(3): 167–72.
43. Chandra DB, Savoldelli GL, Joo HS, Weiss ID, Naik VN. Fiberoptic oral intubation: the effect of model fidelity on training for transfer to patient care. Anesthesiology. 2008;109(6):1007–13.
44. Weaver SJ, Dy SM, Rosen MA. Team-training in healthcare: a narrative synthesis of the literature. BMJ Qual Saf. 2014;23(5): 359–72.
45. Mazzocco K, Petitti DB, Fong KT, Bonacum D, Brookey J, Graham S, et al. Surgical team behaviors and patient outcomes. Am J Surg. 2009;197(5):678–85.
46. Shekelle PG, Wachter RM, Pronovost PJ, Schoelles K, McDonald KM, Dy SM, et al. Making health care safer II: an updated critical analysis of the evidence for patient safety practices. Evid Rep Technol Assess. 2013;211:1–945.
47. Research AIf. Training Guide: Using Simulation in TEAMSTEPPS® Training provides instruction on using simulation-based training when teaching TeamSTEPPS http://www.ahrq.gov/professionals/education/curriculum-tools/teamstepps/simulation/index.html2011.
48. Fletcher G, McGeorge P, Flin R, Glavin R, Maran N. The role of non-technical skills in anaesthesia: a review of current literature. Br J Anaesth. 2002;88:418–29.
49. Fletcher G, Flin R, McGeorge P, Glavin R, Maran N, Patey R. Anaesthetists' non-technical skills (ANTS): evaluation of a behavioural marker system. Br J Anaesth. 2003;90:580–8.
50. Kiesewetter J, Schmidt-Huber M, Netzel J, Krohn AC, Angstwurm M, Fischer MR. Training of leadership skills in medical education. GMS Z Med Ausbild. 2013;30(4):49.
51. Boet S, Bould MD, Fung L, Qosa H, Perrier L, Tavares W, et al. Transfer of learning and patient outcome in simulated crisis resource management: a systematic review. Can J Anaesth. 2014;61(6):571–82.
52. Augustine EM, Kahana M. Effect of procedure simulation workshops on resident procedural confidence and competence. J Grad Med Educ. 2012;4(4):479–85.
53. Sawyer S, French H, Songhier L, Barry J, Johnston L, Anderson J, et al. Educational perspectives: boot camps for neonatal-perinatal medicine fellows. NeoReviews. 2014;15(2):e46–55.
54. Malloy KM, Malekzadeh S, Deutsch ES. Simulation-based ORL emergencies boot camp part 1: curriculum design and airway skills. Laryngoscope. 2013;124(7):1562–5.
55. Kirkpatrick D. Great ideas revisited. Training Development. 1996; 50:54.
56. Mosley CM, Shaw BN. A longitudinal cohort study to investigate the retention of knowledge and skills following attendance on the Newborn Life support course. Arch Dis Child. 2013;98(8):582–6.
57. Avisar L, Shiyovich A, Aharonson-Daniel L, Nesher L. Cardiopulmonary resuscitation skills retention and self-confidence of preclinical medical students. Isr Med Assoc J. 2013;15(10): 622–7.
58. Hubert V, Duwat A, Deransy R, Mahjoub Y, Dupont H. Effect of simulation training on compliance with difficult airway management algorithms, technical ability, and skills retention for emergency cricothyrotomy. Anesthesiology. 2014;120(4):999–1008.
59. Rumball C, Macdonald D, Barber P, Wong H, Smecher C. Endotracheal intubation and esophageal tracheal Combitube insertion by regular ambulance attendants: a comparative trial. Prehosp Emerg Care. 2004;8(1):15–22.
60. Stratton SJ, Kane G, Gunter CS, Wheeler NC, Ableson-Ward C, Reich E, et al. Prospective study of manikin-only versus manikin and human subject endotracheal intubation training of paramedics. Ann Emerg Med. 1991;20(12):1314–8.
61. Cooper S, Cant R, Porter J, Sellick K, Somers G, Kinsman L, et al. Rating medical emergency teamwork performance: development of the Team Emergency Assessment Measure (TEAM). Resuscitation. 2010;81(4):446–52.
62. Nishisaki A, Donoghue AJ, Colborn S, Watson C, Meyer A, Niles D, et al. Development of an instrument for a primary airway provider's performance with an ICU multidisciplinary team in pediatric respiratory failure using simulation. Respir Care. 2012;57(7):1121–8.
63. Sigalet E, Donnon T, Cheng A, Cooke S, Robinson T, Bissett W, et al. Development of a team performance scale to assess undergraduate health professionals. Acad Med. 2013;88(7):989–96.
64. Lubin J, Carter R. The feasibility of daily mannequin practice to improve intubation success. Air Med J. 2009;28(4):195–7.
65. Silverman E, Dunkin BJ, Todd SR, Turner K, Fahy BN, Sukumaran A, et al. Nonsurgical airway management training for surgeons. J Surg Educ. 2008;65(2):101–8.
66. Davis DP, Buono C, Ford J, Paulson L, Koenig W, Carrison D. The effectiveness of a novel, algorithm-based difficult airway curriculum for air medical crews using human patient simulators. Prehosp Emerg Care. 2007;11(1):72–9.
67. Nishisaki A, Donoghue AJ, Colborn S, Watson C, Meyer A, Brown 3rd CA, et al. Effect of just-in-time simulation training on tracheal intubation procedure safety in the pediatric intensive care unit. Anesthesiology. 2010;113(1):214–23.
68. Nishisaki A, Nguyen J, Colborn S, Watson C, Niles D, Hales R, et al. Evaluation of multidisciplinary simulation training on clinical performance and team behavior during tracheal intubation procedures in a pediatric intensive care unit. Pediatr Crit Care Med. 2011;12(4):406–14.
69. Knowles M. The modern practice of adult education: from pedagogy to andragogy. New York: Cambridge, the Adult Education Company; 1980.
70. Issenberg SB, McGaghie WC, Petrusa ER, Lee Gordon D, Scalese RJ. Features and uses of high-fidelity medical simulations that lead to effective learning: a BEME systematic review. Med Teach. 2005;27(1):10–28.
71. Zigmont JJ, Kappus LJ, Sudikoff SN. The 3D model of debriefing: defusing, discovering, and deepening. Semin Perinatol. 2011;35(2):52–8.
72. Dufrene C, Young A. Successful debriefing - best methods to achieve positive learning outcomes: a literature review. Nurse Educ Today. 2014;34(3):372–6.
73. Levett-Jones T, Lapkin S. A systematic review of the effectiveness of simulation debriefing in health professional education. Nurse Educ Today. 2013;34(6):e58–63.
74. Cooper DD, Wilson AB, Huffman GN, Humbert AJ. Medical students' perception of residents as teachers: comparing effectiveness of residents and faculty during simulation debriefings. J Grad Med Educ. 2012;4(4):486–9.
75. Dine CJ, Gersh RE, Leary M, Riegel BJ, Bellini LM, Abella BS. Improving cardiopulmonary resuscitation quality and resuscitation training by combining audiovisual feedback and debriefing. Crit Care Med. 2008;36(10):2817–22.
76. Sawyer TL, Deering S. Adaptation of the US Army's after-action review for simulation debriefing in healthcare. Simul Healthc. 2013;8(6):388–97.
77. Schweller M, Costa FO, Antonio MA, Amaral EM, de Carvalho-Filho MA. The impact of simulated medical consultations on the empathy levels of students at one medical school. Acad Med. 2014;89(4):632–7.
78. Layouni I, Danan C, Durrmeyer X, Dassieu G, Azcona B, Decobert F. [Video recording of newborn resuscitation in the delivery room: technique and advantages]. Arch Pediatr. 2011;18 Suppl 2:S72–8.

Tracheostomy Care: Hospital Management and Transition to Home

Richard Lin, Joanne Stow, Lynn Shesser, and John Tamasitis

The Journey Home with a Tracheostomy: A Roadmap to Success.

Abbreviations

AARC	American Association of Respiratory Care
ATS	American Thoracic Society
CPR	Cardiopulmonary resuscitation
DME	Durable medical equipment supplier
ENT	Ear, nose, and throat
$EtCO_2$	End-tidal CO2
HME	Heat-moisture exchanger
ICU	Intensive care unit
IPV	Intrapulmonary percussive ventilation
LRTI	Lower respiratory tract infection
RT	Respiratory therapist
SSI	Supplemental security income
TSV	Tracheostomy speaking valve
VACHP	Ventilator Assisted Children's Home Program
VAP	Ventilator associated pneumonia
WIC	Women, Infants, and Children

R. Lin, M.D., F.A.A.P. (✉)
Departments of Anesthesiology and Critical Care Medicine, The Children's Hospital of Philadelphia, University of Pennsylvania, Perelman School of Medicine, 34th Street and Civic Center Blvd, Philadelphia, PA 19104, USA
e-mail: linr@email.chop.edu

J. Stow, P.P.C.N.P-.B.C., C.O.R.L.N.
Division of Otorhinolarygology, The Children's Hospital of Philadelphia, 34th Street and Civic Center Blvd, Philadelphia, PA 19104, USA
e-mail: stow@email.chop.edu

L. Shesser, M.B.A., M.S.N., R.N. • J. Tamasitis, R.R.T-.N.P.S.
Children's Hospital Home Care, The Children's Hospital of Philadelphia, Philadelphia,
950 Pulaski Drive, King of Prussia, PA 19406, USA
e-mail: shesserl@email.chop.edu; tamasitis@email.chop.edu

Not all those who wander are lost.—J.R.R. Tolkien, The Fellowship of the Ring.

Frequently, the process of sending a child home with a tracheostomy has been described as a long road, however in reality, it is better described as a journey for the child and family. The principal reasons that a tracheostomy may be recommended for an infant are (1) to provide a safe airway, (2) to give them an airway through which they get chronic mechanical ventilation, (3) to better manage pulmonary secretions, and (4) to bypass extrathoracic airway obstruction. The advantage of a surgical airway is that it allows the patients to be sedation free so they can fully interact with their environment and progress with childhood developmental milestones. It also allows children to be discharged from the acute hospital environment and go home with their parents or caregivers, or go to a transitional care facility if home is not a viable option.

Which Road to Travel?

The journey really starts with a decision about which path to take. The medical team should include families early in the decision-making process when it is first deliberating about whether an infant may benefit from a tracheostomy. The vast majority of families have had little or no exposure to this type of medical device. This lack of knowledge will impact the family's ability to give informed consent, accept the need for a tracheostomy, and comprehend its impact on future home life. The American Academy of Otolaryngology, Head and Neck Surgery, in recently published consensus statements for tracheostomy care, recommends that when possible (patient) and family education should begin before tracheostomy is performed [12].

The reason for tracheostomy impacts both the decision-making process and the timing of the decision. Offering the

J. Lioy and S.E. Sobol (eds.), *Disorders of the Neonatal Airway: Fundamentals for Practice*,
DOI 10.1007/978-1-4939-1610-8_31, © Springer Science+Business Media New York 2015

tracheostomy as a possible therapeutic option should not occur in conjunction with an extubation trial. The family should not be suspicious of the earnestness of the extubation endeavor. The primary principles of "doing good" (beneficence) and "doing no harm" (nonmaleficence) should be in the forefront of discussions between professionals and parents. The treatment option must clearly benefit the child and outweigh the associated burdens and harms [5]. If an infant is severely medically compromised and a tracheostomy does not add to the child's prognosis or quality of life, then palliative care should be discussed as a medical option. Permitting sufficient time between introduction of the tracheostomy as a possible treatment option and the need for a decision to be made by the family allows opportunity for the family to gather information and support. There is no "right" decision or even "best" decision and often the considerations may need to include multiple viewpoints [3]. The decision not to prolong an infant's life with a tracheostomy is emotionally difficult, yet there are cases where this may be the best choice. Parents rely on the medical team to present this option. An explanation of how the infant will be kept comfortable and medically supported during the dying process can help the family manage the devastating experience without guilt.

In most cases the tracheostomy should be explained as a medical device that can help the infant transition to a healthier state. It is important that the need for tracheostomy not be presented merely as a consequence of failure to extubate. The medical team must realize if a tracheostomy is done, the expectation is that the family will either be able to learn the necessary care or be aware that the infant will require placement in a pediatric nursing care facility (when ready for discharge). The placement may be needed only until the family can assume the care or until the child is decannulated and medically stable.

Starting the Journey

The journey home and the necessary discharge planning starts the day the family is in agreement with the recommendation to perform a tracheotomy on their child. Discussion with the family should take place on several different levels. Some opportunities for discussion include bedside rounds, multidisciplinary meetings, interactions with the bedside nurse, or meeting with an experienced ENT (Ear, Nose, and Throat specialist) nurse practitioner or physician assistant. Typically, a mid-level provider within the ENT specialty practice is more accessible than a resident or attending physician and is able to provide very detailed information to the family. It is essential to document and share with the infant's care team all discussions with the family, detailing the topics covered and the family's understanding of them.

Before having a detailed, informative talk with the baby's parents, it is useful to know what they recall having been told by the primary (usually intensive care unit(ICU)) team, and whether they have had interactions with someone who has a tracheostomy. This provides the starting point for the discussion. If possible, this should be a face-to-face conversation in a private area, without distractions, and in an unhurried manner. It is beneficial to bring actual tracheostomy tubes and a doll with a tracheostomy tube in place for parents to see and handle. The conversation should cover several points, many of which are listed below.

- The reason why a tracheostomy is being considered for their infant.
- The benefits to tracheostomy over current airway management (safer airway, more comfortable, less need for sedation, improved nutrition and growth, more opportunity for normalizing development.)
- Basic airway anatomy.
- Basic tracheostomy tube anatomy.
- The tracheotomy surgical procedure, including risks, benefits, alternatives.
- What to expect during the first postoperative week (appearance of site, care of site while healing, need for minimal movement, pain and sedation management, timing of first trach change.)
- Routine care of tracheostomy (site cleaning, trach tube and tie changes, suctioning.)
- Future care when ready for discharge-home versus facility, possible home care nursing.
- Training requirements for family if baby will be going home, including approximate timeline.
- Tracheostomy and communication (varies by child and situation: neurologic status is a factor, some can vocalize around trach, some will learn sign)
- Tracheostomy and eating by mouth (varies by child and situation: will require assessment by Speech Language Pathologist prior to discharge to assess safety.)
- Length of time the tracheostomy will be needed (minimum 1 year or more, until reason for the need has resolved.)

It is helpful to provide the family with some basic information sheets to review independently. The Parent-Family Education manual for tracheostomy care at our institution, which is appropriately titled "Breathe Easy," is accessible online by all staff members. Although available as a complete binder of information, individual pages can be printed from our internal hospital website. This manual provides answers to many commonly asked questions and is written in language that is understandable at a basic 5th grade reading level. Some institutions have information on their websites that families can access at their convenience.

The next phase of the journey towards home requires that:

1. The child is medically stable and his/her care is practical for a home or transitional care setting.

2. Caregivers are trained thoroughly and appropriately to deliver all the necessary care, and
3. Services are in place to assist with home care, including private duty shift nursing, home respiratory care, pharmacy services and a durable medical equipment supplier.

These resources can be mobilized anytime during the hospitalization, even before the child has received the tracheostomy. Ideally, staff will address these activities concurrently, so that all aspects of discharge planning can be well-coordinated and completed in a timely fashion.

Institutions should develop standardized education and training to ensure safe care of the child with a tracheostomy at home. The expectations for the caregivers must be outlined in writing, discussed in full at the beginning of the process, and periodically reviewed by the medical team as training takes place to gauge the competency and comfort of the parents to provide the care. Others have described guidelines for the skills caregivers should be taught and what supports will be needed at home [2, 6]. Ultimately, the success of the transition depends on how comfortable an institution is with helping families on their journey and what infrastructure supports there are in the community.

The program most often used at a full service children's hospital like our own is based on the expectation and standard that a child will go home in the care of a primary caregiver and a back-up caregiver. Frequently both parents are the caregivers. We have been fortunate that most of the families we work with live in the mid-Atlantic area, particularly in the state of Pennsylvania, and qualify for 16–24 h of private duty nursing per day. We are also fortunate that services such as nursing and medical equipment supply are generally readily available. However, we do find that depending on the family's insurance there is variability in the amount of *approved* home nursing services. Some policies do not include a benefit for private duty nursing in the home. Families may be able to use secondary insurance policies, including state Medicaid, to get coverage for private duty nursing. However, if the family's income level is above that of Medicaid eligibility, the family will be able to receive Medicaid assistance through a state waiver program. The flexibility of Medicaid waivers varies from state to state and may have limited enrollment. Families should be encouraged to check requirements with their local Medicaid or county assistance office. In some states, the expectation is that only a single caregiver is trained in the child's care and there may not be availability of trained private duty nursing, particularly with the skill set required for the care of technology-dependent children. An added complication is that some states lack transitional care facilities, requiring children to be moved to a different state should they require these services.

> Today is your day! Your mountain is waiting. So… get on your way.—Theodore Seuss Geisel.

A Steep Climb But a Clear Path

For a successful trek home, the family must manage several obstacles along the path. The largest obstacle, but the one that the family has the most control over, is the mountain known as *Training*. The task requires parents or other caregivers to become experts in their child's care and to be able to deliver that care independently for short periods of time in the event that home nursing is not available. Although it seems Herculean for a lay person to train to a skill level near that of a healthcare professional in a short time period, a vast majority of parents and caregivers are able to meet the challenge. In many cases, family members who are trained caregivers are so successful that they play a significant role in orienting new nursing staff. The hope is also that the trained caregivers are comfortable enough with the child's care that they can train others.

In a full-service children's hospital like our own, a multidisciplinary team is responsible for family education. This team consists of hospital-based physicians, respiratory therapists, physical and occupational therapists, and nurses as well as home care respiratory therapists who collaborate to help the family achieve full competence in caring for their child.

While some institutions may compress their training curriculum into a 2 week period, our caregiver training program spans 8 weeks or more, depending on the patient's medical stability, the availability/schedule of the caregivers and the literacy capabilities of those caregivers. This program includes not only training with written material and classroom sessions but also a substantial amount of bedside "*hands-on*" practice. There is no declared standard for a training curriculum, but organizations such as the American Thoracic Society (ATS) have come up with consensus statements [1]. Occasionally, families require substantially longer than 8–12 weeks to train and may benefit from transitioning to a chronic care facility to complete their training. Figure 1 summarizes our curriculum.

There are several challenges in training family members. They have varied comfort levels in participating in their child's care. Many have difficulty with the complexity of a tracheostomy or a gastrostomy tube, let alone the equipment that might be connected to it. Families are often apprehensive about learning their child's care for fear of causing harm, especially if they and their children have gone through a difficult course in the ICU. Because of these and other factors, the primary and secondary caregivers may train at a different pace. Some "fear" is not necessarily a bad thing. Each caregiver will have a different comfort level with the new facts and terminology as well as varying levels of literacy. Lay caregivers, just like medical caregivers, also have different learning styles; some are more comfortable with reading

The Children's Hospital *of* Philadelphia **38:A:03**
Tracheostomy Education Checklist
(Not a Permanent Part of the Patient's Record)

Please document ALL teaching on Interdisciplinary Patient-Family Education Flowsheet.

Only document on this sheet when competency is demonstrated

Learner's Name: ______________________________

Discharge Process	Date/ Educator's Initials
Respiratory System and Lung Function	
Understand Need for Trach	
Temperature	
Respiratory Rate and Assessment	
Monitoring (Pulse Ox/ETCO2)	
Airway Clearance (Cough Assist/IPV)	
Use of a Speaking Valve	
Respiratory Medications	
Suctioning (Trach, NP, OP)	
Manual Ventilation (Self-Inflating Bag)	
Oxygen Administration	
Trach Care	
Trach String Change	

Trach Tube Change	
1st In	
1st Out	
2nd In	
2nd Out	
3rd In	
3rd Out	

Trach Emergencies	
Plugged Trach	
Decannulation	
Water in Trach	
Unable to Place Trach	

Ventilator Care	
View LTV PowerPoint	
Ventilator Settings	
Ventilator Alarms / Troubleshooting	
Ventilator Circuit Change	
Portability with a Ventilator	

Feeding/Nutrition	
Formula Preparation	
Administration of Feeds via Feeding Tube	

Medications	Date/ Educator's Initials
Medications and Purpose of Each	
Drawing Medications Up in Syringes	
Administration of Medications	

Family Learning Center	
Trach Class Part 1	
Trach Class Part 3	
Trach CPR	
NGT/GT Class	
Feeding Pump	

Family / Team Meeting	
Initial FTM	
Focus FTM	
Discharge FTM	

Car Safety	
Car Seat Test Passed	

Becoming Independent	
Assembling Equipment for Independent Walk	
Walk Off the Unit with Assistance	
Walk off the Unit Independently	
24-hour Stay	
Patient on Home Vent	

Equipment / Home Preparation	
All Equipment Lists Completed and Signed	
Home Inspection Completed	
Equipment Delivered to Home and Checked by Family	

Prescriptions Filled and Checked by Nurse	

Written 1/2009, Revised 5/09, Reviewed 4/12

Page 1 of 1

Fig. 1 Tracheostomy Educational Checklist—this checklist summarizes the basic curriculum that is covered in training caregivers to be able to care for a child with a tracheostomy about facts and tasks while others are more visual and "hands-on." The varied comfort levels, backgrounds and learning styles require different approaches to education. We have found that it is important to appreciate these differences and adjust our teaching accordingly. Yet, there are families on the opposite end of the spectrum who seem to lack an appreciation of how important it is to learn and practice well the new skills required for their child's care.

Although there are defined, discrete tasks and steps necessary to care for a technology-dependent child, we find that it is even more essential that the family learn *how* and *when* and *why* to combine individual steps and apply what they learn in the process of caring for their technology-dependent child. Our emphasis is not just to help them learn individual tasks but also help them understand how they fit in the whole algorithm of care. Often the best way for families to learn how to synthesize tasks and perform assessments is by doing care at the bedside. We find that the most successful families are the ones that can spend the most time at the bedside. They will have the best chance to render care in both ideal and non-ideal circumstances and will have the opportunity to do so with the safety net of our inpatient medical and nursing staff.

At the start of the education process, we provide the families with the "Breathe Easy" binder which includes all of the fundamentals that families need to learn to care for their child at home. The binder's content has been translated and is available in Spanish. For families speaking other languages, we review the content with an interpreter. In some cases, this binder is distributed ahead of the tracheostomy procedure so the family can better understand why the procedure is being done and they get a sense of what to expect. The book is divided into several sections ranging in content from anatomy to discharge planning (Table 1). For consistent and standardized education practices, hospital-based and home care-based clinicians use this "Breathe Easy" binder and equipment manuals during teaching sessions. Many teaching sessions involve the use of the teach-back method.

Mapping the Path

Scaling the training "mountain" starts with understanding the destination. In our hospital, we have a unit that is more focused in caring for technology-dependent children and training families/caregivers for independent care at home, although training can start anywhere in the hospital. We hold a formal interdisciplinary meeting with families to initiate the concept of bringing their child home. During the meeting, we outline the training program and educational milestones, inform families about the multidisciplinary treatment team that will be supporting them, discuss the need~~s~~ for continual and ongoing meetings to review progress, and articulate how training will culminate in an extended bedside stay (most often a 24-h independent stay) as a "*final exam*" or competency assessment (Table 2). This 24-h independent hospital stay occurs after completion of all the training, much of which has involved portable home equipment. During this stay, two trained parents or caregivers are responsible for administering all medications, checking ventilator settings, responding to ventilator and other alarms, weighing, feeding and performing anything else needed for the child.

We emphasize that the discharge process starts ~~at~~ on admission and that the more families practice their child's care, the more comfortable they will be when caring for their child at home. We give them an outline of the eight-week training program, which lists all the steps that are necessary to bring a technology-dependent child home (Table 3). We adjust specifics in the curriculum to the child's individual medical needs. The actual length of training time depends on the child's medical stability, the family's availability for training, and caregiver mastery of the educational materials and accompanying skills. Frequently one or both caregivers have to work or care for other siblings, which can limit their availability to learn care. We ask families to give us a calendar of their availability so we can plan training sessions and ensure we have the necessary nursing or respiratory therapy (RT) staff available for teaching.

The training involved is a combination of classroom education in our centralized family learning center, which helps assure that all caregivers will get the same training, and bedside hands-on training. Staff nurses and respiratory therapists provide hands-on training for most of the care that the family needs to learn. They assess caregiver's learning needs on an ongoing basis. The goal of caregiver-in-training is proficiency in each task without requiring additional reinforcement by the completion of the training. All disciplines track each caregiver's progress on one interdisciplinary form. Once caregivers are deemed proficient, they are encouraged to use that skill to help with the child's care as opportunities arise. Although there is a prescribed number of times that the family must demonstrate ~~a~~ certain tasks, we are careful to emphasize that the goal is NOT demonstrating a skill the requisite number times, but repetition of skills as often as needed to gain comfort in that skill. We also stress critical thinking skills and troubleshooting techniques.

Hiking to the Mountain: Understanding and Seeing Their Child in a New Light

We teach families the basics of airway anatomy (from nose to alveoli), the muscles of respiration, and the role of the respiratory system in the body. Staff also reviews what a

Table 1 Contents of the "Breath Easy" binder

1. The basics	(a) Ventilator
(a) Respiratory system	(b) Tracheostomy only
(b) General tracheostomy information	(c) Safety
• Learning about tracheostomies	11. Managing Emergencies
• Questions parents often ask about a tracheostomy	(a) Critical Airway
2. Discharge Process	(b) Emergencies
(a) Discharge Plan	(c) CPR
(b) Teaching Plan	(d) Artificial Airway Bedside Card
(c) Questions about classes	(e) Contact List
(d) 24 Independent Stay	12. Monitoring
3. Assessment Skills	(a) Pulse oximeter
(a) Taking a temperature	(b) Capnograph (ETCO2)
(b) Fever	(c) Apnea monitor
(c) Respiratory rate and breath sounds	13. Prepare the Home/Home Safety
4. Airway Clearance	(a) Preparing the Home
(a) Chest physiotherapy (PDPV)	• Activities of Daily Living
(b) Mechanical In/Exsufflator (MI-E)	• Safety/Inspection Checklist
5. Tracheostomy Skills	• Home nursing
(a) Suctioning your Child	• General supplies
• Tracheostomy	• Cleaning Equipment—Reusables and disposables
• Mouth/Nose	14. Communication Development
• Suction Equipment	(a) Passy Muir valve
6. Manual Ventilation	15. Additional Information
(a) Stoma Care	(a) Glossary
(b) Changing Trach Ties	(b) Hand Hygiene
(c) Tracheostomy "Go-Bag"	(c) Phone update Information sheet
(d) Changing tracheostomy tube	(d) Discipline
• Routine	
• Emergency	
• Care of the cuffed tracheostomy tube	
7. Humidification	
(a) HME (Heat-Moisture Exchanger)	
(b) Heater/humidifier or T-piece if asleep	
8. Respiratory medications	
(a) MDI	
(b) Nebulized	
9. Ventilator	
(a) Settings	
(b) Alarms and troubleshooting	
(c) Circuit Changes	
(d) Portability	
10. Oxygen in the home	

tracheostomy tube is and what it looks like, the function of a tracheostomy, and what to expect after the initial surgery. There is also a list of frequently asked questions (and answers) in the training materials that parents often have about tracheostomy tubes. The goal is to teach them the purpose of the tracheostomy tube in their child's care and help them appreciate that the facts they are learning are important to their child's well-being (Fig. 2).

Since the ability to do a respiratory assessment in this population is critical, we teach caregivers to do a thorough clinical respiratory assessment. We teach them to count their child's respiratory rate accurately and know the differences between inspiration and expiration. We also teach caregivers to use a stethoscope properly, where to auscultate and how to describe what they hear. We emphasize that it is important for them to know their child's "normal" respiratory status and the value of assessing their child's respiratory status regularly so that deviations from the baseline can be recognized and addressed quickly if appropriate. They are expected to be able to recognize the symptoms of respiratory distress

Table 2 The 24-h stay—the "final exam"

Nurse and Respiratory Therapist Responsibilities	Family Responsibilities
Arrange the 24-h stay Complete the necessary paperwork for the caregivers before the stay. This includes the Daily Care Schedule, the 24-h Stay Checklist and the medication schedule	A trained caregiver needs to be awake at all times Provide *all* necessary care for the child
Review paperwork with all caregivers	Perform paperwork to document that you performed care and certain tasks
Measure vital signs Check ventilator settings Perform assessments as usual Document above care	Measure vital signs three times in the 24-h period unless your child needs more frequent monitoring
Remains alert to all alarms and respond if necessary	Respond appropriately to all alarms
Place the monitor in the *Monitor Pause* mode if nurse call and central monitoring are available on the unit. The patient remains visible on the central monitor at all times but alarms only sound in patient's room. (A doctor's order is required for Monitor Pause for this 24-h time period)	Respond to all alarms. Request assistance as needed
Obtain pulse oximeter Obtain feeding pump if necessary	Monitor child on home equipment
Post medication schedule Double check that medications administered by caregivers have correct name, dose, time, route and indication Give meds to the caregivers upon request if above parameters are correct Watch the caregiver give each medication	Give medications at the correct time according to the medication schedule Ask nurse for the correct medicine at the correct time Understand the indications for all medications Have nurse observe
Respiratory therapy observes respiratory treatments	Perform all respiratory treatments at the correct time and according to schedule Have RT observe
Respiratory therapy observes vent tubing change to assure that it is done correctly	Change ventilator tubing change at some point during the stay. Check the ventilator settings and document this on the 24-h Stay Checklist
Is knowledgeable of time for trach change and available for emergency assistance during trach change	Change trach without help from the staff. Have nurse available in case of an emergency
Double check that the caregivers have all necessary equipment for the walk off the unit. The patient will be on his highest ventilator support	Gather the necessary equipment for an independent walk off the unit and make the ventilator portable Have nurse and/or respiratory therapist check equipment and settings
Evaluate 24-h stay and family's ability to care for child independently	Review/Discuss the 24-h experience with nursing and respiratory staff
Document the caregivers' ability during the 24-h stay in a Progress Note in the chart and on the Interdisciplinary Patient-Family Education Flowsheet	Evaluate success or need for remediation
Reinforce training. Reschedule 24-h hospital stay if first attempt is unsuccessful	Reschedule 24-h hospital stay if first attempt is unsuccessful

such as the presence of retractions, nasal flaring, wheezing and cyanosis. Finally, they are expected to know when to call a healthcare provider and how to describe their observations.

Caregivers are also expected to understand and troubleshoot monitoring devices, including pulse oximetry (which all of our patients go home with) and end-tidal CO_2 monitoring (which many of our patients go home with). Fewer of our patients also go home with apnea monitoring. Pulse oximetry is the mainstay of noninvasive respiratory monitoring since it can be done continuously and serves not only to directly monitor oxygenation and pulse rate but also indirectly monitors ventilation (although its sensitivity to ventilation declines with increasing levels of supplemental oxygen). It should be emphasized that pulse oximetry is NOT a substitute for frequent and direct observation of the child with a tracheostomy since hypoxemia and bradycardia may be relatively late signs of problems with ventilation, particularly due to an occluded or displaced tracheostomy tube. We teach that when the pulse oximeter alarms, parents should check the child first, then the monitor.

End-tidal CO_2 ($EtCO_2$) monitoring is often useful as direct monitor of ventilation in the hospital setting, and can be quite sensitive to occlusion or displacement of a tracheostomy tube. However, the $EtCO_2$ monitors available in-home

Table 3 The "8 week" plan of care—this is the roadmap that many families follow to figure out what they should be doing and when during their training

Timeframe	Task	Responsible parties
Before tracheostomy	Initial meeting to discuss discharge options. Review tracheostomy info	Family with current healthcare team
	Explore shift nursing, therapy and equipment benefits	Case manager
	SSI disability or Waiver application	Family and social worker
	Identify 2 Caregivers, if home is the goal	Family
Week 1 (once medically stable)	Family Focus meeting to set discharge goals/tentative discharge date	Family and healthcare team
	Develop Letter of Medical Necessity for nursing	Nurse practitioner/doctor and case manager
	Obtain *Breathe Easy: Caring for Your Child with a Tracheostomy at Home*	The family learning center
	Develop training plan—schedule on calendar	Family and registered nurse
	Begin training	Caregivers and healthcare team
Week 2	Training continues	Family and healthcare team
	Home Nursing Agencies interviewed	Family
	Durable Medical Equipment (DME) companies interviewed and one chosen	Family (and case manager)
	Initial equipment list submitted	Case manager. Respiratory therapist, nurse
	Home Evaluation by DME scheduled	Family and case manager
	Application for Home Ventilator Program begun (Pennsylvania residents)	Social worker and family
	Application for Handicapped Parking placard	Social worker
	Initiate age-appropriate school planning	Family and social worker
	Consults to therapies for home adaptive equipment—special stroller, wheelchair and other equipment— prescription (Rx) and letter submitted	Physical and occupational therapists and case manager
Week 3	Training continues	Family and healthcare team
	Home nursing agency chosen	Family (and case manager)
	Therapists schedule a home visit, if needed	Family, physical therapist and occupational therapist
	Home evaluation by DME completed	Family and case manager
	DME Report communicated to family	Family, case manager and DME
Week 4	Training continues/documentation reviewed	Family and healthcare team
	Initiate referrals for Outpatient Therapy, if needed	Therapists and case manager
	Wheelchair ordered if needed	Physical therapist
	Home Vent Application submitted (Pennsylvania residents)	Social worker
	Therapists home visit completed; recommendations given to the family	Therapists, family, case manager and social worker
Week 5	Training continues	Family and healthcare team
	Family/Team Meeting to discuss progress, evaluate tentative discharge date	Family and healthcare team
	Review home readiness, (stroller, car seat)	
	Identify Primary Care Pediatrician	Family and nurse practitioner/physician assistant
2 weeks before discharge (~week 6)	Training continues	Family and healthcare team
	Discharge meeting scheduled for Week 7	Family and case manager
	Home Equipment delivered to hospital and vent used	DME, case manager and respiratory therapy
	Review transportation needs	Family, social worker and case manager
	Pre-authorizations for medications obtained; pharmacy chosen	Case manager, nurse practitioner/doctor/physician assistant

(continued)

Table 3 (continued)

Timeframe	Task	Responsible parties
1 week before discharge (~week 7)	Training completed; 24 h stay scheduled	Family and healthcare team
	Submit any changes to home equipment list	Nurse and respiratory therapist
	Home equipment delivery date set	Family, case manager and DME
	Home repairs/alterations completed	Family
	Adaptive equipment needs finalized	Family, therapists and case manager
	Discharge family/team meeting occurs	Inpatient and outpatient healthcare team
	Prescriptions forwarded to pharmacy	Family and healthcare team
	Initiate Early Intervention paperwork	Family and social worker
	WIC application completed and appt made	Family and social worker
Week of discharge	Home equipment delivered and inventoried	Family and case manger
	Letters sent to local emergency response and utility companies	Family, case manager and social worker
	24 h stay completed, home medications reviewed	Family
	Formula preparation reviewed	Family and nutrition
	Discharge transportation plans completed	Family and case manager
	Home Nursing schedule completed and approved by outpatient attending physician	Family, case manager and doctor/nurse practitioner
	Outpatient therapy services confirmed; summaries to parents	Case manager, nurse practitioner and doctor
	Chest X-ray copied for home	Case manager
	Complete plans for Early Intervention or school reintegration	Family and social worker
	Follow up appointments reviewed	Nurse practitioner/doctor/physician

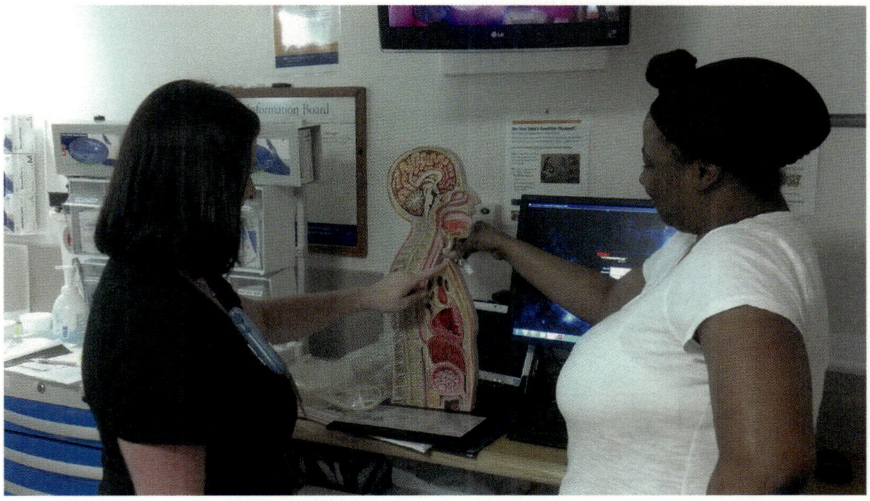

Fig. 2 Nurse and parent review airway anatomy to understand tracheostomy placement

care are not well suited for continuous monitoring. These monitors are frequently sidestream (aspirating), instead of mainstream, and are more prone to failure due to moisture and occlusion with secretions.

Patients on mechanical ventilation at home have additional alarms that may be helpful in detecting airway issues, such as low and high pressure, low minute ventilation and apnea alarms. These are not perfect and may not detect partial occlusion. Also, a high incidence of false ventilator alarms may lead to decreased responsiveness by caregivers, which can be dangerous.

Climbing Up the Mountain: Learning to Do the Care

Since assistance in airway clearance is something this patient population frequently needs, we train caregivers in performing percussion and postural drainage, and targeting different lobes. For those patients who are receiving adjunctive clearance therapies such as cough assist, intrapulmonary percussive ventilation (IPV), or Vest® Percussion systems, we train caregivers in the use of these machines as well.

Our team spends a substantial amount of time in helping caregivers achieve comfort and competence with caring for the tracheostomy tube. We do "hands-on" training after first reviewing the basic concepts of pulmonary anatomy and assessment with caregivers. The first part of training is devoted to suctioning, including how to operate and clean a suction machine and how to suction a tracheostomy tube as well as the nose and pharynx. Many of our patients now go home with in-line suctioning so we review the use of in-line catheters as well as connecting them to the tracheostomy.

Although our hospital standard is to use flow inflating bags, our default home care standard is to use self-inflating bags. The advantage of the self-inflating bag is that it is simpler to use and does not require an external gas source for use. Disadvantages are that it cannot reach the FiO_2 that a flow inflating bag can, is not as effective at maintaining a positive end-expiratory pressure (PEEP), and cannot be left on a breathing patient without assisting the patient. Sometimes we will send families home with PEEP valves to try to ensure some level of positive end-expiratory pressure but these valves will not help if there is a leak around the tracheostomy tube. We train our caregivers in how to use these bags and sometimes will have staff use the self-inflating bag in the care of a patient in the hospital to make sure that it can be used successfully over the course of the patient's care and in the patient's home.

Scaling the Cliff: Conquering the Tracheostomy Tube

Perhaps the part of the care that creates the most anxiety for families is manipulating the tracheostomy tube. We teach this material first in our Family Learning Center and reinforce it with bedside training. Families begin with learning how to care for the stoma and then progress to changing tracheostomy ties (Fig. 3). Much of the emphasis is on the organization required for this task—to get needed supplies ahead of time and to have these supplies laid out ahead of time. This kind of anticipatory planning also helps them to organize and create their own "*Go-Bag*" of supplies that they will need to take their child out of the house. We provide a small travel bag with multiple see-through compartments during the inpatient stay. This "*Go-Bag*" is a hospital standard for all inpatients with a tracheostomy and is required to be with them at all times (Fig. 4a, b).

Among the most critical tasks that we teach families are when and how to change a tracheostomy tube. As with stoma and string care, we emphasize with families that they need to be organized and have their supplies arranged ahead of time. We also train them to do this as a clean procedure and as a two-person team (one removing tracheostomy, verifying proper position and securing the airway, the other inserting and stabilizing the airway, and each

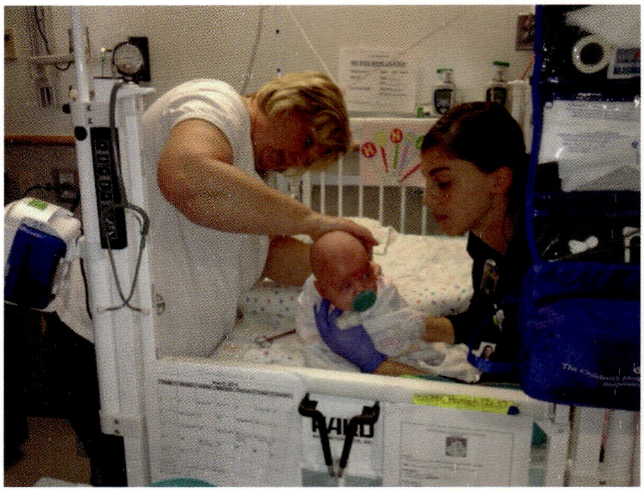

Fig. 3 A grandparent does "hands-on" training with a nurse for string care. Notice that the infant is bundled to make care easier. Because one parent may need to continue to work to get the insurance benefit to pay for private duty nursing, the caregiver team often consists of a parent and grandparent

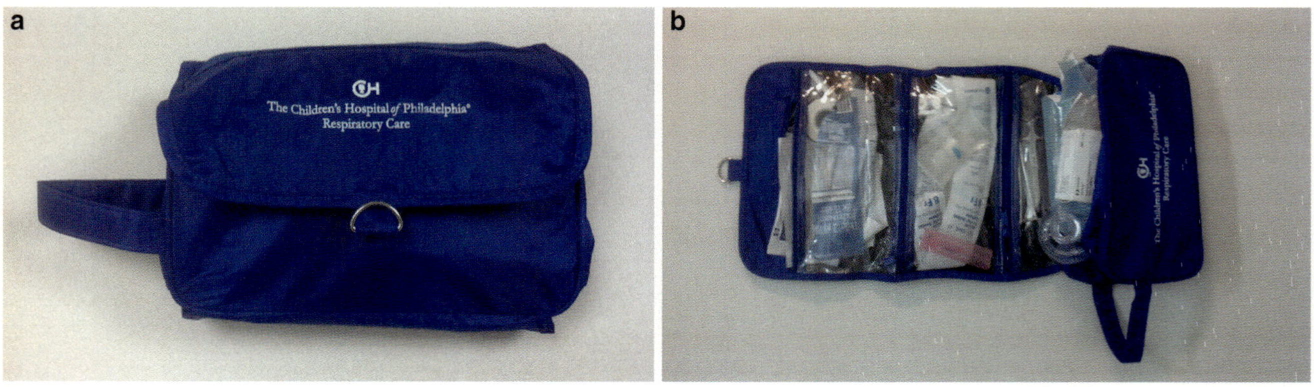

Fig. 4 Tracheostomy supplies bag (the "Go-Bag"). This bag includes all the supplies that would be needed to change a tracheostomy tube, including a backup which is slightly smaller, as well as items to be able to do airway toilet. (**a**) is bag folded and (**b**) is bag unfolded

clearly communicating to the other). They are taught how to inflate and deflate a cuff if that is applicable. We also teach families techniques to master challenging airway insertions, such as using an obturator, positioning their child properly, waiting for the inspiratory phase, use of a smaller size tracheostomy tube, and sometimes even bundling the child to minimize extraneous movement. As caregivers become more experienced with tracheostomy changes, they may be taught "last resort" measures such as inserting a suction catheter into the stoma (attached to oxygen), and mouth to stoma resuscitation, and bag-mask ventilation. The need for these last resort measures would necessitate emergency transport to a hospital for further treatment. There are some programs that train caregivers in a single-caregiver technique of changing tracheostomies, but this requires a cooperative child or the use of a restraint device. Caregivers are initially trained on a mannequin in our centralized Family Learning Center, and are then invited to see a tracheostomy change done by our staff. They eventually directly participate in the tracheostomy change themselves. Although in our routine practice, a tracheostomy change may be done every 1–2 weeks, we often will have families change the tracheostomy tube as frequently as every other day (if deemed medically safe) to ensure they have the opportunity when they are available. The "checklist" goal is for each caregiver to achieve proficiency by the time they do three removals and three insertions, but again our emphasis is not so much the quantity, but the comfort level of each caregiver.

Down the Slope: Things that Connect to the Tracheostomy

In addition we train caregivers in the purpose and practice of providing airway humidification, a necessary skill since the tracheostomy tube bypasses the natural humidification of the nasal, oral, and pharyngeal passages. In our patient population, the default humidifier is a heated humidifier in the ventilator circuit or used in a T-piece or tracheal mask setup. For patients on mechanical ventilation, providing humidification is straightforward since the ventilator provides a source of gas flow to be humidified. For patients not requiring a ventilator, there has to be some other source of gas flow for active humidification to work; in the home environment, this is typically done by using an air compressor (enriched with supplemental oxygen if necessary) to drive flow through the heated humidifier.

For portability, a passive heat-moisture exchanger (HME) device can be connected to the tracheostomy to maintain airway humidification. This device contains absorbent material such as paper or cloth, which traps exhaled water vapor and is also warmed by exhaled gas. The HME works by conserving the exhaled moisture and energy to re-humidify air from the surroundings when the patient inhales. Some HME devices have additional features such as a connector through which supplemental oxygen may be bled in and a port that can be opened so that airway secretions can be suctioned without needing to remove the HME from the tracheostomy.

Many children with tracheostomies have some element of chronic lung disease or reactive airway disease and so will require some sort of aerosolized medication for maintenance therapy or to treat exacerbations of underlying conditions. If applicable, caregivers are trained in the use of devices such as metered dose inhalers or nebulizers with tracheostomies and ventilator circuits.

Verbal communication for a child with a tracheostomy may be challenging since their ability to make sounds largely depends on their ability to move gas across their vocal cords to generate sounds that can be modulated to form the elements of speech. The tracheostomy is a low resistance pathway for air and oxygen to flow into the tracheobronchial tree and lungs, thus gas flow is diverted from the natural airway. Also obstructive pathophysiology such as high grade subglottic stenosis that would require a tracheotomy may also prevent flow across the cords. Finally, the degree of mechanical ventilator support that a child needs may mandate the use of a tracheostomy with a cuff, which will also decrease gas flow through the natural airway.

With time and treatment, the underlying obstructive pathophysiology and need for mechanical ventilator support may decrease, particularly as the child grows. There may be flow that develops around the tracheostomy tube as the trachea becomes larger in diameter or there is less need to use a tracheostomy tube with an inflated cuff. This will become manifest as a "leak" through the nose and mouth that may become evident with ventilator breaths or as sounds coming from the child. To develop or relearn verbal communication skills, it will be helpful to periodically make use of this leak to generate sounds from the vocal cords. This involves the use of a speaking valve (also known as a tracheostomy speaking valve (TSV)—a commonly used brand is the Passy-Muir® valve). These devices are inserted in between the ventilator circuit and tracheostomy (if the patient is on ventilation) or are connected to the tracheostomy directly. These valves are one-way valves: they allow airflow through the tracheostomy on inhalation, but close on exhalation, diverting flow around the tracheostomy tube and through the trachea. The use of these valves requires the presence of a sufficient leak around the tracheostomy tube. This is assessed by checking for a leak pressure by auscultating for sound over the suprastomal trachea and glottis. The pressure needs to be low (typically below 10–15 cm H_2O air pressure) since an inadequate leak will lead to a higher end-expiratory pressure because of breath stacking, causing patient discomfort or even a pneumothorax. The valve can be used on and off mechanical ventilation (a different version is required for use on mechanical ventilation). If the tracheostomy tube has a cuff, then the patient must be able to tolerate having their cuff deflated. TSV use is prescribed by or in coordination with a speech therapist, and is often scheduled in coordination with therapy sessions. The valve is also useful in helping a child with a tracheostomy to learn or relearn how to feed orally as the positive glottis pressure is thought to be helpful in developing coordination of sucking and swallowing.

Not all children with tracheostomies require mechanical ventilation, but for those that do, their families are expected to learn about their ventilator. The vast majority of our patients go home on a Carefusion LTV™ series ventilator, although some go home on a Philips Respironics Trilogy™ series ventilator. Caregivers are expected to understand the different settings of the ventilator (both modes and parameters that are prescribed), what the different alarms mean (such as high pressure and low pressure), how to disassemble and reassemble the breathing circuit, and how to troubleshoot alarms and issues. The reason that this level of detailed knowledge is required is so that families are able to put their children on or take them off of mechanical ventilation, are able to do routine circuit changes, and are able to make them portable for transport outside of the home. They may be expected to be able to change modes or some settings if required. Although there is basic information and diagrams in their handbook, most of the teaching is done at the bedside by staff respiratory therapists and is also reviewed by the home care respiratory therapists and/or durable medical equipment suppliers. We also review mobility and traveling with the child and his/her equipment, and expect that caregivers will take advantage of the equipment's portability by taking their children on walks around the unit (and off the unit once they are signed-off on skills such as tracheostomy changes and cardiopulmonary resuscitation (CPR) in a child with tracheostomy) (Fig. 5).

Some children, whether ventilated or not, may require supplemental oxygen during part or all of their day. We teach caregivers about the different sources of supplemental oxygen (compressed, liquid, and from a concentrator) and how to enrich the oxygen concentration their children are receiving. Selection of sources of supplemental oxygen outside of the hospital will depend on the child's needs and are determined by the medical equipment supplier in collaboration with the child's medical staff. Factors will include the FiO_2 is required, the range of the child's minute ventilation, and portability needs. These factors will help decide what combination of enrichment, compressed gas and/or liquefied gas will best serve the patient's needs. It should be noted that for commercial air travel, a concentrator is the standard for oxygen delivery since this obviates the need to transport compressed gas cylinders. A home care respiratory therapist may select different oxygen systems to meet the physician's orders and the patient's clinical needs. The RT will select

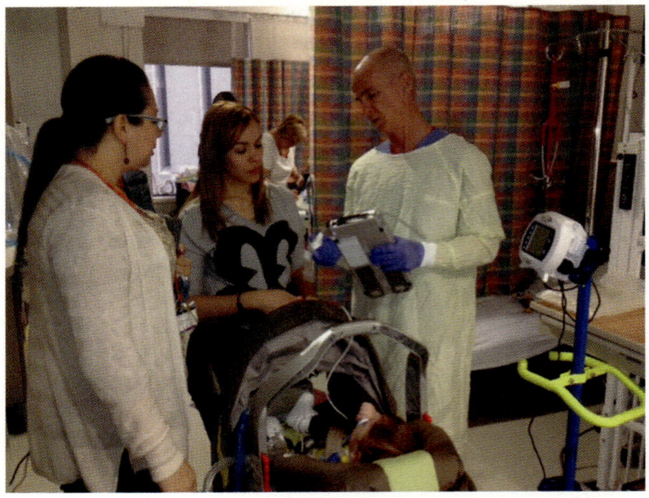

Fig. 5 A mother learns the skills needed to make her son "portable," or transitioned from crib to a stroller. This mother was from the Dominican Republic and spoke only Spanish, so an interpreter was provided for all of her training sessions

different oxygen systems dependent on FiO_2, flow and portability capabilities, and applications.

Supplemental oxygen can be delivered through the tracheostomy using an HME or a speaking valve, via the ventilator, via a transtracheal oxygen catheter, or transiently using a self-inflating bag system. Since oxygen in the home environment is a potential hazard in the home, families who take home children with tracheostomies are also taught principles of oxygen safety that must be observed, ranging from the obvious guidance of "no smoking" to the subtleties of placing oxygen supplies relative to home appliances, which may increase the risk of igniting flammable material (Table 4).

Bumps Along the Path: Learning to Put Skills Together

We teach caregivers the signs and symptoms of respiratory distress and how these might be signals of issues with the tracheostomy tube such as occlusion or displacement. The response to these situations may need to be individualized depending on how severely affected the child's natural airway is. For example, a child who has a tracheostomy for mechanical ventilation but has little obstruction in their natural airway may be able to be supported by mask ventilation through their nose and mouth, but if a child has severe subglottic stenosis or a surgical tracheal diversion, this type of support will not be an option. We teach parents about the natural history of a displaced tracheostomy tube, including the potential for the stoma to close and require a smaller emergency airway to be inserted before the child's standard airway can be reinserted. They also learn about the possibility that a false tract or passage may be encountered on attempts

Table 4 Our home care group's commandments for safe oxygen use

Oxygen safety guidelines
Oxygen must be handled with care. It makes things burn faster and ignite easier. Anything that sparks or catches fire will burn faster with oxygen present. As a Home Care patient, you must follow these safety guidelines to prevent a fire and/or injury to yourself or others
• A sign that says "Warning: No Smoking. No Open Flame. Oxygen in Use" must be posted on the front door or the door used as the entrance to your home. The signs will be provided by Children's Hospital Home Care
• Place a sign that says "Warning: No Smoking. No Open Flame. Oxygen in Use" in your home where you most often use or store oxygen
• DO NOT allow anyone to smoke, light a match or use a cigarette lighter in the home with oxygen in use
• If you or your child is using an oxygen tank while traveling in a car, DO NOT allow anyone to smoke in the car
• The rooms where oxygen is used and stored must be well ventilated
• Keep oxygen tanks at least 10 ft away from space heaters, radiators, gas stoves or other heat sources
• Keep oxygen tanks at least 3 ft away from electrical outlets
• DO NOT use electrical appliances such as electric razors or hair dryers while wearing oxygen
• DO NOT use open flames such as gas stoves, lit candles or lit fireplaces when oxygen is in use
• DO NOT store or use flammable products such as spray cans, nail polish remover, rubbing alcohol, paint thinners and other oil-based lubricants near oxygen
• DO NOT use any oily, greasy, petroleum-based products on your child or near your oxygen. They are highly flammable and can cause burns when oxygen is in use. Make sure to use NON-petroleum-based or water-based products
• Secure oxygen cylinders in stands
• Secure oxygen tubing to avoid tripping and falls
• If there is a fire near the oxygen, turn off the oxygen and carry the child to safety
• Turn off the oxygen when it is not being used
• Notify your fire department that you have oxygen in your home
• If possible, avoid using clothes or bedding made of wool, nylon or other materials that tend to build up static electricity. Try to use cotton materials to limit static electricity
• DO NOT store oxygen in closed vehicles or car trunks
• Liquid oxygen must be stored in a well ventilated area. Liquid oxygen stationary and portable units must be stored in the upright position
• Never touch liquid oxygen, if exposed. Its cold temperature can cause frostbite
• Always be sure to have a functioning back-up oxygen system

to reinsert the airway and that this needs to be recognized if it happens. To be fully prepared for emergencies, we teach caregivers about how to do and coordinate rescue breathing via a tracheostomy while delivering chest compressions when they do CPR.

We review several emergencies scenarios with caregivers-in-training ("*what would you do if your child….*"). At the conclusion of training, it is expected that caregivers successfully respond with trouble shooting activities when quizzed.

Our hospital also trains caregivers of children who are dependent on noninvasive ventilator technologies. We have been successful with this patient population in training caregivers for emergencies using high-fidelity simulation and scenarios, and hope to use this approach in the near future with caregivers of children that have tracheostomies. Our current limitation is that our mannequins do not accommodate a tracheostomy tube.

Other obstacles: Stormy weather…

Technology-dependent children are medically fragile and over the course of hospitalization, may become ill or may be deemed not "stable" enough for transfer home. Among the requirements we have to discharge a tracheostomy- or technology-dependent child home safely are that they are medically stable and their medical care is simplified so it can be safely provided in the home setting. Medical stability is important so that the family has a baseline against which to judge so that will have a way to evaluate when their child is ill and needs medical attention. "Simplifying" medical care may mean that the frequency of therapies such as nebulizer treatments or clearance therapies can be carried out by home care providers, the amount of supplemental oxygen required can delivered at home, or the ventilator settings are judged to be "safe" by the pulmonologist. There are also other practical considerations, such as the limits of pressures and volumes that can be provided by the home ventilator, and whether there is "wiggle room" to temporarily increase parameters in the setting of acute illness.

Some organizations, such as the American Association of Respiratory Care [4] and the American College of Chest Physicians [10] have guidelines for what characterizes a patient as "stable" and "safe" for home care, although there is certainly some subjectivity to these criteria. Some practitioners will deviate from these criteria, depending on the anticipated improvement in quality of life for patient and family that a discharge will bring as well as the comfort level of the medical, respiratory and nursing staff who will be managing care in the home setting. Another consideration, especially in this era, is what the goals of care will be and whether the move home is considered "palliative," where the overarching goal is comfort and maximizing the remaining quality of life.

Whatever the definition of medical stability and simplified care is, a general principle that our team tries to adhere to is not making changes in the care plan for a certain specified window of time prior to discharge. "Last minute" changes in care may make things confusing for the family, home care nursing and respiratory staff, medical equipment suppliers and outpatient pharmacy, and may lead to medical errors. More importantly, the stress of transport and changes in environment have the potential to cause the patient to be clinically different after he/she is discharged. A change in the medical care regimen too close to discharge may also cause a clinical change around the time of discharge, which can add to the confusion.

Caregivers must also have a complete understanding of their child's individualized emergency management plan. First is the environmental plan related to storms, power issues and fire plan; second is an equipment emergency management plan which is developed based on the patient's dependence on particular pieces of equipment; last is a clinical emergency plan based on clinical needs and physician's orders, such as titration instructions for supplemental oxygen in the case of hypoxemia.

Traveling Companions

Just as it takes a multidisciplinary team to get a technology-dependent child through an acute hospital stay, it takes another multidisciplinary team to streamline that child's care, train the family and make arrangements to get the child home.

We remind families that they are not alone in their journey home. Our hospital is fortunate to have helpful sherpas in our social work, case management staff and a home care department. Social work is an invaluable resource that can help families navigate through issues with insurance, applying for medical assistance if the insurance does not have benefits for private duty nursing or home equipment, and putting families in touch with programs in the community such as Early Intervention for development, Supplemental Security Income (SSI), Women, Infants, and Children (WIC) food and nutrition programs, and any other resources that may be available to help support families with tracheostomy and technology-dependent children. Social work can also help direct families how to:

- Notify utilities that their home will need priority for restoring services such as electricity to minimize the threat to their technology-dependent child.
- Contact their local emergency medical service providers to familiarize them ahead of time with their child's medical condition and special needs, and
- Apply for handicapped placards/license plates to decrease the burden of traveling with a child with assistance needs.

Our case managers are incredibly helpful to families in terms of assisting them to understand what their insurance benefits are and what the needs will be relative to staffing, equipment, transportation, medications, and clinical follow up. They also help families recognize what they should be thinking about and what questions to ask when choosing a home care company, durable medical equipment supplier and private duty nursing agency. They are the ringmasters who coordinate the hospital discharge process so that it goes as smoothly as possible.

There are other vital staff members who are travel companions with the family on their journey home. The bulk of teaching and evaluation is done by our nurses and respiratory therapists who, in addition to their clinical duties of patient care, are responsible for training families and caregivers, evaluating their performance, and giving them feedback and suggestions for improvement. Our home care colleagues also participate in discharge teaching, working collaboratively with inpatient clinicians on joint teaching responsibilities from the same scripts, materials and documentation tools (Fig. 6). They also touch on more complex elements such as emergency management, use of portable home care equipment, and traveling safely away from home.

Some of the medical equipment suppliers may also do focused training on pieces of equipment such as the pulse oximeter, suction machine, and ventilator.

Our child life staff addresses the emotional and developmental needs of our patients, making sure they are able to cope with the changes in their lives and that of their siblings as well (Fig. 7). Some also use modalities such as music and art therapies to help them cope with their hospital stay. In this way, they are able to help with coping by providing therapeutic activities for self-expression/emotional expression, developmentally appropriate education for patients and siblings, and providing procedural support to initiate a coping plan for things like tracheostomy care that can be used at home. If siblings need to be brought to the hospital so that a caregiver can be trained, a child life specialist can work with the siblings so they are comfortable with the concept of a technology-dependent brother or sister coming home. Volunteers, under the direction of a child life therapist, may also work with younger siblings to allow caregivers focus on training without the distraction of the other children.

Physical, occupational, and speech therapists not only tend to the rehabilitation and development needs of the patients, but also teach parents and caregivers skills they will need to help their children with his/her development and recovery. They also evaluate the children for specialized

The Children's Hospital of Philadelphia®

IPF-004/005
Rev. 10/10

LAST NAME FIRST NAME
MR# DOB

PLACE PATIENT LABEL HERE OR COMPLETE ABOVE

DO NOT HANDWRITE PATIENT INFORMATION HERE

3-Hole 1/4 4 1/4 c-to-c

INTERDISCIPLINARY PATIENT – FAMILY EDUCATION FLOWSHEET:
HOME MANAGEMENT OF A TRACHEOSTOMY

Page 1 of 6

Check identified learning needs under "Education Plan". Document each teaching session on the rows below. Use the numbers from the key to document in each column.

EDUCATION PLAN	PERSON(S) TAUGHT	BARRIERS/READINESS FOR LEARNING	DISCIPLINE COMPLETING TEACHING	TEACHING METHOD(S)	OUTCOME
☒ 1. Diagnosis	1. Patient	1. No limitations/barriers	1. Nursing	1. Written Info	1. Able to verbalize or demonstrate understanding of content. No review necessary.
☒ 2. Test/Procedure/Treatment	2. Mother	2. Fatigue/Pain/Anxiety	2. Physician	2. Verbal	2. Needs reinforcement. (explain in comments)
☐ 3. Pain Management	3. Father	3. Cultural	3. Social Work	3. Demonstration	3. Poor understanding. Repeat all. (explain in comments)
☒ 4. Nutrition/Diet	4. Family member (name)	4. Language	4. Respiratory care	4. Return Demonstration	4. Family involvement necessary
☒ 5. Medications/Food-Drug	5. Guardian (name)	5. Difficulty reading	5. Pharmacy	5. Videos	5. Unable to teach (explain in comments)
☐ 6. Community Resources	6. Other (name)	6. Cognitive/sensory	6. Nutrition	6. Family Learning Center Class	6. See Progress Notes for additional documentation
☐ 7. Rehab Techniques		7. Religious	7. Pastoral Care	7. Group Class	7. Group Class. Continue with individual education
☒ 8. Health Promotion/Safety		8. Physical	8. Rehab Therapies	8. Language Line/ Interpreter	
☒ 9. Medical Equipment		9. Unreceptive	9. Case Manager	9. Other (specify)	
☐ 10. Homecare		10. Unavailable	10. External agency		
☒ 11. Discharge Process		11. Group Class; identify barriers in individual sessions.	11. Child life		
☐ 12. Other _________		12. Other (specify)	12. Transplant Coordinator		
			13. Admission Coordinator		
			14. Home Care Liaison		
			15. Behavioral Health		
			16. Other (specify)		

Item from Education Plan	Date / Time	Person Taught	Barriers/ Readiness	Discipline/ Initials	Teaching Method	Outcome	Content Taught / Comments (Names of teaching materials used, name of interpreter, other concerns etc.)
(11) Discharge Process	/						PFE 38:B:01C
	/						
	/						
	/						
(1) Respiratory System and Lung Function	/						PFE 21:B:02
	/						
	/						
	/						
(1) Learner will understand need for tracheostomy	/						PFE 38:B:01 a/b
	/						

(Chart continued on other side)

Learner's Name / Relationship to Patient	Teacher's Initials / Signature	Teacher's Initials / Signature
____________ / ____________	_____ / ________________	_____ / ________________
	_____ / ________________	_____ / ________________
	_____ / ________________	_____ / ________________

Fig. 6 Form used to track progress of parents and caregivers as they journey over the training "mountain." A sheet is maintained for each individual learner. Results are summarized on the checklist in Fig. 1

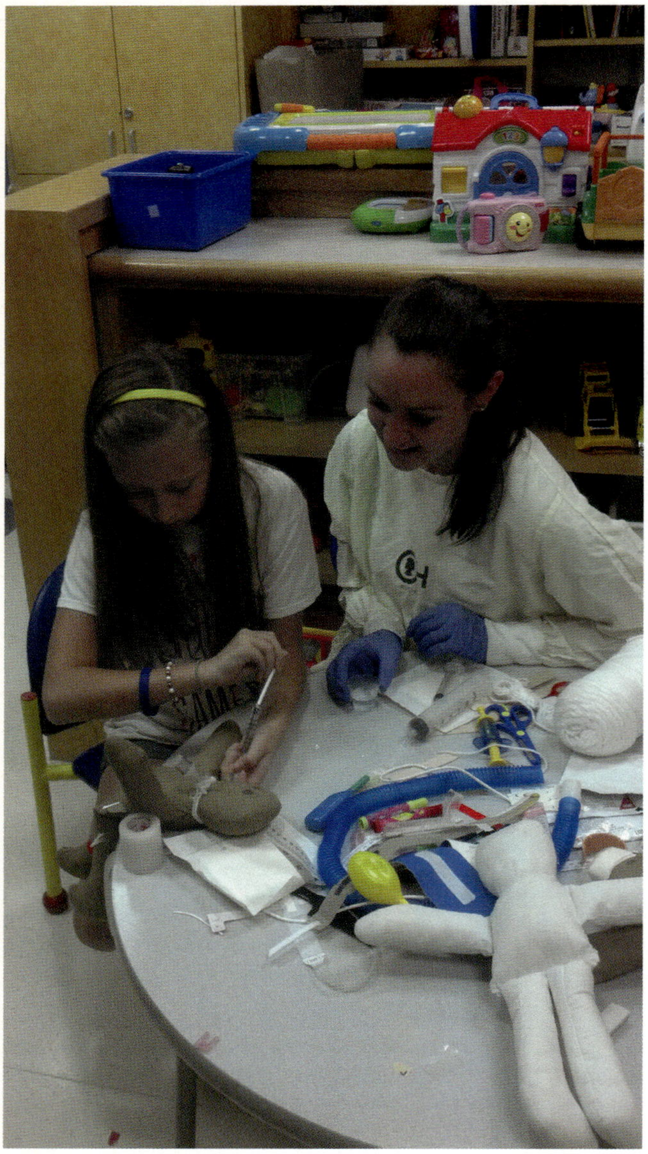

Fig. 7 A child life specialist does an activity with the younger sister of a technology-dependent patient to help her cope with his tracheostomy

equipment that may be required to help with the activities of daily living, assist with completing the necessary prescriptions and letters of medical necessity, and teach parents and caregivers how to use the equipment.

To provide the best assistance to the family along their way, representatives from all disciplines meet weekly to get a medical update on each patient and discuss the progress their families are making, helping us coordinate our efforts.

> It is good to have an end to journey toward; but it is the journey that matters, in the end. —Ernest Hemingway.

Although families go through the tracheostomy journey with the goal of getting home, another journey immediately starts when they get home. It takes a village to support a tracheostomy dependent child in the community. The family will need support services at home, which include private duty nursing services, home respiratory therapy, and a durable medical equipment (DME) supplier as well as coordination with medical specialists, developmental specialists and a pediatrician who is comfortable with a technology-dependent child.

Ideally private duty shift nurses will work collaboratively with the inpatient team and home respiratory therapists prior to and post-discharge to develop a care plan around physician orders. Private duty nursing can be invaluable in helping the family care for a child with a tracheostomy, especially if the child is ventilator dependent. A child with a tracheostomy needs constant supervision, particularly since the monitors available in the home are limited and may not alert the care provider in a timely fashion. Shift nursing gives the family a break from care responsibilities to do their other activities of daily living such as working and caring for siblings. However, when we train families to take children with tracheostomies home, our goal is to make them experts in their child's care because they will have to cover missed nursing shifts and also help acquaint nursing staff with their child's care, as the experience level and skill set of private duty nursing can be variable. There are specific skill sets required for nurses to help care for this population of high risk patients [9]. The selection of a private duty nursing company is determined by the family subject to limitations of their insurance and availability of staff in the area where they live. The parents or caregivers interview agency staff while the child is still a patient in the hospital. Sometimes the duties may need to be shared amongst more than one agency.

Inevitably, children with tracheostomies will have specialized equipment needs in the home. A Durable Medical Equipment (DME) supplier will contact the family ahead of time to make sure that equipment will be available in the home by the time of discharge. Staff from these companies visit the family's home ahead of time to perform safety assessments that address fire safety, fall prevention, and environmental and electrical needs (Fig. 8). It is imperative that the house be evaluated for proper wiring, outlets and current to power any needed equipment. In some cases, the local electric company will need to increase amperage to the home. The safety assessment also checks that there is a functional smoke detector and working telephone, that the home's layout will accommodate any assistive equipment such as wheelchairs and that there are <u>not</u> any issues with pests or pets that need to be mitigated. DME staff may also help the family to deal with the potential need to rearrange the home. The technology-dependent child will have new needs in terms of increased electrical capacity for devices, space for equipment and a place for a home care nurse to work. Frequently the child will have a "day" area where he/she will spend time during the day in addition to his/her own bedroom. Families will have to find places to store the new

CHHC Rev: v4 8/2009 | **Home Safety Assessment** | Page 1 of 1

Home Safety Assessment			
Dwelling is: ☐ House ☐ Apartment ☐ Other: ______________________		List Number of Floors in Dwelling: ______________________	
Emergency preparedness plan reviewed	☐ yes	Telephone available	☐ yes ☐ no
		Enter Phone Number	
Fall risk assessment completed	☐ yes ☐ no	911 Available	☐ yes ☐ no
		List Name of Local Hospital	

O_2 Safety	☐ N/A	Environmental Requirements	
CHHC Oxygen guidelines reviewed	☐ yes ☐ no	Adequate access to HME	☐ yes ☐ no ☐ n/a
No smoking sign posted	☐ yes ☐ no	Door size adequate for HME	☐ yes ☐ no ☐ n/a
O_2 3 ft from electrical outlets	☐ yes ☐ no	Infestation of bugs or rodents absent	☐ yes ☐ no
O_2 10 ft from heat source	☐ yes ☐ no	Obstacles to safe use of HME absent	☐ yes ☐ no ☐ n/a
Spare tank location identified	☐ yes ☐ no	Obstacles to safe mobility absent	☐ yes ☐ no
Storage is appropriate	☐ yes ☐ no	Refrigerator/freezer operational	☐ yes ☐ no
Electrical Requirements		Clean and adequate water supply	☐ yes ☐ no
Electricity supplied to home	☐ yes ☐ no	Heat and/ or Cooling adequate in home	☐ yes ☐ no
Electrical outlets grounded	☐ yes ☐ no ☐ n/a	Environment suitable for home care and/or HME	☐ yes ☐ no
Appropriate extension cords in use on HME	☐ yes ☐ no ☐ n/a	Pets (type):	☐ yes ☐ no
Amperage adequate for HME	☐ yes ☐ no ☐ n/a	Appropriate storage & disposal of medical supplies and sharps	☐ yes ☐ no ☐ n/a

Fire Response/Safety			
Emergency exit procedure reviewed	☐ yes	Fire extinguishers present	☐ yes ☐ no
Smoke detectors present	☐ yes ☐ no	Fire extinguishers functional	☐ yes ☐ no
Smoke detectors functional	☐ yes ☐ no	Fire extinguishers checked in the past 30 days	☐ yes ☐ no
		Family encouraged to purchase fire extinguishers and where they can be purchased.	☐ yes ☐ no
Smoke detector checked in the past 30 days	☐ yes ☐ no	CO Monitor present	☐ yes ☐ no
Family encouraged to purchase a smoke detector and where it can be purchased	☐ yes ☐ no	CO Monitor functional	☐ yes ☐ no
All medical equipment checked for its fire safety	☐ yes ☐ no	CO Monitor checked in the past 30 days	☐ yes ☐ no
Concerns		Family encouraged to purchase a CO monitor and where it can be purchased.	☐ yes ☐ no

Patient/Caregiver informed of all potential hazards identified in the Home Safety Assessment.
☐ yes ☐ no ☐ n/a

Recommendation:

Patient/Caregiver confirms understanding of safety concerns and recommendations to improve patient safety.
☐ yes ☐ no – clinician notified of concerns ☐ n/a

Plan/Follow-Up actions:

CHHC Signature:	**Patient Name:**
Date:	**Date of Birth:**
	Medical Record Number:

Fig. 8 Safety checklist use by our home care company to do home inspections

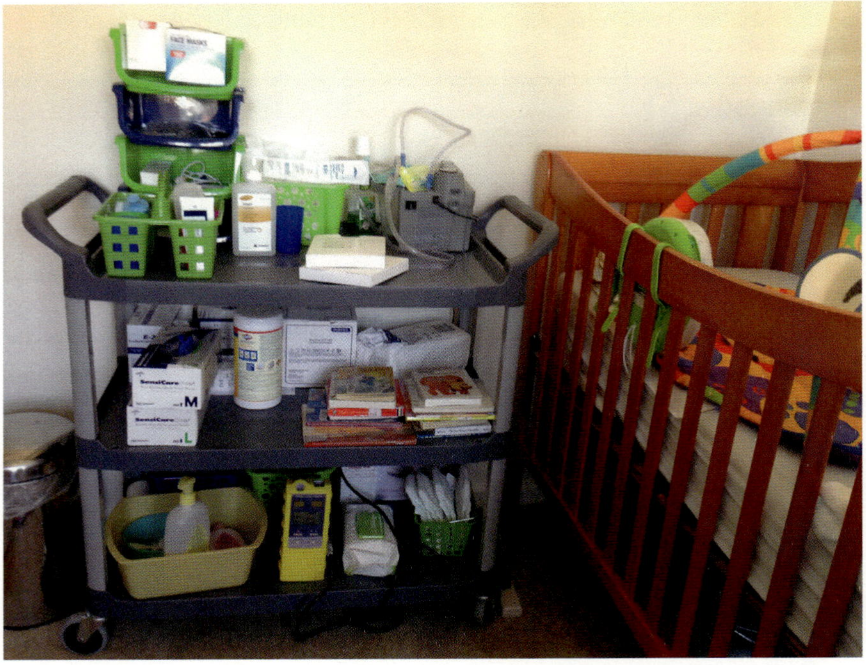

Fig. 9 Home bedside cart and crib setup

equipment they will be using to take care of their child as well as other supplies they will need to keep their medically fragile child's living area clean (hand sanitizer, bleach wipes) and other cleaning supplies (which can include vinegar, peroxide, sterile/boiled water, bleach or isopropyl alcohol), which they will use to clean equipment. DMEs can also give families strategies to keep equipment and supplies organized, using readily available items like stacking bins, shoe racks, and rolling carts (Fig. 9).

In the week prior to discharge, the DME company prepares the home for the child's return. As part of this preparation, a home care respiratory therapist works with the family and shift nurses to identify a safe and convenient location to outfit a room for the child. The goal is to find space that best meets the family's life style and the patient's clinical needs, and makes ergonomic sense for caregivers. At this time, the respiratory therapist also rechecks the home's electrical capacity and/or enhancements made by the electric company as follow-up to the initial electrical inspection. This confirms that the home has enough amperage to power all required equipment.

Just before the child is discharged, the DME company delivers the prescribed medical equipment to the home. Equipment generally includes:

- Back-up ventilator (primary home ventilator is delivered to the patient at the hospital)
- Capnometer
- Pulse oximeter
- Two Heaters/Humidifiers
- Two Suction machines
- Two Oxygen tanks: (Oxygen back-up is a safety requirement per Joint Commission regulations)
- Enteral feeding pump (if needed)

Also before discharge, the home care team holds a case conference with shift nurses, home respiratory therapy and the entire home care team to review patient's care, orders and needs. Then in conjunction with the family, the home care RT reviews discharge orders for completeness, assembles the equipment and sets up the environment. To promote smooth workflow and convenient care, rolling carts and power strips organize equipment and related supplies. The RT checks that all the required equipment functions properly, alarms are audible and oxygen is placed at safe distances from electrical outlets and heat sources.

The End of a Journey...and the Beginning of Another

Also preceding discharge, a home care RT who has been communicating with the family and inpatient healthcare team, and joint teaching with inpatient RTs for nearly two months, formally participates in the final inpatient interdisciplinary discharge team meeting. He/she also makes one last inpatient visit with the family to perform medication reconciliation, and discuss patient/family rights and responsibilities related to home care. At this final inpatient meeting, the caregiver signs consent for home care treatment and together with the home care RT, shift nurse and physician reviews the medication profile, final physician orders, and the *go-bag*, and also develops a home care plan. Once home, the family will have access to a 24-h on-call system for contacting their home care company and/or DME company about clinical and equipment issues. Families that are Pennsylvania residents will also be referred to the Pennsylvania Ventilator Assisted Children's Home Program (VACHP), a program funded by the Pennsylvania Department of Health for over 30 years, which provides consultation and support.

Hospital discharge is an exciting as well as intense time. For the initial discharge to home, the child is almost always transported home by a transport team, generally accompanied by a parent/caregiver. Once at the home, the transport team relays pertinent patient information to the home care RT, home care nurse and private duty shift nurses. The home team reviews medical orders, performs in-home medication reconciliation together and jointly creates/reviews a care plan. Now, this home care team begins to work as a unit just as the inpatient interdisciplinary team worked. Home care personnel will perform ongoing intermittent assessments and teaching at specified intervals. Follow-up plans and visit intervals are based on patient acuity and protocols but our home care department makes daily visits for the first week post-hospitalization. Private duty agency nurses will tend to the child 16–24 h each day. Open and ongoing bidirectional communication with physicians, the home care company and shift nursing is essential for a safe and successful transition to home.

The Journey Continues…

Acute awareness of psychosocial stressors may prompt a social worker referral. Research outlines several principle stressors that these families face. There may be feelings of fear, frustration, fatigue and depression [11] along with issues resulting from the family's complex roles of caregiver, advocate, activist, educator and case manager [8]. Social workers from inpatient units, outpatient clinics, and/or home care agencies support families by helping them achieve a sense of hope and accomplishment.

Costs to care for such technology-dependent children can be a financial burden for many families. Most care for these children is covered by insurance. Patients are generally covered all or in part by their state's Medical Assistance program that covers chronic illnesses. In some regions of the country, there is reluctance for insurors to pay for redundant equipment that may be life-saving, such as a back-up ventilator. Also, associated hidden costs may include:

- Lost wages of mother or father
- Out of pocket expenses for non-reimbursable items
- Co-pays, when only 80 % of fees (and frequently even less) are covered by insurance
- Cost of skilled nursing care

But So Does the Support…

There are many ancillary issues that may be inadvertently overlooked because of overwhelming attention to a medically complex child's basic physiologic needs and safety. These include:

- Support groups for parents to address their mental health needs
- Assistance with respite care and funds
- Advocacy for services and funding to meet the healthcare, developmental and basic social needs of the ventilator-dependent child

Outpatient social workers in primary care or specialty care clinic or social workers in the VACHP can help assist families to access these resources.

There are also agencies to help families make physical accommodations to their homes that will improve accessibility for their ventilator-dependent child. Some are non-profit organizations, many of which have been established by parents of technology-dependent or special needs children. Others are church-based groups.

Although insurance companies will provide case managers to help families manage care in the outpatient setting, most of those managers are unfamiliar with the needs of a technology-dependent child.

Our hospital is fortunate enough to have a home care department that provides not only DME services but also some nursing, pharmacy, nutrition, social work, and other supports as well. The home care team is able work closely with the private duty nursing agency as well as the physicians and specialists who provide follow-up care for the child. Because they are tightly integrated in our healthcare network, they are able work on initiatives to improve care, such as follow-up of hospitalizations and readmissions. When home ventilator program patients become hospitalized, the home care department looks to evaluate and identify the reason for admission, trying to determine if the patient has a lower respiratory tract infection (LRTI) or ventilator associated pneumonia (VAP) that could have been prevented. (This home care company uses its VAP rate as a quality indicator.)

For all patients with VAPs or repeated admissions for other LRTIs, respiratory therapists investigate and make additional home visits to identify the source of infection. As part of infection surveillance activities, he/she may investigate the family's technique for changing circuits, managing humidification, suctioning, hand hygiene or exposures to illnesses. This is always followed by additional education or reinforcement of techniques for performing specific tasks.

Each year with feedback from patients, caregivers and community partners, our home care department works to enhance its program. Early enhancements have been related to organizing communication and educational responsibilities between inpatient and home care respiratory therapists. One of the more recent and very successful enhancements has been an outreach effort. The home care department has created a program to educate private duty shift nursing agencies about shared patients. Local home health nurses are invited to the home care facility, where home care respiratory therapists create simulation experiences that mimic the home environment of a ventilator-dependent child. Two things occur during sessions. The first is that the shift nurses become acquainted with the technology and equipment associated with a specific patient. The second is that the home care respiratory therapy management reviews patient-specific scenarios so that the in-home care team will be prepared for specific events such as desaturation episodes, bradycardia, or abdominal distension after feeding. In this manner, our home care RTs create care paths/algorithms targeted to a specific patient and educate shift nurses about managing unexpected events.

The home care department is continually re-evaluating and enhancing its Home Ventilator Program to provide the safest and most comprehensive up-to-date services. Some additional activities that are being developed include incorporation of high-fidelity simulation training for families and home care health providers, establishing outcomes measures to formally evaluate the effectiveness of home care's services, and a formal survey directed towards the technology-dependent patient population with focus on quality of life, satisfaction with existing services, ideas for additional services and areas for improvement. In addition, the home care department has begun piloting protocol-driven weaning orders that allow an increase in weaning trials based on a patient's clinical status (e.g., change in vital signs, weight gain velocity, tolerance of therapies).

Reflecting on the Journey

To limit burden of care and improve family satisfaction and quality of life, a home ventilator management program must focus on: [7]

1. Safe home environment
2. Early planning for discharge
3. Understanding insurance rules
4. Simplifying care plans
5. Allowing for adequate training time
6. Promoting effective communication and hand-offs
7. Organizing and coordinating follow-up
8. Recommending parent-to-parent support groups
9. Partnership all around

We have been privileged to help shepherd families with infants and children with tracheostomies on their journey home for over 30 years. Our program continues to evolve, but its success stems from three elements: standardization of fundamental components, orchestrated communication, and interdisciplinary collaboration between and among inpatient staff and the home care department, and commitment from personnel.

We strive to provide the same comprehensive program and the same quality care to every patient, every time.

Closed loop communication and complete hand-offs between hospital and home care staff are critical factors to success. Because there are so many players that support discharge of the technology-dependent child, it is essential that all involved remain in the communication loop. This is accomplished through hospital rounds, regular interdisciplinary team meetings at the hospital prior to discharge, inpatient and home care department interdisciplinary care plans, clinical notes in a common electronic medical record accessible by both inpatient and home care personnel, common teaching plans and documentation of competencies, and ongoing phone interactions from the hospital to home care, skilled nursing services agency and the family.

Finally our staff's commitment to problem solving and pursuing the best for each child and family is remarkable, and has contributed to the program's continuous quality improvement.

Our experience has shown that it is medically possible, and in most circumstances socially, emotionally, and financially beneficial, to move the ventilator-dependent child out of the acute-care setting to home. Over the past 30 years, the staff of many children's hospitals have learned how best to support this experience, and have developed a best practice for the community that sets the standard of care. Whether the child goes home or to a transitional facility, the goal is to see that each infant and child progresses as far as their potential will allow (Fig. 10).

> Never measure the height of a mountain until you have reached the top. Then you will see how low it was. —Dag Hammarskjold.

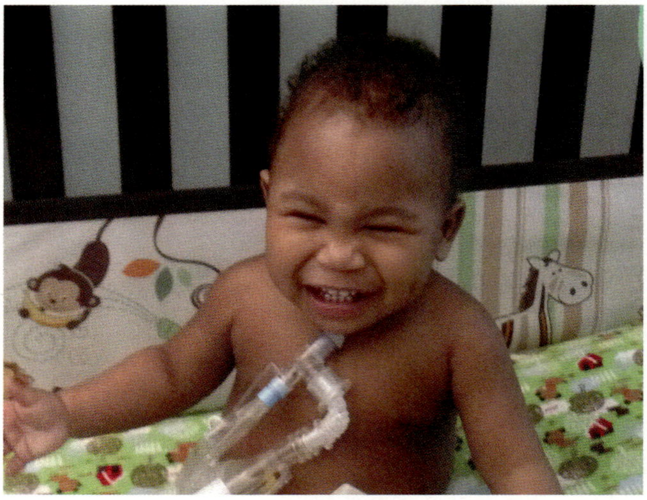

Fig. 10 Another child happy that his family made the journey home…

Bibliography

1. Sherman JM, Davis S, Albamonte-Petrick S, Chatburn RL, Fitton C, Green C, Johnston J, Lyrene RK, Myer C, Othersen HB, Wood R, Zach M, Zander J, Zinman R. American Thoracic Society—care of the child with a chronic tracheostomy. Am J Respir Crit Care Med. 2000;161(1):297–308.
2. Fiske E. Effective strategies to prepare infants and families in home tracheostomy care. Adv Neonatal Care. 2004;4(1):42–53.
3. Simonds AK. Ethical aspects of home long term ventilation in children with neuromuscular disease. Paediatr Respir Rev. 2005;6:209–14.
4. AARC. Clinical practice guideline. Long-term invasive mechanical ventilation in the home—2007 revision and update. Respir Care. 2007;52(1):1056–62.
5. Jackson Allen P, Vessey JA. Primary care of the child with a chronic condition. St. Louis: Mosby; 2004.
6. Noyes J, Lewis M. Care pathway for the discharge and support of children requiring long term ventilation in the community: National Service Framework for Children, Young People, and Maternity Services. UK Department of Health and Barnados, 2005.
7. Lewarski JS, Gay PC. Current issues in home mechanical ventilation. Chest. 2007;132(2):671–6.
8. Boroughs DS, Dougherty J. A multidisciplinary approach to the care of the ventilator-dependent child at home: A case study. Home Healthc Nurse. 2010;28(1):24–8.
9. Boroughs DS, Dougherty J. Decreasing accidental mortality of ventilator-dependent children at home—a call to action. Home Healthc Nurse. 2012;30(2):103–11.
10. O'Donahue WJ, Giovanni RM, Goldberg AI, et al. Long term mechanical ventilation–guidelines for management in the home and at alternate community sites. Chest. 1986;90(1):1–37S.
11. Carnevale FA, Alexander E, Davis M, Rennick J, Troini R. Daily Living With Distress and Enrichment: The Moral Experience of Families With Ventilator-Assisted Children at Home Pediatrics. 2006;117(1):e48–60.
12. Mitchell RB, Hussey HM, Setzgen G, et al. Clinical consensus statement: tracheostomy care. Otolaryngol Head Neck Surg. 2013;148(1):6–20.
13. American Association of Respiratory Care. AARC clinical practice guideline: long-term invasive mechanical ventilation in the home—2007 revision and update. Respir Care. 2007;52:1056–62. www.aarc.org. Accessed 8 Dec 2011.
14. American College of Chest Physicians. Home Mechanical Ventilation Resource Center. 2011. http://www.chestnet.org/accp/article/home-mechanicalventilation-resource-center. Accessed 8 Dec 2011.
15. American College of Chest Physicians. (Patient education guides) Mechanical ventilation: beyond the ICU. 1999. http://www.chestnet.org/accp/patientguides/mechanicalventilation-beyond-icu. Accessed 8 Dec 2011.
16. Amin RS, Fitton CM. Tracheostomy and home ventilation in children. Semin Neonatol. 2003;8(2):127–35. From abstract accessed via EBSCOhost on 22 Apr 2011.
17. Boroughs D. A multidisciplinary approach to the care of the ventilator-dependent child at home: a case study. Home Healthc Nurse. 2010;28(1):24–8.
18. Department of Health and Human Services, Centers for Medicaid and Medicare Services. Durable Medical Equipment, Prosthetics, Orthotics, Supplies (DMEPOS) Quality Standards, Medicare Learning Network. 2011. https://www.cms.gov/MLNProducts/downloads/DMEPOS_Qual_Stand_Booklet_ICN905709.pdf. Accessed 1 Mar 2012.
19. Franco A, Carnevale F, Alexander E, Davis M, Rennick J, Troini R. Daily living with distress and enrichment: the moral experience of families with ventilator-assisted children at home. Pediatrics. 2006;117(1, Suppl):e48–60.
20. Graham R, Fleegler W, Robinson W. Chronic ventilator need in the community: a 2005 pediatric census of Massachusetts. Pediatrics. 2007;119(6):e1280–8. Originally published online 7 May 2007.
21. Hickey EM, Miske LJ, Debrest CL, Markov ML, Chiappa JR. An 8-week protocol decreases time for initial discharge to home of pediatric patient dependent on mechanical ventilation. J Pediatr Nurs. 2006;21(2):129–30.
22. Kopacz MA, Moriarty-Wright R. Multidisciplinary approach for the patient on a home ventilator. Heart Lung. 1984;13(3):255–62. Abstract from EBSCOhost accessed from Medline database on 22 Apr 2011.
23. Lehoux P. Patients' perspectives on high-tech home care: a qualitative inquiry into the userfriendliness of four technologies. BMC Health Serv Res. 2004;4(28):1–9.
24. Lewarski J, Gay P. Current issues in home mechanical ventilation. Chest. 2007;132(2):671–6.
25. Noyes J. Comparison of ventilator-dependent child reports of health-related quality of life with parent reports and normative populations. J Adv Nurs. 2007;58:1–10. doi:10.1111/j.1365-2648.2006.04191.x.
26. Ottonello G, Farrari I, Pirroddi I, Diana M, Villa G, Nahum L, Tuo R, Moscatelli A, Silvestri G. Home mechanical ventilation in children: retrospective survey of a pediatric population. Pediatr Int. 2007;49:801–5.
27. Reiter K, Pernath N, Pagel P, Heidi S, Hoffman F, Schoen C, Nicolai T. Risk factors for morbidity and mortality in pediatric home mechanical ventilation. Clin Pediatr 2011;50(3):237–43. Published online by SAGE Journals On-Line, 2 Dec 2010.
28. Tamasitis J, Shesser L. A hospital-to-home program for ventilator-dependent children sets the standard of care. AARC Times. 2012;36(10):44–52.
29. Tearl D, Cox T, Hartzog J. Hospital discharge of respiratory-technology-dependent children: role of a dedicated respiratory discharge coordinator. Respir Care. 2006;51(7):744–9.
30. Tibballs J, Henning R, Robertson CF, Massie J, Hochmann M, Carter B, Osborne A, Stephens RA, Jones SE, White J, Bryan D. A home respiratory support programme for children by parents and layperson carers. J Paediatr Child Health. 2010;46(1–2):57–62.

Creating an Effective Quality Improvement (QI) Process for Airway Emergencies

John Chuo, J. Thomas Paliga, and Janet Lioy

Overview

Airway emergencies are life-threatening situations that have little tolerance for errors and require immediate responses by qualified surgeons, neonatologists, and support staff. Therefore to ensure patients do not suffer harm from airway emergencies, an airway safety program must not only have rapid and effective response processes that are reliable, but also processes that can identify and mitigate high risk situations. Principles of high reliability organizations (HRO), which include sensitivity to operations, preoccupation with failure, deference to expertise, resilience, and reluctance to simplify [1], are applied to drive a higher state of mindfulness. The goal is to cultivate a workplace culture where all providers become stakeholders and engaged in HRO practices, and eliminate unnecessary variations in healthcare delivery that can lead to miscommunication and suboptimal care. By making practice more consistent amongst providers wherever possible, we are able to better practices for better outcomes. Numerous quality improvement collaboratives have embarked on such efforts and have contributed significantly to understanding factors that affect success [2–5].

J. Chuo, M.D., M.S.
Division of Neonatology, The Children's Hospital of Philadelphia, The Perelman School of Medicine at the University of Pennsylvania, Philadelphia, PA, USA
e-mail: LIOY@email.chop.edu

J.T. Paliga
Division of Plastic Surgery, Department of Surgery, The Children's Hospital of Philadelphia, Philadelphia, PA, USA

Duke University School of Medicine, Durham, NC, USA

J. Lioy (✉)
Attending Neonatologist, Director Neonatal Outreach, Medical Director, Neonatal Airway Program, The Children's Hospital of Philadelphia, Associate Professor of Clinical Pediatrics, The University of Pennsylvania Perelman School of Medicine, Philadelphia, PA, USA
e-mail: LIOY@email.chop.edu

Literature review on system design models that supports quality improvement and patient safety [6–8] appears to illustrate a common theme: such systems are built to accomplish certain goals by synergizing people, process, and tools. Below is an example of an airway safety program that targets improving airway emergency response, perioperative handoff, and bedside airway management. To support this program, a system was built to operationalize functions that drive vigilance, improvement, and safety such as (1) engage frontline in its purpose; communicate effectively amongst stakeholders, and judicious use and feedback of actionable data. Figure 1 is a worksheet that describes such a system, where the people, process, and tools that support each function is detailed.

For the program to succeed, those taking care of the patients must believe in the program's mission and support the methods of its execution. Establishing a decision-making team of six to eight members that represents the gamut of provider types is recommended. This team can reach out to a larger frontline provider group through focus groups and brainstorming sessions [9].

Providing effective avenues for stakeholders to communicate with one another is critical [10]. For example, how will a neonatologist caring for the patient know what the surgeon's concerns are in the postoperative period? How will the overnight nurse inform the morning medical team that they had issues with the airway's security? How will the team ensure that important information on the patient is passed off accurately and completely from shift to shift? From a patient handoff standpoint, the most effective communication mode is live, person-to-person while the least effective is a written note. The choice of using live (in person, phone call, video conferencing) and non-live (email, text messaging) methods depend on (1) the information to be communicated, (2) urgency, (3) whether a response is required and how quickly, (4) number of people/disciplines involved, and (5) whether the team can overcome competing processes that prevent live communication. Periodic monitoring of how well the team is communicating is critical because the contextual environment is not static and

J. Lioy and S.E. Sobol (eds.), *Disorders of the Neonatal Airway: Fundamentals for Practice*, DOI 10.1007/978-1-4939-1610-8_32, © Springer Science+Business Media New York 2015

		Functions		
		Engage frontline	Communicate effectively	Manage actionable data
System	People	Neonatologist and ENT attendings, Fellows, and Nurse practitioners, bedside nurses	Neonatologist and ENT attendings, Fellows, and Nurse practitioners, bedside nurses	Fellows, Neonatologist
	Process	Ask frontline what they think is important in airway safety	Perioperative communication workflow, weekly airway round process	Airway safety log sheet to be filled out during airway rounds, existing process for data acquisition, analytics, and reporting
	Tools	One to one communication	Email, text, phone calls	Paper data entry forms used on rounds and periop handoffs

Fig. 1 Organizational system chart showing components of a successful airway safety program. People, process, and tools make up the system

frequently can introduce process changes that impact communication. For example, if the surgeons are doing more cases, they may be more absent in postoperative handoffs. If the N/IICU adds more beds and expand location, the emergency airway response process will likely need to accommodate the geographical challenges. As the patient census grows and the unit becomes busier, safety rounds may need to happen more frequently and require more leaders to participate (Fig. 1).

Identifying actionable, meaningful data directly related to the active improvement efforts is critical. Allowing important (but extraneous to the effort) metrics to "scope creep" into the monitoring process is discouraged. Regular review of all emergency airway calls can reveal insights into system vulnerabilities often missed with surveys and questionnaires. Furthermore, data must be collected in a manner that is capable of reflecting whether improvements in processes ensure safety. Importantly, monitoring outcome and process metrics at frequent intervals over a wider range of scenarios is more useful that collecting numerous amount of data in one scenario.

Supporting the above operations systems, we describe an airway safety program, centered on airway emergency response protocol, effective perioperative communications, and weekly multidisciplinary rounds.

Improving Airway Emergency Response

Safety and efficacy in response to airway emergencies are critical to the success of any airway program. As such, quality improvement relies heavily on the ability to identify the deficiencies in safety and efficacy of emergency responses. Upon activation of an advanced airway response, the respiratory therapist brings a critical airway emergency cart containing a flexible fiber optic bronchoscope, a video laryngoscope, and other emergency anesthesia and surgical airway equipment to the bedside. At the end of the event, the respiratory therapist completes a questionnaire documenting the type of airway, nature of emergency, time to response, interdisciplinary communication, use of emergency airway equipment including the use of flexible bronchoscope and the final disposition (Fig. 2).

To provide an example of the application of these initiatives, in-house data collected since the beginning of the Children's Hospital of Philadelphia QI program was reviewed retrospectively. Airway emergency response was activated more than 120 times since the start of the program. The average response time was 5.5 min (±3.1 min); critical airway emergency cart was at the bedside 100 % of the times. Otolaryngologists identified themselves to the other caregivers > 85 % of the times. Interdisciplinary communication between the otolaryngologist and neonatologist was noted in >92 % of all instances. Flexible laryngoscope was used in 78 % of all instances. 2.8 mm laryngoscope was used in 60 % of cases, whereas 2.2 mm laryngoscope was used in 40 % of cases. Majority of the airway emergencies (>97 %) were resolved by repeat tracheal intubation (>98 %) via use of either Miller laryngoscope (>60 %) or Benjamin laryngoscope (<35 %). Most (98 %) of airway emergencies were resolved in the N/IICU, whereas <2 % were resolved in the operating room. A multidisciplinary airway emergency response program can improve the quality of care in a cost-

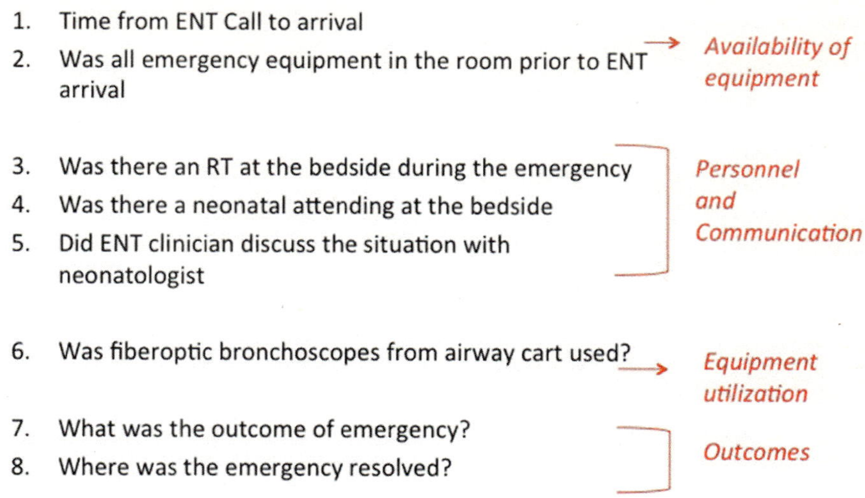

Fig. 2 Emergency airway tracking sheet to be used as a tool to gather information at each airway emergency and create QI metrics for improvement. (Courtesy of Neonatal Airway Program, The Children's Hospital of Philadelphia)

effective manner by improving both the response time, time to tracheostomy, duration of procedure and post-procedural intensive care unit stay.

Improving Perioperative Communications

Poor perioperative communication affects medical decision-making, patient safety, and productivity and invariably leads to surgical delays, patient inconvenience and, sometimes, serious errors. Recent specialization of otorhinolaryngology surgical care in neonates and a growing number of tracheostomies and bronchoscopies performed potentiate an increased risk of experiencing serious errors in perioperative communications. Inadequate handoffs between attending physicians continue to be a problem as growth of staff and patient beds outpace the existing infrastructure.

To identify the deficiencies in perioperative communication during neonatal ENT surgeries and in the large Children's Hospital of Philadelphia N/IICU, two separate initiatives were enacted. The first includes weekly "Airway Rounds" with ENT and neonatology to identify patients. The second involves use of a "Tracking Sheet" for perioperative communication during every procedure and documentation of pre- and post-care communication between ENT and neonatology practitioners. Cell phones and email between all physicians were used as the primary mode of communication. A daily "ENT patient list" was sent out each morning to identify the neonatal patients a "tracking sheet" was completed prior to every procedure documenting all communication, what was learned, and would have been missed without this communication. The construction of a swim lane algorithm was then applied. A 14-question online survey examining many aspects of perioperative communications was sent out to all ENT and neonatology faculty. Responses were received from 100 % of ENT surgeons and 85 % of neonatologists. The following critical information was gained from perioperative communication: unexpected findings on bronchoscopy, unexpected change in size and type of tracheostomy, confirmed genetic diagnosis, need for cardiac anesthesia, critical family issues and resuscitation wishes, and changed date or cancellation of procedure. The data acquired from the physician survey suggested positive benefits with communication, awareness, and collaboration that are achievable and sustainable when all stakeholders share the same goal (Fig. 3).

Airway Safety Rounds

The authors' institution has an extensive neonatal airway program with more than 3,000 consult days per year. There is an active tracheostomy program with upwards of 50 tracheostomies performed annually under 1 year of age. Most of these infants receive their preoperative and postoperative care in the N/IICU or CICU. Notable repeated anecdotal reports of serious errors such as tracheostomy care orders, improper size tracheostomy tube size and cuff volumes recorded in the EMR, led to several "Near Miss Safety Events." As a response to this, weekly airway safety rounds were initiated, which complemented the hospital-wide initiative of patient safety. Airway rounds involved multidisciplinary bedside rounds once a week with a neonatologist, an ENT fellow or advanced practice nurse, a respiratory therapist, and bedside nursing. The team kept a document for each patient and checked for accuracy of orders regarding the proper tracheostomy size, cuff status, cuff volumes, and

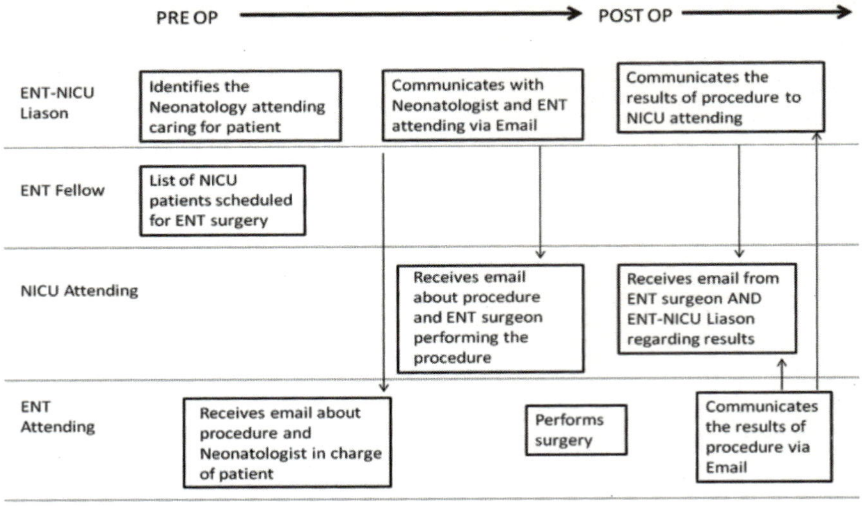

Fig. 3 Flow diagram: perioperative communication map deemed necessary before and after airway procedures to insure effective peer-to-peer communication

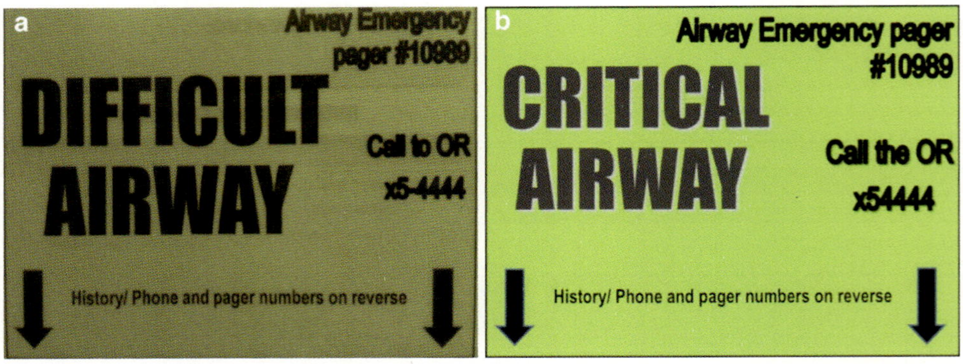

Fig. 4 (**a**, **b**) Difficult; critical airway label cards—kept at the bedside providing visual recognition of infants with specific airway problems. (Courtesy of Neonatal Airway Program, The Children's Hospital of Philadelphia)

presence of emergency replacement tracheostomy tube at the bedside. Lastly, patients were identified as either *DIFFICULT* or *CRITICAL* airways and labeled at the bedside as such (Fig. 4).

The following metrics were organized into a process and outcome metric chart used to assess the effectiveness of the airway safety program QI process (Fig. 5):

Consistent improvement in the outcome metrics was noted over an entire 1-year period following initiation of the airway safety rounds. Substantial improvement showing bedside nursing and respiratory therapist awareness for their patient's tracheostomy tube size and cuff volume improved to well over 95 % of instances. Most importantly substantial improvements in all bedside emergency back up tracheostomy equipment being correct and matching the patient was present in 100 % of instances. Unfortunately, the information on the bedside card regarding the size of the tracheostomy tube, cuff status and cuff volume did not match the orders or documentation in the EMR in over 50 % of the cases. This was found to be the most deficient metric, which was the basis for another rigorous QI project.

Closing Statements

Advances in neonatal medicine have significantly improved the survival of critically ill newborns, including those born with extreme prematurity and those with extensive congenital anomalies affecting the airway. Due to the increased complexity of these patients, neonatal airway emergency remains a life-threatening event commonly encountered in a tertiary care neonatal intensive care unit. Management of neonatal airways is an essential skill for the neonatal physician and is fundamental to the practice of neonatal otolaryngology. There are no specific guidelines for response to airway emergencies in neonates, as compared to pediatric and adult populations, and the NRP guidelines are often used for all airway emergencies.

While adverse events in neonatal airway emergency are rare, the occurrence represents the end result of an interaction of numerous factors including anatomical and physiological differences in the neonatal airway, congenital and acquired causes of upper airway obstruction unique to neonates, practitioner competence in securing the airway,

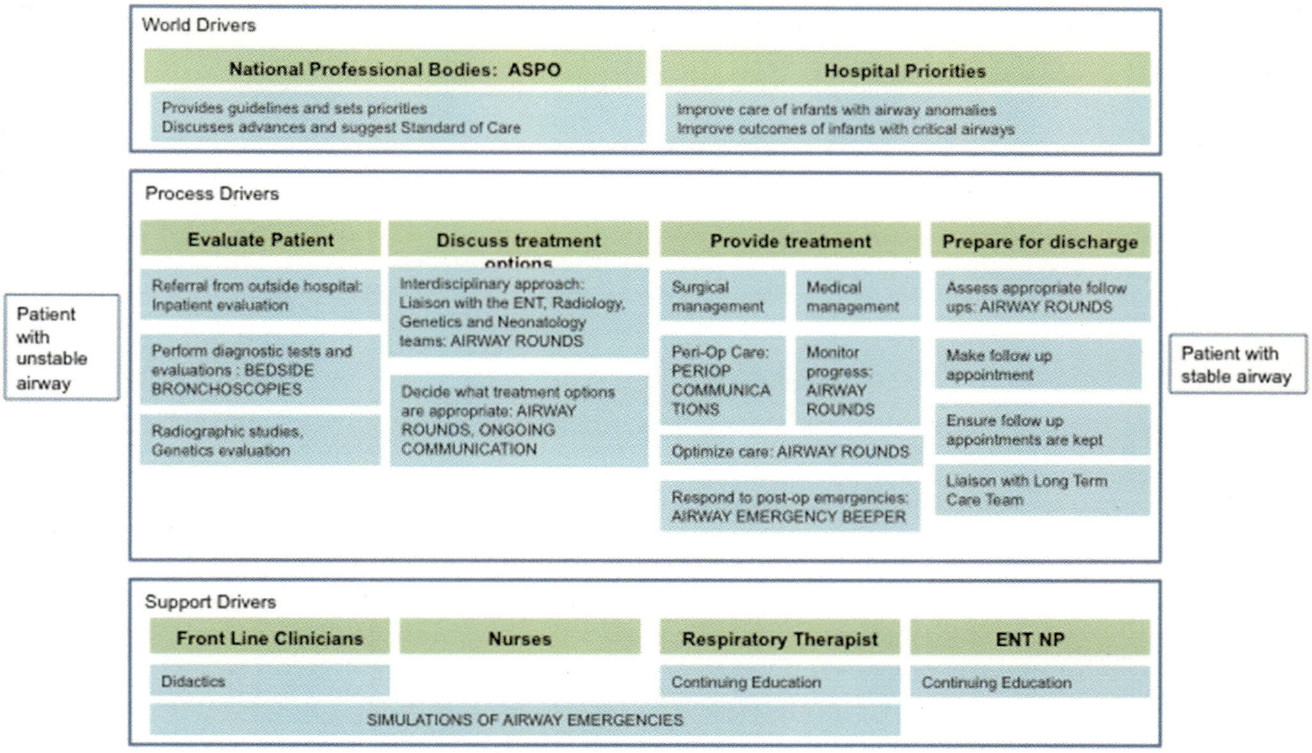

Fig. 5 QI Airway program systems process map—helpful for following the proper pathway of information flow to ensure proper communication

standard practices for response to airway emergencies and specialized equipment. Enhancing safety and efficacy in response to airway emergencies is critical to the success of any airway program and represents a vast opportunity to improve patient safety.

References

1. Hines S, Luna K, Lofthus J. et al. Becoming a high reliability organization: operational advice for hospital leaders. (Prepared by the Lewin Group under Contract No. 290-04-0011). AHRQ Publication No. 08-0022. Rockville: Agency for Health care Research and Quality; 2008.
2. Gurses AP, Seidl KL, Vaidya V, Bochicchio G, Harris AD, Hebden J, et al. Systems ambiguity and guideline compliance: a qualitative study of how intensive care units follow evidence-based guidelines to reduce healthcare-associated infections. Qual Saf Health Care. 2008;17(5):351–9. PubMed PMID: 18842974.
3. Horbar JD. The Vermont Oxford Network: evidence-based quality improvement for neonatology. Pediatrics. 1999;103(1 Suppl E):350–9. PubMed PMID: 9917477.
4. Horbar JD, Carpenter JH, Buzas J, Soll RF, Suresh G, Bracken MB, et al. Collaborative quality improvement to promote evidence based surfactant for preterm infants: a cluster randomised trial. BMJ. 2004;329(7473):1004. PubMed PMID: 15514344. Pubmed Central PMCID: 524548.
5. Payne NR, Finkelstein MJ, Liu M, Kaempf JW, Sharek PJ, Olsen S. NICU practices and outcomes associated with 9 years of quality improvement collaboratives. Pediatrics. 2010;125(3):437–46. PubMed PMID: 20123773.
6. Carayon P, Schoofs Hundt A, Karsh BT, Gurses AP, Alvarado CJ, Smith M, et al. Work system design for patient safety: the SEIPS model. Qual Saf Health Care. 2006;15 Suppl 1:i50–8. PubMed PMID: 17142610. Pubmed Central PMCID: 2464868.
7. Kraft S, Carayon P, Weiss J, Pandhi N. A simple framework for complex system improvement. Am J Med Qual. 2014 Apr 10. [Epub ahead of print].
8. Duvalko KM, Sherar M, Sawka C. Creating a system for performance improvement in cancer care: Cancer Care Ontario's clinical governance framework. Cancer Control. 2009;16(4): 293–302.
9. Chawla NV, Davis DA, Geva A, Gray JE, Pursley DM, Smallcomb JE. Network analysis of team structure in the Neonatal Intensive Care Unit. Pediatrics. 2010;125(6):e1460–7.
10. Dingley CDK, Derieg MK, Persing R. Improving patient safety through provider communication strategy enhancements. In: Henriksen K, Battles J, Keyes MA, Grady ML, editors. Advances in patient safety: new directions and alternative approaches. Rockville: Agency for Healthcare Research and Quality; 2008.

Index

J. Lioy and S.E. Sobol (eds.), *Disorders of the Neonatal Airway: Fundamentals for Practice*,
DOI 10.1007/978-1-4939-1610-8, © Springer Science+Business Media New York 2015

D

O

P

Printed by Printforce, the Netherlands